CHOICES

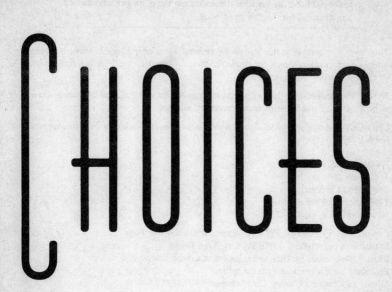

CHOICES

MARION MORRA & EVE POTTS

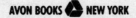
AVON BOOKS ◣ NEW YORK

This book was current to the best of the authors' knowledge at publication, but before acting on information herein, the consumer should, of course, verify the information with an appropriate physician or agency.

NOTE: The designations that treatments are standard or under clinical evaluation are not to be used as a basis for reimbursement determinations.

CHOICES is an original publication of Avon Books. This edition has never before appeared in book form.

AVON BOOKS
A division of
The Hearst Corporation
1350 Avenue of the Americas
New York, New York 10019

Copyright © 1980, 1987, 1994 by Marion Morra and Eve Potts
Illustrations copyright © 1980, 1994 by Avon Books
Interior illustrations by Dick Oden, unless otherwise noted
Published by arrangement with the authors
Library of Congress Catalog Card Number: 94-14927
ISBN: 0-380-77620-0

Library of Congress Cataloging in Publication Data:

Morra, Marion E.
    Choices : realistic alternatives in cancer treatment / Marion Morra & Eve Potts.—
Rev. ed.
        p.   cm.
Includes bibliographical references.
1. Cancer—Miscellanea. 2. Cancer—Hospitals—United States—Directories.
I. Potts, Eve.
RC270.8.M67   1994   94-14927
616.99'4—dc20   CIP

Second Revised Edition: October 1994
First Revised Edition: March 1987
First Avon Books Trade Printing: April 1980

AVON TRADEMARK REG. U.S. PAT. OFF. AND IN OTHER COUNTRIES, MARCA REGISTRADA, HECHO
EN U.S.A.

Printed in the U.S.A.

OPM   10   9   8   7   6   5   4   3   2   1

This third edition of Choices *is dedicated*

to the many cancer patients and their families

who continue to inspire us with their courage

and desire for authoritative information,

to our wonderful family and many friends

who made it possible for us to get the job done,

and especially to Bob Potts,

for his unswerving and loving support

Acknowledgments

This book owes its existence to many people, involved in cancer care through recent history, who have shaped the medical advances of the last decade. It is impossible to acknowledge all of the books and other sources such as articles, original scientific writings, pamphlets, oncology seminars and medical textbooks that made it possible for us to write this latest edition of *Choices*.

The materials from the National Cancer Institute, especially the state-of-the-art statements, and the American Cancer Society's textbooks and research reports have been of inestimable value. Most important to the tone and content of the book have been the insights of the many patients and families who continue to share with us their experiences and the real-life, everyday problems they encounter. From the very start, it has been people living with cancer on a day-to-day basis who have inspired us. We have been enriched by each encounter and by the opportunity to add to our knowledge. From them and from their questions, we have gleaned invaluable material which is the heart of this book.

A group of professionals in the cancer field have been unstinting in reviewing our material for this edition of *Choices*, helping us to avoid medical pitfalls in our writing: Tish Knobf, RN, MSN, Clinical Nurse Specialist at Yale Cancer Center and one of the country's most experienced oncology nurses, and Hilda Karp, RN, MA, of the Cancer Information Service at Memorial Sloan-Kettering, gave an incredible amount of time, expertise and genuine professionalism to the medical aspects of the manuscript.

Donna S. Cox, Program Director of the Cancer Information Service at The Johns Hopkins Oncology Center; Karen Hassey Dow, RN PhD, Nurse Researcher at Beth Israel Hospital, Boston; Diane Erdos, RN, MSN, Clinical Nurse Specialist, Yale Cancer Center; Julie Keany, RN, Cancer Information Service, Memorial Sloan-Kettering Cancer Center; Dr. Diane Komp, Pediatric Oncologist, Yale Cancer Center; Dr. Phyllis Kornguth, Department of Diagnostic Radiology, Duke University Medical Center; Linda Mowad, RN,

Cancer Information Service, Yale Cancer Center; Dr. Wen-jen Poo, Medical Oncologist, Yale Cancer Center; Dr. George P. Pillari, Diagnostic Radiologist, New Hyde Park, New York; Dr. Alan C. Sartorelli, Albert Gilman Professor, Department of Therapeutic Pharmacology, Yale University School of Medicine; Irene Karlsen Thompson, RN, Clinical Nurse Specialist, Swedish Hospital, Seattle; Marie Whedon, RN, MSN, Clinical Nurse Specialist, Norris Cotton Cancer Center, New Hampshire; and Jean Wooldridge, Project Director of the Cancer Information Service at Fred Hutchinson Cancer Research Center, Seattle, were all invaluable in helping review chapters for the book. Others who contributed in their specific areas of expertise: Audri Allred, Donald Stroetzel, Diane Saverance and Cancer Lifeline, Washington State. We also acknowledge Amy Potts Kelly for the information she provided and Abby and Michael Pillari for manuscript deliveries. We are grateful to the members of our family for their encouragement from beginning to end, especially Bob Potts and Mollie Donovan, our other sister, for ongoing assistance and infinite patience.

Though it is through the help of many, many people that this book came to life, we alone take responsibility for any errors or misinterpretations.

Preface

More than eighteen years ago when we first sat down to compile
the first edition of *Choices*, we did so because we were frustrated.
There had been an explosion of new developments in the cancer
field. Chemotherapy was becoming a new science. Treatments for
cancer were becoming more sophisticated. New technology was
being introduced. But none of the information was sifting down
to the consumer, who in this case was someone who needed information to make informed medical decisions. There was an ava-
lanche of written material directed at doctors and nurses—but not
a shred of enlightened material for the patient. The best that could
be hoped for were one-sheet pamphlets prepared with the barest
of information, implying, at least to these observers, that cancer
was a pretty hopeless business. The first *Choices* made its mark by
presenting a wealth of information written in lay terms, and geared
to people with cancer and their family and friends.

This latest edition of *Choices* still uses the familiar question-and-
answer format. Many things have changed over the years, but not
that format—which makes it easy to get a direct answer to a question and to delve as shallowly or deeply as you choose in any one
sitting. The new edition reflects the many changes that have occurred in the cancer and medical field. There have been many
dramatic advances in all phases of the cancer experience, with new
age technology replacing some of the uncomfortable procedures
that were once routine. All the latest techniques and terminology
have been covered in this edition.

All of the treatment information has been updated, using the
NCI's PDQ information system as a base. Each of the many charts
that deals with the stages and treatments available for each kind
of cancer has been simplified and incorporates material that encompasses the latest thinking on the part of the nation's top specialists.

As before, much of the information contained in the pages of
this book is drawn from the experiences of hundreds of people

who have endured treatments and shared with us what they would have liked to have known before starting out on the cancer journey.

We reexamined every piece of information contained in our previous editions, researching, rewriting, reconfirming, and amplifying facts, discussing with patients, nurses and doctors and honing the material to include every kernel that we felt needed to be shared with you. Primarily we tried, as we have from the start, to make this a book written from the patient's point of view. You'll find this edition includes more sophisticated terminology. What struck us particularly in looking back over the past decade is how much more quickly people who have cancer pick up the nomenclature of their disease and treatment. Because the terminology is what is used in hospitals and doctors' offices, we have tried to clarify language throughout the book so that when it is encountered during treatment, it will be understandable. We have tried to define the terms so that in discussions with the medical profession, who use these terms in their daily language, you will be on familiar territory. We hope it will make it possible for you to ask more detailed questions and therefore enter into more meaningful discussions, helping you to become a partner with your doctor in dealing with your cancer problem.

We realize that the book covers a wide range of information from the homey to the high tech—but we know from our discussions with many of you that you appreciate getting the information that your doctor would never think to tell you as well as the information that you are told but that you might not understand. While every cancer case is different, every type of cancer is different and the course of every cancer illness is different from every other, basic information and the questions that need to be explored remain the same. Medical treatment can vary depending upon who performs the treatment, where it is done, and your particular medical condition. We hope that this book will serve as a resource that fills the gap between material available in medical books and journals and the information given to you by your doctor, nurses and other health professionals.

Contents

Contents

Contents

List of Illustrations

CHOICES

chapter 1

Facing the Diagnosis

You have the diagnosis. Your doctor has told you that you have cancer. What happens next?

When a diagnosis of cancer is first made, you have the greatest number of choices concerning the kind of treatment best for you. Each decision may make the critical difference in the outcome. The wrong choices close the doors to other options. In order to make informed decisions, you need information, the kind of information that makes it possible for you to seek out the right doctor and hospital as well as sufficient information to make it possible for you to ask the right questions.

You need to put the whole emotional background of having cancer into perspective before you can deal intelligently with the diagnosis of cancer. For many people, the cancer word, the big C, still carries with it the old fears and myths, left over from the days when cancer was incurable. Today, with nearly five million Americans alive and most considered cured of cancer five years or more after their initial diagnosis and treatment, you need to be aware that cancer is considered and treated, in the majority of cases, as a "chronic" illness that can be managed for many years with proper treatment.

- **Cancer is a major illness but it is not necessarily fatal, contrary to what many people still believe.**
- **You can have cancer and continue to enjoy life.**

Anyone who has had cancer remembers the day the diagnosis was delivered. The mind became a blank. All the nagging fears that had been pushed to the back of consciousness landed in a huge lump in the throat. The mind raced with dark thoughts of death and wills and horror at the possibilities of dreaded treatments and a limited future.

1

There's no question that the diagnosis of cancer is one of the low points in life. The real news is that more than half of the people with cancer are considered cured. For some types of cancer, nine out of ten people diagnosed can be considered cured. Many others will live a very long time before dying of cancer. There is hope for every patient. Some are cured at once, by surgery, chemotherapy and radiation. Some are never cured, but their disease is controlled so they can expect to live for many, many years. Admittedly, there are some types of cancer where treatments may prolong life for no more than a few months.

ABOUT SURVIVAL STATISTICS

Your physician may talk about "five-year survival" rates. Many people misinterpret this to mean that you are expected to live only five years after treatment or that you aren't considered cured even after five-years without cancer. Five-year survival is used as a measure by scientists to compare the value of one treatment against another. Statistics are gathered for a five-year period. In many forms of cancer, five years without symptoms following treatment is the accepted time to consider a patient cured. Actually, depending on the type of cancer, some patients are considered cured after one year, others after three years, while for some it may be longer than five years. One more thing—the statistics are based on treatments that were done five years or more ago. With the fast pace of change in cancer treatment and with increasing successes, those statistics can become outdated quickly.

It is important for you to know at the outset what category your type of cancer is so that you will not be worrying unnecessarily and so that you will be dealing with reality when you make decisions about your treatments and how you will be living your life. You need full information to make certain that you will be getting the very best possible treatment for your cancer as well as for your coping style, personality and living style. The best place to begin in collecting information, of course, is with your doctor. But, you need to search out further information on your own if you plan to be an involved consumer. The best place to start is by getting information from the National Cancer Institute, where ongoing research puts cutting edge information at your fingertips.

FACTS YOU NEED TO KNOW ABOUT CANCER

- Over eight million Americans alive today have a history of cancer.
- Five million Americans are alive who were diagnosed with cancer five or more years ago.
- Most of the five million can be considered cured.
- Cured means that the person has no evidence of disease and has the same life expectancy as a person who never had cancer.
- In 1994, about 1,170,000 new cancer cases will be diagnosed. This figure excludes those who have basal cell and squamous cell skin cancers, an additional 700,000 cases per year.
- Things have changed. In the early 1900s, most cancer patients had no hope of long-term survival. In the 1930s, less than one in five was alive five years after treatment. In the 1940s, it was one in four, and in the 1960s, one in three.
- Today, statistics show that when adjusted for normal life expectancy, a relative five-year survival rate of 52 percent is seen for all cancers.

EIGHT THINGS YOU NEED TO DO BEFORE DECIDING ON CANCER TREATMENT

1. Ask the doctor to discuss all the possible alternatives with you.
2. Call the Cancer Information Service, toll-free, at 1-800-4-CANCER for the latest up-to-date information and facts on your type of cancer. Making this call is one of the most important things you can do for yourself. Trained personnel can talk to you about your kind of cancer and help you decide what steps to take. They also will be happy to supply you with booklets, names of doctors in the area, clinical trials that are being done on your type of cancer and PDQ statements from the National Cancer Institute that give you the latest information on treatments. If you have further questions at a later date, don't hesitate to call again.

(continued)

EIGHT THINGS YOU NEED TO DO BEFORE DECIDING ON CANCER TREATMENT *(cont.)*

3. If a medical library is available to you, look there for information. The Cancer Information Service is a good starting point for information, but you and your friends and family may want to do other research as well. Your home computer can be used to access medical and health resources. So much new research is being done in so many places that you may find an important clue to a treatment that may be helpful to you.

4. Meanwhile, make sure you have the right doctor. The kind of treatment you get depends on how much your doctor knows about your particular kind of cancer. Ask your doctor about clinical trials and the latest PDQ statement from the National Cancer Institute on your kind of cancer.

5. There are doctors (called oncologists) who specialize in treating cancer. Beyond that there are specialists in every kind of cancer, down to specialists who deal exclusively with one cell type of cancer. Get an opinion on treatment from someone who is treating your type of disease on a daily basis.

6. If during your research you find a doctor who has written a paper on your type of cancer, don't hesitate to call and discuss your case.

7. If at all possible, a second opinion should be sought at the start before submitting to any cancer treatment of any kind. The original diagnosis and treatment plan you were given will probably be confirmed but you deserve the right to have your doctor's diagnosis reconfirmed and any other possible treatments explored and explained to you. Take the time to do your homework. A few extra weeks usually will not make any difference as far as the progress of the cancer is concerned but can make all the difference in your future.

8. In many cases, a second pathological opinion is a good idea. The pathology report is the basis on which all future decisions will be made, and although some cancers are pathologically diagnosed without any question, you need to check to make certain this is the case for you.

Once you know you have cancer, you can live in fear, or you can learn to live with the facts and begin to do positive things to help yourself. Knowing the facts and facing them takes a lot of the scare away.

Here are some basics for starters. Check them and see how many coincide with your own thinking.

- The fact that you have cancer cannot be changed. The time that is most important in decision making is right now, at the very start, when numerous alternatives are open to you.
- You must look at all the alternatives. If you make a decision to go ahead with surgery without sufficient testing or a second opinion, you limit the possibility for other choices.
- Unless you stay calm and in control, a decision will be made for you by circumstances that will take it out of your control. Don't be afraid to say: "I'm going to take the time to learn all I can about this cancer and the options I have available to me before I do anything."
- **CAUTION:** This does not mean postponing taking action. It means postponing starting treatment until you are personally assured that you're taking the right steps.

HOW TO PROCEED

- Get a loose-leaf notebook for keeping records. You can divide it into sections in a way that makes sense for you. You may want to have a section for all the information you will gather about your kind of cancer, names and phone numbers of doctors, hospitals, etc.
- Another section may be reserved for all questions that occur to you and notes on what you are told.
- You probably will want additional sections to include information on medications, doctor appointments, payments made, insurance information, etc.
- A tape recorder can be handy for reference purposes. With the approval of the person being recorded, you can keep a record of discussions you have with the various medical professionals you will be seeing.
- Many people find it helpful to have a running narrative or personal account of what is happening to them throughout the treatment.

- As a cancer patient, you must be an activist. You must become a partner with your doctors in the fight so you can live your life in the way that is best for you.
- You have a right to ask questions just as you would as a consumer of any product or service. However, you need to learn what questions to ask, what the terminology means, and what the realistic possibilities are.
- Hope is not the same as denial. Denying you have cancer closes your mind and your resources to all the possibilities that exist for you. You shut off your inner abilities to deal with reality. Denial closes doors. Hope opens the channels for action.
- Without question, the most difficult time you will experience is at the beginning, when the diagnosis is first presented to you. At that moment, cancer becomes an inescapable fact for you. That is the time when you must mobilize yourself and your resources to plan your future intelligently.

ABOUT YOUR FEELINGS

- Expect to feel depressed at times.
- Expect to find that many of your emotions will be at the surface.
- Try to deal with your feelings honestly.
- Don't try to hide your illness and prognosis from your family and friends.
- Accept and welcome the help and concern of others.
- Think about whether quality or quantity of life—how good or how long—is most important for you. You may be faced with some decisions where the answer to this question will determine what choices you will make.
- Once you've done all the background work and embarked on a course of treatment, your own unique style of coping will help you feel in control. You will be able to face your problems if you know what is being done to you, why it is being done, how it will be done and what the prognosis is.
- You will undoubtedly be anxious, may not sleep well, and may lose your appetite. This is normal.
- You may be surprised to find that once you have made your decisions, you will experience a sense of relief, or a feeling of calmness.

DEALING WITH DOCTORS

- Keep a list of questions you want answered and bring them with you when you keep appointments with doctors.
- Take notes whenever talking with the doctor, radiologist, physical therapist or nurse. (Or you may want to ask if it is OK for you to tape-record conversations, then you can play them back for yourself or your family at your leisure.)
- Review your notes and save them for future reference.
- Ask the doctor to explain any medical terms you do not understand.
- Try always to have a family member or good friend with you when keeping your doctors' appointments. It's helpful to have another person with you who can help you remember and interpret what is being told to you.
- Don't hesitate to ask for information about testing, test results and other procedures. You are entitled to all information that the doctor has about your case.
- Let the doctor know that you are planning on getting other opinions before going any further. This is **not** an **unreasonable or unusual** request. Do not be pressured into proceeding before you are confident about what is being recommended.

JUDGING YOUR OWN ATTITUDE TOWARD CANCER	
TRUE OR FALSE	THE REAL ANSWER
_____ You will die if you have cancer.	**False.** Cancer, if discovered at an early stage, is curable in many instances; or chronic in most cases.
_____ Cancer is contagious.	**False.**
_____ Cancer can develop in any part of the body.	**True.** All parts of the body are susceptible—bone, lymph, skin, nervous system, etc.
_____ Half of cancer patients are cured.	**True.** Of the more than one million newly diagnosed cancer cases this year, more than half can be permanently cured, and many more lead normal lives for many years.
_____ The outlook for cancer treatment is hopeful.	**True.** The rate of cure is now almost one in two, as compared to one in four in 1950. *(continued)*

JUDGING YOUR OWN ATTITUDE TOWARD CANCER *(cont.)*

TRUE OR FALSE	THE REAL ANSWER
_____ The doctor can tell how long you have to live.	**False.** Every case is different and doctors' estimates on how long a patient will live are often guesswork and can do a real disservice to the patient.
_____ There are no untreatable cancers.	**True.** There are always treatments that can be prescribed to make a patient more comfortable, although treatments are not always available to effect a cure.
_____ Putting off seeing a doctor can forfeit the possibility of a cure.	**True.** The earlier cancer is found, the more curable it will be. Of those who die of cancer each year, a large percentage die needlessly because of late diagnosis and inadequate treatment.
_____ More people are being diagnosed with cancer than ever before.	**True.** This is mainly because more people are living to an age when cancer occurs more frequently. Also, because diagnostic techniques are better, more cases are being found.
_____ Cancer is more frequent in men and women over 40.	**True.** Cancer is primarily a disease of middle and old age. Less than 1 percent of all cancers are found in children.
_____ A lump in the breast means you have cancer.	**False.** Eighty percent of all breast lumps are not cancer.
_____ Smoking can cause lung cancer.	**True.** Eighty-seven percent of lung cancers are caused by smoking. Two-pack-a-day smokers die of lung cancer at rates 15 to 25 times greater than nonsmokers.
_____ The sun is good for you.	**False.** Almost all of the 700,000 cases of basal and squamous cell skin cancer each year are sun-related. Sun exposure is also a major factor in melanoma, a cancer that is increasing, especially in fair-skinned persons.
_____ Grains, breads, pastas, vegetables and fruits may reduce risk of colon cancer.	**True.** High-fiber diets may help reduce risk of colon cancer.
_____ It's proven that estrogen replacement is harmless.	**False.** The final word isn't in on estrogen. Estrogen to control menopausal symptoms can increase risk of endometrial cancer. Including progesterone helps minimize risk. Continued research is being done on breast cancer and estrogen use.

PUT THESE THOUGHTS INTO YOUR MENTAL COMPUTER

- People have recovered from every type of cancer.
- Cancer is the most curable of all chronic diseases. Cured means that you have the same life expectancy as someone your age who never had cancer. Latest statistics show that about 60 percent of all serious cancers can be cured.
- Cancer patients can expect to live longer than either heart attack or stroke victims.
- It helps to learn about every detail of your kind of cancer.
- A fighting spirit is healthier than stoic acceptance. It also may strengthen your immune response.
- It's better to express your feelings than to bottle them up.
- Consider yourself an equal partner with your doctor in achieving recovery.
- Listen to your body.
- Don't make a career of having cancer.
- Don't save up real living for tomorrow. Live your best today.

**HAVE YOU MADE YOUR CALL TO THE
CANCER INFORMATION SERVICE?
1-800-4-CANCER
Daily hours: 9 AM to 7 PM
PLEASE DO IT NOW!**

chapter 2

Choosing Your Doctor and Hospital

Doctors vary depending on their training, experience and the services they perform. They vary in the way they deal with patients. So finding the doctor who is right for your case isn't simple. Most of us do more research in buying a car than we do in choosing our doctor or the hospital where we will be treated. Often this is true because we don't really know exactly what to look for.

When you are dealing with cancer treatment, it is especially important that you give careful thought to the doctor and the hospital you will be using. A doctor who deals with a specific kind of cancer on a daily basis usually has broader knowledge of the treatment options available than a doctor who sees such a cancer only occasionally. A hospital that specializes in cancer treatment has more services for the cancer patient than a small local hospital which is designed to serve broader community needs.

With the many changes in health care delivery and with more and more doctors becoming involved in health care organizations, the problem of making decisions about doctors and hospitals has become more important and even more complicated than ever before. However, the facts surrounding your decisions about which doctor and which hospital to choose for your medical care have not changed—even though it might be more difficult to achieve your goal.

BASIC FACTS THAT WILL HELP YOU IN CHOOSING A DOCTOR AND HOSPITAL

- When you have cancer, you need to be under the care of someone who specializes in cancer care. Such doctors are known as *oncologists*. There are many different specialists in oncology, such as surgical oncologists, medical oncologists and radiation oncologists. The major point to remember right now is that *you should not feel that you are limited to dealing exclusively with your present doctor.*
- Your doctor should be board certified in his specialty.
- It is important to check out your doctor's credentials. Doctors don't have to be certified in a field to list themselves as a specialist in it. Make sure that if your doctor is listed as an internist or a cancer specialist, the doctor has been certified in that field. Be aware. Don't take the listing in the phone book for granted.
- We recommend that you consider getting a second opinion before making any final decisions on treatment. This is perfectly standard practice and should not offend your doctor.
- If you live near a comprehensive or clinical cancer center that has been so designated by the National Cancer Institute, you should definitely consider getting treatment, or at least a second opinion, there. Again, you need to be an informed consumer. Not all hospitals that call themselves "cancer centers" have necessarily passed the rigorous standards designated by accrediting boards.
- A referral and a consultation are two different things. A referral means that once you see the specialist, you become a patient of that doctor. A consultation is designed to get another opinion from another doctor. The consulting doctor will not be taking over the responsibility for your care but simply will report the findings to your doctor.

What does board certification mean?

The specialty boards are private, voluntary, nonprofit, autonomous organizations founded to conduct examinations, issue certificates of qualifications and improve and broaden opportunities for graduate education and training. Once doctors finish their required residency in a particular specialty, they become eligible to be certified by the board. This requires taking a rigorous written and oral examination given by other doctors who practice in this specialty. Many doctors do not become certified after their first examinations by the board. Some boards require recertification after a specified number of years. A fellowship in the "college" of specialty means that the doctor is qualified to teach others. It is another step up the ladder and earns a more esteemed place among the doctor's colleagues.

Are there good doctors who are not board certified?

Board certification and fellowships are designed to indicate a high level of competence, but there are many reasons why doctors who are equally competent may not be board certified. In the field of cancer, especially, there are many doctors who treat only cancer patients, yet are not board certified in oncology. This is because the boards in oncology are relatively new and were not available to older doctors when they started in practice. Some doctors in practice in the large cancer centers who combine research with patient care are not board certified but are extremely well qualified to treat cancer patients.

What is the difference between a board-certified and a board-eligible doctor?

The doctor who passes the examination for a given specialty is known as a diplomate of the board and is said to be board certified. A physician who has completed a formal training program in the specialty but has either chosen not to take the exams or has not completed the exams is called board eligible (newly trained doctors are board eligible between the time they finish their residency or fellowship and the time they take their boards and get the results). There are well-trained specialists who for good, legitimate reasons are board eligible. These are exceptions. There's no question that it's better to have passed the exams than not to have passed them.

**CALL THIS NUMBER TO SEE
IF YOUR DOCTOR IS BOARD CERTIFIED
OR TO GET NAMES OF DOCTORS
WHO ARE BOARD CERTIFIED
1-800-776-CERT
(American Board of Certified Specialties)**

Are there other ways to check out my doctor's credentials?

There are several directories which list doctor credentials. The *Directory of Medical Specialists* and the *American Medical Directory* are two of the most readily available. Our favorite is the *Directory of Medical Specialists* because it lists only those doctors who are board certified. The listing of doctors in the American Medical Directory is a listing of all doctors who belong to the *American Medical Association*, whether or not they have board certification. If your library does not have either of these books, you can call 1-800-776-CERT to check on whether or not the doctor is certified. In addition, your state or local department of health or medical society can give you information.

What are some of the major specialties?

The specialty areas that pertain to cancer treatment include:

- **Anesthesiology:** anesthesiologists administer drugs for relief of pain during surgery or childbirth. During an operation in which general anesthetic is used, the anesthesiologist is responsible for monitoring and maintaining safe levels of the patient's bodily functions. Some anesthesiologists are also certified in pain management.
- **Colon and rectal surgery:** surgeons who have had additional training in diagnosis and treatment of diseases of the intestinal tract, rectum and anus.
- **Dermatology:** doctors who treat skin diseases and conditions, including skin cancer.
- **Family practice:** doctors specializing in the continuing and total care of the family.
- **Geriatric medicine:** family physicians who have additional training in treating disorders of old age.
- **Internal medicine:** doctors who treat a wide range of medical problems. Internists who take an additional one or more years of "fellowship" are certified for subspecialties such as:
  Cardiovascular disease: treatment of diseases of heart, lungs and blood vessels.
  Endocrinology: disease of organs which secrete hormones into the bloodstream such as the thyroid, adrenal glands and ovaries.
  Geriatric medicine: treatment of illnesses in elderly.
  Gastroenterology (GI): diseases of the digestive tract (mouth to anus, including stomach, bowels, liver, gallbladder).

Hematology: diseases of the blood and blood-making tissues (bone marrow, spleen, lymph glands).

Infectious diseases: difficult cases of infection.

Medical oncology: treat all types of benign and malignant cancers in any organ of the body. Prescribe chemotherapy or may refer patient to radiation oncologists or surgeons.

Nephrology: disease of the kidneys, urinary system and related disorders of metabolism.

Pulmonary: diseases of the lung.

Rheumatology: diseases of joints, ligaments, muscles, bones and tendons.

- **Medical genetics:** diseases that are linked with hereditary disorders.
- **Neurological surgery:** surgery in the nervous system, including brain, spinal cord and nerves.
- **Neurology:** diseases of the brain, spinal cord and nerves.
- **Nuclear medicine:** evaluate functions of all organs in body and treat benign and malignant tumors, and radiation exposure.
- **Obstetrics and Gynecology:** treat female reproductive system; there is a specialty in gynecological oncology.
- **Otolaryngology:** doctors who specialize in medical and surgical treatment of head and neck; called otolaryngologists, head and neck surgeons, or ear, nose and throat doctors.
- **Pathology:** physicians who specialize in study of body tissues, secretions, and fluids to diagnose disease and gauge how far it has spread. There are nine subspecialties in this discipline, including dermatopathology (skin), hematology (blood), cytopathology (cancer cells).
- **Pediatrics:** doctors who care for children up to age 16. Subspecialties are similar to internal medicine and include pediatric hematology-oncology, pediatric endocrinology, pediatric nephrology, etc.
- **Physical medicine and rehabilitation:** known as physiatrists, specialize in evaluating and treating patients with impairments and restoring maximal function.
- **Plastic surgery:** plastic surgeons perform surgery to correct functional and cosmetic deformities of face, head, body and extremities.
- **Psychiatry:** treatment of mental, addictive and emotional disorders.
- **Radiology:** Divided into three categories—radiation oncology (use of radiation in treatment of cancer), diagnostic radiology (use of x-rays, CAT scans and MRI for diagnosis of

cancer), and diagnostic radiology with special competence in nuclear radiology (use of radioactive substances in diagnosis of disease).

- **Surgery:** General surgeons are specialists prepared to manage a broad spectrum of surgical conditions affecting almost any area of the body; specialty in thoracic surgery, including cancers of the lung and esophagus.
- **Urology:** treatment of urinary system, including kidneys, bladder, prostate, adrenal gland and testes.

What other information can I determine from the listings in the medical directories?

You will want to scan the information in the front of the book before using it, so you will be able to decipher all the information given in each biographical listing. The listings are geographical by specialty, so this is a good time to find out and jot down the names and credentials of other specialists in your area—such as surgeons, anesthesiologists, gynecologists, urologists, etc. If no one in your town is listed, look for names of doctors in nearby towns. (Just a tip, it's easier to check the alphabetical listing in the index of the last volume of the book if you have the name of a specific doctor you want to check. It will give you the page number for the listing.)

What should I look for in analyzing the listings?

- Does the doctor have a teaching appointment at a medical-school-affiliated hospital? This indicates the doctor is up-to-date and respected by peers.
- What kind of hospital is the doctor affiliated with? Is it a medical-school-affiliated hospital? Requirements for this sort of hospital are rigid and must be earned through teaching appointments.
- If the doctor is a surgeon, does he have privileges at three or more hospitals? This sounds impressive but it takes so much of the doctor's time that you might be better served by someone who concentrates on one or two hospitals. The quality of the association with the hospital is more important than the number.
- How large is the hospital? If you don't live in an area with a university hospital center, the larger the hospital (200 beds or more) the more equipment and facilities it will have.
- What societies does the doctor belong to? One or more is preferable for these help keep doctors up-to-date on the latest information being developed by others in the specialty.

Can doctors list themselves as specialists?

Yes. Doctors, once licensed, can list themselves as they wish. Even physicians with no specialized training beyond medical school and internship can call themselves gynecologists or internists or dermatologists, etc. They can legally perform operations. That is why it is important to determine whether or not your physician has had additional training, is board certified and is practicing in a legitimate hospital. Four years of medical school after college, plus one year of internship, allow doctors to be licensed to practice under any title they choose to assume. So be sure to check credentials so that you know for certain that your doctor is qualified to be treating you.

What is a medical oncologist?

A medical oncologist is a doctor who specializes in treating cancer with drugs. In the past, this training was often in the treatment of blood diseases (hematology), particularly leukemia and lymphoma, since these were the first tumors to be treated with drugs. More recently, a medical specialty called medical oncology trains doctors exclusively in the treatment of cancer patients. These specialists are certified by the American Board of Internal Medicine, by the American Board of Medical Oncology, and in the case of doctors who treat children, by the American Board of Pediatrics.

What is a radiation oncologist?

The radiation oncologist treats cancer with radiation. This doctor also may be called a therapeutic radiologist or an x-ray therapist. Qualified radiation oncologists should be certified by the American Board of Therapeutic Radiology. There is a difference between a radiation oncologist and a diagnostic radiologist. A diagnostic radiologist is a doctor whose specialty is in performing and interpreting x-rays used in diagnosing illness.

What is the difference between a medical oncologist and a hematologist?

A medical oncologist is a doctor of internal medicine who specializes in the administration of a variety of drugs needed to treat specific cancers. This doctor may also be referred to as a hematologist (one who specializes in blood diseases). The administration of most chemotherapy drugs is very complex. These drugs need to be given under the supervision of a doctor who specializes in this field.

JUDGING YOUR DOCTOR

ASSESSMENT SCORE	KIND OF PRACTICE	SCORE YOUR DOCTOR
+5	Hospital-based office	
+5	One-specialty group	
+5	Multispecialty group	
+2	Loose association with other doctors	
+1	Partner	
−5	Practices alone	

Generally, a doctor who practices with a group that specializes in a variety of disciplines is better as a family doctor. Specialists who practice in a group or in a hospital are subject to constant review by peers.

	HOSPITAL AFFILIATION	
+10	Practices at an NCI-designated Comprehensive or Clinical Cancer Center	
+5	Practices at hospital which you prefer	
+5	University or medical school hospital (part- or full-time staff member)	
+5	On teaching staff of medical school	
+4	Staff, community hospital with 200 beds or more	
+3	Staff, community hospital with less than 200 beds	
+1	Part owner, staff of small private hospital (proprietary)	
−1 or −5	No hospital affiliation (ask why; score depends on answer)	

A doctor who is a part- or full-time staff member at a university or medical school hospital or a larger community hospital has shown his merit. The doctor who practices in a small for-profit hospital may be just as qualified, but should be checked more closely for other credentials.

	BOARDS	
+10	Board certified in specialty, specialist in oncology	*(continued)*

JUDGING YOUR DOCTOR *(cont.)*

Assessment Score	Boards	Score Your Doctor
+5	Board certified and/or fellow of the board	
+4	Board certified	
−5	No longer eligible or not listed	

Board certification is a big plus. It means that beyond training in the specialty field, the doctor has been subjected to the scrutiny of peers in written and oral examinations. A fellowship is an extra flag of distinction. Oncology specialty means that the doctor is skilled in cancer treatment.

	Manner, Personality, Office Efficiency	
+5	Warm, concerned, explains procedures and listens well	
+2	Difficulty communicating, impersonal, but efficient	
+5	Efficient, well-run office, pleasant personnel	
+5	Willing to discuss fees and insurance	
−5	Poor office practices, appointment schedules inefficient	
	Nursing Staff	
+10	Communicative, willing to discuss problems, give helpful solutions, supportive, professional, skilled	
−10	Office assistants but no nurses	

Your own observations about your doctor's manner, skills and office personnel are an important part of your evaluation. The manner in which the physician's office is run tells you a great deal about the doctor's standards and probably also reflects on the doctor's professionalism. While not as vital as professional credentials, when taken in context with other observations, this serves as another guideline for judgment.

Can any doctor prescribe chemotherapy for me?

It is important, if you are living in a community that does not have a medical oncologist, to make sure that your doctor has consulted with a major cancer center, a medical school, or an oncologist to determine which drugs are best for your case, the dose of drug to be given and the side effects to be expected. In most areas, doctors, nurses, and pharmacists work as a team in the administration of chemotherapy.

How do I find a surgeon who specializes in cancer?

Some surgeons have special training and limit their practices to cancer surgery. Although there is no certification that denotes this kind of training, it is important to find out what a surgeon's interest and experience are. While medical oncologists and radiation oncologists deal exclusively with cancer patients, many surgeons have practices where they deal with a variety of diseases. Look for a cancer surgeon who is certified by the American Board of Surgeons

CHECKLIST FOR CHOOSING A SURGEON FOR A CANCER PROBLEM

Ask these questions:

- How many of these procedures have you done?
- How often do you do this procedure? (At least two or three times a week, for major surgery, is a minimum. Studies show that mortality rates are lower at hospitals where surgeons do a procedure frequently.)
- How often is this procedure done in your hospital? (The more often, the more likely it is that other staff members who are assisting and caring for you will be well trained.)
- What is your success rate with this operation?
- What are the complications and aftereffects?
- What happens if I do nothing?
- If it is a new procedure or method, ask: What are the advantages of this procedure over the old-fashioned way? How long have you used this procedure? Is it more costly?
- How do you handle emergencies if I should need to reach you after office hours?
- Who covers for you on nights and weekends? Will that person have access to my records?

or by one of its subspecialty boards such as Neurosurgery, Obstetrics and Gynecology, Orthopedic Surgery, or Urologic Surgery. There are surgical specialists who treat specific parts of the body. You will want to discuss the choice of a surgeon with your medical oncologist or radiation oncologist. People with very rare or difficult kinds of cancer—such as in the head and neck area—should realize that the best treatment may be available in only a few major cancer centers where significant numbers of people with similar tumors are treated.

If my doctor has no hospital affiliation what does that mean?

If your doctor has no hospital affiliation you owe it to yourself to ask the reason. Some perfectly good family doctors confine themselves to an office practice. When their patients need hospitalization, they recommend the specialist they feel has the proper skills. If, however, the doctor was once affiliated with a hospital and no longer has that affiliation, make sure you ask for reasons.

If a doctor is in practice alone, is that a good sign?

Many doctors practice in rural areas and may have no choice but to work alone. However, in general, the doctor who works with other doctors is usually a better bet than one who has a solo practice. If you have such a doctor, you should know what arrangements have been made for coverage when the doctor is away or unavailable. If the covering doctor does not have access to your medical records, there is a great limitation on how the covering doctor can treat you in your own doctor's absence.

Is it a good idea for a group of one kind of doctor to practice together?

If your doctor is part of a group that consists of several other doctors who practice the same specialty, such as a group of internists, this is a real plus. Usually each has a different area of expertise. This gives them, and you, the advantage of other opinions on a specific case.

How can I find out which doctors practice at which hospitals?

The easiest way is to call the hospital's staff office or patient-referral service and ask if the doctor practices there or for the names of doctors in particular specialties who do practice there.

If I have a choice between an equally qualified young doctor and older doctor, which should I choose?

When choosing a doctor in private practice, many people reason that the younger doctor may be more up-to-date as far as technique is concerned, but the older doctor will be more experienced. In the medical academic area, the older doctor is probably both more up-to-date and more experienced. Teaching in a medical school means a physician must stay up-to-date and be ready to explain to students the wisdom of using a particular procedure or treatment.

Why should I consider getting a second opinion?

There are several reasons for wanting to get a second opinion from another qualified physician. Foremost is reassurance that the first opinion is correct and that you have explored all your choices. A

WAYS OF GETTING A SECOND OPINION

- You can ask your own doctor to suggest the name of someone to see for a second opinion.
- You can make the appointment yourself, or you can ask the doctor to make the appointment for you.
- You should always discuss your plans for consultation with your doctor. You will need to bring your original x-rays and tests for the other doctor to use during your consultation. If your doctor is uncooperative, then you have other decisions to make about continuing that relationship.
- You can call the toll-free 1-800-4-CANCER number and ask for information about getting an appointment with a specialist in your kind of cancer at an NCI-designated comprehensive or clinical cancer center near you.
- You can call your nearest medical school and ask for suggestions. A medical school's outpatient clinic, where some of the country's top specialists practice, is also a good place to check.
- Some hospitals have a special telephone line for physician referral—although many simply give names of all the doctors who have privileges to admit patients to their facilities. You can write the director of the hospital of your choice and ask for suggestions.
- You can call the American Board of Certified Specialties at 1-800-776-CERT for names of specialists in your area.
- You can check the *Directory of Medical Specialists* at your library and call the specialist directly.
- You can check the *Directory of Medical Specialists* for the names of two or three doctors in the area and ask your doctor to suggest which one you should see.

second opinion may also be wanted when surgery has been recommended, when you question the evaluation made by your first doctor, when you think the doctor is underestimating the seriousness of your illness, when the doctor seems unable to find out what is wrong with you, or when you think there may be another form of treatment. Getting a second opinion is common practice.

Won't my doctor be offended if I ask for another opinion?

If your doctor is offended, then you have a good reason for finding another doctor. The important point to remember is that most doctors *welcome* a second opinion. A second opinion does not mean you are questioning your doctor's competence. If you have cancer, a decision about how you proceed with treatment is probably the most important decision you will make in your life. You need the best advice you can get before proceeding with a course of treatment. Just as you don't hesitate to check out various makes and models of cars when you are buying, you should not hesitate to check out all the possible angles before making a decision about your health and your future. Remember, the choices you make at the very beginning are the most important ones.

How can I tell my doctor I want a second opinion?

It may be easier for you if you ask a family member to help you do this. He or she can simply explain to your doctor that before going any further you would like to have a confirming opinion. This is not an unusual or unreasonable request. It is a very necessary step for you to take. You may be told that the x-rays and tests are conclusive as far as the doctor is concerned. Do not let that put you off or pressure you into backing down. Explain again that you want a second opinion, that it will strengthen the conclusions already made and set your mind at ease.

What if I decide I want to change doctors?

This is more difficult than asking for a second opinion. If you are not satisfied with your relationship with your doctor, you have every right to choose another doctor. Whatever your reason for wanting to change, whether it is because you want someone with more experience to treat you, whether you have lost confidence in the ability of your present doctor to treat you, or if you wish to make the change for personality reasons, if you are feeling negative about your doctor, it is not in your best interests to continue in the relationship. You should not be afraid to be honest with your doctor about wanting to end the relationship. No doctor likes to lose a patient, but every doctor has had that experience. You might handle the discussion diplomatically by thanking the doctor for what has been done, assure the doctor that you appreciate all the help that has been given to you, but that you would prefer to try to find another doctor who is more suitable for your particular needs at this time. Your doctor is legally obligated to provide your new doctor with any existing records, x-rays and test results.

Who will recommend a specialist to me?

This can work in a number of ways. You might want to discuss the results of your own research for a specialist with your primary doctor, who will usually want to make a recommendation. Sometimes your primary doctor will give you more than one name. You should be sure to determine the specialist's credentials and be sure you have the answers to these questions:

- Why are you referring me to this particular doctor?
- Is this doctor a specialist in doing this operation (or in this field)?
- How often does this specialist perform the particular operation (or service)?
- Is the doctor board certified? On the staff of an accredited hospital?

How do I get an appointment for a consultation?

Sometimes the doctor who refers you will make the appointment for you. If you are calling yourself, explain that you have already had a diagnosis and wish to make an appointment for a consultation. Don't make the mistake of trying to let the doctor think you haven't been to another doctor. Using a specialist on a consulting basis means that you will get a straight answer, since that doctor has nothing to gain from recommending one treatment over another.

What is the difference between a referral and a consultation?

If your doctor decides that your illness requires the attention of a specialist, you will be given the names of one or several specialists for you to see. This is called a referral and differs from a consultation. A referral means that once you see the specialist you become the patient of that doctor. In a consultation, the consulting doctor advises you but does not take over responsibility for treating you.

Is a medical school's outpatient clinic a good place to go for a second opinion?

This is an excellent place to turn for a second opinion. Physicians who practice there are on the faculty of the medical school and are usually using the latest methods of treatment. Because most outpatient departments are divided into specialties, this is where some of the top specialists in the country practice. You can contact the clinic by calling the medical school and explaining that you are interested in contacting a doctor who specializes in the area of your specific problem. Don't be afraid to explain that you want to get a second opinion and to describe your experience to date. Each clinic, of course, has its own setup—but most have appointment secretaries who are very knowledgeable about the clinic and the doctors in their service and will be most helpful in making arrangements for a consultation.

Does having a consultation at a medical school mean I have to go there for treatment?

You have a free choice in the matter. The decision is yours. Sometimes people shy away from getting expert advice from doctors at a large medical center because they feel this will mean that they have to return there for treatments. Many medical and cancer centers diagnose and recommend treatment for patients to be followed by doctors in local communities. If the medical center is a long distance from your home and you do not want the expense and inconvenience of returning there each time you need treatment, you can take advantage of a consultation and continue to be treated by your own doctor and at your local hospital.

What will a consultation cost?

You will be amazed to find that some of the finest physicians in the country charge no more—and sometimes considerably less—than doctors with far less experience and expertise. Part of the reason is that medical school faculty physicians are often salaried and their fees are returned to the medical school.

Who pays for a second opinion?

Many insurance companies now pay for second opinions. Some even require them. Even if your particular insurance company does not pay, the cost of a consultation is considerably less than the first opinion because all the test results and x-rays are already available to the second doctor.

What if the second opinion differs from the first?

Second opinions can be confusing. If the first doctor recommends a course of treatment different from the second, you are left more puzzled than when you started. You have several alternatives in this case. You can ask the two specialists to discuss the case to see if they can resolve the conflict, you can go back to your family doctor and ask for help in making the judgment, you can seek a third opinion and accept the majority decision or you can follow your own instincts about what doctor and treatment are best for you.

What if I want a second opinion and I am already hospitalized?

Getting a second opinion when you are already hospitalized is more difficult to arrange, unless your doctor is agreeable to the need for another opinion. Explain to your doctor that before you go ahead with any further treatment you would like to have another consultation. If there is a specialist on the hospital staff who is qualified, arranging a consultation will be easier than if the specialist is located at another hospital. However, don't let difficulties deter you from seeking a consultation that will give you further insight into what possibilities are open to you. Even when you are hospitalized, it is still your right to demand that your doctor find another physician—even one from another hospital—to give you an independent opinion. Check to see if the hospital has a patient advocate service or ombudsman to help with this kind of situation.

Is it appropriate for me to take notes or tape-record my conversation with the doctor?

It is perfectly acceptable for patients to take notes or even ask to record discussions with physicians. However, it is best to mention to your doctor that you plan to tape the information. Explain that you want to use it as a refresher when you get home, rather than having to call back to ask the doctor to repeat the information for you or your family members. Some doctors, concerned about malpractice suits, may not be entirely comfortable with this, but a taped record can be very helpful to you in reviewing a consultation or it can be used to get feedback from someone who is not present during the appointment.

What is the role of the nurse in cancer care?

The nurse is a very important part of the health team in cancer care. A growing number of nurses in the country are specializing in the cancer field. Some of these nurses work in medical centers with the physicians who are doing investigational work in chemotherapy and radiation therapy. Some work in the offices of oncologists. Others are ostomy nurses or enterostomal therapists who take care of the needs of patients who have had operations in the gastrointestinal areas. Some nurses give chemotherapy drugs under the doctors' supervision. Others are involved with teaching patients how to take care of themselves after leaving the hospital. Many will evaluate how the patient and the family are coping with the illness and managing symptoms such as pain, nausea, vomiting, fatigue, and loss of appetite. When you see the initials OCN after the nurses' names, you know that these nurses have been certified by the Oncology Nursing Society. This designation, similar to board certification for physicians, signifies their special expertise and competence in cancer nursing. Advanced practice nurses, with a master's degree, may have additional certification as certified nurse practitioners. Nurses who are Fellows of the American Academy of Nursing (FAAN) have earned this special status for scholarly contributions, practice and research. Get to know the nurses who are involved with your care. They can be your best allies.

How do I choose a doctor and a hospital if I am in an HMO?

When looking for a doctor within the plan, you'll need to ask the same questions as if you were choosing a private doctor. An HMO is a network of doctors and hospitals grouped together to deliver comprehensive medical care to its members. (HMO stands for Health Maintenance Organization.) The larger HMOs have a large panel of doctors, sometimes numbering in the thousands. Many require you to pick a primary-care doctor from the HMO's directory. This doctor then is responsible for your health care, decides what health care you will receive and what specialists you will go to. If you need hospital care, you'll have to use one of the hospitals in the HMO's network. In many cases, if you go outside the HMO's network, you will have to pay the bills yourself. Some plans have an opt-out or point-of-service feature where the employer pays some of the cost, usually 60 to 70 percent, if you obtain care outside the HMO. As more and more companies move to managed care, insurance plans have a greater effect on the decisions you make in choosing a doctor and a hospital. If possible, you may want to check with someone in the plan with a similar condition to see how things have worked out.

What is a PPO?

A PPO is a network of doctors and hospitals that have agreed to give the sponsoring organization discounts from their usual charges. (PPO stands for Preferred-Provider Organization.) The doctors and hospitals may be the same ones used in an HMO or they may be different. In a PPO, you can go to any doctor in the network whenever you want (although in some areas you need a referral from your primary physician to see a specialist). As long as you use the network doctors, your coverage will pay the stated proportion of the bill. If you go outside, you are paid a smaller percentage. There are also so-called Gatekeeper PPOs, where the medical services are more tightly controlled. In some of these plans, no benefits are paid if members go outside the network. These are known as exclusive provider organizations.

What is an EPO?

EPO, which stands for Exclusive-Provider Organization, resembles an HMO but is usually not regulated under state insurance laws. As a result, this type of plan may lack some consumer safeguards, such as quality assurance programs and the formal grievance procedures found in real HMOs.

What questions should I ask before signing up for an HMO or PPO or EPO?

- When must I notify the plan before going to the hospital and how do I do it?
- Will I be penalized for going to a doctor outside the network?
- Is there a percentage paid for services outside the network? What is the percentage paid and what does it apply to?
- Will the plan pay for a second opinion outside of the network?
- What happens if I see a specialist on my own who is not in the plan?
- Which doctors provide primary care? (Sometimes a highly regarded specialist will join the plan as a consultant in a subspecialty but will not be available to provide primary care.)
- Are all services offered by a doctor in a network covered?
- How is payment made to an outside doctor—am I billed? And who pays if my regular doctor is unavailable and another doctor is covering the service?
- Are doctors in the plan taking any new patients?
- Are the doctors in the plan board certified? Have you checked their credentials? How long have they been involved in the plan?
- Are the doctors satisfied with their involvement in the plan?
- Are the doctors obligated to continue my treatment in the hospital even if they decide to leave the plan?
- Do I need to get a referral from my assigned doctor to go to a specialist?
- Does my doctor have to get approval before sending me to the hospital or to specialists?

- Is there a limit to the number of visits I can have with the specialist once I am referred?
- How long does it take to get an appointment for nonemergency care?
- Are prescription drugs, dental treatment, annual physicals, and eye care covered?
- Is it possible to see nonplan doctors if I am willing to pay some of the out-of-pocket medical costs?
- If you are on Medicare, be sure to ask: Will I still get Medicare benefits if I go outside the plan to a specialist?

What if I am unhappy with the medical care I have received from a doctor or a hospital?

You have a right to complain directly to the hospital where you received treatment or to the local medical society. If you are not happy with the results, you can call your state licensing board. Check Chapter 26 for a listing. For a free information packet on how to file a complaint, write to the People's Medical Society, 462 Walnut Street, Allentown, PA 18102.

CHOOSING YOUR HOSPITAL

It's not always easy to tell a good hospital from a bad hospital—and deciding which hospital to use may not be simple for you. Sometimes it isn't even a decision you realize you have a right to make, since so much depends upon where a doctor practices. Many people feel most comfortable going to a hospital that is closest to home. Some people feel that a hospital with a religious affiliation of their choosing is important. Others judge a hospital by the food it serves.

When you need specialized cancer care, it is essential that you evaluate your hospital's credentials in medical terms to be certain that the hospital delivers the very best and the very latest treatment available. Accomplishing this may take a bit of time and effort—but it is worth thinking about.

It is helpful to know the criteria that distinguish a good hospital from a bad one so that you can evaluate your options in determining where you want to be treated. The hospital's track record in dealing with cancer cases, the range of services offered, the hospital's credentials, its participation in research and education, and overall experience, are all important to the kind of care and treatment you will receive.

Measuring quality care is much harder than measuring the merits of the new car you are going to buy. Though it may be difficult, it's worth the effort to investigate the credentials of the organization which will have a direct impact on the outcome of your treatment.

How can I tell a good hospital from a bad one?

There are many ways of judging a hospital. Some hospitals that give loving care but do not offer expanded facilities may be fine for some types of hospital stays. However, when you are choosing a hospital for specialized cancer treatments, there are other considerations. You'll be interested to know that there are about 7,000 hospitals in the United States. Of these, about 500 are medical school affiliated and another 1,500 have intern/residency teaching programs. On the other hand there are approximately 1,600 hospitals that continue to lack minimum accreditation. In the middle is a group of average hospitals that offer care ranging from superior to substandard. Surveys done among hospital professionals usually list 25 to 50 hospitals in the country that are categorized as superior.

What kind of accreditation is required of hospitals?

Hospitals voluntarily submit to being judged by a number of organizations which rate them on a variety of criteria. The American College of Surgeons has set up a multidisciplinary cancer committee that surveys hospitals and approves hospital cancer programs along with other requirements. This credential is an important one for anyone planning to have cancer surgery. Most hospitals are surveyed by the Joint Commission on Accreditation of Healthcare Organizations, a nationwide authority that accredits hospitals. The JCAHO decides whether a hospital gets, keeps or loses accreditation based on its meeting certain criteria for staffing, equipment and facility safety requirements. If the hospital that you are considering is not accredited, it is important to know why.

Where can I check to see if a hospital is accredited?

You can call the hospital and ask for this information or you can check with the Joint Commission on Accreditation of Healthcare Organizations. Their phone number is 1-708-916-5800.

What is the difference between a comprehensive cancer center and other hospitals?

There are only twenty-eight comprehensive cancer centers designated by the National Cancer Institute, called NCI for short, across the country. Each of the comprehensive cancer centers is devoted to the diagnosis and multidisciplinary treatment of cancer patients,

JUDGING YOUR HOSPITAL

Assessment Score	Type of Hospital	Score Your Hospital
+50	Comprehensive cancer center designated by National Cancer Institute	
+40	Clinical cancer center designated by National Cancer Institute	
+40	Community hospital with a community clinical oncology program grant from the National Cancer Institute.	
+20	Approved hospital cancer center program sponsored by American College of Surgeons	
+20	Directly affiliated with medical school which uses hospital for internship and residency programs	
+15	Teaching hospital, residency and internship training, medical school affiliation, but medical school not located in hospital	
+10	Residency and/or internship program, without medical school affiliation	
+5	Accredited by Joint Commission on Accreditation of Healthcare Organizations as a hospital but without approved internship and/or residency programs	
0	Not accredited	
0	Government-supported (so-called public) hospital (VA, Public Health Service, county, city or state)	
0 or −10	Proprietary or for-profit hospital, owned by individuals or stockholders, including doctors who practice there.	

If at all possible, take advantage of the finest facility within your reach. Use of a comprehensive cancer center, if it is accessible, is a wise choice since that is where the experts are. Hospitals with medical schools generally provide excellent care since they attract top doctors and range of services is extremely broad. If not directly connected to a medical school, facilities are probably good, but not as wide-ranging. Accreditation is a minimum standard ensuring adequate care. About a quarter of U.S. hospitals are not accredited, and

(continued)

JUDGING YOUR HOSPITAL *(cont.)*

therefore are not eligible for Medicaid payments. Government-sponsored and proprietary hospitals vary from excellent to substandard. Proprietary hospitals sometimes are not as well equipped because of efforts to keep costs low and profits high. Local reputation is the key to your score on this.

ASSESSMENT SCORE	NUMBER OF BEDS	SCORE YOUR HOSPITAL
+20	Over 500 beds	
+15	100 to 500 beds	
+5	Under 100 beds	

Of the more than 3,000 hospitals with fewer than 100 beds, only a handful are medical school affiliated, and less than 1 percent offer residency programs. Check yours out. There are a few outstanding exceptions in this category.

	LOCATION OF HOSPITAL	
+25	Within 30 miles	
+15	Within 100 miles	
+5	Within 200 miles	

If your local hospital does not seem adequate to provide you with the services you will need, you should ask your doctor to refer you to a specialist who is affiliated with a hospital which is better suited to your needs. You must weigh emotional support and the burden of traveling in your calculation. Remember that you can arrange to be evaluated by one of the specialists, who can then advise your doctor on treatment.

	GENERAL HOSPITAL SERVICES	
+5	Postoperative recovery room	
+5	Intensive care unit	
+10	Pathology lab	
+10	Diagnostic laboratories	
+5	Pharmacy	
+5	Blood bank	
+5	Sophisticated x-ray equipment, CT scanner, MRI	*(continued)*

JUDGING YOUR HOSPITAL *(cont.)*		
ASSESSMENT SCORE	**TYPE OF HOSPITAL**	**SCORE YOUR HOSPITAL**
+5	Radioactive scanning equipment	
+5	Brain wave equipment (EEG)	
+10	Tumor committee, tumor registry	
+5	24-hour respiratory therapy	
+5	Physical therapy	
+5	Patient advocate services	
+5	Social services	
+10	Anesthesiologists (rather than anesthetists) in operating room	
+10	Adequate nursing staff	
+10	Advanced practice nurses as part of staff	
+10	24-hour-a-day physician staffing	

All of these facilities are part of an up-to-date hospital facility. Depending upon your needs and condition, these are all items that make up a well-run and well-equipped hospital that can serve every need. This chart is designed to allow you to check your hospital on its ability to deliver cancer care. It is not meant to be used to judge your hospital on its adequacy for emergency care, general surgery, etc.

Over 200—Excellent
Over 180—Very good
Over 130—Good
Over 100—Adequate
Under 100—Poor

laboratory research in several scientific fields, a strong program of clinical research and an ability to transfer research findings into everyday practice. They are specifically geared to treating cancer with the most up-to-date methods. Their credentials and programs have been rigorously peer reviewed and designated by the National Cancer Institute as "centers of excellence." If you live near a comprehensive cancer center, you should definitely consider going there for your diagnosis and treatment.

WARNING: Many hospitals use the word *comprehensive* in their titles. However, few of these hospitals have been rigorously reviewed for their expertise by the National Cancer Institute. In addition, there are for-profit groups in various parts of the country that have added the words *comprehensive cancer center* to their titles. These are NOT the same as the NCI-approved comprehensive cancer centers. Many of these for-profit centers are free-standing, not affiliated with medical schools and do not participate in research. They do, however, make available standard care, including chemotherapy and radiation therapy, and have oncologists on their staffs. If the hospital you use is not listed below or cited as an approved clinical and laboratory center (see Chapter 26, "Where to Get Help"), then it is **not** an authentically designated **comprehensive cancer center.**

Where are the NCI-designated comprehensive cancer centers located?
The following hospitals are designated as comprehensive cancer centers by the National Cancer Institute:

Alabama: University of Alabama, Birmingham
Arizona: Arizona Cancer Center, University of Arizona, Tucson
California: Jonsson Comprehensive Cancer Center, University of California, Los Angeles; USC/Kenneth T. Norris Jr. Cancer Center, University of Southern California, Los Angeles
Connecticut: Yale Cancer Center, Yale University School of Medicine, New Haven
District of Columbia: Lombardi Cancer Research Center, Georgetown University Medical Center, Washington, D.C.
Florida: Sylvester Comprehensive Cancer Center, University of Miami, Miami
Maryland: Johns Hopkins Oncology Center, Baltimore
Massachusetts: Dana-Farber Cancer Institute, Boston
Michigan: University of Michigan Cancer Center, Ann Arbor; Meyer L. Prentis Comprehensive Cancer Center of Metropolitan Detroit, Detroit
Minnesota: Mayo Comprehensive Cancer Center, Mayo Clinic, Rochester
New Hampshire: Norris Cotton Cancer Center, Hanover
New York: Memorial Sloan-Kettering Cancer Center, New York City; Kaplan Cancer Center, New York University Medical Center, New York City; Roswell Park Cancer Institute, Buffalo
North Carolina: Duke Comprehensive Cancer Center, Duke University Medical Center, Durham; Lineberger Comprehensive Cancer Center, University of North Carolina School of Medicine,

Chapel Hill; Cancer Center of Wake Forest University, Bowman Gray School of Medicine, Winston-Salem

Ohio: Ohio State University Comprehensive Cancer Center, Columbus

Pennsylvania: Fox Chase Cancer Center, Philadelphia; University of Pennsylvania Cancer Center, Philadelphia; Pittsburgh Cancer Institute, Pittsburgh

Texas: The University of Texas M. D. Anderson Cancer Center, Houston

Vermont: Vermont Regional Cancer Center, University of Vermont, Burlington

Washington: Fred Hutchinson Cancer Research Center, Seattle

Wisconsin: University of Wisconsin Comprehensive Cancer Center, Madison

(More information about comprehensive cancer centers, including addresses and telephone numbers, can be found in Chapter 26, "Where to Get Help.")

Should I go to a comprehensive cancer center for diagnosis and treatment of cancer?

If one of the comprehensive cancer centers is nearby, by all means take advantage of it. You can use its expertise for your care, or you may wish to have your case reviewed by the experts on its staff. If you need help in getting a referral to a comprehensive cancer center, call the Cancer Information Service. The information specialist can give you information on how to make an appointment at the center nearest you.

Is there any way I can benefit from the expertise of a comprehensive cancer center even if I live far away?

You can ask your doctor to refer you for evaluation by one of the specialists, who can then confer with your doctor on your treatment. Or, you can ask your doctor to contact one of the doctors who specializes in your type of cancer to discuss your case. This is especially important if you have a rare type of cancer which your doctor does not see very often.

Can I be treated at the Clinical Center at the National Institutes of Health?

The National Institutes of Health, the federal government's agency for medical research, has a medical research center and hospital—the Warren Grant Magnuson Clinical Center. You can be treated at the Clinical Center only if your case fits into a research project. The Clinical Center provides nursing and medical care without charge for patients who are being studied in clinical research programs. There is more information on the Clinical Center and on clinical trials in Chapter 9, "New Advances and Investigational Trials."

What are National Cancer Institute clinical centers?

The clinical centers are medical centers which have support from the National Cancer Institute, focus on both basic research and clinical research and often incorporate nearby affiliated clinical research institutions into their overall research programs. Many of the leading hospitals in the country are part of this program and can offer many of the same services as a comprehensive cancer center. They include:

California: City of Hope National Medical Center, Beckman Research Institute, Duarte; University of California at San Diego Cancer Center, San Diego

Colorado: University of Colorado Cancer Center, Denver

Illinois: Robert H. Lurie Cancer Center, Northwestern University, Chicago; University of Chicago Cancer Research Center, Chicago

New York: Albert Einstein College of Medicine, Bronx; Columbia University Cancer Center, New York; University of Rochester Cancer Center, Rochester

Ohio: Ireland Cancer Center, Case Western Reserve University, Cleveland

Tennessee: St. Jude Children's Research Hospital, Memphis

Texas: San Antonio Cancer Institute, San Antonio

Utah: Utah Cancer Center, University of Utah Medical Center, Salt Lake City

Virginia: Massey Cancer Center, Medical College of Virginia, Richmond

In addition, there is one other center, known as a consortium cancer center, which specializes in cancer prevention and control research. This center is the Drew-Meharry-Morehouse Consortium Cancer Center in Nashville, Tennessee.

What is a clinical trials cooperative group?

A clinical trials cooperative group, sponsored by the National Cancer Institute, is composed of academic institutions and cancer treatment centers throughout the United States, Canada and Europe. These groups work with the National Cancer Institute to identify important questions in cancer research and to design carefully controlled clinical trials to answer these questions. There are fourteen major cooperative groups, involving more than 2,200 institutions that contribute patients to group-conducted clinical trials. More than 16,000 individual investigators also participate in NCI-supported cooperative group studies.

Who pays for the treatment given to patients in clinical trials cooperative groups?

Most costs of medical treatment in clinical trials cooperative groups are borne by the patient, although medical insurance usually pays for the doctor's visit. Drugs not yet commercially available may be provided free of charge. In some specialized treatments, all costs are paid for. In Chapter 26, "Where to Get Help," you will find the name of the chairman of each clinical trials cooperative group and the phone number for contact. The address listed is not an indication of where these groups are located. It is simply the information center for the specific type of study group. Your doctor or you may contact that person for information on what physicians in your area are involved in clinical trials. The Cancer Information Service (toll-free at 1-800-4-CANCER) can give you information on what clinical trials are being run in your area.

Is it a good idea to go to a research or teaching hospital?

Naturally, this is a personal decision, based on many factors. Certain demands are made on patients in these hospitals which may be disturbing for some and comforting to others. Physicians, nurses, psychologists and social workers often interview patients. Members of the medical staff other than the patient's physician may drop by to examine the patient's condition. Of course, patients always have the option of refusing to be examined by or treated by anyone other than their own doctors (except in emergencies where quick decisions are essential). Some people object to being treated by anyone except their own personal physician. If you feel this way, it is important for you to understand how these hospitals operate. The care in research and teaching hospitals can be very attentive, the staff is very competent, and the patient can be assured that the latest and most up-to-date treatment is available.

If I go to a research or teaching hospital will I become a guinea pig for a cancer-research project?

Many people are frightened at the thought of being used in a research project without their consent. Each patient participating in a research project must sign a consent form which explains both the potential value and the possible risks. All research projects must first be approved by the hospital's research committee (usually called the human investigations committee), which has strict guidelines it follows in evaluating whether or not the project can be carried out at that hospital. Before consenting to become part of a research project, you should consider asking the following questions:

- What is the purpose of the study?
- What kinds of tests and treatments will be done and how will they be done?
- What is likely to happen to my cancer with, or without, the new research treatment?
- What are my other possible choices and what are their advantages and disadvantages?
- Are there standard treatments you might recommend for my case and how does the study compare with these standard treatments?
- What side effects might I expect from these research treatments that differ from what I would expect from standard treatments or from the natural course of the disease?
- How long will the study last? Is this longer than standard treatments?
- Will I have to be hospitalized? If so, how often and for how long?
- What will be the cost on my part? Is any of the treatment given free?
- If I should not respond to the new treatment, what further treatment would be possible?
- What type of long-term follow-up care is part of the study?

There is more detailed information on clinical trials in Chapter 9, "New Advances and Investigational Trials."

Why is a teaching hospital considered to be superior to a hospital which does not have an intern/residency program?

In a teaching hospital, there are more professionals on the job—more doctors on site checking up on the competence of other doctors. In a teaching hospital you are seen on regular daily "rounds" by your doctor and other interns and residents. Doctors who receive appointments to these hospitals are usually tops in their fields. Teaching hospitals attract the finest medical minds in the country.

If you're in a teaching hospital and feel you're being badgered by too many interns and residents, what can you do?

Some patients find it annoying to be "poked at" by countless interns and residents. If you find this to be a problem, you have a perfect right to discuss this with your doctor, and ask how this practice can be limited.

Can I refuse to be examined by a medical student?

You are within your rights to refuse to be examined. However, many a helpful diagnosis or insight has been made by medical students who were doing their jobs as painstakingly as only novices will. It may be to your advantage to allow the services of a soon-to-be doctor. Of course, if you are feeling very ill and find the whole process troublesome, you can request that you not be questioned or examined.

Is size an important factor in considering a hospital?

In the checklist "Judging Your Hospital," you'll notice we have given greater weight to a hospital with 500 or more beds than we have to one with between 100 and 500 beds or one with less than 100 beds. This is a general rule of thumb. We do know of some excellent small hospitals. There are some poor large hospitals. Size is not all—but the number of patients with serious illnesses seen by the staff is an important factor. In a larger hospital, in the course of a week, a doctor will probably treat as many patients with a specific illness as the small hospital doctor will see in a year. Hospital death rates have been estimated to be 40 percent higher in less-than-100-bed hospitals than in larger hospitals. The overall capabilities of a large hospital are greater than those of a small one. Although people may complain that large hospitals are impersonal, the overall capabilities of a large hospital are greater than those of a small one.

What if the doctor sends me to a hospital where I do not wish to go for treatment?

You have a right to go to the hospital of your choice. However, if your doctor does not have privileges at that hospital, you cannot be treated by that doctor in that hospital. That is why, in choosing a doctor, an important consideration is hospital affiliation. Some doctors have admitting privileges at more than one hospital. Therefore, if you have a specific preference for a hospital, be sure to discuss this with your doctor at the outset.

What is the difference between an anesthesiologist and an anesthetist?

An anesthetist is a person who administers anesthetics. An anesthesiologist is an M.D. whose specialty is the administration of anesthesia. For any operation which requires the use of anesthesia, you should make certain that your anesthesia is administered under the supervision of a board-certified anesthesiologist.

What kinds of nurses are involved with caring for me in the hospital?

It is useful to understand the functions of the various nurses. In most hospitals, particularly in larger ones, you will find, in order of authority:

- Director of nursing (responsible for entire nursing staff).
- Clinical director (in charge of major nursing areas).
- Nurse manager (responsible for a particular unit or units).
- Clinical nurse specialists (advanced clinical skills for management of patients and families).
- Staff nurses (direct nursing care).
- Aides (assist nurses in care of patients and in charge of the clinical area).

Staff nurses are registered nurses who have completed a nurses' training program, possess a nursing school diploma or an associate's or bachelor's degree and are licensed by the state to practice nursing. These nurses have fundamental knowledge of most diseases and know how to observe and manage patients. They handle patient care which requires special knowledge such as giving out medication, adjusting medical devices (such as tubes, drains, respirators, etc.), changing intravenous bottles, giving injections, and recognizing problems which need a doctor's care. Licensed practical nurses have completed a training program in nursing and are also licensed by the state. Some also may complete an additional pharmacology course and are qualified to give medication.

Do I have a right to see my hospital records?

Though many nurses and doctors are extremely secretive about hospital records, you do have a right to see yours. You may not be able to understand much of what is in it because it is written in medical shorthand. Usually a nurse or a doctor will be present so that you will not misunderstand or misinterpret the information.

Am I obligated to sign consent forms?

Consent forms are necessary before the doctor can go ahead with any procedure that entails any element of risk—surgery, anesthesia, spinal taps, etc. However, do not sign a blank consent form. Do not let the doctor get away with an explanation that there is some uncertainty as to what the surgical procedure will entail and so is asking you to sign a consent form to be filled in later. Your doctor has an obligation to inform you of the risks and consequences of any procedure and to state the specific procedure for which you are being asked to give your consent. (Specifications for surgery should include the specific area to be operated on and the specific procedure the surgeon expects to perform.) Do not sign any form unless all your questions have been addressed.

How can I guard against medication errors in the hospital?

You should ask and know what medications your doctor has prescribed for you, what they are designed to do, and what they look like. If you have any question at all about a medication, ask the nurse to check the order book to make certain the doctor's orders have been followed or to check back with the doctor in case an error has been made. Many a medical disaster has been averted by a patient who asks, "Is this a new pill?" Be alert to what medications you are taking and why they are being given.

Should I discuss finances with my doctor?

Cancer is a very expensive illness, and you should know what kinds of costs will be involved. You should never be afraid to ask the doctor about office and personal fees, what the laboratory tests will cost, how much the hospital bill will be, and what x-rays and drugs cost. The earlier you have this kind of discussion, the better off you will be. The doctor may not be able to detail all of the costs since office staff usually does the actual billing and tends to accounting services. Ask to speak with the person who does the billing, if this is the case. Nurses and social workers often can be helpful in some instances since they are knowledgeable about coverage, eligibility, services, programs and insurance issues.

chapter 3

What Is Cancer?

> There are over 100 kinds of cancer, and each kind and site has its own distinguishing characteristics. Cancer occurs when cells become abnormal and keep dividing and forming more cells without control or order. Cancer is predominately a disease of middle and old age. It is quite rare in children and young adults.

The human body is made up of some ten trillion cells. Each cell carries out specialized functions and most have the capacity for infinite multiplication—in a very carefully controlled manner. Cells are constantly dying off and being replaced with new cells. When cancer occurs, the cells escape from the normal mechanism and begin to behave in an uncontrolled fashion. They never stop reproducing themselves and soon there are many more of them than of the healthy cells in the tissue surrounding them. When cells escape from regulatory control, they hand down their independence to their descendants and each continues to reproduce at will, cloning an independent colony in rebel fashion.

WHAT YOU NEED TO KNOW ABOUT CANCER

- Precancerous changes in cells can be detected under the microscope. In healthy tissue, each cell is identically shaped, each with its own sharply defined nucleus.

- In precancerous change, the cells lose their uniformity. Cells of different sizes are interspersed with cells of normal size. In many, the nuclei are irregular. At this point, these irregular cells are no more than that. They show no signs of invasion of other tissue or of movement to other parts of the body.

- When any part of the body needs repair, all cells in the immediate vicinity leap into action, dividing rapidly to repair the defect. If a pathologist looks at tissue from a healing wound, the rapidly dividing, immature cells resemble those from a malignant tumor. However, in the case of ordinary wound healing, the well-controlled cells that are involved revert to their normal pattern when the healing is complete, whereas cancer cells continue their rapid division.

- When cancerous cells begin to reproduce, the distortion of individual cell structure is more pronounced, with a tendency for the cells to appear to be more primitive and with the abnormal cells moving from their normal locations to surrounding tissues. This uncontrolled growth of cells is what brings about symptoms—a mass or a lump or bleeding.

- Cancer may behave differently in different people. Learning the basics about cancer will help the person without a medical background to better understand what the doctor is talking about when discussing the diagnosis, treatment and outcome.

- There are many things you can do to prevent cancer, such as stopping smoking, changing your diet, using sunscreen or staying out of the sun.

- There are many studies that are trying to determine the association of environmental issues and cancer, such as DDT, nuclear power plants, and electric power lines. However, the newest research shows that each person is born with various genetic susceptibilities—weak spots in the genetic makeup—that may play the major role in causing cancer.

Do all normal cells look alike?
No, each normal cell has a specialized structure designed to do a particular job in a particular organ. For example, those cells which form the skin tend to be flat. The class of cells which make up the nerves are long and slender. Within each class, all normal cells are quite uniform in size and almost identical in shape. Each class of cells presents different arrangements when they join each other. Glandular cells, for example, form circles which build upon each other like stones lining a well. Skin cells stretch out in sheetlike layers, row on row, like a brick wall. Each type of cell joins together

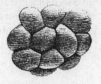
normal cells

precancerous cells

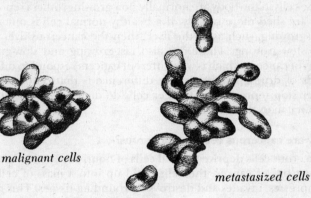

malignant cells

metastasized cells

How cancer grows

with other similar cells to form tissues which arrange themselves in orderly patterns to form the various parts of our complex bodies.

What's the difference between a benign and a malignant (cancerous) tumor?

A benign tumor is a growth that is not cancerous. It can usually be removed and in most cases does not come back. It does not spread to other parts of the body. Most benign tumors do not endanger life, unless they are growing in a confined area such as the brain. Malignant tumors, on the other hand, do not organize themselves into normal patterns, and even though the tissue resembles the tissue of the normal cell, the arrangement is imperfect. Sometimes the cancer cells are so dissimilar from the normal structure that it may be difficult to identify the tissue from which the cancer started. The imperfection of the abnormal cells is the failure of the cancer cells to mature (or differentiate, as the physicians would say). Cancer cells can damage nearby tissues and organs. They also can break away from the malignant tumor and spread to form new tumors in other parts of the body.

Can benign tumors become cancerous?

In most cases they do not. The tumor that begins as a benign tumor usually remains a benign tumor. However, there are lesions that are considered precancerous, such as a thickening of the lining of the mouth or cervix. These should be taken care of before cancer occurs.

Are there fast-growing and slow-growing cancers?

Some cells in the body are normally slow growing; others reproduce and are shed more rapidly. If a healthy normal cell is one that is slow-growing, such as in the liver, then the cancerous liver cell is also slow-growing. There are also fast-growing and slow-growing types of cancers, which is why different cancers respond to different kinds of drugs. The important difference is that cancerous cells never stop reproducing. Cancer cells do die, but their death rate is lower than their birth rate.

Why are cancerous cells so dangerous?

Cancerous cells deprive normal cells of nourishment and space. In most types of cancer, the cells build up into a mass of cells that compresses, invades and destroys surrounding tissues. This mass is often called a growth, a tumor, or a neoplasm (new growth).

Is it true that the more irregular the cells, the more malignant the cancer?

As a general rule, the more irregular or abnormal (the doctors call this undifferentiated) the cells look under the microscope, the more malignant the cancer. The greater the difference in appearance from a normal cell, the more active the cancer is likely to be and the more uncontrollable its course.

What does it mean when the doctor refers to differentiated and undifferentiated cells?

A differentiated cell is a cancerous cell that resembles normal cells. The more differentiated the cell, the more it resembles a normal cell, the less aggressive it is and the more likely it is to respond to treatment. An undifferentiated cell, as you might expect, is more abnormal. The more undifferentiated (or abnormal) the cells appear under the microscope, the more cancerous the cells are and the more active and uncontrollable the cancer is likely to be. Many types of cancer are graded by how differentiated the cells are and this factor is considered when treatment is planned.

How many cells are in a cancerous tumor?

The number varies by the size of the tumor and the type of cell. First of all, you should understand that there is considerable variation in the size of cells making up different parts of the human body. The most numerous of the body cells are so small that it would take between 700 and 800 cells to cover the head of a pin. A one-centimeter lump in the breast, which is a little larger than the size of a pea, is about the smallest lump which you can feel with your fingers. Such a lump contains over a billion cells. This size tumor has undergone about thirty doublings since it first became an abnormal cell.

What does the doctor mean when he says I have a solid tumor?

A solid tumor is a tumor such as carcinoma or sarcoma which forms a mass of growth. Other types (see chart) originate in other types of cells.

TYPES OF CANCERS	
TYPE	**DESCRIPTION**
Carcinoma	Originates from tissues that cover a surface or line a cavity of the body. This is the most common type of cancer.
Sarcoma	Originates from tissues which connect, support or surround other tissues and organs. Can be either soft tissue or bone sarcomas.
Myeloma	Originates in the bone marrow in the blood cells that manufacture antibodies.
Lymphoma	Originates in lymph system—the circulatory network of vessels, spaces, and nodes carrying lymph, the almost colorless fluid that bathes the body's cells.
Leukemia	Involves the blood-forming tissues and blood cells.

What does the term *in situ* mean?

This term is used to describe an early, noninvasive cancer. One of the most constant characteristics of cancer is the invasion of healthy tissues bordering the tumor. However, there appears to be a period before invasion begins. Such growths are called in situ, and the results of removal are more positive than those for cancers which have already begun to invade neighboring tissues. The term also applies to another group of tumors—usually found on surfaces—which have other characteristics of malignancy but in which normal cells may be completely replaced by tumor cells before

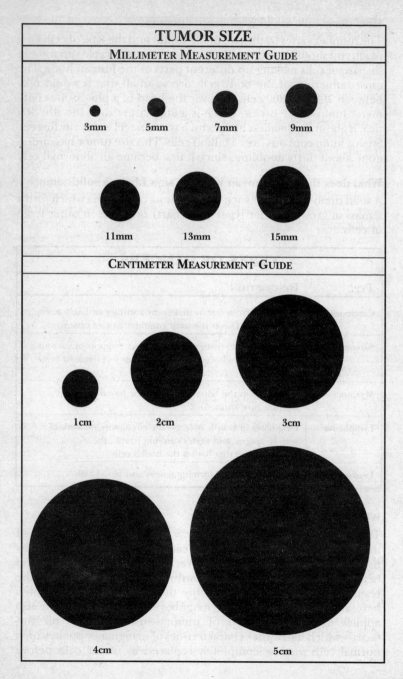

TUMOR SIZE

MILLIMETER MEASUREMENT GUIDE

3mm   5mm   7mm   9mm

11mm   13mm   15mm

CENTIMETER MEASUREMENT GUIDE

1cm   2cm   3cm

4cm   5cm

there is evidence of invasion of surrounding tissues. In most instances, removal of the in situ cancer is considered a cure.

What does it mean when the doctor says my cancer has metastasized?

This means that the cancer is not confined to one area of the body but has spread or has started to spread. (Sometimes the doctor will say that the tumor is disseminated, which means the same as metastasized.) The process by which cancer spreads from where it began (that is, from the primary tumor) to distant parts of the body is called metastasis. Tiny clumps of cells break off from the tumor and are carried in the lymphatic vessels or the bloodstream to a distant part of the body. These "seeds" from the original cancer start growing in the new location. The new tumor is said to have metastasized to the new site, and such a tumor is often referred to as a metastatic tumor. The plural of *metastasis* is *metastases*. Sometimes you will hear the word *mets* used as a shorthand term for metastases.

Where does cancer usually spread?

Different types of cancer have different spreading patterns. Breast cancer, for instance, generally spreads or metastasizes from the breast (primary site) to four places in the body: liver, bone, lung and brain. More rarely, it can spread to the spinal cord, to distant lymph nodes and to other parts of the body. Identifying whether or not a cancer has metastasized is the most decisive factor in the choice of treatment and the success of treatment.

When a tumor metastasizes or spreads, is it called by the name of the organ to which it has spread?

No. This can be quite confusing to most people, but when you understand the way the body works, it makes sense. If the original tumor is in the prostate, for example, and it spreads to the bone, it is not considered or treated like bone cancer. It is prostate cancer that has spread to the bones. The type of cancer cells found in the bones will be the same type as the cancer cells found in the prostate. These cells will grow, reproduce and behave according to the pattern of metastatic prostate cancer (prostate cancer which has spread to other areas) and not like bone cancer. Because of this fact, metastatic cancer of any kind is generally treated in the way the original cancer responds best. Cancer that starts in the prostate and spreads to the bones is not treated in the same way as cancer that starts in the bones would be treated. It is still treated as a form of prostate cancer, because that is what it is.

At what age do persons usually get cancer?

Cancer is predominately a disease of middle and old age. In the United States, 66 percent of cancer in men and 63 percent of cancer in women is diagnosed at age 55 and over. Persons at about the age of 70 account for a higher number of cases than any other age group. Overall, men and women account for about the same number of new cases of cancer.

Is cancer common in children?

Cancer is quite rare in children and in young adults. However, for children under 15, cancer is the second leading cause of death, accounting for one out of twenty-eight deaths. Leukemia is the most common form of childhood cancer, followed by tumors of the central nervous system.

Can a person catch cancer?

There is no indication that cancer can be considered contagious in the popular sense of the word. You should not be afraid that you will "catch" cancer from another person. People who care for cancer patients on a daily basis do not have a higher incidence of cancer than the general population. There is no evidence to suggest that living in the same household with a cancer patient over a long period of time, sharing his or her possessions, kissing or having intercourse with a cancer patient, increases the chances of being diagnosed with cancer.

What are the most common warning signs of cancer?

There are seven basic symptoms:

1. **Unusual bleeding or discharge.**
2. **A lump that does not go away.**
3. **A sore that does not heal within two weeks.**
4. **Change in bowel or bladder habits.**
5. **Persistent hoarseness or cough.**
6. **Indigestion or difficulty in swallowing.**
7. **Change in a wart or mole.**

The specific symptoms for cancer in different parts of the body are given at the beginning of each chapter.

Is it possible to have cancer without any warning symptoms?

It is possible. Often symptoms seem so trivial to most people that they may be ignored. For example, coughs are so common that we do not get alarmed when we have one. Usually you can tell yourself that you have been smoking too much or blame your sinuses or rationalize that everyone you know has a cough. However, coughing can also be the first visible sign of lung cancer. Irregular vaginal bleeding can be due to a whole list of causes, too, which can lull you into not bothering to see a doctor. But irregular vaginal bleeding can also be the first sign of cancer of the uterus. What is important to remember is that you must learn to pay attention to your body's signals. Any suspicious symptom that persists for longer than two weeks should be investigated by a qualified physician.

What new research is being done to learn more about how cancer starts and behaves?

This is an exciting time for scientists, using the tools of molecular biology to follow up clues as to why one person gets cancer and another one does not. The current understanding of how various parts of the cellular system develop is almost completely at odds with beliefs that researchers held only a few years ago. Every day new information is being discovered about how a cell grows and what signals make it divide, as well as how the body rids itself of cancer-causing agents. Words like *cyclins* (proteins that can turn on enzymes stimulating inappropriate cells division) and *adducts* (formed when chemicals stick to DNA; if the damage is not repaired before the cell divides, mutations occur that can cause cancer) are being added to the cancer vocabulary.

What are genes and how are they related to cells?

Genes are the biological units of heredity. Almost every cell in the body contains 50,000 to 100,000 genes. Each gene acts as a blueprint for making a specific enzyme or other protein or for telling the cell to do something. A flaw in a gene can result in diseases, including cancer. The genes are arranged on chromosomes—rodlike structures composed of DNA and protein. Each cell, in humans, contains 46 chromosomes (23 pairs) located within a central structure known as the nucleus.

Does each person's body treat cancer-causing substances in the same manner?

No. New molecular research indicates that people are born with various weak spots in their genetic makeup. Some people, for instance, have genes that allow their bodies to get rid of carcinogens more easily, while others, born with genes that are more slow-acting, allow the chemicals to bind up with their DNA. Other people have defects on important genes, like the tumor-suppressor p53 gene, that causes them to be more vulnerable to cancer. There are two copies of every gene in most cells. One normal copy of a gene is sufficient to prevent the development of cancer. If both copies are damaged or mutated, however, cancer may develop.

What is an oncogene?

An oncogene is a defect in the gene, and is transmitted on the chromosome. Researchers believe that every person carries oncogenes in each body cell and that the oncogenes remain harmless until triggered by something. When that happens, the oncogene can transform some normal cells into malignant ones.

Is cancer inherited?

For many years doctors puzzled over why some families seem to have more cancer than would occur by chance alone. Today scientists are discovering genetic flaws that put some people at higher risk. A gene called p53 is responsible for an inherited cancer syndrome known as the Li-Fraumeni syndrome. People with this inherited disorder are at higher risk for breast cancer, colon cancer, soft tissue sarcomas, bone cancer (osteosarcoma), brain tumors, leukemia and adrenocortical cancer, all occurring at unusually early ages. The risk of certain other cancers, including melanoma, ovarian, testicular, lung, pancreas and prostate, may also be greater, though to a lesser degree. Genes that account for many other illnesses, even those that have complicated genetic patterns, are being discovered at a dizzying rate. This field of research, known as molecular biology, is transforming the way that cancer is detected and diagnosed and also predicting who will get cancer in the first place. (For additional information, see Chapter 9, "New Advances and Investigational Trials.")

Do we know how cancer starts?

Most scientists believe that many cancers come about through a multistep process, in which several events are required to produce cancer. Research in the area of molecular and cellular biology has identified three steps: initiation, promotion and progression. Cancer-causing agents, known as carcinogens, can contribute to the first two stages.

How does this multistep process work?

It is believed that initiators start the damage to the cell, and cause changes that can lead to cancer. Cigarette smoking, x-rays and certain chemicals are considered initiators. Promoters change the cells already damaged by the initiator from normal cells to cancer cells but usually do not cause cancer. Alcohol, hormones, and growth factors, for instance, are considered promoters. During progression, tumors spread from the initial tumor to other parts of the body.

Does tobacco play a large role in causing cancer?

Smoking tobacco, chewing tobacco and snuff, and being exposed to tobacco smoke without actually smoking may account for about a third of all cancer deaths in the United States each year. Tobacco is the most preventable cause of death in this country. Smoking accounts for more than 85 percent of all lung cancer deaths. Smokers are also more likely than nonsmokers to develop several other types of cancer, such as cancers of the mouth, tongue, lip, larynx, esophagus, pancreas, bladder, kidney and cervix.

How is alcohol linked to cancer?

Drinking large amounts of alcohol increases the risk of cancer of the mouth, throat, esophagus and larynx. People who smoke cigarettes or chew tobacco and drink alcohol have an especially high risk of getting those cancers. Alcohol can damage the liver and increase the risk of liver cancer. Alcohol is an example of a classic promoter. It alone does not cause cancer, but it is clearly associated with the development of certain kinds of cancer.

Does diet cause cancer?

Your choice of foods may affect your chance of developing cancer. Evidence points to a possible link between a high-fat diet and certain cancers, such as cancer of the breast, colon, uterus and prostate. Being seriously overweight appears to be linked to increased rates of cancer of the prostate, pancreas, uterus, colon and ovary and to breast cancer in older women. Salt-cured, smoked and nitrite-cured foods have been linked to cancers of the esophagus and stomach. On the other hand, studies suggest that foods containing fiber and certain nutrients help protect against some types of cancer.

Is sunlight a cause of cancer?

Ultraviolet radiation from the sun and from sources such as sunlamps and tanning booths damages the skin. Scientists estimate that sunlight is responsible for almost all of the more than 700,000 cases of basal and squamous cell skin cancer every year and is a major factor in the development of melanoma. Repeated exposure to ultraviolet radiation increases the risk of skin cancer, especially if you have fair skin or freckle easily.

Should I be concerned if I am taking hormone replacement drugs?

Many women use estrogen treatment to control the hot flashes, vaginal dryness and thinning of the bones (osteoporosis) that might occur during menopause. However, studies show that estrogen use increases the risk of cancer of the uterus. Other studies suggest an increased risk of breast cancer among women who have used high doses of estrogen or have used estrogen for a long time. On the other hand, taking estrogen reduces the risk of heart disease and osteoporosis. The risk of uterine cancer appears to be lower when progesterone is used with estrogen than when estrogen is used alone. But some scientists are concerned that the addition of progesterone may also increase the risk of breast cancer. Scientists are still studying and sifting through new information about the risks and benefits of taking replacement hormones.

Is a vasectomy linked to the risk for prostate cancer?

A consensus conference of scientists, who looked at all the data from published and unpublished studies, concluded that the research results on the association between vasectomy and prostate cancer are inconsistent, and since there is no convincing biological explanation for how a vasectomy might cause prostate cancer, it was determined that additional research is needed.

Has exposure to DES during pregnancy proven to be a cancer risk for daughters and their mothers?

DES is a form of estrogen that doctors prescribed from the early 1940s until 1971 to try to prevent miscarriage. In some daughters of the women who took DES, the uterus, vagina and cervix do not develop normally. DES-exposed daughters also have an increased chance of developing abnormal cells in the cervix and vagina. In addition, a rare type of vaginal and cervical cancer has been found in a small number of DES-exposed daughters. Mothers may have a slightly increased risk of developing breast cancer. DES-exposed sons do not appear to have an increased chance of developing cancer, although they may have reproductive and urinary system problems.

Has exposure to pesticides been studied as a cause of cancer?

There have been several studies of the exposure to pesticides, particularly by farmers. In addition, there is a growing body of research that raises concern about the potential risk of breast cancer from exposure to chemicals, such as the now-banned DDT. The National Cancer Institute has found that farmers who used herbicides, especially 2,4-D (2,4-dichlorophenoxyacetic acid), were more likely to have non-Hodgkin's lymphomas than those who didn't use this weed killer. A large study, involving 100,000 farmers, is presently under way, looking at the reasons farmers and their families are at higher risk for leukemia, multiple myeloma and non-Hodgkin's lymphoma, and for cancers of the brain, prostate, stomach, skin, and lip. A study of women in New York City showed that women with high blood levels of DDE, a chemical from the pesticide DDT, were at an increased risk of breast cancer. Researchers at the National Cancer Institute and at the National Institute of Environmental Health Sciences are studying what specific environmental exposures may be contributing to the higher rates of breast cancer deaths in different parts of the country, with six studies funded in the Northeast and mid-Atlantic regions of the United States.

Has Agent Orange been tested?

Agent Orange, a mixture of herbicides used during the Vietnam War mainly to defoliate forest trees and destroy crops, has been studied several times. The studies have been conflicting and inconclusive. However, Vietnam veterans with some cancers (non-Hodgkin's lymphoma, soft tissue sarcomas) have been awarded disability benefits even though the association between these cancers and exposure to Agent Orange has not been proven.

Can asbestos and other substances used in the workplace increase cancer risk?

Being exposed to substances such as metals, dust, chemicals or pesticides at work can increase the risk of cancer. Asbestos, nickel, cadmium, uranium, radon, vinyl chloride, benzidene, and benzene are well-known examples of carcinogens in the workplace. They may act alone or along with another carcinogen, such as cigarette smoke. For example, inhaling asbestos fibers increases the risk of lung diseases, including cancer, and the cancer risk is especially high for asbestos workers who smoke. It is important to follow work and safety rules to avoid contact with dangerous materials.

Is formaldehyde a carcinogen?

The Environmental Protection Agency has classified formaldehyde as a "probable human carcinogen" under conditions of unusually high or prolonged exposure. In industry, under OSHA (Occupational Safety and Health Administration) regulations, the formaldehyde exposure limit is 0.75 parts per million (ppm). There is still a controversy as to whether or not urea formaldehyde foam insulation presents an unreasonable health risk.

Is there a danger living near electric power lines?

The present evidence is not clear. There is a large-scale study under way to examine whether exposure to electromagnetic radiation from electric power lines is linked to the development of childhood leukemia. This study is part of a large investigation to evaluate the risk of acute lymphocytic leukemia associated with a wide range of factors, such as prenatal x-rays, childhood and maternal diseases, maternal drug use, maternal smoking, parental occupations, household chemical exposures and family genetic histories. This same study is examining the potential risk from the nonionizing electromagnetic radiation released by cellular telephones.

Are nuclear facilities responsible for cancer deaths?

There is continuing research under way on this subject by the National Cancer Institute, the Centers for Disease Control and Prevention, various state health departments and other groups. One major study that was done by the National Cancer Institute in 1987 surveyed sixty-two nuclear facilities, all of which had begun operation before 1982. It examined more than 900,000 deaths, using county mortality records collected from 1950 to 1984. The researchers evaluated changes in mortality rates for sixteen types of cancers from 1950 until each facility began operation and from the start of operation until 1984 and compared them to counties within the same geographic region that had similar populations but did not have or were not near nuclear facilities. This study showed no general increased risk of death from cancer for the people living in the 107 U.S. counties containing or closely adjacent to the nuclear facilities.

Can exposure to radiation from medical x-rays cause cancer?

Your risk of cancer can be increased by exposure to large doses of radiation. X-rays used for diagnosis expose you to very little radiation and the benefits nearly always outweigh the risks. However, repeated exposure can be harmful, so it is a good idea to talk with your doctor and dentist whenever x-rays are suggested about the need for each x-ray. You also should ask about the use of shields to protect other parts of your body.

Do my radiation and chemotherapy treatments for cancer cause second cancers?

There have been some studies that show that combinations of drugs and radiation treatments used to treat cancers in the 1970s and early 1980s increased the patients' risk of developing leukemia and other second cancers. Another study, with 41,000 women diagnosed with breast cancer between 1935 and 1982, showed that fewer than 3 percent of the second primary breast cancers that occurred could be attributed to radiation treatment given five or more years before. The risks are very low. As with all decisions, the risks need to be balanced with the benefits.

Does fluoride in the water present cancer risks?

Virtually all water contains fluoride. Currently more than half of all Americans live in areas where fluoride is added to the water supply. The possible relationship between fluoridated water and cancer has been debated at length. The latest survey by the Public Health Service, which reviewed more than fifty human epidemiology studies produced over the past forty years, led the investigators to conclude that optimal fluoridation of drinking water "does not pose a detectable risk of cancer to humans." In addition, the National Cancer Institute scientists examined more than 2.2 million cancer death records and 125,000 cancer case records in counties using fluoridated water. They found no indication of a cancer risk associated with fluoridated drinking water.

Do viruses cause cancer?

Scientists believe that about 5 percent of cancers are associated with some type of virus. Although researchers do not yet fully understand the relationship between viruses and how cancers develop, they do know that some contribute to the change of a normal cell into a cancer cell. In some cases, viruses may cause the cell to lose its ability to control growth so that it continues to reproduce itself, forming tumors. Other viruses may damage the cells of the immune system itself. In some cases, both processes may be at work.

What viruses are involved with the development of cancer?

There are several viruses that appear to be involved in the development of human cancers. They include: human papillomaviruses (a leading factor in some cervical cancers), DNA viruses, such as hepatitis B and hepatitis C (that greatly increase the likelihood of developing liver cancers), herpes viruses, such as Epstein-Barr (linked to Burkitt's and other lymphomas and to nasopharyngeal cancer), RNA viruses, such as HTLV-I (associated with the development of adult T-cell leukemia/lymphomas) and HIV (that can lead to Kaposi's sarcoma, non-Hodgkin's lymphoma and cancer of the cervix).

Does the cat tumor virus cause cancer in people?

Viruses carried by cats, such as feline leukemia and sarcoma viruses, can cause cancer in other cats. However, there is no evidence that these viruses cause cancer in humans. Research carried out by the National Cancer Institute, using laboratory tests of blood samples of pet owners, veterinarians, research workers who handle these viruses, cancer patients with and without pet cats and people from the general population, found that none of these groups showed evidence of infection. Therefore, it has been concluded that these viruses are not considered to cause cancer in human beings.

chapter 4

How Cancers Are Diagnosed

> If it is possible, get a multidisciplinary opin-
> ion on your case, especially if it is a rarer type
> of cancer. This allows the doctors to discuss
> among themselves the best treatment for
> you, and gives you their combined opinion.
> If that is not possible, ask your primary doc-
> tor to play an interpretive role for you.

Cancer diagnosis has undergone many changes in the past ten
years. Newer techniques that make diagnosis easier and less stress-
ful have been introduced. However, one fact remains constant—it
is very important that your cancer be diagnosed correctly. Make
sure you know about the tests that are being ordered. Be certain
you understand who is performing the test, what it will entail and
when you will get the results. All necessary tests must be done before
treatment starts. The findings from these tests will be the basis
for your future treatment. If the diagnosis is not complete or is
uncertain, your treatment may not be appropriate or may be less
than satisfactory.

WHAT YOU NEED TO KNOW ABOUT CANCER DIAGNOSIS

- Many tests for cancer need interpretation by the doctor and
  are thus subject to different interpretations. Medicine is not

an exact science. It is useful to ask for an experienced second opinion on the results of all the diagnostic tests before you begin long-term or difficult treatment.

- Don't be surprised if you get different opinions from different types of doctors. Doctors who work in specific areas, such as surgeons, medical oncologists and radiotherapists, look at cancer and its treatment from different viewpoints and thus may give you a different opinion on what they feel would be best for you.

- Make sure your diagnostic tests are done by competent, qualified physicians and technicians, using up-to-date machines and procedures. This is a sophisticated area that is continually changing.

- It will usually take a few days before the doctor gets the results of your tests. Make sure you have discussed with the doctor how long it will take to get the results of all the tests and when you will be given these results.

- The words *positive* and *negative* are often used in describing test results. Positive usually means that something has been found. In most cases, it is something that is not normally supposed to be there. Negative means that nothing was found as a result of the test. Make sure you understand what the results of the tests mean.

- Tumor markers, measurements of substances in the blood, other body fluids or tissues, are playing a bigger role in cancer. However, at present, they still must be used with other tests in diagnosing cancer since people who do not have cancer also may exhibit the presence of the markers.

- Endoscopy, using a lighted instrument to look into the inside of the body, allows the doctor to diagnose several kinds of cancer without an operation. It is important to have skilled doctors performing these tests, since complications can occur.

- Ultrasound, magnetic resonance imaging, computerized tomography (CT) and nuclear scans, x-rays and cytology also may be used as part of the diagnostic process.

- The biopsy, getting a sample of the tumor, is the only definitive test for cancer. The actual cells must be looked at under the microscope in order to get a definite diagnosis.

- The doctors go through a process known as staging in order to plan your treatment. Staging determines how much cancer there is in the body and where it is located. It is vital that tumors are staged to the fullest extent possible during diagnosis in order for you to have the most effective treatment.

- What is the test for?
- Why do I need this test?
- If I have already had this test done can you use the results?
- What will be learned from this test?
- Is this test necessary to make a treatment decision? How will the results affect my treatment?
- What will the test be like? How long will it take? Who will be doing it?
- How should I prepare for the test? Will I have to stop taking any of my medicine before I can have this test?
- What will the test feel like? Will I be uncomfortable during the test? After the test?
- Will I have to be in the hospital for this test? For how long? Can it be done on an outpatient basis instead? Will I need someone to drive me home after it?
- How much will the test cost?
- What are the risks in doing the test? Is there another test that is less risky?
- When will you know the results of the test? When will you tell me?

What are the kinds of tests used to help detect cancer?

This will depend upon what problems you have, what kind of cancer is suspected and the degree to which it might have spread. The tests fall into the following categories:

- A physical examination, including taking a full medical history.
- Laboratory tests, such as blood analyses, including tumor markers, and urine analyses.
- Endoscopy, inserting a lighted instrument into the body.
- Examination of sloughed-off cells (cytology).
- Imaging techniques, such as ultrasound, magnetic resonance imaging (MRI), nuclear scans, computerized tomography (CT), or x-rays.
- Biopsy, taking a piece of tissue to examine under the microscope.

Do doctors do too many diagnostic tests?

Diagnostic tests are a vital part of the workup for any disease, but especially so in the treatment of cancer. It is of major importance for the doctor to determine what kind of cancer you have, the cell type, and where it has spread. Treatment for different kinds of cancer, or different stages of the same type of cancer, vary. If the cancer has spread, surgery may not be the right choice. A good, thorough workup is vital before treatment of any kind is done for cancer.

Is there a risk in waiting to do the surgery while spending time to do the diagnostic tests?

There is very little conclusive evidence to show that there is harm in delaying a short time (such as two to three weeks) while you are having the diagnostic tests. Occasionally, of course, you may need to have rapid treatment for some specific type of cancer or for specific problems caused by the cancer.

What are some of the things I need to be sure I know about the tests before I have them done?

You need to know what the test is for, what the procedure will be like, what preparations you need to make to take the test, why it is important in light of your symptoms, how the test will affect the decision your doctor will make about your treatment, where you will have the test done, what the test will feel like and what side effects you might have from it, how much the test will cost and when you will be able to learn the results.

What kind of risks are there in the tests done for cancer?

The risks depend on the test and the condition of the person on whom the test is being done. Certainly the more simple ones, such as blood counts, involve little or no risk. X-rays which involve small amounts of radiation are low-risk tests. However, some of the x-rays, as well as some of the other procedures, do involve quite a bit of risk. You need to ask the doctor to discuss the risk versus the benefit of the tests he recommends. Generally in the area of cancer, the benefits of the tests are worth the risk.

Will my doctor be offended if I ask for another opinion?

Most doctors welcome a second opinion. A second opinion does not mean you are questioning your doctor's competence. If you have cancer, a decision about how you proceed with treatment is probably the most important decision you will make in your life. You need the best advice you can get before proceeding with a course of treatment. If your doctor does not want you to get another opinion, you need to think about whether or not you want to change doctors. There is more information on this subject in Chapter 2, "Choosing Your Doctor and Hospital."

Will these tests be painful?

Most of these tests are not painful. You may be given a sedative before some of the tests. An area of your body may be numbed, or you may be given local or general anesthesia. In some of the tests, you may have to be in an uncomfortable position for a period of time. You may want to remember a few simple relaxation techniques to help get you through these periods. If you are relaxed, it will be easier for both you and the doctor.

What are some simple relaxation techniques I can use?

Here are three that might be useful. Try practicing them at home before you go for your tests:

1. Slow rhythmic breathing. Stare at an object or close your eyes and concentrate on your breathing. Take a slow, deep breath in, and let it out slowly. Now begin breathing slowly and comfortably, concentrating on your breathing, taking about six to nine breaths a minute. To maintain a slow, even rhythm as you breathe, you can say silently to yourself, IN, one, two, OUT, one, two.
2. Inhale/tense, exhale/relax. Breathe in deeply. At the same time, tense all your muscles or a group of muscles of your choice. For example, you can squeeze your eyes shut, frown or clench your teeth. Hold your breath and keep your muscles tense for a second or two. Let go. Breathe out and let your body go limp. Relax.
3. Think of a favorite scene, such as the beach. Recall the pleasant warmth of the sun and the tranquilizing sound of the waves. Imagine yourself basking in the warmth and let the sound of the waves lull you into relaxation.

LABORATORY TESTS

What is a complete blood count?

A complete blood count, known as a CBC, is a test to check the number of red cells, white cells and platelets in a sample of your blood. The CBC also checks your hematocrit (portion of blood value made up of red blood cells) and your hemoglobin (blood's oxygen-carrying capacity), along with the red blood cell indices (size and hemoglobin concentration of red blood cells), and white

QUESTIONS TO THINK ABOUT DURING YOUR DIAGNOSIS

QUESTION	COMMENTS
Do I want to know exactly what plans the doctor has for my treatment and what alternative there might be for my type of cancer?	Many people want to participate in the decisions about the treatment of their illness. Knowledge about the treatment plan is important to you if you want to be a part of the decision and how and where you will receive treatment.
Do I want to ask the doctor for a second pathologist to do an independent report?	The pathology report of the biopsy is the basis on which all future decisions will be made. You should think about talking with your doctor about how the pathology report was done, whether it was reviewed by more than one pathologist, whether the doctor talked with the pathologist, whether or not there is any question or doubt about the diagnosis. You may want to request that the pathology be checked at a large medical center.
Do I want to know specifically what kind of cancer I have and the stage it is in?	Some people do. They like to have all the facts so they can do research at the medical library to find out what treatments are being offered. Some want to call the Cancer Information Service and have a search of clinical trials being done on their particular stage of disease. Others do not. However, if you have a rare type of cancer, you should know it, because you need to decide whether you want to go to one of the cancer centers or medical schools specializing in your type of cancer for consultation or treatment. Or you should at least ask your doctor to have a phone consultation with a doctor doing research in the area.
Do I want my doctor to consult with the nearest NCI-designated cancer center or cooperative group about my case?	There are cancer centers and clinical cooperative groups, designated by the National Cancer Institute, conducting controlled studies to determine the best possible treatments. Your doctor needs the latest information to give you the best possible treatment. *(continued)*

QUESTIONS TO THINK ABOUT DURING YOUR DIAGNOSIS *(cont.)*	
QUESTION	COMMENTS
Do I want to go to an NCI-designated cancer center or to a medical school for my treatment?	You need to weigh this decision most carefully. The cancer centers designated by the National Cancer Institute and leading medical schools have doctors on their staffs who are especially trained in the various cancer disciplines. In the course of a week, they will probably be treating more people with your illness than many local doctors see in a year. On the other hand, the practical question of geography and your emotional energy will have to be considered. There are additional details on these issues in Chapter 2, "Choosing Your Doctor and Hospital."

blood differential (percentage of each type of white blood cells). The CBC, most often used as a screening test for infections and anemia, is also used in the diagnosis and treatment of cancer.

How is a complete blood count done?

Usually blood is taken from the tip of your finger or from a vein in your arm. For taking the blood from the vein, the technician will wrap an elastic band around your upper arm tightly enough to stop the flow of blood through the veins, and usually will ask you to make a fist, to make the veins larger so the needle can be inserted more easily. Several small vials of blood may be taken at the same time for the different tests that will be performed. You will usually feel a small pinch as the needle goes through the skin, but no pain as the blood is drawn. You may have a little bruising at the spot where the needle was placed. If you have bleeding or clotting problems, let the technician know before the test is begun.

What does the urinalysis tell the doctor?

The analysis of the urine tells the doctor many things. The degree of concentration of the urine (weight of urine relative to plain water), called specific gravity (SG), indicates urinary obstruction with kidney damage if the count is low or dehydration if the count is high. Using a simple plastic strip with a series of chemically sensitive patches, the doctor, nurse or technician can also check the amount of acidity, protein, sugar and ketones in the urine to diagnose acidosis or alkalosis, kidney damage, diabetes and other diseases. The urine sediment exam checks for red cells, white cells, kidney cells, crystals and microorganisms in the urine that might indicate kidney damage, urinary tract infection or gout.

Is there a blood or urine test that can detect cancer?

There continues to be progress made in identifying substances, called tumor markers, that are found in higher amounts than normal in the blood, other body fluids or tissues of people who have cancer. Presently, most tumor markers can be used as only one of a series of diagnostic tests. For instance, when adults have a higher than normal amount of carcinoembryonic antigen (CEA) in their blood, it may indicate that cancer of the colon or rectum may be present. However, since this protein is also found in the blood of people who do not have cancer, such as smokers and persons with ulcerative colitis, liver disease and lung infection, it cannot be used alone as a definite diagnostic tool, but needs to be used along with other tests. There are a few markers that are presently used in cancer diagnosis, including CA-125 in ovarian cancer, calcitonin in thyroid cancer, CEA in colon and rectal cancer, Philadelphia chromosome in leukemia and PSA in prostate cancer. Many more are being used in clinical trials in an investigational manner. For more information on tumor markers, see Chapter 3, "What Is Cancer?" and Chapter 9, "New Advances and Investigational Trials."

How is the digital rectal examination done?

The doctor, wearing thin gloves, puts a greased finger into the rectum and gently feels for lumps. This examination will detect the presence of any abnormalities in the lowest four inches of the rectum. Any stool on the gloved finger will also be checked for blood.

What is the fecal occult blood test?

This test, also called a guaiac (pronounced "gwi-ak") test, is a simple, inexpensive method of testing stools for hidden traces of blood. Usually stool samples are taken of three consecutive bowel movements so that if there is intermittent bleeding, this can be discovered. To increase the accuracy of the stool analysis, the doctor may ask you to start a meat-free, high-fiber diet (avoiding such vegetables as radishes and red peppers) forty-eight hours before the collection of the first stool specimen and continuing through the next three days. Vitamin C, iron and aspirin also should be avoided during this time to ensure that the test is accurate.

ENDOSCOPIES

What is meant by the term *endoscopy?*

This is the medical term for examination of the inside of the body using optical instruments. There are many kinds of instruments used to do these examinations in different parts of the body. Constant improvements are being made on fiberoptic instruments—tiny flexible fibers that carry a powerful light and a telescope that allows the doctor to peer inside the body. Endoscopy allows the diagnosis of various kinds of cancer without doing a major operation. Sometimes they are used in combination with other tests, such as x-rays, to confirm the diagnosis. You can identify these instruments because they end in the term *scope.*

What kind of doctor will perform endoscopies?

There are specially trained doctors and technicians who specialize in this field, since these tests are delicate, can be difficult to perform and can lead to complications.

How are the endoscopies done?

Endoscopies are individualized procedures and different institutions have different ways of performing the tests. They may be done in an office procedure room, in an operating room or at bedside in a hospital. You probably will start by having blood tests done. Then, about an hour before the endoscopy is to be done, you usually are given an injection to relax you. Sometimes general anesthesia is used. A large machine may be positioned near you to transmit pictures to a TV monitor. Sometimes, you will be able to see what is on the screen. Many times lights in the room are dimmed to allow the doctor to see the lighted area more clearly. The TV monitor is used to help your doctor move the scope to different sections of the organ being looked at. A tiny brush or instrument may be inserted through the scope to collect small bits of tissue for analysis under the microscope.

What is the difference between rigid and flexible instruments used in endoscopy?

The rigid scopes are straight, hollow metal tubes. The flexible scopes are long, thin tubes that contain fiberoptic lighting systems that can send images around bends. The type of scope that your doctor uses depends on many factors. The rigid scopes make it easier, in some parts of the body, to take samples of tissues. The flexible scopes are usually more comfortable for you, are safer, and give a better view of smaller vessels. Often, when rigid scopes are used, you are given general anesthesia.

Is there anything I should tell the doctor before having this test?

There are several things you need to be sure the doctor knows. Your doctor will usually ask if you are allergic to any medicine or anesthetics, if you are taking any medicine, if you have had any kind of bleeding problems, what other kinds of tests you have had recently, and if you might be pregnant.

What should I do to prepare for my endoscopy examination?

It depends on what part of the body is being examined. You may have to fast for eight to twelve hours, stop smoking for twenty-four hours, and have several blood tests. The day of the examination, you may be given a mild drug to relax you, have an IV line put in your vein and have local or general anesthesia. For some endoscopic examinations, the preparations are more complex than for others.

What is a bronchoscopy?

A bronchoscopy is used to diagnose tumors in the lung or other lung diseases. The doctor inserts a lighted instrument through your mouth or nose, after giving you local anesthesia so you will be comfortable as the doctor inserts the scope. Be sure to tell the doctor if you have allergies to any medicine or anesthetics, if you are taking any medicine, if you have had bleeding problems, if you have any loose teeth or if you might be pregnant. You will be asked to remove your dentures, glasses and all your jewelry.

Isn't a bronchoscopy uncomfortable?

The doctor will do everything that can be done to make you comfortable. If the scope is to be put into your throat, the back of your throat probably will be sprayed with anesthetic solution to numb it and to stop you from having a feeling of gagging. Or the anesthesia might be injected into your windpipe. If the scope is going to be put into your nose, the anesthetic is usually swabbed onto your nasal passage. Some people say that their tongues and throats feel swollen and they get the feeling they cannot breathe. Using relaxation techniques from the start, such as taking slow breaths through your nose with your mouth open, can help. The test usually takes thirty to sixty minutes. You will not be able to talk during the test. It might be helpful to discuss with the doctor hand signals to use should the procedure become uncomfortable. Or you may wish to bring along a pad and pencil to write messages.

COMMON TYPES OF ENDOSCOPIES

TEST/PREPARATION	PROCEDURE
Bronchoscopy Lighted viewing instrument inserted through mouth or nose. No eating or drinking for at least 6 to 8 hours before test. No smoking for prior 24 hours. Several blood tests ordered before procedure is done.	General or local anesthesia used. May be given medicine to relax and to dry mouth secretions. IV may be placed in vein. Procedure may be done in sitting or lying position. Test usually takes 30 to 60 minutes. If done as outpatient, need someone to drive you home.
Colonoscopy Lighted instrument inserted in anus and goes through colon. Need to clean colon by one or more of several methods such as liquid diet, laxative, enema, etc.	IV line may be put in vein, used for sedative and pain reliever. Test takes 30 minutes to 2 hours depending on ease of advancing scope. If done as outpatient, need someone to drive you home.
Cystoscopy Lighted instrument inserted into ureter and goes into bladder. If being done under local anesthetic, drink plenty of fluids; otherwise no food or drink for 8 hours before test.	May be given relaxant before test. May have local, spinal or general anesthetic. IV may be put in vein for medicines and fluids. Test takes 15 to 45 minutes. If being done as outpatient, need someone to drive you home.
Laparoscopy Lighted instrument inserted through small cut in abdomen to look at organs in the stomach and pelvic area. Sometimes known as "Band-aid" surgery because of small incision. Do not eat or drink for 8 to 12 hours before test.	May be given relaxant before test. Catheter may be inserted to empty bladder. Instrument may be put in uterus to allow doctor to move it. Usually done with general anesthesia but local or spinal may be used. Test takes 30 to 45 minutes. If done on outpatient basis, need someone to drive you home.
Laryngoscopy Flexible instrument inserted in mouth to check base of tongue, epiglottis, larynx and vocal cords. You will need to remove dentures, jewelry and glasses. You may need to fast for 6 to 8 hours.	Two types used: one is done as office procedure, other in operating room. Test takes from 10 minutes to 30 minutes. If done on outpatient basis, need someone to drive you home. *(continued)*

COMMON TYPES OF ENDOSCOPIES *(cont.)*	
TEST/PREPARATION	PROCEDURE
Mediastinoscopy Instrument inserted into mediastinum through an incision made in the front of your neck. You will need to fast for at least 12 hours before the exam. You will need to remove your dentures, eyeglasses and jewelry.	Done under general anesthesia in an operating room. Tube placed in throat. Procedure takes about an hour. If not staying overnight, plan to have someone drive you home.
Sigmoidoscopy Instrument inserted into anus to view lower intestinal tract. Will need enemas, special diet or a combination of both before the test is done.	Office procedure. Exam takes about 10 to 30 minutes depending on whether polyps taken out or biopsy done.
Upper GI Endoscopy: Esophagoscopy, Gastroscopy, Duodenoscopy Lighted instrument inserted into the mouth and threaded into the area to be examined. Must fast for 8 hours before test. Remove dentures, jewelry and glasses before test.	Done in special procedure or operating room. IV line put into vein for relaxant and sedative. Test takes 15 to 30 minutes. If done on outpatient basis, need someone to drive you home.

Will I have any side effects from my bronchoscopy?

You may have a few. You will need to stay in the hospital or outpatient area for several hours after the test so you can be monitored. You will not be able to eat or drink anything until the numbness in your throat wears off, which will take two hours or more. You may have hoarseness, voice loss or a sore throat for several days. You may need to gargle a salt-water solution or suck throat lozenges. If a biopsy has been done, you may also spit up some matter with blood in it. If you have heavy bleeding, cannot breathe normally, have chest pain or a fever, be sure to call your doctor.

What is a colonoscopy?

A colonoscopy is an examination of the colon by means of a flexible, lighted tube, slightly larger in diameter than an enema tube. It lets the doctor view the entire colon as well as the rectum. The doctor uses a colonoscopy to evaluate symptoms in the bowel, to detect cancer and to check for its recurrence. Fiberoptic colonoscopy is performed with a longer lighted tube that bends around the curves of the colon so that the doctor can see the entire length of the large bowel from the anus to the cecum. The instrument allows the doctor to take a biopsy from any part of the colon. You need to tell your doctor if you are allergic to any medicines, are taking medicine, have had bleeding problems or a history of heart problems, had a recent barium x-ray or might be pregnant.

Do I need to do anything before I have a colonoscopy?

Your colon needs to be cleared before you can undergo a colonoscopy. Several methods are used—being on a liquid diet for several days, taking a laxative, and having enemas. Your doctor will give you instructions on how to do this. Cleansing your colon is an uncomfortable process but is an essential part of this test.

How is the test done?

The colonoscopy is done under local anesthesia. You will be awake but drowsy. You will be lying on your left side, with your knees drawn up. The doctor inserts a thin, lubricated tube into your colon. You may be asked to change your position to help the scope go through the twists and turns of your colon. Your doctor looks at the lining of your colon through the scope and on the monitor. During the procedure, the doctor inserts some air into your colon. You may get cramping, a feeling of pressure, or the urge to move your bowels. Do not be embarrassed if you expel some gas or air. This is perfectly normal. Small growths may be removed or tissue samples taken. It is important to be sure that the doctor is skilled in doing colonoscopy, since perforation and other complications can occur.

Will I have any side effects from my colonoscopy?

You might feel groggy right after the test is finished. You must stay until medications wear off. Be sure to drink fluids after the test to replace those lost in cleansing your colon in preparation for your colonoscopy. You may see some blood in your stools for few days. However, if you have heavy bleeding, severe stomach pain or fever, call your doctor.

What is a cystoscopy?

The doctor inserts a pencil-thin, lighted instrument into your urethra, the tube that brings urine from your bladder, and is able to view the urethra, bladder, kidneys and prostate. This examination is used to diagnose problems in these organs. If you are going to have this test, make sure you tell your doctor if you are allergic, taking medicine, have had bleeding problems or might be pregnant.

How is a cystoscopy done?

You will lie on your back with your knees bent, legs apart and feet or thighs supported. Your doctor will insert a thin, lubricated cystoscope into your urethra and bladder. A sterile solution is put through the scope to expand the bladder and give the doctor a clear view. You may feel cool or fullness and need to urinate. Urine specimens and tissue samples may be taken. Sometimes a catheter is put in to drain urine until the swelling in your urethra subsides.

Are there any side effects to my having a cystoscopy?

You may need to urinate often and you may have a burning sensation during and after urination. Try to drink lots of liquids to prevent infection. You also may have pinkish urine for several days. If your urine is red with blood clots or if you cannot urinate within eight hours of the test, call your doctor. Also call if you have high fever, chills, or pain.

What is a laparoscopy?

A laparoscopy is an examination that uses a lighted instrument to look at the outside surface of the intestines, liver, spleen, uterus, fallopian tubes and ovaries. It is used to evaluate pain or tumors of the stomach or pelvic area. It can also determine whether or not cancer has spread in this area.

How is the laparoscopy done?

You will be under general anesthesia for this examination. You will lie on a tilted table, with your feet higher than your head. The doctor makes a small incision in your abdomen, adds gas to expand your abdomen, and inserts a thin lighted tube through the cut and looks at the area in question. If the doctor needs other instruments, such as to take some tissue for biopsy, it will be done through another small incision farther down in the pubic area. When the examination is finished, the scope is taken out and the gas is discharged. The doctor will take a few stitches or will use a Band-aid to close the cut.

Will I have any side effects from a laparoscopy?

You may have a few side effects from your laparoscopy. You will need to spend some time in the recovery room until the medications wear off and you can walk. You will be a little sore around the area of the incision, may have a dark coloration around your navel, some bloating in the stomach area and feel generally achy for a day or two. You may also have an aching feeling in your shoulder due to the gas that remains in the abdomen, irritating your diaphragm. If you had a tube in your throat, you may have a slight sore throat. You may be able to get back to your regular routine in a day or so, depending on why you had the exam and what was found. Don't do any strenuous activity or exercise for about a week. If you have severe pain in your back or stomach area, if the area around the cut is getting very red or tender, or if your incision is draining, call your doctor immediately.

Will I have a scar from my laparoscopy?

No, there is usually no scar from this examination. If you have stitches, they will dissolve. You will need to keep the area dry for about four days.

What is a laryngoscopy?

This is an examination of areas of the mouth and throat when you have problems such as blood-tinged sputum, difficulty in swallowing, a feeling of a lump in your throat, or a harsh whistling sound when you breathe. Your doctor may use one of two procedures: a flexible fiberoptic instrument that can be used in an office or a straight, hollow, lighted laryngoscope that needs to be used in an operating room.

How is the examination done?

If it is being done in an office, the doctor will apply a numbing solution to your nostrils and the back of your throat. The lighted flexible instrument will be passed through the nostril, down the back of your throat. You will be asked to make several sounds to make your vocal cords move so the doctor can examine them. You will not be able to talk during the exam. You may feel several sensations during this exam. The anesthesia may taste bitter. Your throat may feel swollen, making you feel like you cannot swallow. You may feel like gagging. Try to relax as much as you can, taking panting breaths. If this is being done in the operating room, you will be given a relaxant and general anesthesia. You will be asleep while the instrument is inserted through your mouth, down your throat.

Will there be any side effects from the laryngoscopy?

You may have a sore throat and some hoarseness for a few days. Try gargling with salt water or using lozenges. If you had a biopsy taken, you may spit up a little blood after the examination. If you had general anesthesia, you may feel tired and achy for a few days.

If you spit up a lot of blood, or if you have trouble breathing, call your doctor.

What is a mediastinoscopy?

A mediastinoscopy, which allows the doctor to look at the space between the breastbone and the lungs, can find a tumor in this area and can remove lymph nodes in this area. The examination is done to detect cancer and to determine whether cancer has spread.

How is a mediastinoscopy done?

You will have general anesthesia to put you to sleep and will have a tube in your throat. Then the doctor will make a two to three-inch incision at the base of your neck in the front, just above your breastbone, and will insert a long, thin scope behind your breastbone. You will not feel anything. The doctor will be able to look at the space, and take out lymph nodes or tissue. Then the scope will be taken out and a few stitches will close the cut.

Will I be able to go home right away after this examination?

No, you will need to stay until you are fully awake and able to swallow. You can go home the same day and will be able to keep your normal schedule and diet unless your doctor tells you otherwise. You may feel a little sore where your stitches have been put in and you may have a sore throat from the tube. You may also have a general achy feeling for a few days. Your stitches will be taken out in about two weeks. You will probably have a little scar from this procedure. Call the doctor if your incision starts bleeding or if you have a fever, chest pain, shortness of breath or difficulty swallowing.

What is a sigmoidoscopy?

A sigmoidoscopy is the primary test done to examine the inside of the lower part of the intestinal tract which includes the sigmoid colon, rectum and anus. The test is used in diagnosis when you have unexplained bleeding or pain in the rectum, or change in bowel habits. The doctor can look for tumors, polyps, inflammation, hemorrhoids and other bowel disease.

Will I have to do anything special to prepare for my sigmoidoscope?

To prepare for this examination, the doctor will usually instruct you to have a tapwater enema the night before or the morning of the examination. Some doctors will ask you to have only a liquid diet for a couple of days before the examination along with the enemas. If bleeding, obstruction or diarrhea is present, you will not have to do anything at all before the examination. You will need to undress from the waist down and empty your bladder before the test begins.

How is the sigmoidoscopy done?

The sigmoidoscopy test is usually done in the doctor's office. You will be lying on your left side with your knees drawn up. Some doctors ask you to get on a special table, resting on your elbows and knees, with your buttocks raised. The doctor uses a special instrument, a hollow tube called a sigmoidoscope or proctosigmoidoscope, which is inserted into the anus. Many doctors use a flexible fiberoptic sigmoidoscope, an instrument with a two-foot-long tube that can transmit light around the bends and allows viewing higher into the colon. Sometimes air is inserted through the scope to help clear the path. The doctor may insert other instruments, such as forceps or swabs through the inside of the instrument to remove a small piece of tissue for examination or to take out small polyps. Most people say the thought of this examination is worse than the exam itself. You may be a bit uncomfortable and feel like you are going to have a bowel movement. You also may feel pressure or cramping, but in most instances, you will not feel any pain. Try to relax, taking slow, deep breaths through your mouth. If you need to pass air, don't be embarrassed or try to hold it in.

Will I be able to go right home after this examination?

The doctor will want to make sure you are not dizzy before you are allowed to leave. You may feel some pain in your abdominal area and may pass some gas. If you had a polyp removed or if you had a biopsy, you might have some blood in your stool for a few days. Call the doctor if you have heavy bleeding from the rectum, severe pain in your abdomen or a fever.

What kind of doctor should do the sigmoidoscopy?

This procedure is best done by a proctologist, a gastroenterologist or a physician who is trained in the procedure. Complications from this examination are rare, but an inexperienced doctor could perforate the bowel, causing serious problems.

What examinations are used to view the upper gastrointestinal tract?

There are several examinations done to look at the interior lining of the upper gastrointestinal tract. When the doctor is looking at the esophagus, the tube that leads from the mouth to the stomach, an esophagoscope is used. For the stomach, a gastroscope is inserted. For the duodenum (the first portion of the small intestine), a duodenoscope is the instrument used. Often these three areas are looked at during one combined examination, using a three-foot-long flexible tube that can transmit images around the bends in this area of the body. The doctor can look for inflammation, tumors or bleeding and can take tissue specimens for a biopsy with these flexible lighted instruments.

How are the scopes in the upper gastrointestinal tract done?

You will be given some medicine to relax you and to relieve pain. You will be drowsy but alert during the test. Your throat will be numbed to make it easier to pass the instrument. With you lying on your left side with your head bent slightly forward, the doctor puts the tip of the thin instrument into your mouth and gently moves it down into the area to be examined, while looking though the eyepiece. You may be asked to swallow to help move it along, but you should not swallow during the examination unless you are asked to do so. The doctor may put air or water through the tube to help with the exam. Your saliva may be suctioned from your mouth. Sometimes a camera is used to take pictures. If needed, forceps or brushes may inserted through the instrument to take tissue for biopsies.

Is this an uncomfortable test?

Some people find that the thought of this test is even more uncomfortable than the test itself. You will be drowsy from the medication and may not remember much about the examination. Your throat and tongue will feel numb and swollen. You will not be able to talk during the procedure. Some people say they feel like they cannot breathe with the tube in their throat, but this sensation is caused by the anesthetic. Just remember there is plenty of room for you to breathe. You can help by being as relaxed as you possibly can be. Try to breathe slowly as the tube is being inserted. When the tube is moved or as air is added, you may have some gagging, nausea, bloating or cramping. These are normal reactions.

Will I have side effects from this test?

Very few. You may have the usual aftereffects related to the medication—drowsy feeling, dry mouth, blurred vision—for several hours after the test. Don't eat or drink for a couple of hours while your throat is still numb. The doctor will want to watch you for a couple of hours before you can go home. You may belch and feel bloated from the air that was put into your body. Your throat may be sore, you may have a tickle or cough, and you may be hoarse for several days. You may find it helpful to gargle with salt water or use lozenges. You can go back to your normal schedule and diet. Call the doctor if you vomit blood, have black or bloody stools, have difficulty swallowing, are short of breath or have chest pain, stomach pain or a fever.

What is an endoscopic retrograde cholangiopancreatogram?

This test is a combination of two diagnostic procedures: an endoscope of the upper gastrointestinal area and x-rays of the ducts that drain the liver, gallbladder and pancreas. The endoscope is passed into the duodenum, and a hollow tube is threaded into the opening of the ducts. A dye is injected through the endoscope and the x-rays are taken. This is a test that must be done by an experienced gastroenterologist. It takes about an hour to complete.

CYTOLOGY

What is cytology?

Cytology relates to the formation, structure and function of cells. When it is mentioned in the area of diagnosis for cancer, it is sometimes called exfoliative cytology and refers to the technique of examining cells that have been normally shed or that have been scraped from living tissue. The cells, which cannot be seen by the naked eye, are examined under the microscope, usually by a pathologist or a technician trained to know whether the cells look normal or not.

What kinds of tests are cytological exams?

There are several different tests that use this technique. Among them are:

- Pap test to detect cancer of the cervix; vaginal pool aspiration or endometrial aspiration to detect uterine cancer.
- Sputum tests to detect lung cancer.
- Urine sediment tests to detect cancer of the urinary tract, especially bladder.
- Scrapings from the mouth to detect oral cancer.
- Cell samples from the esophagus, stomach, pancreas or duodenum.
- Fluid tests from areas such as breasts, spinal cord, thyroid, prostate.
- Bone marrow tests.

How are cytological exams performed?

All of these tests are performed in a similar manner. A little fluid or tissue is taken from the area in question, either from cells that have been sloughed off or cells that have been scraped off or that have been taken through a needle. The material is spread on a glass slide, stained with dyes and examined under a microscope. This technique was first used in the Pap test. Today fiberoptic instruments make it possible to obtain smears from less accessible organs, such as the stomach and pancreas.

How is the Pap test done?

The Pap smear is a simple, painless test that can be done in a doctor's office, a clinic, or a hospital. Its purpose is to detect abnormal cells in and around the cervix. While a woman lies on an examining table, the clinician inserts a speculum into her vagina to widen the opening. Living cells are collected in and around the cervix. The specimen is put on a glass slide and sent to a medical laboratory for evaluation. The test is usually done by a gynecologist or other specially trained health care professionals, such as physician assistants, nurse midwives and nurse practitioners. The interpretation of the slide by the laboratory is an important factor in the diagnosis. The percentage of misinterpretations has been shown to be quite high, so it is important to have the test verified before any treatment is undertaken.

Can the Pap test detect cancers in the female tract?

A Pap test can accurately detect cancer of the cervix, but it is not a test for detecting cancer of the endometrium, fallopian tubes, or ovaries. In cases where these types of cancer are discovered through a Pap smear, it is because the cancer cells have passed down into the cavity of the uterus and continued through the cervix and into the vaginal discharge. (See Chapter 18, "Gynecological Cancers," for more information on Pap tests.)

How is a sputum test done?

You are asked to cough deeply to bring up some material, called sputum, from your lungs. The sputum is examined under the microscope to see if there are cancer cells present that have been shed from the inner lining of the breathing passages. The tumor is then located by such techniques as flexible fiberoptic bronchoscopy, because the sputum examination by itself does not tell the doctor where the tumor is located in the bronchial tree.

What is thoracentesis?

Thoracentesis, also called a pleural tap or pleural fluid analysis, is a test in which a needle is inserted through the chest wall to get some fluid that has accumulated between the lungs and the membrane that lines the chest cavity. The fluid will be sent to the laboratory to be tested for cancer cells. You need to be very still during the test, and cannot cough, move or breathe deeply. This is a relatively risky test, since the needle can accidentally puncture the lung.

What are pulmonary function tests?

Pulmonary function tests, also called lung function tests, are given to measure your breathing and evaluate your ability to get oxygen into your blood. The tests measure the amount of air moving in and out of the lungs and indicate if there is an obstruction in the air passages. The tests, which are usually done in a pulmonary function laboratory or a respiratory therapy department, consist of various breathing exercises and can take up to two hours to do. A camera and a computer can be during the test. Pulmonary function tests can be used in diagnosing lung cancer, as well as before surgery.

What is a spinal tap?

A spinal tap, also called a lumbar puncture, spinal fluid tap or cerebrospinal fluid tap, takes spinal fluid out of the spinal canal. The doctor, after numbing the area, inserts a small needle in your lower back to get a sample of the fluid. About two teaspoons of fluid are usually taken out to send to the lab. The test takes about twenty minutes. You will probably have to lie still in bed, not raising your head for twenty-four hours after the test. Some people get a headache that lasts a day or two after the test.

What is a bone marrow biopsy or aspiration?

These are two similar tests. You may be given a mild sedative before the test. The doctor, after numbing your skin, inserts a long, hollow needle into the bone marrow—the soft, spongy center of the bone that produces blood cells. A sample of the marrow is drawn back through the needle. The samples are usually taken from your hip, although the breastbone or the shinbone may also be used. For a bone marrow biopsy, the needle is pushed farther and rotated until there is a piece of whole marrow in it. The tests take about fifteen minutes to a half hour. You will probably have to lie down for ten minutes after the test. If you have been given a sedative, you will need more time to recover. For a few days, you may feel sore at the spot where the needle went in.

IMAGING TECHNIQUES

What are the most common imaging techniques used in diagnosing cancer?

The most common are in three categories: ultrasound, nuclear scans, and x-rays, which include CT scans.

What is ultrasound?

Ultrasound produces an image, called a sonogram, of the inside of your body using high-frequency sound waves that bounce off tissues and create echoes. These are picked up and converted into electric signals. A computer analysis of the signals creates a two-dimensional image that is displayed on a screen like a TV. Ultrasound can differentiate the pattern of blood flow through the abnormal blood vessels that feed a tumor from that of normal blood vessels. It also may be used during an operation to locate tumors in the brain or the abdomen. Ultrasound is in common use in some areas of the body, such as the abdomen. In others, the test is currently being investigated.

Can ultrasound tell a solid tumor from one that is not solid?

A solid tumor looks solid on the screen because echoes are returning from all the particles inside it. But a cyst filled with fluid looks hollow, because fluid does not reflect ultrasound waves.

Can ultrasound tell the difference between a cancerous tumor and one that is not cancerous?

No. Ultrasound can confirm that there is a solid mass. It outlines it and shows the extent of it. But it cannot distinguish a malignant tumor from a benign one. The doctor, looking at the shape and consistency shown by ultrasound and combining it with the medical history of the patient, may be able to say that the tumor is "highly suspicious" of being cancerous.

What are the advantages of ultrasound?

There are several. It is quick, does not hurt, and is relatively inexpensive. It does not use x-ray beams. You need little or no preparation and no needle or instrument will be put into your body.

How is the test done?

You will be in a room especially set aside for ultrasound, either in a hospital or in a doctor's office. A radiologist and a technician will do the test, which will take from fifteen to thirty minutes. You will lie on an examining table. A gel will be put on the area of the test to improve the transmission of the sound waves. The small instrument that emits the high-frequency sounds will be passed back and forth across the area a number of times. You will be asked to hold your breath and be still while each scan is done. You may be asked to change positions so that additional scans can be made. When you are finished, the gel will be wiped off.

What will I feel and hear?

The gel may feel cold and slippery. You will feel a light pressure when the instrument passes over the area of the test. You will not hear the high-frequency sounds.

What is MRI?

MRI stands for Magnetic Resonance Imaging. It is a scanner with a very large cylinder that contains a magnet weighing from five to a hundred tons. It resembles a CT scanner in that it takes sectional images of any part of the body, but rather than using an x-ray beam, it records water molecules within the body. MRI takes advantage of the magnetic properties of protons in hydrogen atoms to create cross-sectional images of organs and structures in the body. When exposed to a magnetic field, these protons line up in parallel rows, and after being knocked out of alignment by a burst of radio waves, give off radio signals as they fall back into place. A computer converts these signals into pictures. MRI can create sectional images of the body, similar to CT scans, but it does not expose you to any radiation.

What is MRI used for?

There are several cancers for which MRI can be used in diagnosis. They include brain and spinal cord, some tumors in the head and neck, lung, liver, bladder, bone, prostate and endometrial areas. It has, in many centers, taken the place of CT scanning in examining disorders of the central nervous system.

Are there people who cannot have an MRI?

Yes. Since the MRI uses a strong magnet, you cannot have an MRI if you have an aneurysm, pacemaker, implanted pump, or any other metallic implant, tattooed eyeliner, surgical clips or metallic monitoring devices. The magnetic pull of the MRI might dislodge an implant, interfere with its operation or even pull it out of your body. However, many implanted ports used by cancer patients are made out of material that may distort the MRI but will not cause them to be dislodged. You need to talk to your doctor and the radiologist to be sure you can undergo an MRI.

COMMON TYPES OF ULTRASOUND TESTS

Type	Preparation	Comments
Gallbladder	Eat a fat-free meal on the evening before the test and fast for 8 to 12 hours.	May be given an injection to make gallbladder contract during test; drug may produce cramping, nausea, dizziness, flushing or sweating.
Kidneys	Lie on back for most of test.	Instrument passed over abdomen.
Liver	No special preparation.	Instrument passed over abdomen.
Ovary	Transvaginal. Still considered investigational test.	Probe inserted into vagina. Waves bounce off ovaries to create sonogram.
Pancreas, spleen	Eat fat-free meal on evening before test and fast for 8 to 12 hours before test.	Instrument passed over abdomen.
Pelvic	Full bladder usually required. You will drink several glasses of water about an hour before test and will not be able to urinate till after test. Remove all clothing.	Instrument passed over abdomen. Tell doctor if you are pregnant, have an IUD, have had difficulty urinating or have had barium enema or upper GI series within past two days or proctoscopy or sigmoidoscopy within past day.
Thyroid	Remove jewelry from head and neck. Remove all clothing above waist.	Instrument passed over neck. Thin needle biopsy usually used instead of ultrasound. Easier to do and less expensive than thyroid scan.
Doppler	No smoking for 30 minutes before test. Depending on area to be examine, clothing must be removed. Blood pressure cuff may be wrapped around one or both legs or arms.	Used to evaluate blood flow through major arteries and veins of arms, legs and neck. If blood is flowing through vessel, reflected sound waves create swooshing sound. Sometimes used instead of arteriography and venography.

What do I do when I am having an MRI?

MRI is usually done in a special room, part of a hospital's nuclear medicine or diagnostic radiology department. You will be asked to take off any metal objects that might be attracted to the magnet. Sometimes, you will be given a contrast dye, through a vein. You will lie on a table, secured by straps. The table will move into a narrow opening, putting you inside the cylinder, with the part of your body to be examined positioned in the center of the magnet. You will need to be very still while the test is being done.

How long does it take to do an MRI test?

The test takes anywhere from thirty minutes to two or more hours, depending on the test being done and on the facility. The cost is about 20 percent higher than an equivalent CT examination. The equipment to do an MRI is usually available only at large medical centers.

Does it hurt to have an MRI?

No, it does not hurt. However, many people complain about feeling closed in because they are literally inside the big cylinder from their head to their thighs, with the wall of the tube only a few inches from their faces. They also say they are uncomfortable, especially when the test takes a long time, because they must lie motionless. In addition, the machine makes loud, continuous, knocking noises. If you think you may have problems or if you have any feelings of claustrophobia, discuss it with the radiologist before you undergo the test. You may need to do some relaxation exercises, or take a sedative before the test.

What are nuclear scans?

Nuclear scans use a radioactive substance, called a radioactive tracer, to diagnose diseases. These scans show the size, shape, and the location of the internal organs in a way not possible with x-rays. Nuclear scans are used in the cancer field to detect cancers, to determine response to treatment and to conclude whether or not cancers have spread to other organs such as the bone, liver or brain. Nuclear scans can often tell the doctor many things that once required more complicated procedures, such as operations. However, the increased use of CT scans has replaced some of the nuclear scans.

How are nuclear scans done?

A small amount of the radioactive material is given to you, usually through an injection into the vein in your arm. The radioactive material accumulates in the organ that has been targeted. The doctor, using a special camera that measures the radiation in the radioisotope, scans your body. A picture or scan is made of the organ being studied. The camera itself does not expose you to any radiation, since it is not an x-ray machine.

What kind of radioactive material is used?

The radioactive material used varies, depending on what test is being done. You may hear the words *radionuclide, radioactive tracer* or *radioisotope,* all of which mean the same thing. The radioactive materials used include technetium-99, radioactive iodine, and gallium citrate.

Are radio-labeled monoclonal antibodies ever used with nuclear scans?

These tests are presently being performed in investigational trials. A monoclonal antibody, targeted against a specific tumor, is combined with the radioactive material. When the material is injected into the vein, the antibody finds the tumor, which lights up on the scanner. This technique is being tested in cancers of the colon, breast, and ovary; and in melanoma and T-cell lymphoma.

What is meant by the term *hot spot*?

There are some radioisotopes that concentrate on the cancerous tissue, forming *hot spots* on the scan. Other radioisotopes accumulate in the normal tissue. In these scans, the areas that are abnormal have less radioactive labeling and are termed *cold spots.*

Are scans difficult to interpret?

You need someone who is skilled and has experience in reading scans. This is a specialized area that requires someone who has been trained in the specialty of nuclear medicine.

Are nuclear scans dangerous?

The amount of radioactive material that is used is very small. Most of it leaves your body within a few days, some within a few hours. Most nuclear scans have the same or less radiation exposure than do major x-rays. These diagnostic tests often give the doctors important information at less risk than other methods. The main issue is whether or not the test is needed to decide on a specific treatment. If you are pregnant or breast-feeding, nuclear scans are not recommended. In addition, they usually are not ordered for babies.

Are nuclear scans painful?

Most nuclear scans are painless. If the radioactive material is injected, you will feel the pinprick as the needle is put into your vein.

On rare occasions, you may have some soreness or swelling in the area where the needle was injected. If you do, put a moist, warm cloth on the area every few hours. Depending on the test and how long it will take, you may feel uncomfortable lying for a long time on the hard table. You may want to ask for a pillow or blanket.

What will I need to do to prepare for this test?

It depends on what part of the body is being scanned. If the doctor is looking at some organs such as the gallbladder, liver, or thyroid, you will be asked to fast for anywhere from two to twelve hours before the test. For some scans, you will need to take laxatives or an enema. You may be asked to drink several glasses of liquid. You will also be asked what medications you are taking and whether or not you have had other scans or tests recently. You will probably be asked to take off all your jewelry and metal objects.

Will I need to stay overnight in the hospital for these tests?

These tests are done without an overnight stay in the hospital. They need to be done by a nuclear medicine physician and a technician, usually in the hospital radiology or nuclear medicine department.

Will I be able to go back to my regular routine after the test?

Yes. In most cases, you will be able to go back to your usual activities and diet after your nuclear scan.

When will I know the results of the scan?

It usually will take a couple of days before the doctor who ordered the scan will know the results. You need to ask the doctor who sends you for the test when you can call for the results.

Why is a bone scan done?

You may need a bone scan to find out whether or not cancer has spread from its original location, such as the breast, to the bone. The bone scan may also be done to see how the treatment being given to you for your cancer is working.

How long does it take to do a bone scan?

The scan itself takes about an hour. However, you will have to wait about two to three hours after the radioactive material is injected, to give the material a chance to get through your body. You will need to drink four to six glasses of water during that time, to flush out of your body the material not being picked up by the bones, but you can be reading or doing your normal routine. Before the scan is done, you will be asked to empty your bladder.

NUCLEAR SCANS USED IN DIAGNOSING CANCER

TEST/PROCEDURE	COMMENTS
Bone Material injected in arm vein, travels through bloodstream to bone. Need to drink several glasses of fluid before scan. You lie on back or change positions as large camera scans back and forth above you.	If you have had barium for x-rays, you may need laxative or enema. Empty bladder needed. Takes 1 hour plus 3 to 4 hours waiting time. Most material leaves body within a day.
Brain Material injected in arm vein. You sit up or lie on back while large camera scans as material goes through arteries in neck to brain.	Scan takes 5 to 10 minutes; second set taken 1 to 2 hours later. Most material leaves body within a day. Not used as often now that CT and MRI are available.
Kidney Material injected into arm vein, travels through bloodstream to kidneys. You sit up or lie on back while large camera scans as material circulates through kidneys. Additional scan shows flow into collecting system, ureters and bladder.	More than one type of radioactive material may be injected, with additional scans taken. Test takes about 1 hour. May need to return in 4 hours or later for additional scans. Need to empty bladder after test.
Liver Material injected into arm vein. You sit up or lie on back while large camera scans as material circulates through liver and spleen. May be asked to hold breath or turn on side or stomach for more views.	No need to fast. Will wait about 10 minutes after material injected before scan taken. Test takes about 1 hour. Most material leaves body within a day.
Thyroid Liquid or capsule with radioactive material is swallowed about 6 hours before test. Need to hold head back while camera scans thyroid area. May sit or lie down. Two different tests may be needed—an uptake study and a scan.	Tell doctor if you are taking any medicine for your thyroid or other problems, including vitamin pills. Also if you have had any other scans or x-rays recently. One test takes about 10 minutes for each measurement. Scan takes about half an hour. Both tests may be done again 24 hours after taking material.

(continued)

NUCLEAR SCANS USED IN DIAGNOSING CANCER (cont.)

TEST/PROCEDURE	COMMENTS
Salivary Gland Material injected into arm vein, travels through bloodstream to salivary glands then comes out through mouth. Camera gives image of glands.	Examines parotid salivary glands located in cheeks and under jaw.
Whole Body (Gallium) Material injected into arm vein. After waiting period, lie on back while large camera moves over body. Need to be completely still during scan.	Laxative taken night before and enema morning of test to clean out bowel. Scans each last 30 to 60 minutes; usually taken several hours after injection of material: 6, 24, 48 or even 72 hours later. Limited use.
PET (Positron Emission Tomography)	Radioactive isotope injected into blood. Expensive equipment—PET machine and cyclotron—needed for test. Used in diagnosing brain cancer. Available in limited number of centers.

What can a brain scan detect?

A brain scan may be done if, due to dizziness, numbness or seizures, the doctor suspects that there may be a tumor in the brain. Sometimes, a brain scan may be used to see how a treatment is working. In many cases, CT and MRI are used instead of brain scans.

Will I have more than one scan taken for my brain test?

Yes. Usually the first set is taken as the radioactive material travels up your neck arteries to the brain. Then, a couple of hours later, a second set is taken. You can expect that the doctor will take several different views of your head. You may have to move into different positions. Each scan takes about five minutes. You will be asked to be absolutely still during that time, then repositioned for the next one.

Why is a scan of the kidneys done?

A scan of your kidneys, also called a renal scan, renogram, renal scintigraphy, or renography, looks at how the kidneys and your urinary system are working. The doctor uses kidney scans, along with other diagnostic tests, to find tumors. The scans are also used if you are allergic to the dyes used in another kidney test, intravenous pyelogram.

Is there more than one type of kidney scan?

Yes. Often two or more of the different types of kidney scans are performed one after the other. You will receive an injection of the radioactive tracer in the vein in your arm. The scan will be done. You will then receive a different type of radioactive material and the scans will be done, often several over a half-hour period.

Do I have to take any special precautions after the test?

The doctor will ask you to empty your bladder after the test. You can then go back to your normal routine and diet. However, for the next day, you should flush the toilet immediately after you urinate to reduce exposure to the tiny amounts of radioactive substance in your urine.

Why is a liver scan done?

This test, which looks at the liver and the spleen, is most often done to find out if your cancer has spread to the liver from another part of the body. A liver scan may also determine whether you have cancer of the liver and how the chemotherapy or radiation treatment in working.

What kinds of thyroid scans are done?

There are two tests, both using radioactive iodine to measure how the thyroid gland is operating. You may need one or both of these tests. One measures the percentage of the iodine that accumulates in the gland after swallowing the radioactive material. The scan shows how the material is distributed throughout the thyroid. If the scan shows cold nodules, you may need a thyroid needle biopsy or an ultrasound to determine what is causing this test result.

Will I need special preparation for the thyroid scan?

About six hours before the test, you will swallow a capsule or a liquid preparation containing the radioactive material. You will be able to go back to your normal diet about two hours after you have taken the material.

Why do I need a whole body scan?

The whole body scan, sometimes called a gallium scan because of the radioactive material (gallium citrate) that is used, may be used in a limited way in Hodgkin's disease, non-Hodgkin's lymphoma and seminoma of the testicle in diagnosis, staging or determining recurrence. The procedure takes several hours of waiting between the time the material is injected and the actual scan and again between scans.

Will I be able to go back to my normal schedule while waiting between whole body scans?

You will need to wait at the hospital or nuclear medicine center for the first scan, usually done six hours after the material is injected. Then you can usually go home, go back to your normal schedule and diet and then come back for the later scans to be taken.

What is PET?

PET stands for Positron Emission Tomography. A radioactive substance is injected. PET produces three-dimensional images of the body's metabolic and chemical activity by detecting positrons emitted by radio-labeled substances that are taken up by tissue. This procedure is done only in large medical centers because of the expensive equipment needed—a PET scanner and a cyclotron. In the cancer field, it is used in diagnosing brain cancer.

X-RAYS

What kinds of x-rays are used in diagnosing cancer?

It depends upon the part of your body that needs to be studied by the doctor. You may have a regular x-ray, such as a chest x-ray. You may have a contrast x-ray, where a substance, such as a chemical dye, air, or radioactive material, is put into the body in order to get more detail. A barium study is an example of a contrast x-ray. Or you may have a CT scan, which uses a scanner and a computer to make images. Since CT scans, ultrasound and nuclear scans have replaced some of the regular x-rays that were once performed, we have covered only those x-rays normally used in diagnosing cancer.

What is digital radiology?

Digital radiology, a technique that is still being studied, records x-ray images in computer code instead of placing them on film. Using computer software, the radiologist enhances subtle variations in the image, making tumors easier to spot. Digital radiology also can be sent anywhere electronically.

How much radiation will I get from my diagnostic x-rays?

You need to discuss this with your doctor. Some of these tests will give you a low dose of radiation, while others give quite a high dose. You also can ask the technician where you are having the test done what dosage the machine is giving, since machines in different offices and institutions can give different dosages, depending on the age of the machine and its calibration. When properly taken and read, x-rays are an important tool. However, the benefits must be weighed against the risks. What is most important is that you ask the right questions so that you can assure yourself you are in the hands of a skilled and competent practitioner.

Why are lead shields used?

Shielding can help reduce the amount of scattered radiation absorbed, especially by the reproductive organs. There are several kinds of shields, such as lead aprons, lead-lined panels, and scrotal cups. The newer machines have built-in shields to avoid scattering.

What are CT scans?

CT stands for Computerized Tomography. Sometimes this test is referred to as a CAT scan (computerized axial tomography). A scanner passes a pencil-thin beam of x-rays through a selected part of the body, creating a 360-degree picture of that slice in a few seconds. The information is processed in a computer, which shows the image on a TV screen. Information from several slices of the body can be combined to create views from different angles. The pictures are much more detailed than regular x-rays. CT scans can be taken of parts of the body that previously were difficult or impossible to see.

For what kinds of cancer are CT scans used?

CT scans can be used to detect cancer in the lungs, the space between the lungs (mediastinum), kidneys, liver, pancreas, adrenal area, spine and brain.

How is a CT scan done?

The test usually is done in the diagnostic radiology department of a hospital or an office. It needs to be performed by a qualified diagnostic radiologist, with an x-ray technician. You will lie on a table. The part of your body to be tested will be positioned in the middle of a large ring. You will be alone in the room, but you will be able to talk to the technician, who will be watching through a window in the room. You will be asked to lie very still while the

X-RAYS USED IN DIAGNOSING CANCER

TYPE	COMMENTS
Abdominal Can look at large and small intestine, stomach, spleen, kidney, and diaphragm.	You lie on back on table; may need to change positions for other views, with machine above you. Need to hold your breath and be still. Takes 5 to 10 minutes. Ovaries cannot be shielded. Can shield testes.
Arteriogram Can look at arteries anywhere in body, including brain, lung.	You lie on back on table, with machine above you. Local anesthesia used. Contrast material injected through long thin flexible tube threaded through artery to area to be tested. Takes 1 to 3 hours plus 4 to 6 hours of rest after test. Involves risk and can have complications. Major procedure. Make sure you understand what will be done before you have it.
Chest	Usually two views taken, one from the front and one from the side. You stand with hands on hips (for front view) or with arms forward or over head (for side view). You will be asked to take a deep breath and stand very still while the x-ray is being taken. Takes about 10 minutes.
CT Scans Computerized tomography or computerized axial tomography (CAT). Can be used to detect cancer in the lungs, the space between the lungs (mediastinum), kidneys, liver, pancreas, adrenal area, spine and brain.	If contrast material used, will need to fast for 4 hours before test. You lie on table with part of your body to be tested in middle of a large ring. Table moves every few seconds, as the machine takes a new slice of pictures. Large scanning machine moves around you. If in brain area, head will be in doughnut-shaped ring. Need to lie very still while images are being taken. Takes about an hour.
GI Series, Lower: Barium Enema X-ray of large intestine. Liquid barium enema used to make area tested visible on x-ray. Uncomfortable procedure.	Must clean intestine before test, usually using liquid diet, laxative, and enema. You lie on table, x-ray film taken, enema tube inserted in anus and barium inserted. X-rays taken from various positions. You need to be completely still and hold breath while x-rays are taken. You expel barium in bathroom. If air-contrast test done, air will be added through tube and additional x-rays taken. Takes 30 to 45 minutes. *(continued)*

<div align="center">**X-RAYS USED IN DIAGNOSING CANCER** (*cont.*)</div>	
TYPE	**COMMENTS**
GI Series, Upper: Barium Swallow, Esophagram Can look at throat, esophagus, stomach, duodenum, jejunum and ileum. Endoscopy has replaced this test in some cases.	If lower GI series also ordered, should be done before this test. Must fast and abstain from smoking and chewing gum for 12 hours before exam. You lie on a table that will be tilted to various positions as x-rays are taken. You swallow barium several times during test. X-rays taken from different angles. Depending on part of body being tested, can take from 30 minutes to 6 hours.
Intravenous Pyelogram (IVP). Can look at urinary tract—kidney, ureters, and bladder.	May need to fast and take laxatives before test. You will lie on back on x-ray table for preliminary film; then contrast material put in vein in arm. You will need to be still while x-rays taken, usually at 5-minute intervals.
Lymphogram, also called **lymphangiogram** Can look at lymph nodes, small lymph vessels and lymph glands. Used in diagnosis of lymphomas, and to evaluate treatment. CT scans may be used instead of or in addition to lymphograms.	May need to fast or have liquid diet for several hours before test. You will sit on specially constructed chair or lie on table. Blue dye will be injected into webs between toes. Local anesthetic given and small cut made in each foot where contrast material slowly put in. X-rays taken after contrast material has spread, 24 hours later and possibly 48 and 72 hours later. Test takes up to 5 hours first day and 30 minutes on successive days.
Mammography In diagnosis, used to evaluate breast lumps, calcifications or other symptoms. Can also see early breast cancer before it can be felt.	No deodorant, perfume, powders or ointment used under your arm or on your breasts. You will need to undress from waist up and remove any jewelry from your neck. Breast rests on flat surface. Compressor pressed firmly against breast to help flatten out breast tissue. You will be asked to hold your breath while x-ray is being taken. Several views may be taken of area in question. Takes about half an hour.

pictures are being taken. The table will move a little bit every few seconds, as the machine takes a new slice of pictures. A large scanning machine moves around you. You may hear a buzzing or a clicking sound. When the test is finished you should be able to go back to your normal routine and diet.

Will I need to do anything to prepare for my CT scan?

You will need to take off your clothes and put on a gown. You need to take off any jewelry or other objects in the area being tested. Depending on what part of your body is being tested, you may need to fast for four hours before the test. You may need to swallow contrast dye, have it injected into your arm vein or get it through an enema. If you need to swallow the material, it may have an unpleasant taste. Some people say they get a flushed feeling when the dye is given. Others complain about a metallic taste in their mouths. All of these symptoms last only a few minutes. Usually, if you receive the contrast material, you will have one scan, receive the dye and then have a repeat scan.

Will there be any difference if the CT scan is of my brain?

There are a few differences. You will be asked to take off your dentures, hearing aids and any other objects, such as earrings or hairpins, that might come in the path of the x-ray beam. Your head will be placed in a headrest in the middle of a doughnut-shaped scanner ring. Your head may be secured with a special device to keep it still. Your face will not be covered.

Are there any aftereffects from the CT scan?

Usually there are none. Some people may have a reaction to the contrast material, such as itching or wheezing. Be sure to tell your doctor if you have any allergies of any kind or if you have been sensitive to iodine.

What is an intravenous pyelogram?

An intravenous pyelogram can look at your kidneys, ureters and bladder. First, a preliminary x-ray will be taken. Then contrast material will be put in the vein in your arm. The doctor then will take several x-rays, usually five minutes apart.

When I have my intravenous pyelogram will I be alone in the room?

The doctor and technician will be with you while preparing you for the test and while the contrast dye is being injected. However, you will be lying on the table, alone in the room, while the x-rays are taken and probably for several five-minute periods between the x-rays. During this period, you probably also will not be able to move. Many times several x-rays are taken during the five minutes after the dye has been put in. Then a belt might be put on your stomach area to keep the dye in the kidneys. X-rays are again taken every five minutes for another fifteen minutes.

Will I feel pain during my intravenous pyelogram?

Probably not. You may have a flushed feeling or a burning sensation in your arm after the dye has been injected. You might feel some pressure from the belt, and be uncomfortable lying on the table waiting between x-rays. After the test you might be lightheaded because you have been without food for several hours.

What is a lymphogram?

A lymphogram is used in the diagnosis of Hodgkin's disease and non-Hodgkin's lymphomas. It can look at lymph nodes, small lymph vessels and lymph glands. A small incision is made in each foot where contrast dye is injected. In some institutions, CT scans are used in addition or instead of lymphograms.

Is the lymphogram a painful test?

You will probably feel a little bit of pain from the needle given to you at the beginning of the test, but should not feel pain during the test itself. Your feet will be cleaned with an antiseptic solution. A small amount of blue dye, which is sometimes mixed with a local anesthesia, is injected into the webs of your feet. You will feel the sting of the needle. Within fifteen minutes or so, you will be able to see the blue dye in the lymph vessels on the tops of your feet. At that time, you will get a local anesthesia so you will not feel the doctor making a small incision in each foot, where the contrast dye will, over the next hour or two, be injected into your feet. You might have a feeling of pressure when the dye is put in. You may find it hard to sit or lie for such a long time while waiting for the dye to go through your body. The doctor will be checking the spread of the dye through x-rays or a TV monitor. When all the dye is in your body, the incisions will be stitched up and covered. Then the x-rays will be taken, usually of your chest, stomach area, and pelvis. The x-rays are repeated 24 hours later and sometimes 48 and 72 hours later.

Will I have any side effects from my lymphogram?

You will probably have to stay on a liquid diet until all the x-rays have been taken. You may have some pain and swelling in your feet where the incisions were made. Keep your feet up for 12 to 24 hours after the test. Talk to the nurse about what you should do if you have swelling in your feet. Sometimes icepacks are recommended to reduce the swelling, which may last up to a month after the test. Your urine and stool may have a bluish tinge for a couple of days. Your skin may look bluish and your eyes may see things with a bluish tone for about a week. You need to keep the area where the cuts were made dry. The stitches will be taken out in a week or ten days. If you have a cough, fever or shortness of breath or if the area around the cuts is tender, red, or has a discharge, call the doctor.

Is a lower GI series the same as a barium enema?

The barium enema is part of the lower GI series. It is done in order to make it possible to take the x-rays of the lower gastrointestinal (GI) tract. For this test, a white liquid called barium, that appears white on the x-ray film, is inserted as an enema into the colon. The barium coats the inside of the large intestine and x-rays reveal any polyps, growths or constricted or displaced areas. Air may be pumped into the colon during the test to expand the bowel and make small tumors easier to see. This technique is called an air-contrast or double-contrast barium enema. The barium enema feels much like an ordinary enema, causing a feeling of fullness.

What preparation should be made before these tests?

Many people feel this is the worst part of the test. Your bowels must be cleared as completely as possible. The doctor will provide you with exact instructions, which usually include a liquid diet and laxatives to help clear the colon of waste so that all areas of the colon can be inspected. You will have many bowel movements, which can be tiring and debilitating. Your anal area may become sore. A warm bath can help with the soreness.

Will I be embarrassed or feel pain during the lower GI series?

Some people do feel embarrassed but the doctors and nurses who do this test often are aware of the problems and will help you get through them. You may be afraid you can't hold the barium in and that it might leak out on the table. If you are, mention it before you start the test and ask what the results will be if this happens. As the barium goes into your colon, you may feel like you need to have a bowel movement. Take slow, deep breaths through your mouth to help you relax. You probably will not feel pain, but you may feel uncomfortable. You may have some cramping or gas pains.

Will I have any side effects after the lower GI series?

You may have some soreness or irritation around your anal area. You should drink large amounts of fluid to keep the barium that remains in your system from getting hard and causing constipation. For a few days after the test, you may see some white or pink material from the barium on your bowel movement. If you have any bleeding from your rectum, pain in your stomach area or fever, call your doctor.

What does the barium that I need to swallow for an upper GI series taste like?

Many people don't like the taste of the barium. It has a thick, chalky consistency, usually sweetened with some flavoring like strawberry or chocolate.

Will I be uncomfortable during the upper GI test?

You will probably feel uncomfortable when your stomach is compressed, by either the use of the technician's hand or a belt. In addition, you may feel uneasy when the table is tilted at different angles.

Will I have any aftereffects from the upper GI series?

Your stool will look whitish for a couple of days after the test. You need to eliminate the barium or it can harden. So if you don't see the whitish color in three days or if your bowel habits change drastically, call your doctor.

What is the difference between a diagnostic and a screening mammogram?

In a screening mammogram, two views of each breast are taken to see if any signs of early cancer are present. A diagnostic mammogram is taken when you have specific symptoms or when an irregularity is found on your screening mammogram. The technician will take different views, from several different angles. The area in question may be magnified to allow the doctor to see the details more clearly so that an accurate diagnosis can be made. All mammograms should be taken on machines that are used only to do mammography and not for x-raying other parts of the body. There is information on screening mammograms in Chapter 11, "Breast Cancer."

What preparations are necessary before having my mammogram?

There are no special diets or other procedures. However, on the day of the examination, you may be asked not to use any deodorant, perfume, powders, ointment or preparation of any sort in the underarm area or on your breasts, since these might obscure the results. Also, it is more convenient to wear a skirt or slacks with a blouse or sweater, since it is necessary to undress to the waist for the examination.

What is meant by the term *microcalcification*?

This means there are tiny specks of calcium in the breast. When these specks form a certain pattern it is called a cluster. A cluster signifies to a doctor that the tissues surrounding the calcium specks may be cancerous. If the pattern is not clear, the doctor may advise you to have another mammogram in three to six months. If the pattern of calcifications looks suspicious to the doctor, you will have a biopsy. About half of the cancers detected by mammography are seen as these clusters on the mammogram.

What are macrocalcifications?

These are coarse deposits of calcium in the breast. They usually result from the aging of breast arteries, from old injuries or inflammations. Macrocalcifications are usually not cancer and do not need to be biopsied. About 50 percent of the women over 50 years of age have macrocalcifications.

Can a mammogram tell whether or not cancer is present?

Mammograms may indicate to a trained doctor a suspicion that cancer is or is not present. They can be used by surgeons to locate the site of the tumor and to check if there are additional tumors in the breast. However, they cannot be used alone to definitely tell whether there is cancer in the breast. Only the pathologist, looking at cells under a microscope, can tell whether they are cancerous. In addition, a negative mammogram **does not** guarantee that there is no cancer in the breast.

Does it hurt to have a mammogram done?

When you have a mammogram, your breast must be squeezed between two flat plates in order to get a good picture. While most women feel that the squeezing of the breast is uncomfortable, it lasts for only a few seconds. A few women complain that the mammogram is painful. It is a good idea to schedule your mammogram between your periods, when your breasts are less likely to be tender.

BIOPSIES

What is a biopsy?

A biopsy is the procedure in which a piece of tissue is obtained and examined under the microscope to determine whether cancer or other disease is present. This microscopic examination of the biopsy specimen is accepted by doctors in determining the nature of a tumor with complete accuracy. Therefore, whenever possible, a doctor insists on obtaining a sample of every tumor that could be cancer before treatment is attempted. The biopsy provides the most reliable basis for a diagnosis of cancer.

Who determines if the biopsy cells are cancerous?

The biopsy is "read" by a pathologist—a physician who specializes in the study of normal and diseased body tissues.

What kind of training does a pathologist have?

In order to be certified by the American Board of Pathology, the person must be a licensed doctor of medicine or osteopathy and have four years of training in both clinical and anatomic pathology or three years of training in either specialty or eight years of practical experience under circumstances acceptable to the board. The doctor must also successfully complete the examinations administered by the board. The pathologist is a vital member of the healthcare team, especially in the field of cancer. In these days of changing technology, with new instrumentation and new testing mechanisms, such as tumor markers, it is essential that the pathologist be well trained and expert in the cancer field.

Are all pathologists skilled in diagnosing cancer from these specimens?

As in all other specialties, the skill and competence of pathologists vary. A decision regarding whether cancer is the disease in the tissue being examined depends on the interpretation one individual pathologist makes of the cellular structure of the biopsy. Often, the specimens are sent to experts in larger institutions for consultation, especially by pathologists practicing alone in small communities. (The Armed Forces Institute of Pathology in Washington, D.C., is used by many pathologists for biopsy review.) If your diagnosis of cancer is based on the single pathological report of a single pathologist in a small community, be sure to ask that a consultation with other pathologists be arranged. As important is the relationship between the patient's doctor and the pathologist. They need to be talking with each other and working together as a team.

How can the pathologist tell if cells are benign?

When looked at under the microscope, normal cells have an orderly appearance. They possess the distinctive features of the organ from which they came. The cells from the thyroid gland, for example, look very different from those of the skin. Normal cells from different organs carry genetic "messages" that determine their structure and function.

What does the pathologist look for when reading the biopsy?

The pathologist does many things. First is to look to see if the specimen is malignant or benign. If malignant, the next step is to identify the specific type of cancer cells present in the tumor and determine just how fast they reproduce themselves. With special stains and fixes, the pathologist can tell much from the tissue samples, such as whether the blood vessels or lymph channels have been invaded. With some kinds of tumors, the pathologist may test for dependency on hormones or other substances. All of this information will help your doctor determine the proper treatment for your cancer.

TYPES OF BIOPSIES	
TYPE	**DESCRIPTION**
Needle aspiration or **core needle**	Fluid or tissue is removed from lump, using a fine or a wide needle. The needle biopsy can be guided by touch or by an imaging technique, such as CT scan.
Endoscopic	Fluid or tissue is obtained by using long instruments, usually with a needle or knife; the optical instrument allows the doctor to see into the body cavity.
Incisional	Part of tumor is cut out to be looked at. Used if suspicious mass is large.
Punch	A punch is used to remove specimen.
Excisional or **total**	The entire tumor is removed for examination. Used when tumor is small, tissue has been identified as cancerous, or if there is strong suspicion that part of tumor may be or may become cancerous.
Stereotactic	Uses a scanning device to find the location of a tumor that is difficult to see. CT or MRI establish the perimeters of the tumor before the biopsy. Used for brain and breast tumors.

What is an incisional biopsy?

In an incisional biopsy, a part of the tumor is cut out and looked at microscopically. This method is usually favored if the suspicious mass is a large one. The object is to get as large a sample as possible, cutting down on the chances of getting a false reading from a bit of tissue that is not representative of the whole.

What is an excisional biopsy?

In an excisional biopsy, the tumor is removed totally. This method is selected when the tissue has been identified as cancerous, when strong suspicion exists that part of it may be or may become cancerous or when the tumor is small. Many skin tumors, for example, are totally removed before the biopsy is performed. When a punch is used to remove the tissue, this is called a punch biopsy.

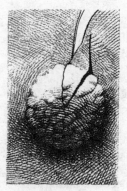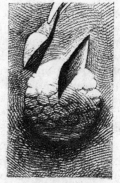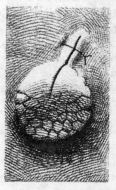

Incisional biopsy

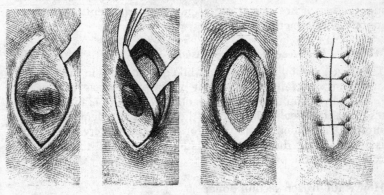

Excisional biopsy

What is a needle aspiration biopsy?

In a needle aspiration biopsy, also called a fine needle biopsy, a needle is used to extract either fluid or tissue from a suspicious mass to be looked at under the microscope. It can be used in diagnosing many kinds of cancers, such as breast, eye, lung, liver, gallbladder, and thyroid.

What is a core needle biopsy?

This is similar to a fine needle biopsy, but it uses a wide needle through which a tiny tool can be inserted for cutting out the sample of tissue to be looked at under the microscope.

What is a stereotactic biopsy?

The stereotactic biopsy, sometimes called a stereotactic needle-guided biopsy, is a procedure that uses a scanning device to locate the site of the tumor that cannot be seen. The radiologist will use imaging equipment to locate the area to be biopsied. The biopsy samples can be taken with either a fine needle or a core needle. Stereotactic biopsies can be used in diagnosing breast and brain cancer.

What is a frozen section?

A frozen section refers to the procedure of preparing the tissue for the pathologist to read. There are two ways of preparing the tissue—via frozen section, which is a quick procedure taking ten to twenty minutes, or via a permanent section, which takes several days. The frozen section is a quick-reference method of determining whether or not cancer is present. The permanent section is a more accurate method.

When is a frozen-section biopsy used?

The frozen section is performed while the patient is in the operating room. Generally, it is used when a suspicious mass cannot be reached to obtain tissue by means other than an operation. It can also be used to determine whether the margins are adequate during surgery. The patient is prepared for the major surgery. The tissue is obtained, but the surgeon waits to proceed until the report is relayed from the pathologist.

How is the frozen section done?

The surgeon sends the section of tissue to the pathology laboratory, where it is quickly frozen and cut into razor-thin slices. The slices are placed on slides, fixed and stained. The slides are then looked at under a microscope. The frozen-section slides are used to look quickly at the structure of the tissue. The entire procedure takes ten to twenty minutes.

How does the permanent section differ from the frozen section?

The permanent section biopsy takes considerably longer than a frozen-section biopsy. In this process, the tissue is put through a time-consuming multistage procedure that is highly complicated and that gives a high-quality slide. The tissue is put through a series of solutions to take out the water and fatty substances from it. It is then saturated with warm liquid paraffin. When it has cooled and hardened, the tissue in paraffin is sliced into thin slices. The slices are placed on slides and stained so that the tissue can be studied under the microscope. Proper staining, which brings out cell formations and their nuclei, requires exact timing.

What are the advantages and disadvantages of the frozen and the permanent sections?

If the tumor is in an area where a permanent section cannot be done under local anesthesia, a frozen section eliminates a second operation. However, in the frozen section, there can be some distortion of cells because of the process used, although today's techniques have greatly improved the quality of frozen sections. The permanent section tissue is fixed better in the formaldehyde solution, the tissue shrinkage is more uniform and the slower process reduces tearing of the tissue and distortion of its structure. The tissue cuts thinner and takes up the stain better than the frozen section. The pathologist has the whole tissue block available for cutting samples at a later date. The definition and character of a single cell is much clearer and more precise than in a frozen section. A permanent section is always done, even when a frozen section already has been completed.

Have there been advances in the kinds of microscopes being used by pathologists?

Yes, there have been substantial advances. For instance, the electron microscope sorts out tumor cells by exposing fine structures visible only at magnifications at least ten times as high as a light microscope provides. It gives information which the standard microscope cannot give and permits the pathologist to tell the difference between primary and metastatic tumors and often to identify where in the body the cancer began.

Can the pathologist always tell where the tumor originated from the biopsy?

No, in about 9 percent of the cases, the pathologist can confirm that the tissue contains cancer cells but is not able to tell where the primary tumor originated. The doctors call these "unknown primaries" or "tumors of unknown origin." Often the pathologist can identify the cell type, or uses tumor markers or hormone receptor analysis to try to determine the kind of cancer, so that treatment can start.

What is meant by staging a tumor?

Staging is the process doctors go through to tell how much cancer there is in the body and where it is located. It is necessary for the doctor to have this information to plan your treatment. Staging is also a "language" used to characterize your specific case.

Why is staging needed?

The doctor needs to determine the amount of cancer in your body and where it is located in order to give you the right treatment for your specific case. The treatment for breast cancer, for instance, at one stage of the disease is different from that at another stage. Your doctor also needs to anticipate the course your disease is likely to take. Staging also makes it possible to compare the results of the different treatments being used by different doctors in different parts of the country and of the world.

What is the doctor looking for when staging cancer?

The doctor wants to know basic information about the original tumor—or the primary tumor, as the medical professional refers to it. Information such as the size and cell type, whether it has spread to areas around the original site and whether it has spread to other organs of the body, away from the original site.

Are the answers to these questions important?

They are vital. Tumors must be staged at the beginning of the diagnosis to the fullest extent possible in order to give you the most effective treatment. For example, if the doctor finds that the cancer that began in your lung has already spread to other parts of your body, your treatment might involve radiation therapy and chemotherapy.

Are all kinds of cancer staged the same way?

No. There have been systems designed for specific kinds of cancer. Most staging has developed through time, as new knowledge has been acquired. Some staging systems are named after organizations, such as the FIGO classification for gynecologic tumors, or after persons who have developed them, such as Clark's and Breslow's classifications for melanoma. However, the most widely used system is the TNM method of the International Union Against Cancer and the American Joint Committee on Cancer.

What do the initials TNM stand for?

These initials are used in the staging system: T = tumor, N = nodes and M = metastases.

T, plus the numbers 1 to 4, is used to describe the size and the level of invasion. The higher the number, the larger the size of the tumor and the depth or amount of involvement in the local area of the tumor.

N, plus the numbers 1 through 4, indicates whether or not there is evidence that the tumor has spread to the regional lymph nodes, the size of the nodes involved and the number of nodes involved.

M, plus a zero or a plus sign, indicates the absence or presence of distant metastases (cancer that has spread to other parts of the body). A letter is sometimes added to the M to show the other areas that are involved. P, for instance, could indicate "pulmonary," indicating that the cancer has spread to the lungs.

An X added to any of these letters means that it cannot be assessed. Therefore, TX means the tumor cannot be assessed. A zero added to any of these letters means there is no evidence—N0 means lymph nodes are not demonstrably abnormal.

What is meant by Stage I disease?

Stage I means your cancer is the most curable. In lung cancer, for instance, Stage I is T1, N0 and M0—the tumor is three centimeters or less in size and is not in the main bronchus, the regional lymph nodes are not involved and there are no metastases.

Do the letters and numbers mean the same thing for every kind of cancer?

Each tumor type has its own classification system. However, a Stage I is always the most curable and a Stage IV is the least curable. The definition of the size of the tumor varies from site to site and of course the treatment will differ. The variation depends upon what the doctors know about each kind of tumor, how it spreads, what treatments are most effective at each stage and what the prognosis is. Some cancers do not as yet have an agreed-upon classification. Others, such as the lymphomas, use a different system from the one just described.

What is meant by tumor grade?

Grading takes into account the structure of the cells and their growth patterns. Because of the differences in appearance and behavior in different tumors, the grading criteria vary. However, there are some basic principles that apply, describing the extent to which the cells conform to the normal tissue. There are two kinds of grading in cancer—histologic and nuclear.

What is meant by histologic tumor grade?

Histologic grading refers to how much the tumor cells resemble normal cells. This is also called differentiation. The lower the grade, the more the tumor cells resemble normal cells. Thus, Grade 1 refers to cells that are well differentiated, whose features and growth patterns nearly resemble normal cells. Grade 2 indicates that the cells are moderately well differentiated—there have been some changes in both the features of the cells and in their growth patterns. Grade 3 cells are poorly differentiated, with features and growth patterns that are abnormal. Grade 4 are undifferentiated and have very abnormal features and growth patterns. The doctor may refer to a tumor as being high grade, with a high number, or low grade.

What is meant by the nuclear grade of a tumor?

Nuclear grade refers to the rate at which the cancer cells in the tumor are dividing to form more cells (called proliferation). Cancer cells that divide more often are faster growing and more aggressive than those that divide less often. The nuclear grade is determined by the percentage of cells that are dividing. A nuclear Grade 1 means that the cells are dividing slowly, with nearly normal nuclei. At the other end is a Grade 3, with fast-dividing cells and abnormal nuclei.

How long does it take to establish a diagnosis?

Ask your doctor about the time it will take. It will depend upon several factors—and the slightest delay will seem like an eternity because you will be living in fear of the unknown. A full evaluation can take from several days to two or three weeks—or may even have to be postponed because a decision cannot be made for any of a number of reasons. Don't be in a rush. Allow time for as many diagnostic procedures, additional consultations and reviews as you can. This is the point in your treatment that is most important to you—because what happens at this point sets the stage for determining much of the future course of your disease.

What should I be evaluating during the period of my diagnosis?

You should ask yourself the following questions:

- Do I have enough information and understand enough to make a judgment?
- Is this the right doctor for me? Do I feel comfortable with this doctor? Is the doctor giving me enough information? Am I happy with the hospital the doctor will send me to?
- Should I have a second opinion?
- Should I go to a major medical center for my treatment?

chapter 5

Treatment

> A number of different methods—alone or in combination—are used in treating cancer. Surgery, radiation and chemotherapy are the most common treatments. Treatments vary depending upon the kind of cancer you have, the extent of your disease and how it is progressing, your physical condition, and how you respond to the treatment.

Most times more than one kind of treatment will be used for cancer. Your operation can be followed by radiation or chemotherapy. Or you might be given chemotherapy or radiation first to shrink the tumor, with the operation following it. Among the treatments being used are:

- **Surgery:** taking out the tumor by operating on it.
- **Radiation:** the use of x-rays or radium.
- **Chemotherapy:** the use of drugs.
- **Hormonal:** the use of hormones.
- **Biologicals:** boosting the body's own defenses against cancer.
- **Investigational treatments:** new treatments or new ways of using older treatments being studied in a scientific manner.

QUESTIONS TO ASK YOUR DOCTOR ABOUT TREATMENT

- What treatments are available?
- What treatment do you recommend?
- Is this treatment necessary for me?
- Are there any other alternatives? What are they?
- Why do you think this treatment is preferable?
- What do you expect the results to be?
- How safe is the procedure?
- What are the side effects of the treatment and what can be done to relieve them?
- Can I be put on a program that doesn't interfere with my work schedule?
- How will we determine how well the treatment is working?
- When can I call you to ask further questions?
- Are there specific times when I can call and talk directly with you?
- Do I have a type of cancer that would be better treated at a specialized center?
- Whom would you recommend for a second opinion?

How will my specific treatment be determined?

Your doctor will consider many factors in determining the treatment for your cancer. Among them are:

- What kind of cancer you have and its pattern of growth and spread.
- Aggressiveness of the cancer.
- Predictability of the spread of cancer.
- The sensitivity of your cancer to specific drugs or other modes of treatment.
- Morbidity and mortality of the treatment procedure.
- Cure rate of the treatment procedure.
- The areas of your body affected by your cancer.
- Your physical state.

Are there standard treatments for the various types of cancer?

For most kinds of cancers, there are standard, state-of-the-art treatments that are used. These treatments are those considered more effective for the specific type and stage of cancer. Many times, there are several standard treatments for a particular type and stage of disease. That means that one treatment does not appear to be better than another.

If there is more than one standard treatment for a particular type and stage of cancer, how does the doctor decide which one I will get?

The doctor will choose the one that is determined to be best for you, depending on your general physical condition and on other factors in your case. Sometimes, if the doctor feels that more than one kind of treatment is equally effective, you will be given all the treatment options and asked to make the choice you prefer. You need to ask questions about different kinds of treatment so that you can be a partner in making these treatment decisions, particularly if there is a choice between two equally effective ones.

Is there a difference between standard treatment and state-of-the-art treatment?

In cancer treatment, the two terms mean the same thing—the best treatment currently available for a specific type and stage of cancer.

What are the advantages of surgery?

Surgery, which is the most common treatment for cancer, allows the doctor to see the extent of the cancer and to define the cell type. Surgery removes the tumor by using a cutting instrument. The disadvantages of surgery are that both normal and cancerous tissues are taken out and, in some instances, the entire body part may be removed. Surgery cannot cure cancers that have spread.

When is radiation used in cancer treatment?

Radiation is used in about 50 percent of all cancer cases. It can be used before or after surgery, for those tumors that are sensitive to it. Radiation can cure some localized tumors and control those that are more advanced. It can have side effects that develop over the length of the treatment.

What are the advantages of chemotherapy?

Chemotherapy, which uses drugs and hormones to destroy cancer cells, works on rapidly dividing cells. Usually used after surgery or radiation as a secondary or preventive treatment, it can cure some cancers that have spread. Its side effects often develop soon after treatment has begun.

When is hormonal treatment used?

Hormonal treatment is used in cancers that depend on hormones for their growth. The treatment either removes or adds hormones to the body. It may include the use of drugs to block the body's

TYPES OF TREATMENT

TYPE	HOW AND WHEN USED	ADVANTAGES AND DISADVANTAGES
Surgery	Removes the tumor by cutting; most often used if tumor is small, if it is limited to a single area of the body and if cancer has not spread to other parts of the body. It is the most frequently used method.	*Advantages:* May cure localized tumors. Allows the doctor to assess the extent of the cancer and to define the cell type. *Disadvantages:* Normal and cancerous tissues are equally destroyed. You may lose body parts. Cannot cure cancers that have spread.
Radiation	Uses x-ray or iridium for cancers that are sensitive to radiation. When cancer is localized, used as an attempt at cure. Often used before or after surgery. Used in about 50% of cancer cases.	*Advantages:* May cure localized tumors and control more advanced disease. Minimal risk of visible deformity. *Disadvantages:* Both normal and cancerous tissue destroyed. May develop side effects over time. Must be available to go every day for 5 or 6 weeks. Some tumors not sensitive to radiation. Can cause cancer.
Chemotherapy	Uses drugs to destroy cancer cells. Usually used after surgery or radiation as a secondary or preventive treatment. Used when cancer has spread within body system rather than localized in one spot. Used to control growth and for palliation. Often combined with surgery or radiation.	*Advantages:* works on rapidly dividing cells. Can cure some cancers that have spread and can eliminate micrometastasis. *Disadvantages:* Resistance to tumor may develop. Affects good cells as well as cancer cells. Has side effects. Can cause cancer. Less effective for large tumors. Some tumors not sensitive to drugs.

(continued)

TYPES OF TREATMENT *(cont.)*		
TYPE	HOW AND WHEN USED	ADVANTAGES AND DISADVANTAGES
Hormonal therapy	Uses or manipulates hormones. Hormones can be natural or synthetic. Can be given by injection or orally. In some cases, surgery is done to remove hormonal organs.	*Advantages:* Can be used to prevent cancer cells from getting hormones they need to grow. *Disadvantages:* Can cause a number of side effects, depending on specific drug or surgical procedure.
Biologicals	Use the body's own defenses against cancer. Boost, direct or restore normal defenses. Use agents occurring naturally in body or made in laboratory.	*Advantages:* Enhance the body's own immune system. Can make cells more sensitive to destruction by body's system. *Disadvantages:* Considered primarily experimental. Often produce major side effects.
Investigational (Clinical Trials)	Includes all kinds of treatments, combinations of different treatments and newly discovered methods. Compares standard treatments with new ones.	*Advantages:* Patient gets latest available treatment. Payment for parts of treatment may be covered by study. *Disadvantages:* Can have unknown risks and side effects. Usually must be done at major cancer centers, sometimes far away from home.

production of hormones or surgery to remove the hormone-producing organs.

What is biological treatment?

Biological treatment uses your body's own defenses against the cancer. It tries to boost, direct, or restore the body's normal defenses. Biologicals include both naturally occurring agents and those made in the laboratory. This treatment is still investigational.

Are any of these treatments ever combined?

Yes. Often several types of treatment are given to the same patient in order to achieve better results than with one type of treatment alone.

Are the different kinds of treatment given one at a time or all together?

It depends on many factors, including the tumor and the extent of disease. Sometimes the different treatments are given one after the other. Other times, two or more treatment modes are intermixed. Sometimes, radiation therapy or chemotherapy is given first, before the operation. For other kinds of tumor, surgery is the first treatment used.

What are the newest types of treatments for cancer?

The newest treatments for cancer involve using biologicals to trigger the body's own defenses against cancer. These cancer-fighting methods, now in clinical trials across the country, are using substances called biological response modifiers. They include monoclonal antibodies, tumor growth factors, gene therapy, differentiation and maturation factors, colony-stimulating factors, tumor necrosis and interleukins. Many of them occur naturally in the body while others are made in the laboratory. Many of these new treatments are still years away from being used for ordinary treatment. Doctors are just beginning to experiment with ways of combining various biologicals with each other and with standard treatments for more effective use. More information on these and other investigational treatments will be found in Chapter 9, "New Advances and Investigational Trials."

What are tumor markers?

A tumor marker is a substance that is found in higher amounts than normal in the blood, other body fluids or tissues of people who have cancer. Tumor markers can be used to monitor patients during treatment and to check for recurrence. For instance, a reduced amount of CEA (carcinoembryonic antigen) in the blood may indicate a favorable response to treatment, while an increase in CEA level may be an indication of a recurrence of colon or rectum cancer. Many tumor markers are being used in clinical trials in an investigational manner. For more information on tumor markers, see Chapter 3, "What Is Cancer?" and Chapter 9, "New Advances and Investigational Trials."

Where are these newest treatments being done?

Many of these treatments are available only at the comprehensive or clinical cancer centers designated by the National Cancer Institute. Some are available in local communities through clinical cooperative groups or through the community clinical oncology program. Some treatments are being done only at the National Institutes of Health Clinical Center. Chapter 26, "Where to Get Help," gives information and lists of key contacts for these resources.

With so much new information about cancer and its treatment, how does the ordinary doctor keep up with what is going on?

It is a serious problem, of concern to the doctors, the patients and the National Cancer Institute (NCI), the federal government's principal agency for research on cancer prevention, diagnosis, treatment, and rehabilitation. The NCI has created a computerized data base to tell doctors of the latest and best treatments for cancer patients. Called PDQ, for Protocol Data Query, it gives information on the state-of-the-art treatment for each type and stage of cancer, as well as information on more than 1,000 active investigational treatment studies under way in the United States.

How can I, an ordinary cancer patient, take advantage of the newest treatments?

It depends upon what kind of cancer you have and the stage of your cancer. Many of the newest treatments are available only to patients with advanced cancer for whom all other treatments have failed, since they are still considered experimental. A first step would be to discuss with your doctor the treatment in which you are interested. You can call the National Cancer Institute's Cancer Information Service, a toll-free telephone line (1-800-4-CANCER), where you can get information on treatment. Trained information specialists can give you information on the kinds of treatments available for your specific type and stage of cancer and, if appropriate, can conduct a PDQ search for those treatments being studied and where they are being conducted.

What is PDQ?

PDQ is a computerized service of the National Cancer Institute which lists the latest information on treatment for cancer patients. It has state-of-the-art treatment statements on more than 100 kinds of cancer. There are two versions of these statements—one written in simple language for patients and one written in medical language for the health professionals. The information specialist can send you the state-of-the-art statement that gives you information on treatment. PDQ also gives information on the investigational treatment studies under way.

How can I get a PDQ search done for my kind of cancer?

You can ask your doctor to do it. Or you can call the Cancer Information Service. If you want to have a PDQ search done, you will need to know the kind of cancer you have, the cell type, the stage of disease, the kinds of treatments you have already had and when you had them. You can also access the data base yourself. (See Chapter 26, "Where to Get Help.")

How can the doctor measure the effectiveness of the various kinds of treatment on the tumor?

Different people respond in different ways to treatment. Different kinds of cancers respond in different ways. The doctor uses several measurement tools—physical exams, x-rays, scans and various laboratory tests—to measure each person's response to the treatment. The doctor will check to see whether the signs and symptoms of the disease have disappeared, whether you feel better, have increased strength and decreased fatigue, whether your appetite has improved and you have gained weight and whether your pain has gone away.

What if the treatment the doctor has chosen for me does not work?

There are usually other treatment programs that can be used. One may result in controlling your cancer even after another has failed to do so adequately.

Why are there so many different kinds of treatments?

Since no two cancers are truly alike and since people respond differently to treatments, two people with seemingly identical diseases may receive different treatments. Each type of cancer has its own way of growing and spreading. It also has its own way of responding to treatment. The treatments must be tailored to your individual cancer, to its size and its location in your body, to your physical condition and to how you respond.

What is meant by adjuvant forms of treatment?

An adjuvant treatment is one that is being used **in addition to** a primary form of treatment.

What is meant by palliative treatment?

A palliative treatment is a treatment that is intended to improve the condition of the patient. It might be used to relieve pain or to eliminate symptoms of the cancer. It is also used to prevent further complications or to give a psychological uplift.

Can I withdraw from a type of treatment once I have started it?

If you decide to stop the treatment, it is your choice. However, before you begin any kind of treatment you should make sure you understand what you are getting into. Your doctor should explain in detail the pros and cons of your recommended treatment as well as alternative forms of therapy which might be available to you. Of course, the final decision is yours, but you should understand that if you stop treatment, you may be losing valuable time that can never be regained.

What is meant by the term *informed consent?*

Informed consent is a legal standard that defines how much a person must know about the potential benefits and risks of treatment before being able to agree to undergo it knowledgeably with legal responsibility for the result. The question of informed consent is a very controversial and complex one, particularly if you are talking about surgery or other treatment procedures that carry some risks. Basically, you have the legal right to know everything you want to know about a treatment that is being proposed for you. If you should become involved in a clinical trial, informed consent is part of the process. You will be asked to sign a paper that explains the pros and cons of the treatments before they are done. In most cancer treatment, however, it is up to you to ask about the major risks involved versus the benefits that are expected.

What is meant by the term *prognosis?*

Your prognosis is a prediction of what the outcome of your disease will be. A doctor bases the prognosis on your general physical condition plus the accumulated information about the disease and its treatment. A prognosis is only a prediction.

What is meant by the term *quality of life?*

This term is often used when talking about cancer treatment. It means how good the life is that you will be leading after treatment. Some people feel that they would rather live a shorter period of time than undergo disfiguring operations or long periods of painful treatment. Influencing your quality of life are such things as your general health, the side effects of your treatment, your ability to function normally, pain, your personal attitude, how you think about yourself (self-esteem), your spirituality, your family, work and social roles, sexuality, economic status and your physical condition. Each of these items needs to be examined as you assess your treatment for cancer.

chapter 6

Surgery

> In most cases, surgery that is needed for cancer can wait while you get a second opinion. Make sure you understand all your biopsy and treatment choices before you agree to a scheduled time for surgery. Remember: once you have the operation, it's too late to change your decision.

Surgery, removing diseased tissue or an organ with some kind of cutting device, is the most often used treatment for cancer. You may need surgery for your biopsy, to take out a tumor that might be cancerous, to relieve pain, or to remove a tumor that is the result of spread of the cancer. It can also be used for diagnosis and prevention. Surgery is often the first step in your treatment plan when cancer is suspected. It is important to be certain that all the necessary diagnostic tests have been done before the operation is planned. Choose your surgeon carefully. It is important to ask questions before your surgery so that you know the reasons for the treatment, exactly what will be done, the expected results and any possible complications.

WHAT YOU NEED TO KNOW ABOUT CANCER SURGERY

- Many biopsies can be performed with means other than surgery. Be sure that the operation you are having is necessary.

You can find more information on biopsies in Chapter 4, "How Cancers Are Diagnosed."

- You are more likely to have a well-qualified surgeon if you choose one who is a fellow of the American College of Surgeons and is board certified in the field of specialty. Doctors who specialize in cancer surgery are known as surgical oncologists, although oncologic surgery is not a board-certified specialty.
- Many of the operations that, only a few years ago, required a stay in the hospital are now being done either in an outpatient area of the hospital or in a surgical center.
- You need to understand exactly what is going to be done, where the operation is going to take place and how long you will be recovering before you agree to having surgery.

QUESTIONS TO ASK YOUR SURGEON BEFORE YOUR OPERATION

- **What is this surgery for? Why do you feel I need it?**
- **Exactly what do you plan to do? Please explain it to me in simple terms, show me what parts of the body are involved and tell me how extensive it will be.**
- **What are my chances for cure with the surgery?**
- **Will I have a scar from it? How long will it be and exactly where will it be? How disfiguring will it be?**
- **What other kind of treatment can be used instead of surgery?**
- **Is this surgery dangerous? What are the risks and what are the benefits?**
- **Do I have time to have a second opinion? If not, why do you feel this operation needs to be done on an urgent basis?**
- **Can I postpone having this surgery? What will happen if I do?**
- **Will I have to go to the hospital or can it be done as an outpatient procedure?**
- **How long will the operation take?**
- **When, following the operation, will you let my family/ friends know the outcome? Where will they meet you? (At this time, if there are specific instructions about how you want family/friends told, you should discuss this with your doctor.)**
- **Will I have to stay overnight?**
- **How long will the recovery period be?**

- How disabling will the operation be? Temporarily? Permanently?
- Will I have drains, catheters, or intravenous lines?
- Will I need a blood transfusion? Can I bank my own blood?
- What are the possible aftereffects of the operation?
- How many times have you performed this operation?
- Whom do you recommend I see for a second opinion?
- How much will the surgery cost? Does that include all the costs?

Is surgery always the first treatment for cancer?

Surgery is usually the initial treatment. However, there are some cases where chemotherapy or radiation therapy is done first, followed by surgery.

Is surgery ever used alone as a treatment?

Some cancers, such as basal or squamous cell skin cancers, are still treated by surgery alone. However, surgery is a local treatment, working only in one part of the body, and thus is limited in what it can accomplish. Many kinds of cancer that in the past were treated with surgery alone, such as cancer of the breast, colon and head and neck, now have additional treatments, such as chemotherapy or radiation, either before or after surgery.

Is surgery dangerous?

All surgery has some risk to it. How much risk is involved depends on many factors: the kind of operation being performed, the physical condition of the patient, the skill of the surgeon and the team performing the operation (including the skill of the anesthesiologist) and the caliber of the hospital and its facilities. You must weight the benefits against the risks. It is certainly a subject you should discuss with the doctor before going ahead with the operation.

Is there a special kind of surgeon who works with cancer patients?

There are doctors known as oncologic surgeons who specialize in performing surgery on cancer patients, although oncologic surgery is not a board-certified specialty. Before you have an operation, you should know whether or not your doctor has had special training in cancer treatment and experience in treating your kind of cancer. There are no easy guidelines, but one or two cases of treatment of a particular kind of cancer each year does **not** qualify as extensive experience. Each cancer has its own special history of how it grows and where it spreads. The choice of a surgeon is a very critical part of cancer treatment. It is very important that the doctor know how your cancer might spread so that the proper operation can be done. For more information on specialties of doctors and their training, see Chapter 2, "Choosing Your Doctor and Hospital."

Are there any guidelines for choosing a surgeon?

Most of the time, your primary doctor will give you suggested names of surgeons. Moreover, whatever health plan you belong to might limit your choice. It is important that you take the time to check out the surgeon's credentials and check out the hospital where the operation will be done, as has been described in Chapter 2, "Choosing Your Doctor and Hospital." Remember these basic points:

- It is best to have a surgeon who is board certified and a Fellow of the American College of Surgeons. Although this professional accreditation is just a guide, it tells you that the doctor is well trained and that those qualifications have been verified.
- It is best to chose a doctor who has performed the operation many times. Although this does not prove the doctor is competent, as a general rule, the more experienced the surgeon is, the more competent.
- It is best to be in a hospital that is affiliated with a National Cancer Institute comprehensive cancer center, that is directly affiliated with a medical school or whose cancer program has been approved by the American College of Surgeons. At the very least, the hospital should be accredited by the Joint Commission on Accreditation of Healthcare Organizations (JCAHO) or the American Osteopathic Association.
- It is best to choose a surgeon who is willing to answer your questions and to give you the time and attention you feel you need. Check your understanding of what the doctor has told you about the operation by repeating it to the doctor in your own words.
- Ask the doctor to tell you the risks of the surgery based on your particular physical condition added to the statistical evidence (both national and local) compiled over the years for the particular operation you will have. You should also ask what the risks are if you do **not** have the surgery.
- It is best to have a surgeon who knows and can work with your general practitioner or internist. Remember it is the

surgeon who will be in charge of your care while you are in the hospital.

- It is best to choose a surgeon who is part of a group or who is hospital based, since this will probably offer you the best total care both before and after surgery.
- If you are getting a second opinion, it is best to get it outside of the particular group practice where your primary physician or surgeon is located.
- The time to get a second opinion is before making arrangements to have the surgery done.

What determines whether the doctor will operate or whether another type of treatment will be used?

There are several factors which the doctor considers before the decision to operate is made. Among them are the following:

- Is surgery the treatment of choice for the site and cell type of the cancer?
- Can similar results be obtained from a different kind of treatment?
- What is the risk of the operation? Are the potential results worth the risk?
- Is it technically feasible to remove the primary tumor and a reasonable margin of surrounding healthy tissue?
- Is there any indication that the cancer may have spread outside the primary site?
- Is the person's physical condition good enough to withstand the operation?

When is preventive surgery done?

There are several factors the doctor takes into consideration when deciding whether or not to do preventive surgery, such as if you are at high risk for cancer or you have a condition that is known to be precancerous, whether the tissue or organ to be taken out is vitally needed, the seriousness of the operation, and whether doing the surgery will put you at a much lower risk for developing cancer or a recurrence. For example, removing a polyp in your colon or a mole on your skin is a relatively simple procedure that can reduce your risk of cancer. On the other hand, removing a breast as a preventive measure is a much more difficult decision. You need to be sure you understand the risks involved, the type of procedure that will be done, the anticipated results and the success rate before you have any surgery.

TYPES OF SURGERY	
TYPE	DESCRIPTION
Preventive	Removal of tissue or an organ not presently malignant. Used when person is known to be at high risk, the tissue or organ is not vital and removal lessens possibility of cancer.
Diagnostic; also may be called biopsy or staging	Removal of tissue to determine whether it contains cancer cells. Used when your symptoms or tests are suspicious for cancer.
Exploratory	Looking at the organ or area suspected, to determine the cause of the problem.
Treatment	Taking out the tumor, organ or tissue to cure or control the cancer or improve the person's quality of life. May be used alone or as part of a sequence with other therapies.
Ambulatory or Outpatient	Done in an outpatient area of the hospital or in a surgical clinic. Person does not need to stay in hospital overnight. Tests are done a day or so before the operation.
Emergency	Must be done immediately. Essential to save person's life, to preserve function of organ or limb, to stop hemorrhage or remove damaged organ.
Urgent	Must be done as soon as possible, usually within 24 hours.
Planned	Surgery can take place within a few weeks. Many operations for cancer fall into this category.
Elective	Not absolutely necessary, but better off if done.
Reconstructive	Correcting functional or cosmetic defects that result from the original surgery. May be done immediately or many years after original surgery.
Palliative	Treating complications incidental to cancer. Used to relieve problems or pain.

What kind of surgery is used for diagnosis?

There are several types of procedures that are used in diagnosis and staging of cancer, such as endoscopies and biopsies. Depending on the site, the doctor may do several procedures to determine how extensive the cancer is before taking out a tumor, especially if the surgery will be radical or alter the way you look or the way your body functions. The diagnostic and staging surgeries are described in Chapter 4, "How Cancers Are Diagnosed."

What is exploratory surgery?

Exploratory surgery is done so that the doctor can see the organ or area suspected of causing the problem which cannot be resolved through the use of diagnostic tests.

Are most cancer operations urgent surgery?

Most operations for cancer are not urgent. Rather they fall into the planned or elective categories. You normally have time to arrange for a second opinion and to think through the procedures you will be having before the operation needs to be scheduled.

What is radical surgery?

Radical surgery involves removal not only of the tumor but also of nearby tissues and organs that may have been invaded by the cancer cells. In addition, lymph nodes in the vicinity of the tumor may be removed for staging the cancer to determine prognosis and treatment.

When is reconstructive surgery done?

Reconstructive surgery tries to restore a person to as near normal as possible following surgery for cancer. The use of surgery for rehabilitation is fairly recent. It can achieve not only cosmetic improvement but also increase function and self-esteem. In order to achieve the best results, it is wise to consider and prepare for reconstructive surgery before the primary surgery is done so the plastic surgeon will be part of the planning team.

What kinds of palliative surgery are performed on cancer patients?

Palliative surgery is sometimes necessary to treat complications incidental to cancer, such as abscesses that are a result of the tumor. The surgeon may sever nerves to relieve pain. Palliative surgery is done to relieve suffering, or minimize the symptoms of the disease, improving the person's quality of life even if cure is not possible.

Does it make any difference what day of the week I go into the hospital for surgery?

You may not have a choice. Normally you are scheduled to go when there is any empty bed. However, you should be aware that it is better not to go into the hospital before a weekend or a holiday, when the hospital may not be as fully staffed as during the normal weekday.

What kinds of tests will I have before my operation?

You will need to have the routine tests, such as a chest x-ray and an EKG to test lung and heart functions. Your blood also will be tested. You will be asked questions about your medical history. Make sure you discuss any chronic health problems or allergies you have, any medicines you are taking for any reason, no matter how unrelated to your surgery it may seem. Any of these items could interfere with your anesthesia. Usually, all of this is done on an outpatient basis a few days before the operation.

Will I need to sign a consent form for my surgery?

Before an operation can take place, you will need to sign a consent form. Make sure you take the time to read it over and that you understand what is going to be done and what alternate procedures your doctor has in mind should the intended one not work out.

What kinds of things should I know in order to make an informed choice about the operation?

There are several things you should know if you want to make an informed choice. Among them are:

- The likelihood of being cured, or that your condition will be improved by the operation.
- The benefits and risks of *not* having the operation.
- The alternative kinds of treatment available.
- How disabling and disfiguring the operation is going to be.
- The risk of death or serious disability from the operation or from its complications.

Will I need to bank my blood for my operation?

This is an important question. **You need to ask the doctor whether or not there is a possibility that you will need to have any blood transfusions during your cancer operations.** If your doctor thinks you will need blood transfusions during your operation, it would be wise to make plans to bank your own blood. Depending on how much blood you need to bank, you may need a few weeks before your operation to do it. Blood can usually be donated from 42 days to 72 hours before surgery.

Will I have drains, catheters and intravenous lines after my operation?

What will be needed will depend on the location and the extent of your operation. Many times, these procedures are routinely done as part of surgery. If you are informed, you and your family will not be alarmed after surgery.

If I have ambulatory surgery, will I be able to go home right after my surgery?

Yes, but you will need to be accompanied by someone. According to the results of a large, long-term study on the aftermath of outpatient surgery, more than one-third of serious postoperative complications occur more than 48 hours after the procedure. It's a good idea to have someone with you when you leave the outpatient area and at home for 24 hours or longer. Refrain from driving, drinking or making important decisions for at least a day. Be sure you have the telephone number of the doctor who performed the procedure, the anesthesiologist (if one was involved) and the center where the procedure was done. You should also have written instructions about medications to take or avoid, what to eat and drink, activity level, bathing instructions, wound care and what to do in case of an emergency. Don't forget to ask which postoperative symptoms are normal and which warrant medical attention.

Are there different ways, besides using a cutting tool, for removing diseased tissue?

There are a number of different techniques. See the chart below.

What is cryosurgery?

Cryosurgery uses extreme cold to freeze and kill the cancer cells. It uses liquid nitrogen, which is applied through a cryoprobe or

SURGICAL TECHNIQUES

Type	Description
Cryosurgery	Use of liquid nitrogen or carbon dioxide to destroy a tumor by freezing.
Laser	Use of intense, narrow light beam to shrink or destroy a tumor.
Electrosurgery	Use of high-frequency current.
Chemosurgery	Use of chemotherapy drugs on tumor before or instead of surgery.
Stereotactic surgery	Uses computer-assisted techniques to allow the surgeon to remove tumors in areas that are normally difficult to reach.
Intraoperative radiotherapy	Use of radiation treatment during the operation.

with a special spray device. The liquid nitrogen freezes and kills any abnormal tissue. Cryosurgery has been used to treat skin cancers. Today, teamed with ultrasound, it is sometimes used to treat cancers of the prostate and liver. Depending upon the location of the tumor and the type of cryosurgery used, the procedure is done either in an operating room, using local or general anesthesia, or in a doctor's office. The treated area sloughs off the dead cells and leaves a sore that eventually heals.

What is laser treatment?

Laser (*light amplification by simulated emission of radiation*) treatment uses a narrow, intense beam of light to shrink or destroy tumors. Lasers are more precise than scalpels, shorten operating times, and allow surgeons to reduce the use of anesthesia. Since laser heat seals blood vessels, there is less bleeding, swelling or scarring and healing time is often shortened. Lasers also bring fast and effective treatment to previously inaccessible areas. The disadvantage to laser treatment is that the equipment is expensive and relatively few surgeons are trained in the techniques. There is more information on the use of lasers in cancer treatment in Chapter 9, "New Advances and Investigational Trials."

What is electrosurgery?

Electrosurgery, or electrocautery, uses an electric probe or needle to burn and destroy tissue.

What is chemosurgery?

Chemosurgery is the use of anticancer drugs to shrink the tumor before surgery or to remove the tumor instead of operating.

What is intraoperative chemotherapy?

Intraoperative chemotherapy is an investigational treatment. A single, high dose of chemotherapy drug is given directly to the tumor or the area of the tumor during the operation.

Is stereotactic surgery used in treating tumors?

Stereotactic surgery uses computer-assisted techniques to allow the surgeon to locate and remove deep or difficult-to-reach tumors in areas such as the brain or head and neck. CT scanning and MRI, attached to special computer-assisted stereotactic instruments, allow a tumor to be reconstructed and viewed in three dimensions.

How is radiation used during an operation?

The surgery is begun and after the tumor is exposed or taken out, the patient is given radiation therapy directly to the area. The operation is then completed. This is called **intraoperative** radiation therapy. Intraoperative radiation can deliver a single high dose directly to the tumor, because surrounding organs sensitive to radiation, such as the skin, intestines and liver, can be held aside or shielded. The exposed tumor can also be felt or seen directly, rather than viewed on a scan or x-ray. This treatment is still being studied through clinical studies.

Will the radiation treatment be done right in the operating room?

It depends on the hospital. Some have an operating room in the radiation department. In others, you are moved to the radiation therapy area and then returned to the operating room.

QUESTIONS TO ASK THE ANESTHESIOLOGIST

- What kind of medication will I be given before I am taken into the operating room?
- Who will be administering the medication and anesthesia? How will they be given to me?
- Are you an anesthesiologist or an anesthetist?
- Will my allergies be a problem?
- What kind of anesthetic are you going to give to me? What are the side effects?
- What are the risks?
- How long will the operation take?
- How long will it take before I regain consciousness?
- Will I go to a recovery room after the operation?
- What are the fees for your service?
- If you do not want to be fully unconscious during surgery, are elderly or have lung problems, ask: Is general anesthesia absolutely necessary or is there another choice?

Who gives the anesthesia?

Anesthesia should be given either by an anesthesiologist or under the direction of an anesthesiologist. An anesthesiologist is a doctor specializing in anesthesia—the physician who can choose the most appropriate type of anesthesia to be used—who during surgery is responsible for maintaining all the body's vital functions.

What is an anesthetist?

Anesthetists are not M.D.s. Usually they are specially trained nurses who give anesthesia under the direction of a doctor. A hospital's department of anesthesiology, besides being responsible for the administration of anesthesia during surgery, usually sets the standards for the way in which the operating room and the recovery room are run.

Will I meet the anesthesiologist?

Many times, you will meet the anesthesiologist before surgery. Make sure you talk about any chronic health problems, allergies or drug sensitivities you have, any medicines you are taking for any reason no matter how unrelated to your surgery it may seem. Any of these items could interfere with your anesthesia. Of course, the information is also available to the anesthesiologist from your medical history and other available medical records as well as by consulting with your surgeon.

Can I decide what kind of anesthesia I would like?

The decision on the kind of anesthesia to be used is usually made by your anesthesiologist and surgeon. However, if you have preferences, you should discuss any feelings and needs you have with the doctors. If you prefer to be asleep instead of awake during the surgery (even though you will not experience any pain in either case) you should talk to the doctor about your preference.

How long can a person stay under anesthesia?

It varies depending upon the kind of drugs used and the condition of the patient. Surgeons are not under the same pressure to hurry through operations as they once were, mainly because of advances in methods of anesthesia and better monitoring of patients during surgery.

How does the anesthesiologist decide what kind of anesthesia to use?

It depends upon the kind of operation, what the surgeon needs during the procedure and the physical needs of the patient.

What will the anesthesiologist do during the operation?

The anesthesiologist will be present during the operation and after it, monitoring your condition, watching your blood pressure, pulse rate, temperature and the electrocardiographic recording of the action of your heart. The anesthesiologist can administer glucose, plasma, whole blood, and various other drugs as needed.

Does the anesthesiologist work only in the operating room?

The anesthesiologist works mainly in the operating room and in the recovery room. It is the responsibility of the anesthesiologist to alleviate pain, relieve anxieties before the operation, increase the safety in the operating room, provide the best conditions for the surgeon during the actual operation, and help ensure complete and comfortable recovery afterward. Advances in anesthesiology have made it possible to operate on patients who not long ago would have been considered poor surgical risks because they were too young, too old, or too feeble.

TYPES OF ANESTHESIA	
TYPE	DESCRIPTION
Topical	Sprayed or painted directly on the area involved.
Local	Limited to a certain part of the body. Used in most minor operations. Patient awake during procedure.
Regional	Affecting a larger part of the body than local anesthesia. Patient awake during procedure.
General	Affecting the whole body. Used for most major operations.

Is anesthesia painful?

Not with today's procedures. Probably an hour or so before the operation, you will be given something to make you drowsy and relaxed. You may also be given medication to dry up mucous and salivary-gland secretions, which will help in the anesthesia. The anesthesia will be given in the operating room. Anesthesia, even types that were once painful, is now an almost painless procedure.

What is topical anesthesia?

An anesthetic is sprayed or painted onto the surface of the area. Topical anesthesia can be used for the eye, nose, and throat procedures. Sometimes it is followed by injections of local anesthetics. It can also be used when tubes are being put into the trachea (windpipe) or esophagus (food passage).

When is local anesthesia used?

Local anesthesia is used for minor operations when a small area needs to be numbed or temporarily deadened. It is injected directly into the tissues at the site to be operated on. Only a small area is made insensitive.

What is regional anesthesia?

Regional anesthesia is injected into the nerves that transmit pain sensations from a particular area. A larger area can be made insensitive than with a local. If regional anesthesia is used, you will be aware during the entire procedure, although you may be given a sedative injection or intravenous medication to help you relax. The affected area may continue to be numb for some time after the operation. The advantage of regional anesthesia is that your heart, lungs, blood pressure and general condition are not greatly affected because only specific nerves are blocked. This means that some poor-risk patients can be operated on who could not withstand general anesthesia.

How is general anesthesia used?

With general anesthesia you are put into a drug-induced sleep. The anesthesiologist aims at producing a sleep of just enough depth to permit safe surgery. The anesthesia may be light for a superficial procedure. Or you may be given a deep anesthesia so that an operation on the heart, lungs or abdomen can be carried out.

Is general anesthesia dangerous?

Although anesthesia entails some risks, it is necessary for surgery. In the case of many cancers, general anesthesia is used so that you will be asleep and relaxed during the operation.

How is general anesthesia given?

After you reach the operating area, the anesthesiologist will probably insert an intravenous (IV) needle into your arm so that any drugs needed during the operation can be injected easily. If you are to be asleep during the operation, a drug will be injected and within seconds you will be sleeping. If a mask is to be used or an endotracheal tube is to be inserted, it will be done after you are asleep so you will not be aware of it. Sometimes, you will be given a short-acting muscle relaxant to make it easier to insert a tube. Muscle relaxants may also be given during surgery to decrease the amount of general anesthetic needed. If you are having spinal anesthesia, a needle is inserted into the spinal canal, the area surrounding your spinal cord, either in the middle (just below the waist), lower down (saddle block) or at the base (caudal).

QUESTIONS TO ASK IN THE HOSPITAL OR SURGICAL CENTER

- Why is this blood test/x-ray being taken? What will this test determine?

- Why am I being given this drug? What will it accomplish?
- What drugs have been prescribed for me and what is their purpose?
- How long do I need to stay here?
- Can I get out of bed and walk around?
- When can I go home?
- Will I need to stay in bed at home? For how long?
- Will I need help? Will I be able to take care of myself?
- When will I be able to go back to my normal activities? (Ask specific questions based on your case: When can I drive a car? When can I play tennis? When can I do my household chores? When can I resume sexual activities?)
- What symptoms, if any, should I report to you? If I have a problem, when can I reach you on the phone? Who else should I call if I cannot reach you?
- What symptoms can I ignore?
- When can I safely go back to work?
- What medications should I continue to take?
- What exercises will I be permitted to do? When?

Are there any special procedures that need to be done the night before an operation?

It depends on what operation you are having done and the particular procedures that your doctor follows. Any of the following may be needed:

Fasting: You will usually not be allowed to eat or drink for about twelve hours before an operation so it can be done on an empty stomach. You will probably be told to have a light evening meal and then nothing by mouth after midnight the night before surgery.

Enema: You may need an enema before some operations because there may be temporary interference with normal functioning of the intestines and the bowels may not move for several days.

Sedative: You may be given a sleeping pill to take so that you will have a good night's sleep before the operation. An hour or two before you go to the operating room, an injection is usually given so that you will be in a calm, semiconscious state.

Shaving: Depending on the location of the operation, you may have a wide area shaved and cleansed before the operation.

Stomach tube: If you are having an operation in the area of the stomach you may need to have a thin tube inserted so that the stomach and bowels will be empty and free of fluids and gas. It is inserted in the nostril and slid down the throat to the stomach. You may be given some anesthetic to numb the area. The tube is usually put in the night before or the morning of the surgery and left in place throughout the operation and for a number of days after it to help suction off fluid and gas.

Urinary catheter: For some operations, especially those in the pelvic and bladder area, a catheter (a flexible, narrow tube) is inserted so that the bladder will be empty. This may be done in your room or in the operating room.

Who will be in the operating room during the surgery?

Several people help with the operation, no matter how minor. The team depends upon the extent of the operation. It may include the surgeon, one to three assistant surgeons, anesthesiologist or anesthetist, chief operating room nurse, nurse in charge of surgical supplies, scrub nurse who handles the instruments, circulating nurse who gets additional supplies, and any additional required personnel.

How can the doctor determine during the operation if the tissue is cancerous?

If the type of cancer and the degree of malignancy are not known definitely before the operation, the doctor takes out a piece of the tumor (or the whole tumor if it is small) and sends it to the pathologist. The pathologist does a frozen-section biopsy. The results come back from the pathology laboratory in fifteen to twenty minutes, allowing the doctor to know the results and continue with the operation as necessary.

What determines how radical the surgery will be?

Different kinds of cancer have different tendencies to spread. The surgeon must understand the history of the kind of cancer being operated on, the growth rate and how the tumor spreads. The doctor must also take into consideration whether or not the lymph nodes are involved and whether there is any indication that the cancer has spread to other parts of the body. The physical condition of the patient is also a determining factor. The surgeon gathers as much information as is possible about the cancer before the operation. But in most cases, all the questions cannot be answered until the doctor actually looks at and examines the diseased area. Doctors usually try to remove the visible cancer tissue plus some of the surrounding tissue, even if it seems normal. This is done in case the nearby tissue contains cancer cells that could later lead to the recurrence of the cancer.

What is meant by the term *clean margins*?

This means that in the area around the tumor no cancer cells are present and all the cancer has been removed from the area.

What is tumor debulking?

This term, used in cancer surgery, means removing as much of the tumor as possible, if the entire tumor cannot be removed.

What is lymph node dissection?

A lymph node is a small bean-shaped organ which is part of the lymph system, the part of the body responsible for fighting infections. Lymph nodes are found throughout the body—under the arms, behind the ears, in the groin, in the stomach area, behind the knee and in many other areas. A lymph node dissection takes out some of the lymph nodes in the area of the cancer, so that they can be looked at under the microscope to evaluate whether or not the cancer has spread. This procedure, which can also be done separately, is called a lymph node biopsy or a lymphandectomy. When you are told this is part of your surgery plan, you should be sure to ask the doctor exactly what this means in terms of scars and how the loss of the lymph nodes will affect the lymph drainage in that part of your body.

What if the doctor finds the tumor has spread too far to remove it all?

The doctor's decision in that case will depend on the kind of operation being done, the condition of the patient, and the history of the disease. For some cancers, like lung cancer, the lung itself may not be removed. Radiation and chemotherapy will then be used. In other kinds of cancer, the doctor may remove as much cancer as possible and then treat the patient with radiation or chemotherapy.

How long do operations generally take to perform?

The location and complexity of the tumor, the procedure being used and the surgeon's dexterity all have a bearing on the length of time involved. Some operations are complete within an hour or two. Others may take many more hours. This is a question you can ask the doctor when you are being scheduled for surgery.

Should I make arrangements for the doctor to talk with someone I designate as soon as the surgery is completed?

If you want someone to be able to talk to the doctor after your operation, be involved with any decisions that might be necessary, or to be there when you come back to your room, make sure you tell your doctor who that person is, ask where the person should wait and how long the procedure will take. Some hospitals and surgical centers have a special waiting room while others will tell you to have family and friends wait in your room. Also, if you feel strongly that someone should not be told anything until you are alert, be sure to explain this to your doctor beforehand. These are all things you should discuss before the operation.

Does the length of time I spend in the operating room indicate the seriousness of the operation?

It depends on the individual case. There are several situations that can make your time in the operating room longer but have no bearing on your own operation. For instance:

- You were taken from your room some time in advance of the actual operation.
- The anesthesiologist may make some additional preparations that last thirty minutes or even an hour.
- The surgeon takes longer than expected on the operation before yours, thus starting on your operation later than scheduled.
- You could spend more time than anticipated in the recovery room.

The people who are waiting for you should understand that they should not judge the length or seriousness of the operation by the amount of time you spend in the operating room.

Will I need to go to a recovery room after my operation?

It depends upon the kind of anesthesia given and the length and seriousness of your operation. If you had topical anesthetic and a simple skin cancer removed, you would not go into the recovery room. However, for most other procedures, you will be watched and checked by the medical team until you are stable enough to move. The recovery room has equipment for monitoring your heart action and respirators for assisting you in breathing if you need them. You can get intravenous fluids and blood in the recovery room. Normally the recovery room is run by a physician anesthesiologist so that you can be monitored when you wake up from the anesthesia. Respiration therapists will probably help you cough and inflate your lungs as soon as you wake up. If you have had general anesthesia, you may spend several hours in the recovery room.

Will things seem hazy as I come out of general anesthesia?

Sometimes they do. Voices may seem very loud or they may seem like they are coming from a long way off. People may seem to be moving differently from the way you think they should. You will probably feel groggy, your arms and legs may feel like lead and you may feel cold. Vision, hearing and sense of balance can all be affected by anesthesia and it takes time for the effects to wear off. You will be half asleep, and until your vital signs are stable and there is no apparent problem, you will be kept in the recovery room.

How long does it take for the anesthesia to wear off after an operation?

Once the operation is finished, it can take anywhere from minutes to hours before you wake up, depending upon the kind of anesthesia you are given and the dose. Some people find that after general anesthesia, they are light-headed for as long as a few days. Don't worry, it will pass and there will be no permanent effect from it.

Is it wise to have someone waiting in my room when I get out of the recovery room?

It is a good idea because someone who knows you may be able to spot problems more quickly. It will also be a comfort for you to know that someone is there even if you are drowsy or sleeping most of the time.

Will I be able to get painkilling drugs after the operation if I need them?

You will probably experience some pain immediately after surgery and for a few days following. How much pain you have and how severe it will be depends on what was done and where in the body your operation was done. There are many painkilling drugs that can be used with perfect safety. In some hospitals, patient-controlled units are available so that you can have pain medicine whenever you need it. If you are having pain, be sure to inform the nurse so that you can get pain medication. If you have any problems, talk with your doctor about it, telling where the pain is, how long the painkillers are lasting, what kind of pain it is, how often it comes back and what relieves it. There is considerable detail about pain and pain medication in Chapter 24, "Living with Cancer."

What are the general procedures that are followed after an operation?

It depends on your doctor, the hospital, the operation performed, and your own physical condition. There are some common procedures that will probably be followed:

- When you return to your room from the recovery room, you will probably spend some time lying flat in bed. You will be encouraged, after you recover from the anesthesia, to change your position and move your legs often, to stimulate your circulation. You may be given a little machine to blow into to make you breathe deeply so you will not get pneumonia.

- Your dressings will be checked often and changed if necessary. If you have a drain coming out of your incision, it will be checked and removed as soon as possible.
- Unless you had surgery of the stomach or intestinal tract, you will usually be given sips of water within a few hours after your operation and a bland diet the next day.
- The next day, you will probably be allowed to get out of bed and walk a little. This speeds your recovery and minimizes the complications from surgery.
- If you are having trouble with stomach gas, you will be encouraged to move about and walk as much as you are able. A record will also be kept of how much fluid you get and how much you urinate.
- Depending on the operation, you may need intravenous fluids and medications, antibiotic drugs, blood transfusions and enemas.

What will the nurses be checking on during my first day after surgery?

They will be checking your general color and appearance, your blood pressure, pulse, temperature and the rate of breathing. They will observe if your reflexes are getting back to normal and if you are swallowing properly. They'll come in to give you your medicine and help you with other things you may need. They will make you move in your bed, sit up, dangle your legs over the side of the bed, and help you to walk. They will be checking for proper elimination of both urine and stool.

Why is deep breathing important?

It is important that you begin deep breathing early after an operation to prevent pneumonia and other complications. If your breathing is shallow, the air sacs around the edges of your lungs don't fill out. You may be asked to blow into a special machine to help you with deep breathing.

What if I have soreness around my incision?

You can expect to have some soreness around the incision but if it is unusually painful, let your doctor or nurse know at once.

When will the stitches be taken out?

Some doctors use stitches made out of a material that will dissolve and do not need to be taken out. Ordinarily stitches are taken out between the sixth and tenth day after the operation. If there is an area that has tension on it or if it is not healing firmly, stitches may be left in for a longer time. You will feel only a slight tugging but usually no pain when the stitches come out. If metal clips were used instead of stitches they are usually taken out on the fourth to sixth day.

How long will I be in the hospital?

Most people go home from the hospital very quickly these days. You may be in overnight or for a few days. Many times you will be sent home with your drain in and instructions on how to monitor it. You need to be sure that you discuss with the doctor and nurse what kind of support you have at home, and what needs you may have for help, before you are discharged from the hospital. If you need help, ask for appointments with the social worker and the discharge planner. They are employees of the hospital who are there to try to aid you in getting assistance if you cannot take care of yourself when you go home.

Is it common to have sexual problems following cancer surgery?

After surgery, many people find that it is some time before they are able to resume their normal sexual activities. The whole process of hospitalization, surgery, scars and tenderness of the areas that have been disturbed may make sex uncomfortable. Worry and concern about the future do not make for a happy atmosphere for sexual pleasures. But as time goes on, most people find that sexual desire returns and sexual activity is again a satisfying part of life. In some cases, accommodations must be made for the changes made in the body by surgery. Losing a body part may make you feel embarrassed. Naturally, the changes vary depending on where surgery was performed. Each type of surgery in each area of the body can affect your sexual being in a different way. Women who have had breast cancer and women and men who have had surgery in the reproductive area have very specific problems. Those who have had to have a colostomy or urostomy face a whole other set of circumstances. Facial cancer, limb amputations and laryngectomy all make it necessary to deal with changes in appearance, which have a bearing on how you feel about yourself. Pain can be a common problem, often related to changes made by the surgery or by pain in some other part of the body. Some of these problems are discussed in the chapters relating to operations in the specific areas involved. Other information about dealing with sexual problems, feelings and pain can be found in Chapter 24, "Living with Cancer."

What is lymphedema?

Lymphedema is an accumulation of lymph fluid in the arms or legs and causes swelling. Not being able to drain, the lymph fluid remains in the soft tissue, where infections can develop. People who have had lymph node dissection, the removal of lymph nodes during cancer surgery, are at greatest risk. Lymphedema is most commonly seen in women who have had axillary nodes removed during breast cancer surgery. However, lymphedema also occurs when the pelvic and inguinal groups of nodes in the legs are removed. Those with melanomas in the arms, thigh or leg may be subjected to lymphedema as well. Men who have had surgery (or radiation) for prostate cancer, women who have had radical surgery and node dissection for gynecologic cancers, or those who have ovarian, testicular, colon-rectal, pancreatic, or liver cancer which has spread to the lower area of the abdomen are all at risk for lymphedema. Curiously enough, not everyone who has lymph node surgery has lymphedema. Lymphedema, however, can occur soon after surgery or even as many as fifteen years after surgery.

How important is it to get immediate care?

Immediate care is essential. Untreated, the condition can result in a permanently swollen arm or leg. Awareness of the possibility of lymphedema and the need for immediate medical attention may help to keep the problem from becoming chronic. Obesity, immobility, poor nutrition, prior radiation or surgery, concurrent medical problems such as diabetes, hypertension, kidney disease, cardiac disease or phlebitis can all be contributing factors to the onset of lymphedema. Those who have any of those problems should be extremely aware of the symptoms and the need for lifelong adherence to the do's and don'ts for prevention and control of lymphedema.

Does lymphedema mean my cancer has spread?

Many people fear that lymphedema means that the cancer has spread or returned. Another fear is that the swollen, nonfunctional limb may be permanently disfigured. It is important to discuss your fears with the health care professionals in your life, so that they can help you to learn the necessary measures you need to take to keep lymphedema under control. Positioning, massage, exercise, special garments and pumps are all used in treating lymphedema.

How can you tell if you have lymphedema?

About half of patients who have lymphedema report a feeling of heaviness or fullness in the affected arm or leg. A slight indentation may be visible when the skin on the arm or leg is pressed. Depending on how extensive the problem is, a deeper fingerprint may take anywhere from five to thirty seconds to return to normal. At the extreme, the arm or leg may swell to one and a half to two times its normal size. You should always be aware of any signs of infection in the involved area—redness, pain, heat, chills, swelling, or fever. Infections can move quickly and become serious very rapidly. (See Chapter 11, "Breast Cancer," for further discussion of lymphedema.) The same information pertains, regardless of whether your arm or your leg is affected.

chapter 7

Radiation Treatment

> You will hear many terms for this type of
> treatment—external beam, brachytherapy,
> linear accelerator, interstitial, x-ray, co-
> balt—to name a few. All refer to the fact that
> some type of treatment using radiation will
> be given.

More than half of all people who have cancer will receive some
type of radiation treatment, either alone or in combination with
other treatments.

Radiation treatment had its beginnings in the late 1800s, when
x-rays were discovered in 1895 and radium in 1898. Within a
few years, scientists found that x-rays were capable of damaging
body tissues. Subsequently researchers uncovered the curious fact
that x-rays and radium did more damage to cancerous tissue
than to normal, healthy tissue. Although radiation therapy is not
a new field, research and improved technology, especially in the
past twenty years, has made it a major treatment for cancer. It
is an area that is rapidly growing and changing, with new equipment, advances in use of computers in planning treatment, and
new procedures, such as radio-labeled antibodies and radiosensitizers. The intricate details of the effects of these powerful types
of radiation on living cells, especially cancer cells, are still being
studied.

WHAT YOU NEED TO KNOW ABOUT RADIATION TREATMENT

- Radiation is used to kill cancer cells, which are growing and dividing more rapidly than most of the normal cells around them. Sometimes radiation is used to shrink tumors.
- You may have radiation before you have an operation, during it or after the operation. Sometimes, your radiation will be combined with chemotherapy treatments and biologic response modifiers.
- There are many advances in the manner in which radiation therapy is given, along with sophisticated instruments that are now being used in defining the area of treatment.
- If you are having external beam radiation treatment, you will probably have a treatment every weekday for about six weeks.
- When undergoing radiation, you will need to take special care of your skin in the treatment area.
- If you are having internal radiation, you may spend some time in the hospital. Newer high-dose brachytherapy treatments have shortened the treatment time from several hours to several minutes and allow patients to go home the same day.
- You may have some side effects from the treatment, depending on the area of your cancer and the method being used. Talk with your radiation oncologist and nurse about steps you need to take to minimize side effects.

QUESTIONS TO ASK YOUR RADIATION ONCOLOGIST BEFORE YOU HAVE RADIATION TREATMENTS

- Exactly what type of radiation treatment will I be getting?
- Who will be responsible for coordinating my radiation treatment? For giving my treatment?
- If I have questions about my radiation treatment who should I ask?
- Can I continue to work during these treatments?
- Is there a more convenient place where my treatments can be given?
- How long will it take for each treatment? For the whole series?
- Will I be able to drive myself to my treatments?
- What side effects can I expect?
- What should I do if these side effects occur?
- What side effects should I report to the radiation oncologist?

- How much will it cost? Is it covered by insurance?
- How much of a risk is involved?
- Will I be having other kinds of treatment in addition to the radiation?
- Are there any alternatives to radiation treatment?

What is radiation treatment?

Radiation treatment consists of using high-level x-rays, tens of thousands of times the amount used to produce a chest x-ray, to destroy the ability of cells to grow and divide. Both your normal cells and the cancer cells will be affected, but most normal cells are able to recover quickly. Radiation oncologists carefully limit the amount of normal tissue being treated to lessen the effects on these cells.

When is radiation treatment used?

Radiation can be used before your operation to shrink a tumor. It may be used after the operation to stop any cancer cells that remain from growing. Sometimes, instead of having an operation, you may be given radiation along with chemotherapy drugs to destroy the cancer. Radiation is also used to treat symptoms of cancer, such as to reduce pressure, bleeding or pain.

Is radiation treatment ever used alone?

It can be used alone in some kinds of cancer. However, many treatments for cancer include more than one form of therapy and radiation is often used in combination with surgery or chemotherapy.

What does the term *radiosensitive* mean?

This term refers to how much a cell is affected by radiation. Some kinds of cancer are more susceptible to destruction by radiation than others. The radiation oncologist takes this fact into consideration when planning your treatment.

Is radiation more successful with some cancers than with others?

Yes. There are many cancers where radiation has been very successful. Hodgkin's disease, breast cancer and some lymphomas respond well to radiation, especially when the disease is diagnosed and treated in the early stages. Certain cancers of the head and neck and cancer of the cervix have had good cure rates with radiation. Early cancers of the bladder, prostate and skin, and certain brain and eye tumors respond well to radiation. For some cancers, radiation is better than surgery because it gives a high potential for cure with little or no loss of function. Psychologically, radiation may be a better choice in cases where surgery might change appearance.

What is meant by the term *radioresistant*?

This term refers to cells that are not affected by radiation treatment. Some kinds of cancer are more resistant to this kind of treatment than others.

Are there cancers that cannot be treated with radiation?

Yes, sometimes because of the location of the tumor, previous treatment or radiosensitivity, radiation therapy would not be the best treatment. Every kind of tissue, each kind of cancer and each patient have a different sensitivity to the effects of radiation. Different cancers spread and grow in different ways. Some kinds of radiation treatment work better for some cancers than others. The general theory in using radiation is that the radiation dose must be large enough to destroy the cancer cells but not so great as to seriously damage surrounding normal tissues. Sometimes the dose required to kill the cancer would also do permanent damage to the surrounding normal tissue. This is the major limitation in the use of radiation in the treatment of cancer and an important consideration when treatment is recommended.

Why does radiation treatment work for some people and not for others?

For many different reasons. Sometimes the tumor is too large for the radiation to have any real effect. Or the tumor may be resistant to radiation. In some cases, the cancer may have already spread too far for the radiation treatment to be effective.

Does a tumor ever continue to grow while radiation treatment is being given?

Not usually, but it depends on what kind of cancer the person has, the exact area being treated and whether the treatment is given to cure that disease or to relieve other symptoms. Some kinds of cancer continue to grow for a short time during radiation, but then shrink or disappear altogether. Sometimes the cancer will continue to grow outside the area being treated (known as the field of treatment) even while it is shrinking where the treatment is being given. Sometimes the radiation is given because of symptoms such as pain. The treatment makes the person feel better, even though the cancer may continue to grow elsewhere. There are cases where a particular tumor in a particular person proves not to respond to radiation treatment. Of course, this cannot be predicted before the treatment starts. In these instances, other forms of cancer treatment, such as chemotherapy, may be used.

Are children's radiation treatments different from adults'?

Yes, as is true for all radiation treatment planning, the dose of radiation is planned especially for the person receiving it. The radiation oncologists and physicists also take into consideration the fact the child is still growing. Particular areas of concern are the bones and organs, such as the breast or ovary, which need to be carefully shielded. Accurate markings and treatment for children are particularly important to prevent unnecessary long-term complications.

Will I have a choice as to where I have my radiation treatments?

Your surgeon or the radiation oncologist who is planning your original treatment will refer you to a radiation oncologist. It is a good idea for you to have a frank discussion with your doctor about why a specific radiation oncologist or radiotherapy department is being recommended. You may want to explore whether it would be advantageous for you to use a larger medical center versus a small hospital or private office closer to home. A large radiation center will have several types of equipment and beams to use for treatment whereas a smaller general hospital or private office may be limited to equipment that is easier to use and maintain. You must weigh for yourself the advantages of convenience versus the technology and expertise a larger medical center may have to offer. Radiation treatment is a science in which many advances have been made both in technology and in application. The radiation team and the equipment will be playing an important part in your treatment.

Will I be able to drive myself to my treatments?

Some people are able to drive themselves to their treatments. Others prefer to have their family and friends drive them. Often it depends on where on the body you receive the treatment, how well you feel in general and the side effects of the treatment for your specific cancer. You need to discuss these issues with your nurse and radiation oncologist before you decide on your transportation needs. If you need help with transportation, discuss it with the nurse at the radiation facility or with the discharge planner where you had your original treatment. Many times you can get rides through services in your own community, such as the American Cancer Society, the American Red Cross, community groups such as FISH, senior citizen transportation services or civic organizations.

What kind of doctor will I go to for my radiation treatments?

Radiation is a very specialized field, requiring treatment from a team especially trained in therapeutic radiology. The radiation oncologist, sometimes called a therapeutic radiologist, heads the team and plans the treatment.

What does the radiation oncologist do?

The radiation oncologist will examine you, take your medical history and study all the pertinent information about your case to evaluate whether or not radiation treatment would be of benefit to you. The radiation oncologist is experienced in the natural history of cancers, when radiation can be used for treating cancer and how much to use to produce the best results while causing the least amount of damage to normal tissues. If you are to have radiation treatment, the radiation oncologist will decide what treatment should be used, supervise its administration and evaluate you at intervals during the course of the treatment to see whether it is working.

Who are the other members of the team?

This will vary from place to place, but there are usually several other people who work with the radiation oncologist. The *radiation physicist* and the *dosimetrist* help in calculating the dose, planning the exact treatment field, creating special blocks or shields and devising other treatment setup aids. They use a computer to plan the treatment and to calculate the distribution of the radiation dose. The *radiation therapist* (sometimes called a *radiation technologist*) is the person who is responsible for following the plan, getting you ready for your treatment and giving your daily treatment under the direction of the radiation oncologist. The *radiation therapy nurse* is an oncology nurse with specialized training in your care during radiation and in helping to manage any side effects, both emotional and physical. The nurse may also coordinate complex treatment schedules and protocols. A dietitian, a physical therapist, a social worker or other health care professionals may also be part of the team's services.

What will determine what kind of radiation treatments I will receive?

The radiation oncologist will take many factors into consideration in planning your treatment, including the cell type of your cancer, where it is located, what stage it is in, how it might spread, your age and general health, what side effects the treatment may give you, the kind of equipment needed to carry out the treatment.

Is there more than one kind of radiation treatment?

Radiation treatment is usually divided into two basic kinds: external beam radiation, where a machine is used, and internal radiation, where the radiation is placed in or near the affected area. Most people have external beam radiation, although some have both internal and external radiation.

TYPES OF RADIATION		
TYPE	**DESCRIPTION**	**WHEN USED**
External radiation; also called **x-ray, external beam, electron beam, cobalt treatment**	Machine, such as a linear accelerator, delivers x-rays or gamma rays to tumor on or in your body. Machine is usually some distance from your body. Neutron beam is a new experimental type of external beam treatment.	Most often used kind of x-ray.
Internal radiation; also called **radium implant, interstitial radiation, intracavitary, brachytherapy**	Radioactive material, such as iridium, is placed on the affected tissue, or in the body near the tumor. It is either sealed in a container and inserted into a body cavity or given orally or injected into the bloodstream or the affected area.	Can be used for a variety of cancers.
Intraoperative radiation	External radiation given during an operation. Investigational treatment done at major centers and hospitals.	Being used for cancers of the breast, colon, rectum, stomach, brain, pancreas and gynecologic organs.

What is the difference between a rad and a gray?

Both are terms for describing radiation dosage, the amount of radiation that is absorbed by the tissues in the body. Rad stands for **r**adiation **a**bsorbed **d**ose and had been used for many years by radiation oncologists to describe doses of radiation. In 1985, the International Commission on Radiation Units and Measurements officially adopted the term *gray* as the unit of radiation dose to replace the term *rad*. One gray equals 100 rads or 100 centigrays (cGy). One rad equals 1 centigray.

EXTERNAL RADIATION

What is external radiation?

When external radiation is used, a machine directs high-energy rays or particles at the cancer and at normal tissue near the cancer.

What kind of radiation beams are used in treatment?

There are several kinds of beams used: x-rays (produced by specially designed equipment), gamma rays (emitted by radioactive materials), electrons (produced by an x-ray tube), neutrons (produced by radioactive elements), heavy ions (such as carbon and neon), and negative pi-meson (small, negatively charged particles). X-rays, gamma rays and electrons are known as low-LET (Linear Energy Transfer) radiation. Neutron beams, heavy ions and negative pi-mesons (pions) are known as high-LET radiation. Facilities for high-LET radiation are limited. Although clinical trials have shown there are some advantages to this type of radiation, the cost of the facilities and of the sophistication of the personnel needed to carry it out has restricted this treatment to selected referral centers for carefully selected cancer patients.

What machines are used to give radiation treatments?

Several machines, with different characteristics, are used for giving radiation externally. They are usually defined by the amount of energy they emit. Kilovoltage and orthovoltage machines give out low-energy rays, less than one megavolt. This type of equipment has limited use today, usually used only for surface skin cancers. Megavoltage equipment, such as linear accelerators and cobalt units, emits energy greater than one megavolt and directs a more precise, intense beam to a tiny target area in the body with less scattering of radiation to surrounding normal tissue. These machines, which give the maximum dose beneath the skin rather than on it, allow much higher doses of radiation to be given to deeply-lying tumors. Linear accelerators are the most widely used machines, found in most hospitals as well as in some private radiotherapy offices. Cobalt units, once the most common equipment, are easier to operate and maintain than the linear accelerators, but take longer to give the treatment.

Are there any new types of particle radiation being tested?

There are several new types that are being tested in clinical trials, including fast neutrons, deuterons, helium ion beams and negative pi-mesons. Most of these have limited application and are very expensive. Their use is presently confined to a small proportion of cancer patients in clinical research studies.

Is heavy ion treatment being conducted in the United States?

The heavy ion accelerator at the Lawrence Berkeley Laboratory in Berkeley, California, that had treated some 400 patients since the 1970s, was closed in 1993. It had been built mainly for high-energy physics. The first large accelerator in the world dedicated solely to cancer treatment, located outside of Tokyo, has begun treating patients. There are plans to begin using a heavy ion accelerator in Germany and a cooperative European accelerator is also under way. In the United States, proton beam treatment is being used instead of heavy ions.

Where is proton beam radiation being done?

There are two places in the United States that have proton beam accelerators for patient treatment: the Massachusetts General Hospital in Boston and Loma Linda University Medical Center in Los Angeles.

What is stereotactic radiosurgery?

Stereotactic radiosurgery is an investigational treatment that uses high-energy x-rays to destroy deep-seated tumors and other lesions in the brain. It can be performed with a roentgen knife or with a gamma knife, a delicate, costly device. Several advanced mechanical technologies can be combined with the roentgen knife, including CT scan, angiography and linear accelerator.

What are hypoxic cells?

Hypoxic or anoxic cells are cells that have a reduced oxygen supply. Tumors with cells that are well-oxygenated are more sensitive to radiation. Those tumors with hypoxic cells are less sensitive to radiation.

What is a radiosensitizer?

A radiosensitizer is a substance or a procedure that makes cancer cells more susceptible to the effects of radiation treatment. A number of different agents are under investigation. Chemotherapy drugs also are used as radiosensitizers.

Are radio-labeled antibodies used to treat cancer?

Yes, they are. Radioactive isotopes are attached in the laboratory to antibodies produced from cells taken from a patient's tumor. The antibodies, reinjected into the patient and carrying the radioactive isotopes, travel through the bloodstream to the tumor. The isotopes attach to the tumor and attack and kill cells. There is more information on radio-labeled antibodies in Chapter 9, "New Advances and Investigational Trials."

What is a radioprotector?

Radioprotectors are chemical compounds that may be able to protect normal cells against short-term radiation damage. They allow the normal cells to repair themselves while the tumor cells are still being treated. Radioprotectors allow radiation oncologists to give higher doses of radiation than would normally be safe for the surrounding tissues. They also may eliminate the problem of second cancers sometimes induced by radiation treatment. There are radioprotective substances presently being tested in clinical trials.

Is radiation ever used before an operation?

Sometimes radiation is done before an operation to shrink the tumor. In some special cases, radiation is used both before and after an operation, with a large single dose given twenty-four to forty-eight hours before surgery, followed by radiation sometime after the operation. This is sometimes referred to as a "sandwich" technique.

Is external beam radiation ever used during an operation?

Yes. This is called intraoperative radiation therapy. The surgery is begun and after the tumor is exposed or taken out, the patient is given radiation therapy directly to the area. The operation is then completed. Intraoperative radiation can deliver a single high dose directly to the tumor, because surrounding organs sensitive to radiation, such as the skin, intestines and liver, can be held aside or shielded. The exposed tumor can also be felt or seen directly, rather than viewed on a scan or x-ray. Sometimes, the intraoperative radiation is given in addition to external radiation. Intraoperative radiation therapy is being used with cancers of the breast, colon, rectum, stomach, brain, pancreas and gynecologic organs. This treatment is being studied in clinical trials at selected institutions.

Will the radiation treatment be done right in the operating room if I am having intraoperative therapy?

It depends on the hospital. Some have an operating room in the radiation department. In others, you are moved to the radiation therapy area and then returned to the operating room. These issues are also being studied in clinical trials at selected institutions.

Is hyperthermia ever used with external radiation treatment?

Some centers are using hyperthermia—raising the temperature of the area of the tumor—before radiation treatment on an investigational basis. Hyperthermia can be applied locally (only to the site of the tumor), regionally (to the tumor site and the surrounding tissue), or to the whole body (elevating the core temperature of the body). There is more information about hyperthermia in Chapter 9, "New Advances and Investigational Trials."

What is meant by the term *boost* or *conedown*?

Once the regular radiation treatment is finished, an additional high dose may be given to a smaller area where the tumor was found. This is referred to as a "boost" dose in a "conedown" or reduced area. It may also be called "shrinking field technique." It is used to help avoid excess radiation to radiosensitive organs that are in the area of the tumor.

PLANNING YOUR TREATMENT

What steps will the radiation oncologist take in planning my external radiation treatments?

The radiation oncologist will thoroughly examine you and study your x-rays, CT scans, pathology slides, hospital records, and any other pertinent information about your case. Then the radiation oncologist will discuss the recommendations on the type and duration of radiation treatment. The next step probably will be a treatment planning session.

Will I have my first treatment at my first appointment with the radiation oncologist?

It is highly unlikely that you will have your first treatment during your first appointment, because your treatment plan needs to be set up. Treatment plans are different for each patient, so it may take several visits before your treatment actually begins. Timing of your first treatment depends on the kind of cancer you have, the kind of treatments you have already had, the stage of your particular disease, your physical condition and how complicated your treatment plan will be.

What is meant by simulation?

Simulation is another term for the session that determines your treatment plan. This is the process in which the radiation oncologist, working with the physicist, determines the area to be treated, the methods to be used, and the positions of the machines. You will be asked to lie very still on a table below a special x-ray machine, called a simulator, which outlines the area to be treated, called the treatment field. This x-ray will be used to define the precise areas where the treatment will be directed, called the treatment port. Some simulators give three-dimensional views of the tumor and surrounding areas. Others include ultrasound devices that produce images of internal structures. Sometimes information on the contour of your body is fed into a computer to help guide the planning process. During this planning session, those areas that need to be shielded will also be pinpointed.

How long does the simulation session last?

Depending on where your radiation is going to be given and how complex the planning is, the session may last from fifteen minutes up to two hours, with one hour being an average. You may find this procedure long and exhausting. If you have just had an operation, you also may find that the simulation session is uncomfortable. Once the simulation is completed, you will be given an appointment to start the treatment.

How are the casts, forms or molds made?

You are put in the position you will assume during treatment. The mold or the cast is made right on your body, using whatever material has been chosen, such as plaster, plastic or Styrofoam. Small windows are cut into the mold to allow the beam to be directed to the precise area to be treated. The radiation oncologist can use the mold over and over again to be sure the beam is always directed to the correct area.

How is the dose of radiation decided upon?

The dose varies with the size of the tumor, the extent of the tumor, the tumor type and grade and its response to radiation. Computers are used to determine the treatment volume and the distribution of the dose within that volume. Several plans may be generated from which the radiation oncologist will select the one that provides the desired distribution of the dose.

Will my normal cells be affected by radiation?

All cells are affected by the radiation, whether they are normal or malignant. The normal tissues have a greater capacity to recover from the damage induced by the radiation than do the cancer cells. The radiation oncologist plans the treatment so that normal tissues are irradiated as little as possible. In addition, some areas will be shielded and protected from the radiation.

Why is the radiation treatment sometimes given from different angles?

One way of giving the maximum amount of radiation to the tumor and the minimum amount to normal tissue is by aiming radiation beams at the tumor from two or more directions. The patient or the machine is rotated. The patient and the machine are placed so that the beams meet each other where the tumor is located. The tumor thus gets a high enough dose of radiation to be destroyed but normal tissues escape with minimum radiation effects since the beams take different pathways to reach the tumor.

Why is the radiation given over a period of time instead of all at once?

The radiation must be strong enough to kill the tumor and still allow the normal tissues to heal. The radiation oncologist determines the total radiation dose necessary and divides it into the number of single-treatment doses that will add up to the total dose by the time of the last treatment. This process, dividing the doses of radiation, is known as fractionation. Fractionation is a very important part of planning and delivering radiation since it affects both the tumor and the normal tissues.

What is accelerated fractionation?

When a radiation oncologist gives you the regular dose of radiation in a shorter time, it is known as accelerated fractionation or hyperfractionation. Hyperfractionation uses the same amount of time but increases the total dose by giving it two or three times a day, usually separated by several hours. There are several studies looking at how best to plan radiation treatment to get results with the least damage to normal cells.

Will I need to remain in the same position for my treatments?

Usually, you will be lying in exactly the same position each day so that you will get the precise amount of radiation to the target site. During the simulation process, retaining or positioning devices, such as bite blocks, casts, or molds may be designed especially for you. Headrests, armboards or handgrips may also be used to assure accurate positioning. Sometimes, especially for children, a custom-made body cast may be used.

What is a bite block?

A bite block is a specially made dental impression that you bite into for positioning during radiation treatment. The bite block is attached to a stabilizing device to hold your head in the right place.

It will be used throughout the course of your treatment to make sure you are in the same position each time the treatment is done. In addition, other devices such as plastic or plaster forms may be made to help you stay in exactly the right place.

How will I be shielded from unnecessary radiation?

There are many safeguards to protect you from unnecessary radiation to the parts of your body that do not need treatment. All the machines are shielded so that the large amounts of radiation are given only to a specific area. The treatment field is usually lit with a light that outlines the surface through which the radiation will pass. A series of safeguards in the machine limits the radiation to this lighted area of your body. Shields, usually made out of lead blocks, are used to shield small areas of your body not needing treatment.

What parts of the body are covered with these shields?

That depends upon where the radiation is being given. Lead cases and blocks, and plastic or plaster molds, are custom-made, based on your own anatomy. They will be used throughout the course of your treatment to protect your vital organs and to keep you in the proper position for radiation. For example, in giving radiation to the ovary, your kidneys would be shielded. The ovaries may be shielded or moved, for instance, in women of childbearing ages who are getting radiation for Hodgkin's disease.

What are portal films?

Portal films, sometimes also called port or beam films, are taken through the treatment machine to confirm that the treatment field and the blocks are in the correct position.

How will the spot where the radiation is to be given be marked?

Once the location has been decided, the radiation oncologist or the radiation therapist will draw marks on your skin. Marking pens, indelible ink or silver nitrate may be used. You will be asked not to wash away these markings. After your first week of treatment, you may have permanent markings put on your skin. Usually a small pinpoint tattoo placed on the corners of the treatment field is used.

How is the permanent tattoo done?

Usually it is a very simple process, which substitutes for the ink markings used for your original treatments. A drop of India ink is placed on your skin, and with a needle, a tiny permanent black dot is made on the skin itself. For sites that are most visible, such as on the face, a mask or head holder may be made of plastic and the markings placed on it rather than on the skin itself.

Is the treatment plan ever changed?

Your original radiation treatment plan may be added to, subtracted from or changed, as the radiation oncologist feels is appropriate. There are a number of reasons for making changes as the treatment goes along. Do not be alarmed if the plan is changed. It does not mean that the disease is getting worse or that the disease has progressed.

GETTING YOUR RADIATION TREATMENT

Can I wear my own clothes while I am having a radiation treatment?

It depends upon where on your body the treatment is being given. You will probably have to undress, so wear clothing that is easy to get on and off. You might even want to bring your own robe. Some people wear old underclothing during this time because sometimes the colored ink used to mark the treatment area comes off.

What will happen during my treatment?

Depending upon where on your body the treatment is given, you may need to undress and put on a robe or a hospital gown. Then you will go into the treatment room and sit in a special chair or lie on the treatment table. The marks on your skin will be used to locate the treatment area. Special shields will be placed between the machine and the parts of your body to help protect your normal tissues and organs. The plastic or plaster casts will be put in place to help you keep your position during treatment.

Will I be alone in the room during treatment?

The radiation therapist will leave the room and will control the machine from the control room. You will be watched on a television screen or through a window in the control room. The machine, which is very large, will make a steady buzzing noise when the beam is on. Some treatment machines rotate around you, making a noise as they move. If you are concerned about what will happen in the treatment room, make sure you discuss it with the radiation therapist or the radiation oncology nurse before you begin your treatments.

What is the actual treatment like?

Most people say that they feel nothing while the treatment is being given. A few say that they feel warmth or a mild tingling sensation.

You will feel no pain or discomfort and it will be unusual if you have any kind of sensation. If by any chance you do feel ill or very uncomfortable during the treatment, tell the radiation therapist. The machine can be stopped at any time. You need to remain very still during treatment, but you can breathe normally. Try to relax. Some people bring their headsets and soothing music into the treatment room with them. You may feel cold in the treatment room, since the temperature is kept cool for the proper operation of the machine.

Will the radiation I am getting make me radioactive?

No. External beam radiation does not cause your body to become radioactive. There is no need to avoid being with other people because of your treatment. You can hug, kiss and have sexual relations with others, without any worry.

Is it safe for a pregnant woman to accompany me to my daily radiation treatments?

Basically, the levels in the radiation department waiting room should be safe for all.

Why can't the radiation therapist stay in the room with me while I am having my radiation treatment?

The machine, although it pinpoints the beam at a specific part of the body, does scatter some of the radiation. Although the amount of radiation outside the beam is tiny during any one radiation treatment session, over months and years, it could add up to a dangerous amount for the treatment personnel. It is important for the staff who are working with radiation all day long not to be exposed to these scattered beams. All personnel who are working with radiation must be carefully monitored with badges which measure their accumulated doses, so that they will be able to tell when the maximum amounts, set by the Food and Drug Administration, have been reached.

How many radiation treatments will I get?

The number of radiation treatments depends upon the kind of tumor, the extent of the disease, the dose involved and your physical condition. For some kinds of cancer, a few treatments are needed over a few weeks. For other kinds, the treatments may last longer. Sometimes the radiation is given over several days. Sometimes there will be a treatment followed by several days or weeks with no treatment.

How long do the treatments take?

The actual treatment lasts from one to five minutes. You are usually in the treatment room for five to fifteen minutes for each treatment. The most usual schedule is to have a treatment each day for five days, with weekends off. Usually you do not have treatments on holidays.

Will the treatment plan be changed during the course of the treatment?

It might change. The plans for treatment depend on how you as an individual respond to the treatment as well as on other factors. Interruptions to allow for rest periods are common. The initial estimate of the time required to complete a series of treatments should not be taken as a rigid or fixed number of days.

What will happen if I miss one of my treatments?

It is better to continue your treatments on a regular basis because the treatment program is precisely planned. If you have important events that you need to attend or a vacation planned, you need to discuss it with your radiation oncologist to see if it is possible to modify your schedule.

Will I have tests each time when I go for my radiation treatments?

There may be some tests during the course of the treatment, but not each time. It will depend on your treatment plan. Usually tests such as blood counts are taken so that the radiation oncologist knows whether the radiation is doing damage to other structures. Sometimes x-rays and other tests are needed to determine if the radiation oncologist should change the treatment plan.

How can the radiation oncologist tell if the radiation treatment is working?

After you have had several treatments, your radiation oncologist will begin checking you to find out how well the treatment is working. For some cancers, the radiation oncologist can use regular x-rays to see whether the tumor is shrinking and can do other tests to find out whether the radiation is causing any damage to normal cells. For instance, you may have blood tests to check the level of white blood cells and platelets, which may be reduced during treatment. Your own reports of how you feel may be one of the best indicators of the treatment's progress. You may not be aware of changes in your cancer, but you will be able to notice any decrease in pain, bleeding, or other discomforts you may have had.

What is total body radiation?

This means that the whole body is treated with radiation. It is used in preparation for bone marrow transplantation.

What is hemibody radiation?

In hemibody radiation, a large single dose of radiation is given in a single treatment to about half of the body, either the upper or lower half. It is usually used if there is a large amount of local disease in the gynecologic area or the abdomen. It may also be used in cancers of the lung, esophagus, prostate and digestive system.

Can radiation be used to treat pain?

Sometimes radiation is used to treat cancer pain, especially in the bone. It has been shown to be useful in treating pain due to pressure on nerves or lymphedema associated with several types of cancers, including colon, rectum, kidney, ovary and other gynecologic organs, lung, and metastases in the liver and bone. Often treatments that last two to three weeks give rapid and sustained pain relief without any major disruptions in quality of life.

MANAGING SIDE EFFECTS FROM EXTERNAL RADIATION

Does everyone have side effects from radiation?

The extent of side effects from radiation varies greatly. The side effects range from slight in some people to severe in a few instances. They depend on the intensity of the treatment, the location of it, and your tolerance and condition. Some people go through their radiation treatments with very little suffering from side effects. Others do have serious problems. Most side effects begin after the second or third week of treatment. We have listed the side effects that have been experienced by people getting radiation treatment. It is important to understand that no one experiences all of them, that the radiation oncologists and nurses can help you minimize some of them and that your own attitude may play a role in determining how severe your side effects will be.

Will I be very sick from radiation?

Most people do not get very sick from radiation treatment, although many people do complain about being tired. Most people are able to work, keep house and enjoy some leisure activities while having radiation treatment. Some people prefer to take a few weeks off from work while they are having their treatments. Others work fewer hours. This is a subject you need to discuss with your employer. You may also want to ask family and friends to help you with daily chores, housework, shopping, taking care of the children or driving.

Are there any specific problems I should report to my radiation oncologist or nurse during radiation treatment?

Your radiation oncologist will tell you what problems, if any, you need to watch for and how you should deal with them. As a rule, you should contact the radiation oncologist or nurse if you have any cough, sweating, fever or unusual pain over the course of your treatment. As soon as any of the side effects discussed in this chapter begin, you should tell your radiation oncologist, radiation therapist or nurse so they can help you to control the problems.

Will I get sick enough from side effects to stop treatment?

Very few people are unable to complete their entire treatments because of side effects. Of course, this depends on your own physical condition, the reason for the radiation treatments, how long they are going to last and where they are being given. Sometimes the radiation oncologist will give you a rest from treatment if you are having a severe reaction, or the radiation oncologist may decide to change the treatment. It is very important that you discuss side effects with your health care team.

Are there some general do's and don'ts for people getting radiation treatment?

Yes, there are some general guidelines. Nearly all cancer patients having radiation treatment need to take a few extra steps to protect their overall good health and to help the treatment succeed. Later in this chapter there are comments on specific areas of radiation. But if you are getting radiation to any part of your body, here are some general recommendations.

- Be sure to get plenty of rest. Sleep as often as you feel the need. Your body will use a lot of extra energy over the course of the treatment.
- Eating well is important. Try to maintain a diet that will prevent weight loss.
- Do not remove the ink marks from your skin. Do not draw over the faded lines at home. After the first week, you may get small, permanent tattoo marks.
- Tell the radiation oncologist about any medicine you are taking before you start treatment. If you need to take medicine, even aspirin, let your radiation oncologist know before

POSSIBLE SIDE EFFECTS OF EXTERNAL RADIATION TREATMENT

POSSIBLE SIDE EFFECT	THINGS YOU SHOULD KNOW
ALL SITES: Ink marks on skin where treatment is given	• Don't wash off the ink marks; they must stay on. After the first week of treatment, more permanent marks may be made. These marks show the radiation therapist where to aim the treatment.
Dry or itchy skin; redness, tanning, sunburned look; skin may turn a shade darker than normal	• When taking a bath or shower, use lukewarm water only, no soap, gently sponge your skin and pat it dry. • Don't put salves, deodorants, powders, perfumes, bandages, medications, cosmetics, suntan lotion or other self-remedies on your skin during treatment or for three weeks after treatment, unless ordered by the radiation oncologist giving you radiation. Stay away from talcum powder because it contains an abrasive; use cornstarch instead. Ask the nurse or radiation therapist to suggest what you should use during and after treatment. • Keep the treated areas out of the sun. Be sure to prevent sunburn during treatment and after completion of treatment. After treatment, the use of a sun block is recommended for the skin that has been radiated to prevent further damage. You will always have to be careful about protecting the treated area from the sun. If treatment is to head and neck area, wear a wide-brimmed hat when outdoors. • Do not apply hot or cold objects to the skin without the radiation oncologist's permission. Do not use hot-water bottles, ice packs, hot-water compresses, electric heating pads, hot packs or heating lights on treatment areas. Heat or cold may further shock your sensitive skin. • Try not to rub, scrub or scratch the treatment area. Do not wear tight-fitting or irritating clothes over the treated areas —no corsets, girdles, belts or other articles of clothing that leave a mark on your skin. Check with the radiation oncologist or nurse about shaving in the treatment area. Use soft shirts and loose collars if radiation is in the head and neck area. • If skin blisters or cracks or becomes moist be sure to tell the radiation oncologist and nurse. Ask them what to do for treatment. Remember these skin reactions are temporary and should disappear within a few weeks after treatment is completed.

Hair loss	Depends on the site of radiation. If hair is present within the area being treated, loss may occur. Areas affected are scalp, beard, eyebrows, armpits, pubic and body hair. Hair usually grows back, starting about two months after treatment has ended. It may be a little thinner.
Feeling weak and tired; extreme fatigue	A natural reaction to radiation treatment. One of most common complaints. Get extra rest. Don't try to force yourself to do things if you feel tired. Limit activity. Rest for an hour or so a day; go to bed early. Get help with daily chores.
Loss of appetite	See eating hints in Chapter 24, "Living with Cancer."
Sluggish bowels	See hints in Chapter 24, "Living with Cancer."
Sexual	Other side effects such as being tired or feeling sick make it difficult to have intercourse. May not enjoy sex or desire to have it. Depending on location of treatment, may have problems having erection or orgasm. May become sterile. Women may have decreased lubrication or shrinking of vaginal tissues.
HEAD, NECK, UPPER CHEST, MOUTH AND THROAT	
Thick saliva	Usually begins during third or fourth week of treatment. Rinse with club soda, which will refresh your mouth and thin out the saliva. Check your local pharmacy for Xerolube (put two or three drops on your tongue and work it through your mouth). Use it as often as you need it.
Dry mouth	Usually occurs near end of treatment and lasts from several months to several years. See hints in Chapter 24, "Living with Cancer."
Sore throat, red tongue, white spots in mouth, sore mouth, unable to wear dentures, lumplike feeling when swallowing (rare)	Usually begins two to three weeks after treatment starts. Symptoms usually begin to lessen after fifth week of treatment and end four to six weeks after treatments stop. Make sure you report it to your radiation oncologist. See hints in Chapter 24, "Living with Cancer."

(continued)

POSSIBLE SIDE EFFECTS OF EXTERNAL RADIATION TREATMENT *(cont.)*

POSSIBLE SIDE EFFECT	THINGS YOU SHOULD KNOW
Loss of taste or change in taste	Usually occurs during third or fourth week of treatment and returns to normal from three weeks to three months after treatment is completed. The x-rays may have destroyed some of the tiny taste buds on your tongue. Many patients prefer egg and dairy dishes instead of meat.
Problems with your teeth	If you have dentures, expect to take them out before each treatment. Have a complete dental examination before radiation treatment begins. Brush your teeth after every meal or snack with a soft toothbrush. Use fluoride toothpaste with no abrasives. Floss once or twice a day. Apply fluoride every day.
Earaches	Ear and throat are closely related—sometimes ears can be affected by treatment. If your ears bother you, tell the radiation oncologist. Sometimes ear drops will be ordered. Sometimes radiation to brain results in hardening of ear wax, which can impair hearing.
Drooping or swelling skin under chin	Fatty tissue under the chin sometimes shrinks after treatment, leaving loose skin which droops or swells. If you notice lumps or small knots on side of neck or in shoulder, tell the radiation oncologist.
Loss of hair	Whiskers, sideburns and chest hair may disappear temporarily or permanently, depending on the dose and area treated. Do not use razor blades for shaving; you may shave with an electric shaver but not more than once a week. Radiation to brain area sometimes causes some hair loss. This is usually a temporary condition. Use a hairpiece or wig temporarily. See Chapter 8, "Chemotherapy," for information on wigs.

BREAST Dry, tender, moist or itchy skin in armpit (axilla), under breast, or breast area	Can occur during third or fourth week of radiation treatment. If itchiness continues, ask the radiation oncologist or nurse for something to put on it. If area is moist, be sure to talk with the radiation oncologist or nurse, who can give you something to put on it. You will probably also need to let the air get at the area several times a day. Sometimes the side effects of radiation continue for four to six weeks. Do not be alarmed, but do discuss them with your radiation oncologist or nurse. You might have a sore breast or swelling in the treatment area. Make sure you contact the radiation oncologist to report these effects. Breast swelling can continue for up to one year. If you have had a breast removed, it is best not to wear an artificial breast (prosthesis) until a month or so after radiation treatment has ended.
UPPER ABDOMEN Nausea, vomiting, feeling of fullness	See Chapter 24, "Living with Cancer."
LOWER ABDOMEN Diarrhea, feeling sick to your stomach, cramps, rectal burning with bowel movement (rare), inflamed bladder (rare)	Usually occurs during third or fourth week of treatment. Varies from one to two soft stools a day to as many as ten watery stools a day. It is best to start diet with foods that are low in fiber early in treatment and not wait until you have this problem. See Chapter 24, "Living with Cancer," for further information.

you start. You also need to tell the radiation oncologist if your medicines are changed during your treatment. If you are a diabetic and you are eating less while you are having treatment, your insulin dose may need to be changed.

- Do not bare treatment areas to the sun during treatment.
- Expect your skin to turn a shade darker than its normal color. This is usually a temporary condition.
- Hair loss is not normally a side effect of radiation treatment unless hair is present within the area being treated. Areas that may be affected are the scalp, beard, eyebrows, armpits and pubic and body hair.
- If you are having problems with nausea and vomiting, ask your radiation oncologist and nurse about antivomiting medicine and about how often you should be taking it. Read the information in Chapter 24, "Living with Cancer," for more eating hints.
- If your throat or mouth is sore, tell your radiation oncologist. You can get a mouthwash medication that, when swallowed or gargled, can numb your mouth so you can eat normally.

What kind of clothing should I wear?

Loose-fitting clothing is the best. You need to stay away from clothes that increase friction in the treated area. Watch out for belts, girdles, high shirt collars, bras (especially underwire), heavy seams in denim or corduroy pants and shirts, and groin bands on men's briefs. Use cotton underwear because it encourages the exchange of air and decreases moisture. Women who are having radiation in the pelvic region also should not wear nylon pantyhose. It is best if you wash your clothes with soaps used for babies' clothes, since they have fewer chemicals in them.

What should I do if my skin gets irritated?

Because the skin in the treatment area is more sensitive, you need to take steps to try not to irritate it. Don't scrub it with a washcloth or a brush. Don't use soaps, creams, lotions or powders on it without first checking with the nurse or radiation therapist. Don't apply anything hot or cold to it. Don't scratch or rub the skin in that area. Do not use adhesive tape because your skin is sensitive and may come off with the tape. Don't expose it to the sun. Wear loose-fitting clothes. If you do see an irritation, or if your skin looks like it's going to blister or crack, be sure you report it to your radiation oncologist immediately.

Does it make any difference what kind of soap I use?

Your nurse can give you advice. Many soaps irritate sensitive skin. Wash with warm water or warm water and mild soap. If you use soap, make sure it is thoroughly rinsed from your skin. Pat your skin dry with a soft, clean towel.

Will my skin get dry or itchy?

Again, it depends on many factors. Some people will have dry skin or itchiness during treatment. Do not scratch. Trim your fingernails to prevent damaging your skin unconsciously while you sleep. If you have allergies, try to stay away from substances that normally cause itching. Use tepid water when bathing to reduce the loss of oils from the skin. Pat your skin dry. Do not rub skin with a towel or have massages. Stay away from soaps that dry the skin or have perfume or detergent in them. Do not use talcum powder because it contains an abrasive. You may use cornstarch for itchy skin, but do not use it if you have a moist reaction on your skin. If you have dry skin, it may help to drink more water and juices. Talk with your radiation oncologist and nurse about medicine you might take to reduce the itchiness.

Why can't I use lotions on my dry or itchy skin?

Many products you can buy in the store, such as lotions or petroleum jelly, leave a coating that can interfere with your radiation treatment or healing. If your skin does become dry, ask the nurse or technician to suggest what you should use during and after treatment.

Why should I be careful about using hot compresses or ice packs?

Do not apply anything—hot or cold—to your skin without asking your radiation oncologist. Skin that has undergone radiation is less able to adapt to extreme temperatures. Do not use ice packs, hot-water bottles or compresses, heating pads, heat lamps or sunlamps on your treatment areas. If you are in a cold climate, make sure you wear warm clothing. Heat or cold may further irritate your already sensitive skin.

Will my skin get darker or redder?

It depends on the condition and color of your skin, the area and kind of radiation, your age and physical condition, medicine you might be taking and the other types of treatment you may be getting. Most people do not see any changes during the first two weeks of treatment. Some people get little reaction at all. Others find their skin looks light pink or red, sunburned or tanned. Sometimes it turns a bit rough and might even peel slightly. You may find that your skin is not as flexible or as movable as before. Tell your radiation oncologist or nurse when you first note reddening of your skin. If you are taking any medicines, make sure you tell the radiation oncologist and nurse what they are, so that they can decide whether they need to watch your skin more closely during treatment.

What happens if my skin feels wet?

You should report this immediately to your radiation oncologist. The area may be painful, bright red and moist. This can happen, especially after many radiation treatments and in areas where the skin creases. This is called "weeping" of the skin, because the upper layers have shed. It is not a burn. Your radiation oncologist may stop the treatment for a while, block the area that is affected or treat a different area. You will get medicine to prevent infection and to reduce the pain. The nurse will teach you how to do soaks (there are several kinds that can be used) or to apply moist dressings to the area, and how to keep the area clean. The goal will be to minimize the loss of fluids, prevent infection and make you as comfortable as possible while the skin heals. Depending on the size of the area, it can take from one to three weeks for the skin to heal.

Do most people get severe skin reactions?

Most people do not get severe skin reactions from the radiation because of skin-sparing effects of modern equipment. However, there are a few instances in which patients may get severe reactions due to the need for high doses of radiation for a particular situation. Even if you have a severe reaction, you can expect your skin to heal well.

Will the skin reactions go away after my treatment ends?

Most of the skin reactions will disappear a few weeks after treatment is finished. In many cases, however, your skin in the treated areas may remain dark. Call your radiation oncologist immediately if your skin cracks, blisters or becomes moist after your treatment ends.

Will I be able to shave or use deodorants?

Not in the treatment area during treatment. Shaving can result in small cuts that can get easily infected and can also lead to the moist skin reaction. If you must shave, use an electric razor but check with the radiation oncologist, nurse or radiation therapist. Deodorants can affect the radiation treatment. Cornstarch may be used instead of deodorant. You should wait several weeks after your treatment has ended to use roll-on deodorants or to shave skin in the treatment area because these activities may pull on the skin and cause damage to it.

May I go swimming while I am having my radiation treatments?

You probably can, as long as it does not cause your skin to dry. You need to rinse your skin well with fresh water if you have been swimming in salt water or in a pool with chlorine in it.

Will I need to do anything to take care of my skin after the radiation treatments have ended?

Yes. You should use some kind of lotion or moisturizer on your skin in the treated area two to three times a day. Use something that will wash away with water (petroleum jelly is not recommended, for instance) and that does not have any perfume.

Will I be able to go out in the sun after my treatment is finished?

Do not expose the treatment area to the direct sunlight for at least a month after you have finished radiation. If you expect to be in the sun for more than a few minutes during that time you will need to be careful, making sure the area is covered. After that you will need to be cautious when you go out in the sun—be it at the beach, on a boat, working in your garden, riding in a car, at a picnic, or skiing. Protect your treated skin with a cover-up, a shirt, and a broad-brimmed hat. Don't use thin, gauzy materials for your cover-up fabric. If you sunbathe, use a number 15 sunscreen and stay in the direct sun only for a few minutes each time. If you see any reaction, such as redness or irritation, stay out of the sun until it goes away. Do not take foolish chances. Ask your radiation oncologist or nurse about using sunblocking lotions.

Will radiation affect my blood counts?

Sometimes it may. The radiation oncologist may find you have low white blood cell counts or low levels of platelets, which can affect your body's ability to fight infection and to prevent bleeding. If your blood tests show these problems, you may have to go off treatment for a week or so to allow your blood counts to come back up.

Will I feel tired from the radiation?

Probably, but it depends on the person, the dose and the area of radiation, what treatments you have had before or during your radiation, and your general physical condition. Most people, after a few radiation treatments, find they tire easily. Some people complain of feeling tired a few hours after treatment. Some who take their treatments every day say they feel tired all the time. The stress related to the treatment plus your trips to the treatment center also can add to your tired feeling. If you feel tired, you should rest and take naps if you can. The feeling should gradually begin to wear off within a few weeks after your treatment ends. The following should help:

- Eat when you feel tired. Sometimes a small amount of food will give you the extra energy you need.
- Rest when you feel tired. Some people get tired more quickly and need more rest during this time. Try to get more sleep at night. Rest during the day if you can. Don't feel you must keep up your normal schedule of activities if you feel tired. Use your leisure time in a restful way.
- Reduce your activities. You may wish to take some time off from work, or work a reduced schedule for a while.
- Don't be afraid to ask others for help. Family, friends and neighbors can help you in shopping, child care, housework or driving.

Does my diet have to change during treatment?
No, your diet does not need to change, unless you are having treatments in the area of your stomach and your intestines. However, it is important for you to eat well to speed tissue repair. You should try to maintain your normal weight through a well-balanced, nutritious diet and have sufficient rest. Your appetite may be affected, but it is important that you eat properly. You should be careful to have both good nutrition and plenty of rest to help your body repair and replace the normal cells. Radiation oncologists have found that patients who eat well can better withstand both their cancer and the side effects of treatment. Try also to keep emotional stress to a minimum. There are further diet tips in Chapter 24, "Living with Cancer."

Can I continue my usual activities during treatment?
Continue as much of your normal activity as you can without feeling tired and strained. Many people find they can continue to work during the treatment period. Others find they can continue some activity but less than the normal amount. This is a time to listen to your body and to take good care of yourself. In addition, your radiation oncologist may suggest that you limit some activities, such as sports, that might irritate the area being treated.

Does radiation treatment put patients at risk for lymphedema?

Radiation treatment alone does not put you at risk for lymphedema, or swelling in your arms and legs. However, if you have had an infection following your surgery, radiation combined with other treatments, such as surgery or chemotherapy may put you at risk for lymphedema if you have some types of cancer. These include breast cancer, malignant melanoma of the arms or legs, prostate cancer (if whole pelvic radiation is given), soft tissue and bone sarcomas and some gynecologic cancers. There is more information on lymphedema in Chapter 6, "Surgery."

Will radiation treatment affect my emotions?

It is not unusual for people who are having treatment for cancer to feel upset, depressed, afraid, angry, frustrated, alone or helpless. These feelings are due to many things, including the changes in their everyday living, their fear about cancer or the fact that they can't do everything they could before. Radiation treatment may add to these emotions, either because of fatigue or from the strain of traveling to radiation treatments every day. However, the treatment itself does not cause mental distress. Some people tell us they feel depressed or nervous during their treatments. You may want to ask your radiation oncologist or nurse about meditation or relaxation exercises that you can use during treatment. Some people find it soothing to listen to audio cassettes during treatment. If you are having some problems with coping, it may be useful for you to talk about them with someone—a nurse, a social worker, a good friend or a chaplain. Or check with your radiation oncologist's office about support groups that might be run in the facility where you are having your treatment or by an organization such as the American Cancer Society or the Leukemia Society.

OTHER SIDE EFFECTS IN THE HEAD AND NECK AREA

Is there anything special I should know about getting radiation in the head and neck area?

There are several things you should know and some things you can do to minimize the changes in your system if you are getting radiation to any area of the head and neck—including the brain, mouth, throat, neck and upper chest.

- Be sure you check with a dentist experienced in treating cancer patients before you begin radiation treatment.

- You may experience some soreness in the area of the mouth and throat.
- You may notice that your tongue is red and that there are white spots in your mouth. You might have a hard time swallowing, feel a lump in your throat, or feel your food sticking in your throat due to irritation of the tissues in the area of the throat and swallowing tube (esophagus). You might not be able to eat with your dentures. All of these are temporary side effects that usually begin two to three weeks after treatment starts and usually begin to decrease after the fifth week of treatment. They usually end some four to six weeks after treatments finish. Of course, you should report any of these problems to your radiation oncologist.
- Smoking and drinking irritate your mouth and throat, especially during treatment. Don't use tobacco, alcoholic beverages, or hot, spicy, rough or coarse foods like pepper, chili powder, nutmeg, and vinegar, since they can irritate your mouth.
- Stay away from coarse foods such as raw vegetables, dry crackers and nuts.
- Don't eat sugary snacks. With the production of less saliva, sugar promotes more tooth decay than usual.
- Don't breathe in strong fumes, such as paints and cleaning solutions.
- Brush your teeth and tongue with a soft, narrow toothbrush within thirty minutes after you eat and at bedtime. Dip the brush bristles into hot water to make them softer. If you regularly use dental floss to clean between your teeth, be gentle so that you do not damage the gums. Massaging your gums can help to improve circulation, clean the teeth and stimulate saliva.
- Use a fluoride toothpaste with no abrasives. You may need to use a solution or tablet after brushing to show whether you have missed any plaque. Rinse your mouth well with a solution of salt and baking soda after you brush (two tablespoons of salt and/or baking soda in a pint of water). Do not use commercial mouthwashes, since they contain alcohol and may cause burning. If you wear dentures, soak them in diluted hydrogen peroxide (and rinse with water) at least weekly to clean. Apply fluoride every day. Moisturize your lips with petroleum jelly, K-Y jelly or aloe gel.
- Don't shave with razor blades in the areas being treated. You may shave with an electric razor. You may find that whiskers, sideburns, eyebrows, head hair, hair in your armpits or chest hair fall out temporarily, depending on the dose of radiation

and the area being treated. Some men with a great deal of hair on their chests who have chest radiation will find that the hair in the treated area falls out within a few weeks. It may grow back in two months after the treatment is ended, sometimes a little thinner than originally.

- Wear a cap, wide-brimmed hat or scarf when you are out in the sunshine, if you are having radiation in the area of your head. Don't use any sunburn products on your skin during the course of your treatments.
- Don't use starch in your collars if you are having radiation in the head and neck area. Wear soft shirts and loose collars to prevent irritation to the treated area.
- You may have earaches, caused by hardening of the wax in your ears.
- You may have swelling or drooping of the skin under your chin. There may also be changes in your skin texture.
- See Chapter 24, "Living with Cancer," for hints about eating during this period.

Why do I need to see a dentist before I begin radiation treatments to the head and neck area?

You need to take special care of your teeth and mouth before, during and after radiation because the treatments can affect your teeth. You should visit your dentist or a dentist who has had experience treating persons who have had head and neck radiation. Before your treatment starts, the dentist will probably take x-rays, examine your mouth and try to do any major work that is necessary or will become necessary within the next year. Ask your dentist to discuss with your radiation oncologist any dental work you need before treatments begin. If your dental work includes taking out teeth, it must be done at least ten days before you start your radiation treatment. The dentist will also explain the special care you should take to protect your teeth and mouth. Your dentist will probably want to see you often during the time you are having treatment. Young people, especially, need to be closely watched to ensure that the radiation does not lead to abnormal development of teeth that are still in the formative stages.

Is there anything I can do for my dry mouth?

Dry mouth is a difficult side effect for people who are having radiation to the head and neck area. Your glands may be producing less saliva than usual, making your mouth feel dry. It may be helpful to suck on ice chips and sip cool drinks, such as water or carbonated beverages, often throughout the day. Sugar-free candy or gum may also help. You will probably need to increase the amount of liquids you drink and perhaps use a humidifier. There are also a number of artificial saliva products that may help. These products have different properties, are semiliquid or gel, come in spray or liquid forms and are usually used after rinsing, brushing, flossing and at bedtime. There are also moisture-stimulating toothpastes, and chewing gum that can be used to stimulate saliva. Talk to the nurse or radiation oncologist about these products. The radiation oncologist also can prescribe drugs that help stimulate the flow of saliva.

Will my loss of saliva be permanent?

If you had a low flow of saliva before you began treatment, you may be left with permanent dryness. Younger people are more likely to recover some of their saliva flow than are older people. Loss of saliva flow makes it even more important to take special care of your teeth, both during and after treatment.

Will my taste buds change?

You may find that you have a loss of taste or change in the way foods taste as a result of radiation to the head and neck area. This usually happens during the third or fourth week of treatment. It may return to normal by three months after treatment. The radiation may destroy some of the tiny taste buds on your tongue.

What can I do for a sore mouth?

Some people who have radiation treatments to the head and neck area suffer from painful sores or swelling of the membranes in their mouths. The soreness may appear in the second or third week of radiation therapy, and decrease from the fifth week on. It will probably end a month or so after your treatment ends. It may make eating, speaking or swallowing difficult. Ask your radiation oncologist or nurse about rinsing with baking soda and water to keep the area clean and to prevent infection. Also ask about relief measures such as medicines that will numb the area so that you will be able to eat and swallow. You may need to take antibiotics if you get any infections as a result of mouth sores, or pain pills to relieve the discomfort.

Will I be able to wear my dentures?

You may notice that your dentures do not fit as well. This may be due to swelling of your gums caused by the radiation. You may need to stop wearing your dentures until the radiation treatments are finished. Discuss this with your radiation oncologist, nurse, and dentist. It is important not to let your dentures cause gum sores that might become infected.

Will I recover my sense of taste after my radiation treatments to the head and neck area?

Usually people who lose their sense of taste recover it within one to three months after treatment. However, you might not recover all of your taste qualities. Salt and bitter are those taste qualities most severely affected by radiation treatment, with sweet and sour least affected.

Will I lose my hair as a result of my radiation treatment?

It depends on where the radiation treatment is being given. For instance, if your scalp area is being treated, you will lose your hair on your head. You can also lose your beard, or eyebrows, if you are being treated in those areas. Usually hair begins to grow back two months after you have finished treatment, but it might be thinner. If you are going to lose the hair on your head, you might wish to buy a hairpiece before you begin treatment. See Chapter 8, "Chemotherapy," for information on wigs.

Should I do something special to protect my skin if I lose my hair?

The area may be somewhat tender. If your scalp is affected, you may want to cover your head with a hat, turban or scarf while you are in treatment. Of course, if you are in the sun you should wear a protective cap or scarf. If you plan to buy a toupee or a wig, try to do it before your hair falls out so you can match your color and style. You should use a mild shampoo (baby shampoo is the mildest) and use a cool setting on your hair dryer. For more information on selecting wigs and hairpieces, see Chapter 8, "Chemotherapy."

Will my hair grow back?

Usually your hair will grow back. The amount of hair will depend on how much radiation you received and the type of radiation treatment you had. It may not start to regrow for a few months following the end of your treatment. Your hair may have a different texture or a different color and may be thinner than before.

OTHER SIDE EFFECTS IN THE BREAST AND CHEST AREA

Is there anything special I should do if I am getting radiation in the breast and chest area?

You should watch for dry, tender, moist or itchy skin in the area of your armpit and under your breast or breast area. If you get a fever, notice a change in the color or amount of mucus when you cough or feel short of breath, be sure to tell the radiation oncologist right away.

Will I have soreness in my breast from radiation treatments in that area?

Some patients who get radiation treatment after a lumpectomy or mastectomy have sore breasts or swelling in the treated area. These side effects should disappear in four to six weeks, but sometimes swelling may persist for several months. It is a good idea to go without a bra during the time you are having radiation treatment in this area. It will help reduce the irritation to your skin. Your skin may stay slightly darker, and the pores may continue to be enlarged and more noticeable.

Will I have the same feelings in my breast as before the treatment?

Some women say the skin on their breast is more sensitive after radiation treatment while others say it is less sensitive. The skin and fatty tissue on your breast may feel thicker. Your breast may be firmer than before. Although many women have little change in size, some women's breasts may be larger or smaller after radiation treatments.

For how long will I see changes in my breast after the radiation treatments are finished?

You should not see any new changes related to the radiation treatment about a year after your treatment is finished. If your breast changes in size, shape, appearance or texture after this time, you need to see your radiation oncologist.

What is radiation pneumonitis?

Radiation pneumonitis is an inflammation of lung tissue, usually resulting from radiation to the lung. It normally occurs several months after treatment is finished. People who have had a lung problem, such as bronchitis, are more apt to get it. It can be painful and may cause breathing problems. It usually lessens in time, although for some people, the inflammation may cause permanent scarring.

OTHER SIDE EFFECTS IN THE ABDOMINAL AREA

Will I have any other side effects from radiation in my abdominal area?

You may have some problems with an upset stomach, a feeling of fullness, or nausea. Depending on where the radiation is being given, you may also have diarrhea or cramps. Rare side effects include rectal burning with your bowel movements or an inflamed bladder. If you are going to have treatment in your digestive area, it is best to start a diet with foods that are low in fiber early in your treatment cycle and not wait until you have diarrhea. You need to discuss these side effects with your radiation oncologist or nurse. You also may need medicines prescribed to help you relieve these problems. See Chapter 24, "Living with Cancer," for more information on managing these side effects.

Is there anything special I should do if I am getting radiation in the pelvic area?

If you are getting radiation therapy to any part of the area between your hips, known as the pelvic area, you may experience some of the problems discussed in the question directly above. You may also find that you need to urinate often or that it might be uncomfortable to urinate. Increasing the amount of fluids you drink may help you. Talk to your radiation oncologist about medication that might help you with this problem.

SEXUAL SIDE EFFECTS

Will I have problems having sex after my radiation treatments?

It depends on where the radiation was given, the dose and the duration. You may have some side effects that may be temporary or some that are permanent. Both men and women who have had radiation treatments can have problems. For instance, they may not enjoy sex as much, may not desire to have sex, or have some problems in having an erection or an orgasm. Other side effects such as being tired or feeling sick may make it difficult to have sexual intercourse. Women who receive radiation treatments in the pelvic area also may have decreased lubrication and some shrinking of vaginal tissues. Men who have radiation in the pelvic area can have reduced sperm production or become sterile.

Male Sexual Problems

Can I father a child while having radiation treatments in this area?

It depends on the area being treated and the dose of radiation being given. If the radiation area includes the testes, your sperm will be reduced both in number and in strength. Since this does not mean that you cannot father a child, make sure you discuss the use of birth control methods with your radiation oncologist.

Will I become sterile from radiation treatment?

This will depend on the dose of radiation and the location of treatment. If your sexual organs are in or close to the field of radiation,

POSSIBLE SEXUAL SIDE EFFECTS OF RADIATION TREATMENT

POSSIBLE SIDE EFFECT	WHO AFFECTED, FREQUENCY AND TREATMENT
Infertility or **sterility**	Often in men and women if treatment is in pelvic area. Sperm banking, blocking or moving and shielding of ovaries may be considered.
Dryness in vagina	Often in women with treatment in pelvic area. Use of vaginal lubricant.
Reduced size of vagina	Often in women with treatment in pelvic area. Stretching walls of vagina three times each week.
Painful intercourse	Often in women with treatment in pelvic area. Use of lubricant, changing positions, relaxing vaginal muscles.
Weak orgasm or **trouble reaching orgasm**	Sometimes. Practice of teasing techniques; delaying orgasm until excited.
Erection problems	Sometimes. Check for hormone imbalance; use of medications or implants.
Low sexual desire	Rare in men and women. Check for depression, anxiety, pain or other causes.

the treatment may cause sterility. Radiation therapy for cancers of the prostate, testicle and penis can affect fertility since the body often stops producing sperm. Sperm production can begin again within six months to several years after treatment, although radiation therapy close to sexual organs can sometimes cause permanent sterility. Be sure to check with your doctor about whether sterility is a possible side effect so that you can make decisions about how you wish to deal with that possibility.

What can be done if the doctor says I may become sterile?

You may want to explore the possibility of having semen frozen and stored at a sperm-banking facility so that you may be able to have children later on.

Does radiation therapy cause erection problems?

Most men who have radiation therapy find there is no change in their ability to have erections. The one-third of men who do have a change find that it develops gradually over the year or two following radiation. Radiation can affect erection by damaging the arteries that carry blood to the penis. As the area heals, internal tissues can become scarred, and the walls of the arteries may lose some elasticity, causing the erection to be less firm. Radiation may also hasten hardening of the arteries, which may narrow the pelvic arteries. Men who have high blood pressure or have been heavy smokers may be at higher risk for erection problems because of prior damage to the arteries.

Should I have my testosterone level checked?

A few men may not produce as much testosterone after having radiation treatment in the pelvic area. If you notice that you have problems with erection or lose the desire for intercourse, discuss with your doctor the possibility of having a blood test to check your testosterone level. You may need to take replacement testosterone. (If you have prostate cancer, you will not be able to take replacement testosterone.)

Is painful ejaculation caused by radiation?

After radiation to the pelvic area, some men ejaculate only a few drops of semen. Toward the end of radiation treatments, you may feel a sharp pain as you ejaculate. The pain results from irritation in the urethra; it should fade within several months after treatment.

Will my erection problems be permanent?

Many of the sexual problems that men experience after cancer treatment are temporary. Pain that occurs with erection after radiation usually lessens or disappears. One way of judging whether the change is permanent or temporary is to test if your reactions vary depending upon circumstances. Do you have trouble getting or keeping an erection every time you have sex? Are you able to do better when you stimulate yourself? Yes answers indicate that the problem may be temporary. If your sleep erections are firm and long-lasting, you will know that physically you function well and the problem probably lies with stress or psychological pressures. There is more information on sexuality in Chapter 12, "Prostate and Other Male Cancers," and Chapter 24, "Living with Cancer."

Can internal radiation treatment in the prostate cause any sexual aftereffects?

Internal implants in the prostate usually result in few long-term aftereffects. Once healing is complete, the quality of male erection is generally unaffected by the procedure.

Female Sexual Problems
Will I continue to get menstrual periods during radiation treatment to the pelvic area?

It depends upon the dose of radiation, where in the pelvic area it is given, length of the treatment, and your age. Your periods may stop temporarily, especially if you have a lower dose of radiation, or your ovaries are moved and shielded. Often, however, your loss of periods will be permanent.

What changes will I notice if my periods stop?

The changes will probably be more abrupt and intense than those of people who have natural menopause. You may have hot flashes, dryness or irritation of your vagina among other possible symptoms. If you have already gone through menopause, you may notice little or no change.

Will my vagina be swollen?

If you have radiation in the pelvic area, the sensitive tissues in the area of the vagina may become pink and swollen. Your vagina may feel tender. After treatment is finished, there may be less elasticity in the vaginal area. The tissues of the vagina may develop scar tissue, narrowing the passage and making it difficult for you to have a vaginal exam or intercourse. Your radiation oncologist or nurse will discuss vaginal stimulation, which usually begins about two weeks after treatment is completed, to help prevent the narrowing of the muscles and tissues that form the walls of the vagina.

How is vaginal stimulation done?

It can be done either with intercourse or with the use of a dilator. Intercourse and the physical movement associated with lovemaking will stretch the vaginal tissues and muscles and help prevent scar tissue formation. If you are sexually active and have intercourse at least three times per week, you will probably not need to use a dilator.

What is a dilator?

A dilator is a tube, usually made out of plastic, that is used to keep the vagina open. It comes in different sizes and you may need to change sizes as your vagina relaxes. Your radiation oncologist or nurse may supply you with a dilator, or give you a prescription for one. You will probably be told to use the dilator three times a week unless you have sexual intercourse at least three times a week.

How do I use a vaginal dilator?

You apply a water-soluble lubricant to the rounded end of the dilator, lie on your back in bed with your knees bent or stand with one foot up on a step or the toilet. Insert the rounded end of the dilator into the vagina gently and as deeply as you can without causing discomfort. Let it stay in place for ten to fifteen minutes. Withdraw and clean the dilator with hot, soapy water, rinsing it well. Do not be alarmed if slight bleeding or spotting occurs following dilator use, especially the first few times you insert it. If you are unable to insert the dilator easily, have pain or increased bleeding, check with your radiation oncologist or nurse.

What can be done to prevent pain during intercourse?

There many be several causes of pain—the sexual activity itself, the shortening or narrowing of the vagina, or the lack of lubrication. Spread a generous amount of water-based lubricating gel around and inside the entrance of your vagina before having intercourse or use a lubrication suppository that melts during foreplay. There are also vaginal moisturizers that you can use to keep your vagina from becoming dry and irritated. Make sure you are fully aroused before you have intercourse. It is only when you are highly excited that your vagina expands to its fullest length and width and the walls produce lubricating fluid. Let your partner know if any kind of touching causes pain. Show your partner the positions that are not painful. Try different positions, such as kneeling over your partner with your legs on either side of the body or facing each other while lying on your side.

Is there a way to teach myself to relax my vaginal muscles?

Once you have felt pain during intercourse, without realizing it you may tighten the muscles that ring the entrance to the vagina each time you have intercourse, making it more painful. If you become aware of these muscles, you can learn to control them. They are the same muscles that control your flow of urine. Try starting to urinate, then shut off the flow for a few seconds, then start again. Notice that when you relax the muscles, the urine starts to flow again. Practice tightening and relaxing these muscles when you are not urinating once you understand how it feels. To exercise the muscle, tighten to the count of three and then relax. You should practice this tightening and relaxing action ten times, one or two times a day. Then during lovemaking, when you are both aroused and ready for intercourse, take a few seconds to tense your vaginal muscles and then let them relax as much as possible before penetration. If you feel any pain, you can signal your partner so you can stop a moment to tighten up and then relax your vaginal muscles.

Are there any medications that would be helpful in making me relax my vaginal area?

Medications, including antispasmodics and analgesics, are sometimes used to help relax the body before intercourse and prevent the tightening of the pelvic muscles. You should consult your radiation oncologist or a sex therapist to determine if medication might be helpful to you.

Is it unusual to have bleeding after intercourse?

Radiation to your vagina can make the lining more fragile. You may find some light bleeding after intercourse. It may be several months after your radiation treatments are completed before full healing takes place.

Can I have sexual relations if I am having radiation treatment in the pelvic area?

It depends. Some radiation oncologists advise women not to have intercourse during the treatment period. Other women find that intercourse is painful. However, some radiation oncologists encourage sexual activities to prevent the narrowing of the walls of the vagina. You need to discuss this with your doctor.

Can I get pregnant during radiation treatment?

Radiation oncologists are still not sure how radiation treatments affect fertility. Most feel that you should not get pregnant while you are having radiation to the pelvic area because the radiation may injure the fetus. If you are already pregnant, discuss with the radiation oncologist what steps can be taken to protect the fetus. If you are of childbearing age, make sure you talk about the use of birth control methods with your radiation oncologist.

Will I be able to have children after having had radiation treatments?

It depends on where the radiation has been given, the dose of the radiation, how long the ovaries were exposed to it, and your age. Some women are sterile temporarily. For others, it is a permanent condition. It may be possible to move the ovaries out of the radiation field (this is called oophoropexy) and shield them. Women may be able to have children after this procedure.

INTERNAL RADIATION

What is internal radiation?

The radiation oncologist places a radioactive material, such as iridium, directly into or on the area to be treated. The material can be implanted in tissues or inserted into body cavities, administered orally or intravenously. The materials are absorbed or metabolized by the body. Internal radiation allows the radiation oncologist to give a higher dose of radiation to the area, while not harming most of the normal tissue around it. Because the radiation is concentrated in the tumor, it is possible to expose cancer cells to a higher dose during a shorter period of time than would be possible with conventional radiation sources. Sometimes, this is called a radium implant, interstitial or intracavitary radiation or brachytherapy.

What kinds of materials are used in internal radiation?

Some of the substances include iridium, cesium, gold, cobalt, iodine, phosphorus, radium, radon, strontium, and tantalium. The devices used to contain the radioactive materials come in several different forms, such as wires, ribbons, tubes, capsules or needles. Sometimes a seed gun is used to inject grains or seeds into the area of the tumor. The radiation oncologist chooses the best source according to the site to be treated, the size of the tumor and whether the implant is temporary or permanent.

What is brachytherapy?

The term *brachy* is a Greek word for "short." In radiation, it means that the container of radioactive material is placed on the surface or inside the body near the tumor or a short distance from the affected area. Sometimes the radioactive source is delivered to the tumor through tubes. This is called remote brachytherapy. The term *brachytherapy* is often used to describe any form of internal radiation treatment.

QUESTIONS TO ASK YOUR RADIATION ONCOLOGIST ABOUT INTERNAL RADIATION

- Why is internal radiation being recommended?
- What kind of radioactive material will you be using?
- How will the radioactive material be put in my body?
- Will I need surgery to have radiation implanted?
- Will I need anesthesia? Will it be local or general?

- Will I need to be in the hospital for this procedure? For how long?
- Will I have to stay in bed during this time?
- Will I be able to have visitors? Will there be any restrictions on the visitors?
- Will the implant be permanent or temporary? Will I need anesthesia when the implant is removed?
- Will I be radioactive while the implant is inside me? For how long?
- What side effects should I expect?
- When will it be safe to have intercourse?
- When will I be able to get back to my normal routine?

How is interstitial radiation done?

The radioactive materials are put into small metal tubes, needles or containers and implanted within or near the cancerous tissue. After the required radiation dose has been given, usually in one to six days, the container is generally removed. High-dose brachytherapy allows the radiation to be given in a few moments, with the patient being able to return home the same day.

What is intracavitary radiation?

The radioactive material is placed in a container and put into a cavity of the body, such as your uterus or vagina, as close to the tumor as possible. The implant may be temporary or permanent. Intracavitary radiation is most often used in the treatment of gynecologic cancers.

Is the radioactive material ever swallowed?

Some radioactive material comes in liquid form and may be swallowed or injected into the bloodstream or into a body cavity. When the radioactive substance is injected, it is not sealed in a container.

Will I need to have anesthesia for my internal radiation treatment?

It depends upon which type you have. For most of the implants, you will need to be in a hospital and will get either local or general anesthesia, so that the radiation oncologist can place whatever container is being used into your body.

What is meant by the term *afterloading*?

The container for the radioactive substance is positioned in your body through an operation. The radioactive material is inserted into the container at a later time, after the proper position has been checked by x-ray and you are back in your room. In some institutions, specialized equipment allows for remote afterloading. A catheter may be placed in the body using an endoscope. The radiation is delivered through the catheter, which is connected to the treatment machine. A computer is used to direct the radiation source through the tubing to the area of the cancer. The high-dose-rate sources produce the same effect as do the low-dose-rate sources, but in a shorter period of time. Remote afterloading requires a multidisciplinary team, including radiation oncologists, radiation therapists, physicists, nurses and trained operating room personnel.

Will I need to stay in the hospital if I am having the treatment using afterloading?

It depends on the type of treatment you are having. For some kinds of cancer, you will need to stay in the hospital for a few days. If you are in a center that is using the high-dose remote afterloading technique, you may be able to go home after you have spent an hour or two in the recovery room.

How long is the implant left in the body?

It depends on the kind of cancer, where it is located, the amount of radiation that the radiation oncologist needs to treat you and the type of implant being used. Some implants with a low dose rate may be left in for from one to seven days. Others with a high dose rate may be removed after a few moments.

Are the high-dose implants done in a different way?

Yes. Hollow tubes, called catheters, are placed in or near the tumor. The catheters are connected to the delivery system and the radioactive material is given via catheter for the prescribed period of time. This allows the radiation oncologist to give a high dose of radiation over a short period of time to an exact tumor site within the body.

Are some implants left in permanently?

Yes. There are some implants that are left in permanently. Usually these are put into the body through a hollow needle, hollow tube or seed gun. The implant loses some energy each day. You usually have to take some precautions for a few days after you leave the hospital.

Will the implant spread radiation to others?

It depends on the implant. The radioactive substance in your implant may transmit rays outside your body. Usually if the implant is in a sealed source, such as a needle or a hollow applicator, neither you nor any of your body excretions, such as blood, urine or stool, become radioactive. Items you touch, such as bed linens, also do not become radioactive. However, if your treatment uses radioactive material that is unsealed, your urine and stool may contain some radioactive materials.

Will I get regular hospital care when I have a radioactive implant?

Your hospital care will be a bit different than usual. The nurses and other hospital personnel are limited as to how long they can remain in your room and how close they can come to you and your bed. You might notice that they come into your room more often but for shorter periods of time. Your bed may be close to the window wall. The nurses will probably not come close to the side of your bed, but will talk with you from the foot of the bed or from the doorway. They will probably be wearing film badges to measure the radiation. Housekeeping personnel may be changing your linens less often or only when soiled. Naturally, the restrictions for hospital personnel depend upon what part of your body the implant is in, the kind of radioactive material used, and the dose. Pregnant nurses may not be allowed to take care of you. Most times, you will be assigned to a single room. Although personal contact is limited because of the radiation implant, you should not hesitate to call a nurse if you need one for any reason.

What if I need help?

Your bedside table, call bell and television controls will be put within easy reach so that you can be as self-sufficient as possible. If you need help, you should ask for it. But you will notice that the nurse will work quickly, concentrating on doing what needs to be done in the shortest period of time possible.

Will I be allowed to have visitors?

It depends on what hospital you are in. Most will restrict visitors to persons over 18 years old and persons who are not pregnant. Visitors are usually asked to sit at least six feet from your bed. They will probably have to limit their visits to less than thirty minutes each day.

Will I be alone most of the time?

Yes, you will. Make plans for activities you can do while you are in bed or in the room alone, such as reading, handwork, puzzles, listening to the radio or music, using a portable computer or watching television.

Will I be in pain as a result of my implant?

Most of the time you will not have severe pain. However, you might be uncomfortable, especially if you have an applicator containing the radioactive material. If you have an applicator in the gynecologic area, you may have some low back pain. Depending on the location of your implant, you may have to stay in bed and restrict your movements so that the radiation source will not become dislodged and harm sensitive organs. You may be given sleeping pills or other medication to relax you. If you feel you need medicine for pain, be sure to let your nurse and radiation oncologist know.

Is it dangerous for me to touch the implant while it is in me?

It is important that you do not touch the implant while it is in your body. Although the container is sealed, touching it could cause radiation damage to your skin.

Will I have any side effects from this treatment?

If you have had general anesthesia, you may feel drowsy, weak or nauseated for a short time after your operation. Be sure to tell your nurse if you have any burning, sweating, or other unusual symptoms. Depending on what kind of implant you have had and where it is located in the body, there may be some other side effects.

Will I be able to eat while the radiation implant is in my body?

Yes, you will usually be given a special diet with lots of fluids. The nurses will place the food where you can manage it without having to move your body. If your implant is in the vaginal area, you will be given pills to discourage bowel movements while the applicator is in your body. If you have an implant in the head and neck area you will have difficulty in eating and in talking.

How is the implant removed?

This is usually done right in your room. You will be given some pain medication about half an hour before the radiation oncologist comes in to take out the applicator. Once the implant is removed, you will then be allowed to get out of bed. Usually the nurse will help you move around until you are steady on your feet.

Is internal radiation used alone?

Sometimes internal radiation is used alone. Other times it is used in addition to external beam radiation, either before or after the internal radiation treatment.

COSTS OF RADIATION TREATMENTS

How expensive is radiation treatment?

Radiation treatment, with its complex equipment and sophisticated staff, can be very expensive. The cost will depend on the type, the complexity and the number of treatments that you will have. Although most health insurance policies pay for radiation treatments, you need to talk with the staff of the radiation department to find out how much of the cost will be covered under your specific policy.

What items are included in the cost?

You will probably see costs for a variety of items, such as initial consultation, treatment planning, simulation, dosimetry calculations, physics consultation and weekly treatment fees.

Do Medicare and Medicaid pay for radiation treatments?

Both Medicare and Medicaid cover the major portion of the cost of treatment. For Medicare, if the radiation oncologist is a participating physician (one who has agreed to accept the charges established by Medicare), the physician will be paid 80 percent of the recognized charge. You will pay the other 20 percent. If you have a Medigap insurance policy, it will usually cover the 20 percent copayment. Be sure you are not confused by the "billing balance" that some radiation oncologists who are not participating physicians add to your copayment bill. For instance, if Medicare pays $100 as the "reasonable" charge, a nonparticipating radiation oncologist may charge $120 for the procedure. Medicare would pay the patient or physician $80. If you pay the $20 copayment, $20 will remain as the billing balance. You should be aware that some states have legislated against the practice of this kind of balance billing.

chapter 8

Chemotherapy

> **Most people are afraid of chemotherapy, and especially of its side effects, fearful that the cure is worse than the disease. But not all who have chemotherapy get nauseated or lose their hair. For many, it's a difficult treatment to get through, but most will tell you that it is worth the effort.**

Chemotherapy means the use of drugs to treat cancer. To most people, chemotherapy is frightening because of the side effects that are sometimes caused by the use of the potent drugs needed to disrupt the cancer cells' ability to grow and multiply. Over the past several years, great progress has been made, both in preventing some of chemotherapy's most serious side effects and in lessening and minimizing those that do occur. Chemotherapy treatment also has proven itself to be very effective—more than 50,000 cancer patients are being cured each year with cancer drugs, used alone or combined with other kinds of treatment.

WHAT YOU NEED TO KNOW ABOUT CHEMOTHERAPY

- Your chemotherapy may be given in several ways—in pill, capsule or liquid form, by applying it to the skin, by injecting it into a muscle, in a vein or through an internal or external pump.

- Often a variety of drugs are given. Each drug acts on the cell in its own way and at different times in the cell cycle.
- How fast your cancer cells will be destroyed by the drugs varies with the medication and the type of cancer.
- You will be given your chemotherapy drugs one at a time, in sequence or in combination. Your treatment may be weekly, monthly or even daily. You normally have some rest time between treatments, to give your normal cells a chance to rebuild and regrow.
- Sometimes the treatment lasts for long periods of time—up to one or two years. Some people may be on and off chemotherapy for several years.
- Most people worry about the side effects of chemotherapy treatment. Side effects vary greatly from drug to drug and from person to person. Every person doesn't get every side effect and some people get few, if any at all. If you do have side effects, there is much you and the health care team can do to help lessen and relieve them.
- Chemotherapy is a serious treatment that must be given carefully by experienced medical professionals. Medical oncologists are the physicians who most often prescribe and supervise the treatment. Nurses play a major role in the administration of the drugs and in treating and dealing with side effects.
- There are many clinical trials in the area of chemotherapy. These trials are designed to test new drugs, gauge the addition of growth factors to stimulate your own system for cell regrowth, analyze how well combining chemotherapy with other treatments works or what different combinations of drugs and different schedules are most effective.

QUESTIONS TO ASK YOUR DOCTOR BEFORE YOU HAVE CHEMOTHERAPY

- **What chemotherapy drugs will be used? Why a combination of drugs? What is each drug supposed to do?**
- **Who will be responsible for giving me my treatment?**
- **What are the possible side effects?**
- **What is the treatment schedule? How will the drugs be given to me? How long will it take for each treatment? How many treatments will I get?**
- **What are the possible side effects? What should I do if these side effects occur? Which ones should I report immediately? To whom?**

- May I take other medication at the same time? May I drink alcohol?
- Is there any special nutritional advice I should follow?
- Are there any special precautions I should take while I am on chemotherapy?
- Can I have an immunization shot while I am taking these drugs?
- If I have questions about my chemotherapy who should I ask?
- Can I continue to work during these treatments?
- Will I be able to drive myself to my treatments?
- How much will it cost?
- How much of a risk is involved?
- Will I be having other kinds of treatment in addition to the chemotherapy?
- Are there any alternatives to chemotherapy?
- What if I don't have this treatment at all?

What is chemotherapy?

Chemo means "chemical" and *therapy* means "treatment." Thus, chemotherapy is simply the treatment of cancer using chemicals (drugs).

What does chemotherapy do?

In simple terms, the chemicals destroy the cancer cells, either by interfering with their growth or by preventing them from reproducing. Most times, chemotherapy uses a variety of drugs. They may be given during the same treatment or on different days. The various drugs work in different ways to interrupt the cell life cycle. Some affect the cycle during one or more of its phases of growth but have no effect on the cell during the other phases. Others affect the cell throughout the whole cycle. The idea behind the use of chemotherapy is to slow down the multiplying of cancer cells or to destroy the cancer cells themselves.

When is chemotherapy used?

Chemotherapy is used for many different reasons:

- It can cure some kinds of cancer.
- It can be used to keep cancer from spreading.
- It can be used to achieve long-term remissions in some kinds of cancer.
- It can be used before surgery to reduce a large tumor.

- It can be used after surgery to kill the cells that may have been left behind or are in another part of the body.
- It can be used with radiation therapy, either before, during or after the radiation treatments.

Is chemotherapy ever used alone as a treatment?

Like other treatments for cancer, chemotherapy is sometimes used alone. Many times, however, chemotherapy is used in combination with another kind of treatments—usually surgery or radiation therapy.

What does chemotherapy do that is different from the other kinds of treatments?

Chemotherapy is known as a systemic treatment. This means that it goes through your whole body system, unlike surgery or radiation, which concentrates on one specific part of the body. The drugs used in chemotherapy enter the bloodstream either by being injected directly into it or by being absorbed through the tissues. Therefore, the drugs reach wherever tumor cells may be growing. Chemotherapy is used when there is the possibility that cancer cells may be deposited in a different place from the primary tumor or may be circulating throughout the body via the bloodstream.

What effects does chemotherapy have on cancer?

Chemotherapy can cure some cancers. In some cancers, chemotherapy makes the tumor shrink. When this does not happen, the drugs at least stop the tumor from growing or make it grow more slowly. Sometimes, the drugs stop the growth for a period of time. There are times when chemotherapy is used to relieve pain and other symptoms, which allows the person to live a longer, more comfortable life. There are some types of cancer, however, in which chemotherapy has little or no effect on the growth of the cancer.

What are the different kinds of chemotherapy?

Chemotherapy drugs are classified by their structure and function. They fall mainly into the following classifications:

- **Alkylating agents** are called non-cell-cycle-specific agents because they attack all cells in a tumor whether the cells are resting or dividing—that is, any phase of the cell cycle. They work by stopping or slowing down cell growth.
- **Antimetabolites** are drugs that interfere with the cells' ability to replicate. These drugs are designed to starve cancer cells

by interfering with vital life processes. They fool the cell by introducing the wrong building elements or blocking synthesis of the right ones.

- **Natural products** include plant alkaloids and antibiotics. Plant alkaloids stop cell division at one of its phases. Antibiotics are made from molds like penicillin but are stronger and do not act in the same way as regular antibiotics. Rather, they interfere with cell division and damage more cancer cells than normal cells.

- **Hormones** are naturally occurring substances in the body that stimulate or turn off the growth or activity of specific cells or organs. In cancer treatment, the environment is changed by either adding or removing the hormones, thus antagonizing the growth-stimulating hormones that promote growth of cancer cells in certain tissues.

- **Miscellaneous agents** are those that don't fit into any of the other categories and act against cancer cells in a variety of ways.

How many different kinds of chemotherapy drugs are now in use?

There are about 100 different chemotherapy drugs that are presently in use in the treatment of cancer. Some of them are still under investigation. The National Cancer Institute sponsors an international cooperative chemotherapy program, involving many research laboratories of the federal government, the universities and medical schools, and the pharmaceutical industry. This program encourages scientists of all kinds to search for drugs to cure cancer. Chemotherapy is one of the most heavily studied areas in cancer treatment. Scientists are creating new chemical compounds, studying plant specimens and extracting antibiotics from natural fermentation products and soil samples. At the same time, many of the world's top chemists are searching for ways to improve the activity of known drugs. There is more information on new chemotherapy agents and the clinical trials that test them in Chapter 9, "New Advances and Investigational Trials."

Who prescribes chemotherapy?

We cannot stress strongly enough that chemotherapy should be prescribed by a doctor who has had special training in the use of drugs and drug combinations for the treatment of cancer. This may be a medical oncologist, who is a specialist in internal medicine with special training in the overall care of the cancer patient, or a hematologist, who is a physician who specializes in blood diseases. Some chemotherapeutic drugs may be prescribed by other doctors, but it is important that the doctor have special training in treating cancer patients. Most chemotherapy drugs are too risky to be prescribed by general physicians without special training.

Do nurses play a role in administering the chemotherapy drugs?

Nurses play a major role in the actual administration of the drugs. There are specially trained nurses in most parts of the country, both in doctors' offices and in hospitals and outpatient facilities, who actually give the majority of the chemotherapeutic drugs under the supervision of a doctor. These nurses are well trained in the administration of the drugs and know what side effects to look for and how to cope with them. In most institutions, the nurses must be certified in chemotherapy administration, usually using national standards produced by the Oncology Nursing Society. Most state boards of nursing have enacted rules that require adherence to the national standards.

Why is it important to have specially trained personnel dealing with chemotherapy drugs?

Chemotherapy, and especially combination chemotherapy, in which more than one drug is used, may be dangerous if the person getting it is not closely monitored. In addition, it is a field of medicine that is continuously changing. New forms of treatment may not always reach the doctors who are not specializing in this field. If you are living in a community that does not have a specialist to administer the drugs, you should make sure your doctor seeks a consultation with a cancer center, a medical school or a large medical center for guidance from experts who know the latest drugs in use, the administration technique, how to adjust doses and what the side effects are on normal cells.

Where will I get my chemotherapy?

You may get it in one of several places—in your doctor's office, your hospital's outpatient department, a clinic, a hospital, or even in your home. It depends on the drugs you are being given, their potential side effects, your physical condition and your doctor's preference. For some drugs that have serious side effects, the first doses of the drugs are given in the hospital so that the health care team can monitor your reactions to them and make minor modifications if needed. This usually involves a short-term stay, with the remaining drugs given in another setting. If the drugs need to be given intravenously over a long period of time, you may need to stay in the hospital.

How does the doctor decide on what kind of drug to use?

The doctor takes many things into consideration, such as the type of tumor you have, the extent of its growth, how it is affecting you, and your general condition. Also evaluated are the responses of chemotherapy in similar patients and what kind of drugs are most likely to damage or kill the cancer. However, individual differences among patients and the effects of the anticancer drugs on various kinds of tumors make this an inexact science. The medical oncologist cannot always specifically predict how the drug will affect the tumor of any given patient, although the major side effects of any particular drug can be anticipated.

Does each patient get the same dose of drug?

The doses are most often calculated according to the patient's body surface area (per meter squared) and occasionally by weight (in kilograms). The patient's body surface area is determined by a formula using height and weight. When more than one drug is used in a combination treatment plan, the dose for each drug is usually lower than when the drug is used alone. What the doctor is trying to do for each person is to give the "maximum tolerated dose"—that is, the amount of the drug which will give the greatest anticancer effect with the least amount of damage to normal cells.

Are there any new developments in chemotherapy drugs and the way they are administered?

The following techniques and developments are currently under investigation:

- Attaching a drug to monoclonal antibodies or other structures that will find and kill cancer cells, leaving normal cells alone.
- Using implanted, refillable pumps to deliver anticancer drugs directly to affected organs.
- Isolating cancer cells from a patient's tumor in the laboratory and testing different drugs against those cells before chemotherapy is begun on the patient. It is hoped that this will allow doctors to match drugs more closely with an individual's disease.
- Using biological drugs—that is, those made by the body itself.
- Using more intensive drug treatments, in sequence, for shorter periods of time to make sure that the patient gets full doses of each drug as quickly as possible, and adding

growth factors to help overcome the side effects of the more intense doses.

There is more information on new developments in cancer treatment in Chapter 9, "New Advances and Investigational Trials."

How often will I get the chemotherapy and for how long?

The length of time and how often you will be having treatments depend upon the kind of cancer you have, the drugs being used, how long it takes your body to respond to the drugs and how well you tolerate them. Treatment schedules vary widely. Chemotherapy may be given daily, weekly or monthly. Some drugs are given every four to six weeks, with other drugs given weekly in between. There are also drugs that may be given every day for a short time or drugs that may be taken in pill form once or twice a day over a long period of time. Many times, you are given a rest period in between treatments to allow your body to build healthy new cells and regain strength.

How is chemotherapy given?

Chemotherapy can be given in several ways:

- It can be put on your skin (topical).
- You can swallow it just like any other medicine, either a pill, a capsule or liquid (PO).
- You can have it injected into your vein through a thin needle, usually in your arm or on your hand (intravenous—IV) or into your artery (intra-arterial or IA).
- You can have it injected through a thin needle into a muscle in your arm, buttocks or thigh (intramuscular—IM), beneath the skin (subcutaneous—SQ) or directly into a cancerous area in the skin (intralesionally—IL).
- It can be delivered to specific areas of the body, such as your liver, using a catheter (long thin tube) that is put into a large vein and stays there as long as is needed.

How is topical chemotherapy used?

The drug, usually in a cream base, is applied to the area once or twice a day with cotton swabs or a special applicator. The area will become red and tender, the skin will die and shed, and healthy skin regrows. You need to be careful to apply the drug only to the area affected and to treat the area gently while the treatment is progressing. Topical chemotherapy, using nitrogen mustard and fluorouracil, is one of the treatments used for some skin cancers.

Are there any precautions when taking chemotherapy pills or tablets?

You need to be careful to make sure you are taking the right amount of the drug. Take the amount that has been ordered, nothing more and nothing less. It's a good idea to have a calendar with the doses marked on it and space for you to record taking the drugs. Most of the drugs are taken on an empty stomach with water, although a few need to be taken with food. Discuss with the nurse and doctor what to do if you miss a dose. Also be sure to tell them what other medicines you are taking, including over-the-counter drugs. Don't take any new medications without checking with your doctor and nurse.

Are there any drugs that I can inject myself?

There are some that are injected under the skin, or as the health professionals say, subcutaneously, that you can give yourself at home. The steps are similar to those that diabetics use when giving themselves insulin. If you are to do the injections yourself, the nurse will instruct you.

Does it hurt to get a chemotherapy drug?

If you are taking your drug in a pill, capsule or liquid form or applying it as an ointment, it is no different from taking any other medicine in this manner. If you are getting a drug injected into your muscle, you usually just feel a pinprick, like you would if you were getting an antibiotic shot. If you are taking a drug that needs to be injected into the vein, the process takes longer, but usually does not involve pain. Depending on the drugs being used, it may take anywhere from a few moments to several hours when given intravenously. Some people say they feel a temporary burning sensation in the area of the injection. Others feel warmth throughout the body. Some people say the needle insertion hurts. If you have any pain, burning or discomfort that occurs during or after an IV treatment, be sure you report it to your nurse.

How is the drug injected IV?

IV stands for intravenous. It is the most common method for giving chemotherapy. The drug or drugs will be injected into your vein through a thin needle, usually in your arm or on your hand.

What is meant by central venous access?

The term *central venous access* describes the use of a soft plastic catheter, a flexible tube, in giving chemotherapy drugs. The catheter is placed in one of the larger veins in the body, rather than a hand or arm vein, and remains in place for a long period of time. There are three major types of devices used for central venous access in cancer treatment—peripherally inserted central catheters, central venous tunneled catheters and implanted ports.

What is a peripherally inserted central catheter?

This is a device, usually referred to as a PIC catheter, that can be put into a vein by a specially trained nurse or a doctor, without surgery, can be easily removed and can remain in place for twelve to thirty days, until the treatment is completed. The PIC needs care at the external site and requires flushing.

What is a central venous tunneled catheter?

This catheter is implanted into one of the central veins, tunneled through tissue and comes out at either the chest or abdomen. You need general or local anesthesia when it is put in. This catheter can stay in from months to years. The most commonly used brands are the Hickman catheter, Raaf Cath and Groshong catheter. They require care at the external site and need routine flushing.

What is an implanted port?

An implanted port is a hollow housing, made out of steel, titanium or plastic, that is connected to a catheter that is inserted in a major vein. The port is implanted under the skin surface, most commonly in the chest area, by a surgeon in an operating room. It can remain in place and be used for many years. It does not need care at the external site. Taking it out requires another surgery.

What is meant by continuous infusion?

Continuous infusion is giving chemotherapy over a long period of time, usually taking more than two hours. Usually continuous infusion drugs are given using a central venous tunneled catheter, such as a Hickman catheter or an implanted port.

Can drugs be given directly into the artery to reach the tumor itself?

There are two different ways this can be done. You may have a catheter that attaches to an external pump. You will lie flat while the drugs are infused. Or the doctor can implant a drug delivery system, usually in the stomach area, consisting of a stainless steel chamber and a catheter. The catheter is placed in the artery, then attached to the pump which has been put into a surgically created pocket. This requires major surgery and hospitalization and is usually done only if it is needed for three or more months of treatment.

What is meant by giving a drug by depot?

A depot is a site in the body where a drug may be accumulated, deposited or stored. The drug is distributed into the body from the depot.

How will the doctor decide what method to use?

Some drugs can be given in only one way. For instance, most drugs are given IV (injection into the vein) because they are better able to reach the cancer cells everywhere in the body. If the drug can be given in different ways, the decision will hinge on the necessary dose, preferences of the doctor and the patient, what kind of cancer is being treated and the location of the cancer.

Will it make a difference if I have to miss a treatment?

If you are unable to make a treatment, call the doctor and discuss how you can reschedule it so that it doesn't interfere with the effectiveness of the treatment.

Will I be able to drink wine and cocktails while I am on chemotherapy?

Usually you can drink in moderation with your doctor's permission. That means one or two cocktails daily or wine with your dinner. In some circumstances, however, you may be told not to have alcohol. If your platelet count falls, for example, or if you develop bleeding, your doctor may advise you not to drink alcoholic beverages.

Can I take other pills or drugs during treatment?

There are some medicines that may interfere with how your chemotherapy works in the body. To be safe, you should tell your doctor about any medicine that you are taking, regardless of whether it is prescription or over the counter. Make a list, with the name of the medication, how often you are taking it and the dosage. Bring it with you so the doctor can look at it before you start treatment. If you begin to take new medicine while you are on chemotherapy, be sure to tell the doctor.

What are some of the drugs that can alter how chemotherapy drugs work in the body?

Such drugs include aspirin, antibiotics, anticoagulants, antiseizure pills, barbiturates, blood pressure pills, cough medicine, diabetic pills, hormone pills, sleeping pills and tranquilizers, and diuretics (water pills). It is important that your doctor know what you are taking since whether or not the medications interfere with your treatment depends on what chemotherapy drugs are being given.

Will I be able to have dental work done while on treatment?

You usually will. Again, it depends on the drugs you are taking. Regular cleaning and cavity repairs are usually not a problem. However, be sure to tell your dentist that you are on chemotherapy. If the dentist is going to perform oral surgery, take out a tooth, or give you an injection, tell your doctor so that blood counts can be taken a few days before the dental work is going to be done. If your blood counts are normal, you can have minor dental surgery.

Will I be able to continue working while I am having chemotherapy drugs?

Most people find they are able to continue working while they are being treated. If you wish, you may be able to schedule your treatments so that they cause the least disruption with your work schedule—late in the day or just before the weekend. Some people feel very tired when they are going through treatment and find they need to alter their normal schedules.

How will the doctor know whether or not the drug is working?

There are several ways of measuring how well your treatments are working. You will have physical exams, laboratory tests, scans, x-rays, blood counts and blood chemistry tests. Don't be surprised by the number of tests that will be done while you are having treatments. Some, like the blood counts, will be used by the doctor to help adjust the doses of drugs. Your nurse can explain why the various tests are being done. Do not hesitate to ask your doctor about the results of the tests and what they are showing.

Do chemotherapy drugs ever stop being effective?

Sometimes drugs lose their effectiveness against the particular cancer. Scientists believe that in some cases the cancer cells are multiplying more quickly than the drug can kill them. Other times, the cancer cells undergo change and are able to survive and even grow rapidly in the presence of a drug that previously was effective. When this happens the cells are called ''drug resistant.''

How do cells become drug resistant?

Some cancer cells make genetic changes and learn to produce a large amount of an enzyme that overrides a drug's usefulness and allows the cancer to grow again. In other cases, the cell membrane changes in a way that allows it to block the entry of the drug into the cell or reduces the time the active drug remains in the cell. Scientists are working on ways to overcome drug resistance, including different ways of administering drugs or giving other drugs that may overcome the membrane changes.

What is meant by combination chemotherapy?

When more than one drug is being used for treatment it is called combination chemotherapy. Many times two to five drugs are used in combination in an attempt to kill cells in different phases of their reproductive cycle and to delay or prevent resistance of the tumor to the drugs from occurring. Sometimes, several drugs are given during the same treatment. Sometimes the drugs are given sequentially: first one drug is given for several weeks, followed by the next drug. There are hundreds of different combinations of drugs. Many of them are known by their initials, usually made up of the names of the drugs that will be given. For instance, the combination chemotherapy regimen MOPP, used in lymphoma, stands for **m**echlorethamine, **o**ncovin (vincristine), **p**rocarbazine and **p**rednisone. ABVD, another combination used in lymphoma, stands for **a**driamycin (doxorubicin), **b**leomycin, **v**inblastine and **d**acarbazine.

Why are female hormones used to treat prostate cancer and male hormones used to treat breast cancer?

Cancers that start in tissues such as the breast in women and the prostate gland in men depend on the presence of the hormones for their growth. Scientists feel that treatment with hormones may affect these cancers by changing their normal environment. Thus androgens, male hormones, are sometimes used to treat women with breast cancer. Female hormones, estrogens, are used to help suppress the growth of cancer of the prostate. Other hormones that are used in cancer treatment include corticosteroids, such as cortisone and prednisone, for certain types of leukemia and lymphomas. Doctors also sometimes remove glands that secrete hormones, such as the ovaries or testicles, to help slow down malignant growth.

What androgens are used in cancer treatment?

There are several, including testosterone propionate (Neohombreol, Oraton), fluoxymesteron (Halotestin, Ora-Testryl), nandrolone decanoate (Deca-Durabolin), calusterone (Methosarb), and dromostanolone propionate (Drolban, Masteril, Macleron, Permastril).

MAJOR CHEMOTHERAPY DRUGS AND HORMONES, THEIR USES AND MOST COMMON SIDE EFFECTS

Name and Use	Common Side Effects	Occasional Side Effects
Aminoglutethimide (Cytadren, Elitpen) An aromatase inhibitor used in adrenal and prostate cancers. May be used as medical adrenalectomy in breast cancer. Given as tablet.	Skin rash with fever, sluggishness and tiredness (usually goes away slowly 4 to 6 weeks after treatment is finished).	Dizziness, swelling of face, weight gain, leg cramps, fever, chills and sore throat, loss of appetite, mild nausea and vomiting, leg cramps.
Asparaginase (Colaspase, Elspar) An enzyme used mostly in leukemias. Usually given in muscle.	Nausea and vomiting, and loss of appetite. You may need to drink extra liquids to prevent kidney problems.	Difficulty in breathing, fever, chills and sore throat, joint pain or inability to move arm or leg, puffy face, skin rash or itching, stomach pain, unusual bleeding or bruising; drowsiness, confusion, seizures; or hallucinations, severe headaches, mouth sores, swelling of feet or lower legs, unusual thirst, yellow skin or eyes.
Bleomycin (Blenoxane) An antitumor antibiotic used in squamous cell carcinoma, Hodgkin's disease, sarcomas, melanoma, cancers of the thyroid, testicle, kidney, esophagus and ovary. Given IV, in muscle or under skin.	Darkening or thickening of skin, changes in fingernails or toenails, skin rash, peeling redness or tenderness. Coughing, shortness of breath, or other chronic lung problems.	Fever and chills, nausea, vomiting and loss of appetite, sores in mouth, headache, swelling and pain in joints, unusual taste sensation.

Drug	Description	Side Effects
Buserelin (Buserelin acetate, HOE 766, Suprefact). A luteinizing hormone-releasing hormone (LHRH) analogue used in prostate cancer. Injected under skin or inhaled.	Pain at injection site, hot flashes, impotence and breast enlargement (males), lack of or irregular menstrual periods and spotting, bone pain, difficulty urinating.	Infrequent nausea, vomiting, diarrhea, and constipation; headache, muscle weakness, depression.
Busulfan (Myleran) An alkylating agent used for chronic myelogenous leukemia, polycythemia vera and bone marrow transplant. Given as a pill or, for bone marrow transplant, IV.	Nausea and vomiting, when given at high dose for bone marrow transplant. If you miss a dose, do not double the next dose; talk with your doctor.	Fever, chills or sore throat, unusual bleeding or bruising, darkening of skin, pain in joints, side or stomach, sores in mouth, swelling of feet or lower legs, diarrhea, dizziness, missing period, breast enlargement, impotence, sterility, eye problems.
Carboplatin (Paraplatin, CBDCA, carboplatinum, JM-8, NSC-24120). An alkylating-like agent. Used for cancer of the ovary. May also be used in cancers of the testes, head and neck, cervix and lung. Given IV.	Nausea and vomiting (usually preventable with antinausea medicine), anemia, fever, chills and sore throat.	Skin rash, hair loss, tingling of hands and feet, blood in urine, pain at injection site, hearing loss, eye problems.
Carmustine (BCNU, BiCNU) An alkylating agent used for multiple myeloma, Hodgkin's disease and non-Hodgkin's lymphomas, melanoma, cancers of the brain, colon, rectum, stomach and liver. Given IV.	Nausea and vomiting, hair loss and darkening of skin, redness, burning, pain or swelling where injection is given, lung problems.	Fever, chills, cough and sore throat, unusual bleeding or bruising, shortness of breath and flushing of face, mouth sores, diarrhea, difficulty in swallowing, dizziness, eye problems.

(continued)

MAJOR CHEMOTHERAPY DRUGS AND HORMONES, THEIR USES AND MOST COMMON SIDE EFFECTS *(cont.)*

Name and Use	Common Side Effects	Occasional Side Effects
Chlorambucil (Leukeran) An alkylating agent used in leukemias and lymphomas, multiple myeloma, cancers of the breast, ovary and testicle. Given as a pill.		Nausea and vomiting, diarrhea, loss of appetite, loss of hair, fever, chills or sore throat, mouth sores, seizures, cough, shortness of breath, joint, stomach or side pain, skin rash, changes in period, sterility, itchiness, eye problems, second cancer (leukemia).
Cisplatin (Platinol, Platinol-AQ, platinum, *cis*—platinum) An alkylating agent used in lymphoma, sarcoma, cancers of the testicle, ovary, bladder, brain, adrenal glands, breast, cervix, uterus, endometrium, head and neck, esophagus, lung, skin, prostate, and stomach. Given IV with intravenous fluids.	Nausea and vomiting may last up to 3 days. Loss of appetite, diarrhea. Numbness and tingling in fingers, toes or face. You need to take antinausea medicine for first 24 hours and for following 4 days. You need to drink extra liquids to prevent kidney problems.	Hair loss, dizziness, loss of taste, blurred vision, change in ability to see colors, difficulty in hearing, ringing in ears, sores in mouth, fast heartbeat or wheezing, fever, chills and sore throat, decreased urination, swelling of feet or lower legs, unusual bleeding or bruising.

Drug	Common side effects	Serious/other effects
Cyclophosphamide (Cytoxan, Neosar, Endoxan) An alkylating agent used in lymphomas and Hodgkin's disease, myeloma, neuroblastoma, retinoblastoma, sarcomas, Wilms' tumor, cancers of the ovary, breast, prostate, head and neck, lung, bladder, cervix, stomach and uterus. Given IV or as a pill.	Nausea, vomiting, loss of appetite, loss of hair. You need to drink extra liquids to prevent bladder problems. If you miss a dose, do not double the next dose; talk with your doctor.	Blood in urine, pain when urinating, black tarry stools, fever, chills, nasal stuffiness and sore throat, cough and shortness of breath, dizziness, confusion, fast heartbeat, sterility (may be temporary), skin darkening, metallic taste during injection, blurred vision, cataract, second cancers (leukemia, bladder).
Cyclosporine (Cyclosporin A, CsA, Sandimmune). An immunosuppressant agent used in bone marrow transplant. Given with other drugs to reverse multidrug resistance. Given IV.	Headache, tremor, hypertension, hairiness (women), kidney problems.	Diarrhea, loss of appetite, nausea and vomiting, hiccups, constipation, confusion, depression, facial flushing, shortness of breath, wheezing, enlargement of breasts, hearing loss.
Cytarabine (Ara-C, Cytosar-U, arabinosyl, Tarabine) An antimetabolite used in the leukemias and the lymphomas. Given IV or, less commonly, under the skin.	Nausea and vomiting, diarrhea, anemia.	Mouth sores, loss of appetite, black tarry stools, ulcers, dizziness, headache, lung problems, tiredness, bone, joint or muscle pain, heartburn, irregular heartbeat, fever, chills and sore throat, numbness or tingling in fingers, toes or face, reddened eyes, mouth sores. *(continued)*

MAJOR CHEMOTHERAPY DRUGS AND HORMONES, THEIR USES AND MOST COMMON SIDE EFFECTS *(cont.)*

Name and Use	Common Side Effects	Occasional Side Effects
Dacarbazine (DTIC, DTIC-Dome, imidazole carboxamide) An alkylating agent used in melanoma, Hodgkin's disease, soft-tissue sarcomas, neuroblastoma and islet cell carcinoma. Given IV.	Nausea and vomiting (may be severe but lessens with each additional daily dose), burning pain at injection site.	Fever, chills and sore throat, mouth sores, metallic taste, sensitivity to sun, flushing of face, skin rash, diarrhea, hair loss, confusion, blurred vision.
Dactinomycin (Actinomycin-D, Cosmegen) An antitumor antibiotic used for Wilm's tumor, sarcomas, leukemias, melanoma, cancers of the testicle, uterus, endometrium and ovary. Given IV.	Nausea and vomiting (may happen about one hour after a dose and may last several hours; may get worse as treatment continues), hair loss.	Mouth sores, skin rash, acne, loss of appetite, diarrhea, fever, chills and sore throat, redness, pain or swelling at place of injection, tiredness, anemia, hair loss, black tarry stools, mouth sores, stomach pain, liver problems, darkening of skin, may activate skin reactions from past radiation.
Daunorubicin (Daunomycin, rubidomycin, Cerubidine) An antitumor antibiotic used for acute nonlymphocytic leukemia in adults and acute lymphocytic leukemia in adults and children. Given IV.	Nausea and vomiting (may happen about one hour after a dose and last for several hours), red urine (usually lasts one or two days after each dose), burning pain at injection site, hair loss.	Fever, chills or sore throat, shortness of breath, joint or stomach pain, skin rash or itching, mouth sores, darkening or redness of skin, liver problems.

Drug	Instructions	Side Effects
Doxorubicin (Adriamycin, Rubex, Adriamycin RDF, PFS or MDV) An antitumor antibiotic used in leukemias, lymphomas, Wilm's tumor, neuroblastoma, multiple myelomas, sarcomas, cancers of the breast, ovary, bladder, thyroid, stomach, cervix, endometrium, liver, esophagus, head and neck, pancreas, prostate, testes and lung. Given IV.	Nausea and vomiting, red urine (usually lasts one or two days after each dose), hair loss, loss of appetite, heart problems.	Mouth sores, darkening of soles, palms or nails, may reactivate skin reactions from past radiation, fever, chills and sore throat, diarrhea, eye problems, fast or irregular heartbeat, shortness of breath, pain in joint, side or stomach, burning pain at injection site.
Estramustine (Emcyt) A hormone used in prostate cancer. Given as a capsule.	Nausea and vomiting. Do not take more or less than your doctor ordered or more often than ordered. If you miss a dose, do not double the next dose; talk with your doctor. Do not take within an hour before or two hours after you have had milk, milk formulas or other dairy products.	Diarrhea, shortness of breath, slurred speech, vision changes, breast tenderness or enlargement, skin rashes, fever, chills and sore throat, sudden severe or sudden headaches, sudden loss of coordination, pains in calves of legs.
Etoposide (VP-16, Vepesid, VP-16-213, EPEG, NSC 141540, epipodophyllotoxin) A plant alkaloid used in cancers of the testes, lung, prostate, brain, bladder, stomach, uterus, and breast, lymphoma, leukemia, trophoblastic tumors, and sarcomas. Given as IV or capsule.	Nausea and vomiting (more common when taken as capsule), hair loss, loss of appetite.	Lung problems, fever, chills and sore throat, mouth sores, stomach pain, diarrhea, unpleasant taste in mouth, constipation, local pain at site of injection, sleeplessness, tiredness, headache, eye problems, muscle cramps, second cancer (acute myeloid leukemia). *(continued)*

MAJOR CHEMOTHERAPY DRUGS AND HORMONES, THEIR USES AND MOST COMMON SIDE EFFECTS *(cont.)*

Name and Use	Common Side Effects	Occasional Side Effects
Floxuridine (FUDR, 5-FUDR) An antimetabolite used in gastrointestinal adenocarcinoma metastatic to the liver. Usually given IV into the liver.	Loss of appetite.	Nausea and vomiting, diarrhea, mouth sores, stomach pain and cramps, hair loss or thinning, itching, swelling or soreness of tongue, ulcers, fever, chills and sore throat, scaling or redness of hands or feet.
Fludarabine (Fludarabine phosphate, Fludara, 2-fluoro-ARA, AMP, FAMP, NSC-312887) An antimetabolite used in leukemia, lymphoma, and multiple myeloma. Given as IV.	Fever, chills and sore throat, nosebleeds.	Anemia, nausea and vomiting (can be prevented by antinausea drugs), loss of appetite, constipation, stomach cramps, mild hair loss, sleeplessness, tiredness.
Fluorouracil (Adrucil, 5-FU, 5-Fluorouracil, Efudex) An antimetabolite used in cancers of the stomach, colon, rectum, breast, pancreas, bladder, cervix, endometrium, esophagus, head and neck, liver, lung, ovary and skin. Usually given IV, except for skin, where a cream is used.	Nausea, mouth sores, diarrhea, skin darkening (sensitive to sun).	Mouth, tongue or lip sores, hair loss, skin rash or dryness, vomiting, poor muscle coordination, swelling of palms and soles, nail loss or brittle nails, eye irritation, increase of tears, blurred vision, headache, euphoria.

Fluoxymesterone (Halotestin, Ora-Testryl) An androgen used in breast cancer. Given as a tablet.	Acne, yellowing of eyes and skin, swelling of arms and legs; voice deepening, hoarseness, menopause, and vaginal dryness (in women).	Patchy hair loss, breast swelling (in men).
Flutamide (Eulexin) An antiandrogen used in prostate cancer. Given as a capsule.	Nausea and vomiting, breast enlargement, breast tenderness, impotence. If you cannot swallow capsule, open it and mix the contents with applesauce, pudding or other soft foods. Do not mix in liquid because it does not dissolve well in water.	Anemia, diarrhea, pain.
Goserelin (Zoladex, ZDX, ICI 118,630, NSC-606864) Luteinizing hormone-releasing hormone (LHRH) analogue used in prostate and breast cancer. Given by depot (pellet of drug is injected beneath skin of abdomen, where it is slowly released) or implanted	Hot flashes, impotence, breast enlargement in men; spotting, irregular or lack of menstrual periods, bone pain, retention of urine.	Nausea and vomiting, diarrhea, constipation, discomfort where pellet is implanted, headache.

(continued)

MAJOR CHEMOTHERAPY DRUGS AND HORMONES, THEIR USES AND MOST COMMON SIDE EFFECTS *(cont.)*

Name and Use	Common Side Effects	Occasional Side Effects
Hydroxyurea (Hydrea) An antimetabolite used in leukemia, melanoma, head and neck, prostate, and ovary. Given as a capsule.	Mild nausea, vomiting. Do not take more or less than your doctor ordered or more often than ordered. If you miss a dose, do not double the next dose; talk with your doctor. If you cannot swallow capsule, open it and dissolve the drug in water. Discard the white powder that does not dissolve and is floating on top of the water. You may need to drink extra liquids to prevent kidney problems.	Skin rash and itching, mouth sores, itching, diarrhea or constipation, hair loss, loss of appetite, drowsiness, redness of face.
Ifosfamide (Isophosphamide, Ifex, IFF, NSC-109724) An alkylating agent used in lymphoma, sarcoma, melanoma, leukemia, cancer of ovary, pancreas, testes and lung. Given IV. Mesna (Mesnum, Mesnex, uromitexan, NSC-113891) is given before and after this drug to protect bladder.	Nausea and vomiting (may be prevented by taking antinausea medicine), loss of appetite, bladder infection.	Fever, chills and sore throat, hair loss, constipation, diarrhea, confusion, disorientation, seizures, drowsiness, tiredness, burning pain where drug was injected, stuffy nose, sterility, mouth sores, darkening of skin, skin rash, lung and heart problems, anemia.

Drug		
Leuprolide acetate (Leuprorelin acetate, Lupron, LEUP) A gonadotropin-releasing hormone (GnRH) analogue used in prostate, breast and islet cell cancers and endometriosis. Injected under skin or in muscle; pellets inserted into skin.	Loss of appetite, nausea, constipation, taste change, diarrhea, dry mouth, itchy or dry skin, acne, hair loss or growth, hot flashes, impotence, breast tenderness or enlargement, loss of sexual desire, decrease in size of testicle, irregular or lack of periods, vaginal dryness, decreased bone density.	High blood pressure, swelling of arms and legs, sleeplessness, headache, dizziness, depression, anxiety, blurred vision, tiredness, sluggishness, mood swings, pain at site of tumor.
Lomustine (CCNU, CeeNU) An alkylating agent used in Hodgkin's disease and non-Hodgkin's lymphoma, melanoma, multiple myeloma, cancers of the brain, lung, colon, rectum and kidney. Given as a capsule.	Nausea and vomiting (may happen but usually does not last more than 24 to 48 hours), loss of appetite. You may have need to take two or more different types of capsules to get the right dose. If you take capsule on a empty stomach at bedtime, you may have less stomach upset.	Mouth sores, hair loss, anemia, shortness of breath, tiredness, fever, chills and fever, irregular menstrual periods, darkening of skin, skin rash or itching, awkwardness, confusion, slurred speech, second cancers (leukemia).
Mechlorethamine (Mustargen, nitrogen mustard) An alkylating agent used in Hodgkin's disease, sarcomas, leukemias, cutaneous T-cell lymphoma, bronchogenic carcinoma and brain tumors. Given IV or used topically prepared in an ointment.	Nausea and vomiting (may be severe; usually begins one hour after IV given), irritation of veins, hair loss, burning pain at incision site.	Painful rash and itching, irregular menstrual periods, fever, chills and sore throat, shortness of breath, wheezing, loss of hearing, vein discoloration (where drug administered), ringing in ears, mouth sores, confusion, diarrhea, drowsiness, headache, loss of appetite, metallic taste. *(continued)*

MAJOR CHEMOTHERAPY DRUGS AND HORMONES, THEIR USES AND MOST COMMON SIDE EFFECTS *(cont.)*

Name and Use	Common Side Effects	Occasional Side Effects
Melphalan (Alkeran, Alkeran IV, L-PAM, L-phenylalanine mustard) An alkylating agent used in multiple myeloma, melanoma, cancers of the ovary, breast, thyroid, testes and bone marrow transplants. Given as a pill usually, higher doses IV.	Nausea and vomiting (especially if given IV in larger doses). Do not take more or less than your doctor ordered or more often than ordered. If you miss a dose, do not double the next dose; talk with your doctor.	Mouth sores, diarrhea, skin rash or itching, fever, chills and sore throat, missed menstrual periods, cataracts, second cancers.
Mercaptopurine (Purinethol, 6-MP, 6-Mercaptopurine) An antimetabolite used in leukemia and non-Hodgkin's lymphoma. Given as a tablet. IV is investigational.	Occasional nausea and vomiting. Do not drink alcohol without discussing it with your doctor. You may need to drink extra liquids to prevent kidney problems.	Skin rash and itching, mouth sores, diarrhea, fever, chills or sore throat, joint, side or stomach pain, darkening of skin, headache, yellowing of eyes and skin, anemia.

Methotrexate (Folex, Folex PFS, Mexate, Mexate-AQ, Abitrexate, Rheumatrex) An antimetabolite used in choriocarcinoma, hydatiform mole, multiple myeloma, leukemia, lymphomas, sarcomas, cancers of the breast, head and neck, lung, bladder, brain, cervix, esophagus, kidney, ovary, prostate, stomach and testes. Given IV most commonly, in the muscle, or as a tablet.	Mild nausea and vomiting, diarrhea, mouth sores. Do not take more or less than your doctor ordered or more often than ordered. If you miss a dose, do not double the next dose; talk with your doctor. You may need to drink extra liquids to prevent kidney problems. Do not take aspirin or other medicine for swelling or pain without first checking with your doctor. When very high doses are given, it is followed by the drug leucovorin calcium to counteract life-threatening side effects (called leucovorin rescue).	Loss of appetite, stomach pain, yellowing of eyes or skin, fever, chills and sore throat, cough, shortness of breath, blood in urine or dark urine, hair thinning, headache, dizziness, blurred vision, drowsiness or confusion, joint pain, skin rash, reddening of skin (sensitive to sun), anemia, flank pain, blurred vision, confusion, seizures.
Mitomycin (Mutamycin, mytomycin C) An antitumor antibiotic used for leukemia, cancers of the stomach, pancreas, bladder, breast, cervix, esophagus, gallbladder, head and neck, and lung. Given IV.	Nausea and vomiting, loss of appetite, burning pain at injection site, fever, chills and sore throat.	Hair loss, fatigue and tiredness, diarrhea, mouth sores, blurred vision, blood in urine, numbness or tingling in fingers and toes, purple-colored bands on nails, skin rash, kidney or lung problems. *(continued)*

MAJOR CHEMOTHERAPY DRUGS AND HORMONES, THEIR USES AND MOST COMMON SIDE EFFECTS *(cont.)*

Name and Use	Common Side Effects	Occasional Side Effects
Mitotane (Lysodren, o,p'DDD) An adrenal cytotoxic agent used in adrenal cancer. Given as a tablet.	Nausea and vomiting, loss of appetite, depression, dizziness or vertigo. Do not take more or less than your doctor ordered or more often than ordered. If you miss a dose, take the missed dose as soon as you remember. If it is almost time for the next dose, skip the missed dose, go back to your regular schedule and do not double the next dose; talk with your doctor. Do not stop taking this medicine without first checking with your doctor. You may get dizzy, drowsy or less alert than normal. Make sure you know how you react to this medicine before you drive, use machines or do other jobs that need an alert mind.	Diarrhea, skin rash, tremors, blurred or double vision, skin rash, light-headedness, shortness of breath, wheezing, flushing, muscle twitching, lethargy, drowsiness, headache, hypertension, fever, chills and sore throat, loss of appetite.
Mitoxantrone (Mitoxantrone hydrochloride, Novantrone, DHAD, DHAQ, NSC-301739) An antibiotic used for leukemia, lymphoma, breast and liver cancers. Given IV.	Nausea and vomiting (usually can be prevented with antinausea medicine), mouth sores, hair loss (usually mild), blue-green urine (may last for 24 to 48 hours).	Diarrhea, abdominal pain, skin rash, dry skin, chest pain, problems with breathing, cough, headache, liver problems, blue streaking in or around the vein.

Drug		
Plicamycin (Mitracin, Mithramycin) An antitumor antibiotic used for leukemia and cancer of the testes. Given IV.	Severe nausea and vomiting, diarrhea, loss of appetite, burning pain at injection site.	Bloody or black tarry stools, nosebleed, liver or kidney damage, mouth sores, fever, chills and sore throat, headaches, depression, nervousness, drowsiness, flushing, redness or swelling of face, skin rash or small red spots on skin, anemia.
Procarbazine (Matulane, Ibenzmethyzin, Nutulanar) An alkylating agent used in Hodgkin's disease, non-Hodgkin's lymphoma, multiple myeloma, melanoma, brain and lung cancers. Given as a capsule.	Nausea and vomiting, loss of appetite, constipation. When taken with certain foods and drinks can cause very dangerous reactions. Do not eat foods containing tyramine, such as ripe cheeses (especially cheddar), spicy sausages, chicken livers, pickled herring, foods that are aged or overripe. Do not drink alcohol, including beer and wine. Do not take any other medicine unless prescribed by your doctor, including over-the-counter medicine. You may also be drowsy. Make sure you know how you react to this medicine before you drive, use machines or do other jobs that need an alert mind.	Anemia, diarrhea, weakness, dizziness, trouble sleeping, nightmares, depression, headache, muscle pain or twitching, sweating, visual disturbances, hallucinations, seizures, frequent urination, blood in urine, sterility, breast enlargement, irregular menstrual periods.
Streptozocin (Zanosar) An alkylating agent used in cancer of the pancreas, carcinoid tumors and Hodgkin's disease. Given IV.	Nausea and vomiting (usually occurs within two to four hours after receiving a dose and may be severe), liver and kidney problems, second cancers.	Diarrhea, mild anemia, bone marrow depression, confusion, depression, anxiety, nervousness, shakiness, redness or pain at place of injection, diabetes.

(continued)

MAJOR CHEMOTHERAPY DRUGS AND HORMONES, THEIR USES AND MOST COMMON SIDE EFFECTS *(cont.)*

Name and Use	Common Side Effects	Occasional Side Effects
Tamoxifen (Nolvadex, taxomifen citrate) An antiestrogen used in breast cancer. Given as a tablet.	Hot flashes, vaginal discharge. Do not take more or less than your doctor ordered or more often than ordered. If you miss a dose, do not take the missed dose at all and do not double the next dose; talk with your doctor. You should use birth control measures while you are taking it, but do not take birth control pills since they may change the effects of the tamoxifen. Talk to your doctor right away if you do get pregnant while on the medicine.	Vaginal bleeding, dryness or itching, nausea, and vomiting, loss of appetite, irregular menstrual periods, hot flashes, endometriosis, bone and tumor pain, visual changes, skin rash and itchiness, dizziness, loss of hair, depression, light-headedness, confusion, fluid retention, headache, anemia, swelling of legs, loss of appetite, blood clots, increased risk of uterine cancer.
Taxol (Paclitaxel) A plant alkaloid used in cancer of the ovary, breast and lung. Given IV.	Fever, anemia, hair loss (usually 14 to 21 days after treatment starts, sudden and complete; flushing, shoulder, muscle and joint pain, mouth sores (occur 3 to 7 days after first dose; get better 5 to 7 days after).	Chest, stomach or leg pain, fever, chills or sore throat, burning sensation in feet, loss of feeling in feet, mild nausea and vomiting, diarrhea, fatigue, headache, alterations in taste, pain at injection site.

Teniposide (VM-26, Vumon, PTG, thenylidene-lignan-P, NSC-122819). A plant alkaloid used in lymphoma, leukemia, melanoma, cancers of lung, breast, kidney, ovary, brain, and bladder. Given IV.	Mild hair loss, fever, chills and sore throat.	Nausea and vomiting, loss of appetite, flushing of face, dizziness, mouth sores, loss of muscle coordination, diarrhea, sluggishness, confusion.
Thioguanine (6-Thioguanine, 6-TG, aminopurine-6-thiol-hemihydrate, NSC-752) A antimetabolite used in leukemia. Given as tablet. IV is investigational.	Diarrhea, mouth sores, fever, chills and sore throat, skin rash, unsteady gait.	Nausea and vomiting, jaundice, loss of appetite.
Thiotepa (TESPA, TSPA, Triethylenethiophosphoramide, NSC-6396) An alkylating agent used in lymphoma, cancer of the breast, ovary, bladder, and lung. High dose used with bone marrow transplant. Given IV. May also be given in artery, in muscle or put into specific areas of body.	At high doses: mouth sores, infections, nausea and vomiting, fever, chills and sore throat, hives, skin rash, dry skin.	Headache, allergic reaction, dizziness, burning at injection site, hair loss, stomach pain, bloody urine, frequent urination, weak legs, loss of appetite, diarrhea, impaired fertility, second cancer (leukemia).

(continued)

MAJOR CHEMOTHERAPY DRUGS AND HORMONES, THEIR USES AND MOST COMMON SIDE EFFECTS *(cont.)*

Name and Use	Common Side Effects	Occasional Side Effects
Vinblastine (Velban, Velsar, Alkaban AQ) A plant alkaloid used in Hodgkin's disease, non-Hodgkin's lymphoma, cutaneous T-cell lymphoma, Kaposi's sarcoma, choriocarcinoma, leukemia, melanoma, neuroblastoma, cancer of the testes, breast, kidney, bladder, cervix, head and neck, ovary and lung. Given IV.	Decreased ability to make red and white blood cells and platelets.	Nausea and vomiting, hair loss, mouth sores, loss of reflexes, fever, chills and sore throat, shortness of breath, burning pain, redness or swelling at injection site, severe constipation, skin rash (sensitive to sun) and itching, mental depression, headache, diarrhea, pain in jaw, joints, bones, muscles, back or limbs, pain in testicles, mouth sores, double vision, drooping eyelids.
Vincristine (Oncovin, Vincasar PFS, leurocristine) A plant alkaloid used in leukemia, lymphomas, sarcomas, neuroblastoma, Wilms' tumor, melanoma, multiple myeloma, cancers of the colon, rectum, brain, breast, cervix, ovary, lung and thyroid. Given IV.	Hair loss, numbness or tingling in hands or feet.	Pain in arms, legs, jaw or stomach, pain in testicles, mouth sores, fever, chills and sore throat, severe constipation, metallic taste, hoarseness, agitation, confusion, light-headedness, dizziness, drooping eyelids, jaw or joint pain, blurred or double vision, anemia, stomach cramps.

Note: A listing of other, less common, chemotherapy drugs is found at the end of this chapter.

What estrogens are used in treating cancer?

The estrogens that are used in treating cancer include diethylstil-bestrol (DES), diethystilbestrol diphosphate (Stilphostrol, Stilbestrol diphosphate), chlorotrianisene (TACE), ethinyl estradiol (Estinyl) and conjugated equine estrogen (Premarin).

Are antiandrogens used in treating cancer?

Antiandrogens, used to block the function of the male hormones in the body, are sometimes used in treating prostate cancer. Fluta-mide (Eulexin) is the antiandrogen currently being used.

Is progesterone used in treating cancer?

Progesterone is used in treating cancers of the breast, kidney and endometrium. Some progesterones that are used include medrox-progesterone acetate (Provera, Depo-Provera) and megestrol acetate (Megace, megestrol).

What biological response modifiers are being used in treating cancer patients?

There are several types that are being used, including interferons, interleukins, tumor necrosis factors, and colony stimulating factors. Sometimes these biological response modifiers are combined with chemotherapy. There is more information on the use of these substances in Chapter 9, "New Advances and Investigational Trials."

SIDE EFFECTS

Do all chemotherapy drugs produce some side effects?

The extent of side effects varies greatly from patient to patient and from drug to drug. The side effects range from slight in some people to severe in a few instances. Some drugs have more noticeable side effects than do others. Some people go through their entire chemotherapy treatment without suffering side effects. Others do have serious problems. We have listed the side effects as known for each drug. It is important to remember that no one experiences all of them. Remember too that doctors and nurses can help you minimize many of them. Sometimes your own attitude can play a role in determining how severe your side effects will be. There is some research that shows that techniques such as relaxation can help you experience milder side effects. (See Chapter 24, "Living with Cancer.")

Why do you get side effects from chemotherapy?

Many of the drugs kill the fast-growing cancer cells. They also can harm the normal ones, especially those cells that are growing fast or are not fully developed. Your mouth, stomach and intestines, the roots of your hair (hair follicles) and the bone marrow are areas of the body that normally have fast-growing cells. Thus, they may be affected by the chemotherapy. When they are, side effects may result. To allow the normal tissues to repair themselves, drugs are generally given in cycles, with rest periods in between. Normal cells repair themselves faster than do the cancerous ones.

What are the most common side effects?

The most common side effects of chemotherapy are nausea and vomiting, hair loss, a feeling of tiredness and the decreased ability of the body to make red and white blood cells and platelets (bone marrow suppression).

Are the side effects of all the drugs the same?

Each drug has its own potential side effects. When drugs are combined, the side effects can change. You should talk with your doctor and nurse about what side effects to expect for the kind of chemotherapy drugs you will be getting.

What can be done to minimize side effects?

First of all, great progress is being made in preventing some of the most serious side effects of chemotherapy. Many new drugs and techniques are being used to increase the powerful effects of chemotherapy on the cancer while decreasing its harmful effects on healthy cells in the body. In addition, many things can be done to help minimize or lessen side effects, if you get them. There is, for instance, a wide range of drugs that can help curb nausea and vomiting. Do not hesitate to discuss any side effects with your health care team. If the side effects are severe, your drugs or treatment schedule may need to be changed. There are suggestions on ways of treating side effects in Chapter 24, "Living with Cancer."

How long do the side effects last?

Some of the side effects, such as nausea and vomiting, can occur with each treatment and last for a relatively short time. Others, like tiredness, come on gradually and go away in the same manner.

How long does it take to recover from the side effects of chemotherapy?

The time it takes to get over all the side effects and regain your former energy varies from one person to another, and depends on the kinds of drugs you have been getting as well as on your own physical condition. When your chemotherapy treatments are completed, most normal cells recover quickly and the side effects disappear as the healthy cells have a chance to grow normally.

Do the side effects mean that the drugs are working?

There does not seem to be any relationship between the side effects and what is happening to the tumor. Neither the appearance of side effects nor their absence seems to have any relation to the effectiveness of the drug. One person may have no side effects and yet the drug may be making the tumor shrink greatly. Another person's tumor may also be shrinking with the person experiencing considerable side effects. It depends upon the body's tolerance to the drugs being given and the responsiveness of the cancer cells to them.

Are there any serious side effects I should report to the doctor immediately?

You should promptly report the following symptoms to your doctor:

- Fever over 100°.
- Any kind of bleeding or bruising.
- Development of any rash or allergic reaction, such as swelling of eyelids, hands or feet.
- Shaking chills.
- Marked pain or soreness at the chemotherapy injection site.
- Any pain of unusual intensity or duration, including headaches.
- Shortness of breath or inability to catch your breath.
- Severe diarrhea.
- Bloody urine.

Any other new, unexpected symptoms that arise should be reported promptly to the doctor.

When does nausea and vomiting usually occur?

Nausea and vomiting can begin as early as an hour after the treatment is given or as late as eight to twelve hours later. It may last for just a few hours or as long as three or four days. Some people feel mildly nauseated most of the time. Others become severely nauseated for a limited time after the treatment. Some even begin to feel nauseated before the treatment starts (called anticipatory nausea). Be sure you tell your nurse and doctor if the nausea or vomiting has lasted more than a day or has been so bad you cannot even keep liquids down.

What can be done to help control my nausea and vomiting?

Drugs called antiemetic agents are used to help lessen nausea and vomiting. They are usually given before the chemotherapy treatments begin. Among the drugs that may be prescribed are Compazine, Marinol, Norzine, Reglan, THC, Thorazine, Tigan, Torecan, Valium, or Zofran. They are given IV, orally, intramuscularly or rectally. Many times they are used in combination form.

Can relaxation techniques be used to help relieve my nausea and vomiting?

Studies have found that some people's nausea and vomiting can be helped with methods that are used to cope with stress. There are several methods that you might wish to try, including rhythmic breathing, biofeedback, imagery, visualization and hypnosis. There are additional details about these methods in Chapter 24, "Living with Cancer."

Is marijuana being used to reduce nausea and vomiting?

There has been much interest in the use of marijuana to treat chemotherapy-induced nausea and vomiting in cancer patients. Dronabinol is a synthetic form of the active marijuana constituent THC (delta-9-tetrahydrocannabinol). It is currently available by prescription for use as an antiemetic for mild nausea and vomiting under the trade name Marinol.

Is dronabinol effective?

Scientists at the National Cancer Institute feel that dronabinol is probably not as effective as certain other antiemetics or combinations of antiemetics in controlling nausea and vomiting caused by the initial courses of anticancer drugs. The absorption of dronabinol and its effectiveness vary among patients. However, it may be useful for a limited number of cancer patients.

Is there something I can do about my lack of appetite when I feel nauseated?

It is important for you to eat well—especially a diet high in protein—during your treatment period. Your appetite may be poor, but you need to make sure you are eating a balanced, high-protein diet in order to maintain your strength, to prevent body tissues from breaking down, and to rebuild the normal tissues that have been affected by the drugs. There is additional nutritional help in Chapter 24, "Living with Cancer."

Will I lose my hair?

Not all drugs cause hair loss, but it is a common side effect of many drugs. The rapidly growing cells that make up the hair roots (follicles) are sensitive to chemotherapeutic drugs. If you do have hair loss, it may become thinner or it may fall out altogether.

Will I lose my hair in places other than on my head?

The hair follicles of the beard, mustache, eyelashes, eyebrows, armpits, chest, legs and pubic area are all rapidly growing cells and are sensitive to some of the drugs used in chemotherapy. Sometimes the loss is partial. Many times, while there is a complete loss of scalp hair, hair loss in other body areas is much less common.

Will my hair fall out gradually or all at once?

Hair loss differs from patient to patient and from drug to drug. It may fall out gradually or in clumps. Your scalp may become sensitive, flaky or irritated. Use a soft bristle brush to lessen pulling on the hair. If you have long hair, cut it short before it begins to thin—the weight of long hair may hasten the loss. Avoid using a curling iron or rollers, or teasing your hair. Use a mild or moisturizing shampoo.

What should I do to prepare for losing my hair?

You need to think about what would make you most comfortable—wearing a wig or a hairpiece, a turban, scarf, cap, leaving your head uncovered or a combination of any or all of these alternatives. Try some hats and scarves to see how they might look. You also need to think about ways to conceal lost eyebrows. Some people find that horn-rimmed glasses or other glasses that are fitted with rims coming just in front of the eyebrows can help. You may need to practice using eyebrow pencil and false eyelashes.

Are there any general hints about buying wigs and hairpieces?

- Buy the wig before you start losing your hair. If you can, get the wig before you start having chemotherapy treatments. Get your first wig the same color as your natural hair so you can start wearing it as your hair begins to thin.

- Buy the wig yourself. Bring a friend along for moral support, but don't send someone else to do it for you. It is essential that the wig or hairpiece fits you well, is comfortable to wear, is flattering on you and pleases you. Many people find it useful to buy more than one wig, especially if they need to wear it for more than six months.
- You might want to consider borrowing a wig or hairpiece. Some hospitals and some American Cancer Society offices have wig banks where you can get them free.
- Wigs are tax-deductible medical expenses and may be covered by some medical insurance policies. You need to get a prescription from your doctor.
- A good synthetic wig washes better, is less expensive to maintain, is cooler and costs less than a real-hair wig.

Will my hair grow back the same as it was before?

When your hair begins to regrow it will be thick and soft and sometimes even better than before. It usually begins to grow back once the chemotherapy is stopped. Occasionally, it will begin to regrow while you are still under treatment.

What can cause my urine to change color while I am on chemotherapy?

Some drugs can temporarily change the color of your urine. Some may turn it red, orange, bright yellow or blue-green, or cause it to take on a strong or medicinal odor. Your doctor or nurse can tell you if your drug can cause this side effect. This side effect is temporary.

Why does the doctor tell me to drink more fluids?

Some of the drugs can affect your kidney and bladder. You will be advised to increase the amount of liquids in your diet—water, juice, coffee, tea, soup, soft drinks, broth, ice cream, soup, Popsicles, and gelatin—to ensure good urine flow and help prevent problems.

Are there any signs I should watch for if the drugs I am taking can affect my kidney and bladder?

If you see any of these signs, you need to inform your doctor:

- Pain or burning when you urinate.
- Frequent urination.
- A feeling that you must urinate right away.
- Reddish or bloody urine.
- Fever or chills.

Will the drugs damage my bone marrow?

Many types of chemotherapy, while stopping the growth of the tumor cells, also stop the growth of cells in the bone marrow that is responsible for producing most of your blood cells. Since bone marrow cells duplicate rapidly in order to maintain normal blood counts, these cells are particularly sensitive to the drugs. Among the cells involved are white blood cells that help fight fungal and bacterial infections, red blood cells that help carry oxygen to various parts of the body and platelets that help blood to clot. Three types of drugs usually have this side effect: alkylating agents, antimetabolites and antitumor antibiotics. When your bone marrow is not producing enough red and white blood cells, the condition is referred to as bone marrow depression.

What is a drop in blood count called?

If the drop is in the white blood cell count, it is called leukopenia. In the red blood cells it is called anemia. In the platelets it is called thrombocytopenia. If all of them drop, it is called pancytopenia.

When is my blood count checked?

If you are taking drugs in these categories, your blood count usually will be checked before you are given each chemotherapy treatment. If your counts are slightly low, your treatment may be held up for a few days until your count comes back up again.

What if my blood count is very low?

If your blood count falls very low, you will be carefully followed. A serious drop in white blood count makes you susceptible to infections. A serious drop in your platelet count puts you at risk for bleeding. In some cases, you may need to have a transfusion of blood cells, either red cells or platelets.

What flulike symptoms do some people have?

Some people report that they feel as if they have the flu a few hours to a few days after they have had their chemotherapy—muscle aches, headache, tiredness, nausea, slight fever, chills, sore throat and little or no appetite. Usually, these last for a few days. However, since these symptoms also can be caused by an infection or by the cancer itself, be sure to report them to your doctor.

Will I get tired?

Many people do get tired during treatments. One of the reasons is the lack of red blood cells. This can cause you to feel tired, weak, dizzy, chilled, and sometimes short of breath. The tired feeling usually begins to wear off a few weeks after your treatment ends and will gradually go away. The following also should help:

- Eat well, including plenty of iron-rich foods, such as green leafy vegetables and red meat. Sometimes a small amount of food will give you the extra energy you need.
- Rest when you feel tired. Some people get tired more quickly and need more rest during this time. Try to get more sleep at night. Rest during the day when you feel you need it.
- Don't feel you must keep up your normal schedule of activities if you don't feel like it. Use your leisure time in a restful way.
- Reduce your activities. You may wish to take some time off from work, or work a reduced schedule for a while.
- Don't be afraid to ask others for help. Family, friends and neighbors can help you in shopping, child care, housework or driving.
- To prevent dizziness, get up slowly from a seated or lying position.

What are the side effects of a low platelet count?

Too few platelets can affect the blood cells that help stop bleeding by making your blood clot. You may bruise and bleed more easily than usual, even for a small cut. It is best to avoid situations that might result in an injury—such as contact sports. Be careful when you use sharp tools or knives. Use heavy gloves when you reach in the oven or work in your garden or workshop. Blow your nose gently and avoid forceful sneezing. Use an electric razor for shaving.

Are there any signs I should report to the doctor that signal low platelet counts?

There are several things you need to report to your doctor:

- If you bruise yourself unexpectedly.
- If you see small red spots under your skin.
- If you have pink or reddish urine, or black or bloody bowel movements.
- If you have any bleeding from your gums or nose.

What kind of problems will I have if my white blood count is too low?

A low white blood count makes it difficult for your body to fight infection. Many parts of your body, including your mouth, skin, lungs, urinary tract, rectum and reproductive tract are susceptible to infection. You should take several precautions:

- Try to stay away from crowds and people who have colds, flu or any other disease you can catch, such as the measles or chicken pox. This is particularly important the first ten days after you receive your drugs because your white blood count will automatically drop before it goes back up.
- Clean cuts and scratches with warm water and an antiseptic, and keep them clean until the sore heals. Don't scratch or squeeze sores, such as pimples.
- Be careful not to cut or nick yourself when working with knives and scissors. Don't cut or tear the cuticles of your nails. Use an electric razor when shaving. Protect your hands with gloves when doing heavy work.
- Wash your hands often during the day, especially before you eat and before and after you go to the bathroom. Clean your rectal area gently but thoroughly after each bowel movement.
- Take warm (not hot) showers and baths. Use lotion on your skin to prevent dryness and cracking.
- Do not get immunization shots without first checking with the doctor.
- Inspect your body for signs of infection in your nose, on your lips, in your eyes or in the genital or rectal area. If an infection should develop, tell the doctor about it right away.
- If you get a cold or the flu, call your doctor. Do not take any medicine that has not been prescribed by the doctor, including aspirin, cough medicine, vitamins, antibiotics, painkillers or any other types of medicine.

What are the signs that I might have an infection?

You need to check the following and call the doctor if they occur:

- Fever.
- Chills, cough, sore throat.
- Sweating.
- Loose bowels (may be due to the drugs), burning feeling when you urinate.
- Unusual vaginal discharge or itching.
- Redness or swelling, especially around a sore, pimple or boil.

What can I do about the sore spots inside my mouth?

Some drugs can cause sores in the mouth and throat, make the tissues dry and irritated and cause them to bleed. It is important to take steps to prevent these sores from becoming infected by taking good care of your mouth and teeth. Brush your teeth after each meal, using a soft toothbrush. If your gums are extremely sensitive, use a cotton swab or gauze. Make sure that your toothpaste does not contain abrasives. Or you can use a paste of baking soda and water. Rinse your toothbrush well after each use and store it in a dry place. Do not use a commercial mouthwash that contains a large amount of salt or alcohol. Ask the nurse about using a rinse made out of baking soda or glycerin and water. You might want to use a numbing medication, such as those used for teething babies, to soothe your pain. Ask the doctor to prescribe one that you can use before meals. See Chapter 24, "Living with Cancer," for information on dealing with mouth sores.

Is the metallic taste in my mouth a common side effect?

It is not common but it can happen to some people who are getting chemotherapy drugs. Try sucking on sugar-free hard candy (peppermint seems to work especially well) or rinsing your mouth frequently to mask the taste.

Will chemotherapy affect my teeth?

Certain chemotherapy drugs cause a reduction in saliva in your mouth. Saliva protects your teeth against tooth decay. It is important, if possible, to go to the dentist before you start chemotherapy and to do any dental work that may be needed. You should also ask the dentist to show you the best ways to brush and clean your mouth while you are having treatment. The dentist might prescribe the daily use of a fluoride gel in a small tray that fits over your teeth. Fluoride mouth rinse may also be recommended. It is important to be under the care of a dentist who has experience in treating people undergoing chemotherapy.

Will I experience diarrhea?

Some chemotherapy drugs, the antimetabolites or antitumor antibiotics, affect the cells lining your intestines and may cause you to have soft stools, or diarrhea. If it lasts more than twenty-four hours or if you have pain and cramps along with the loose stools, you need to talk with your nurse or doctor. You should try a diet that is low in roughage (avoid foods such as raw vegetables, bran, beans, fresh fruit) and high in low-fiber foods (such as yogurt, mashed potatoes, chicken, turkey, white rice and noodles). Diarrhea can easily cause you to lose fluids and become dehydrated. Make sure you drink plenty of clear liquids (apple juice, clear broth, water, ginger ale) and that you eat foods that are high in potassium (bananas, oranges, potatoes). You should not take any medicine for your diarrhea without discussing it with your doctor. There is additional information on dealing with diarrhea in Chapter 24, "Living with Cancer."

Will constipation be a problem for me?

It may be, since some of the chemotherapy drugs can cause constipation. In addition, you may be eating differently or be less active than you were before. Try to prevent constipation by drinking lots of fluids (at least eight glasses a day), such as water, juices, or broth. Warm drinks work especially well to help loosen the bowels. Eat fruits and vegetables if your diet allows. A glass of prune juice or a few tablespoons of bran in the morning may help. Keep active with light exercise such as walking. If you do become constipated, discuss it with your doctor or nurse. You may need to take a laxative or a stool softener but only with the approval of your doctor or nurse. There is additional information for dealing with constipation in Chapter 24, "Living with Cancer."

Do people on chemotherapy have problems with retaining fluids?

The drugs themselves, hormonal changes due to the drugs or the cancer itself may cause your body to retain fluids. If you notice any swelling or puffiness in your face, hands, feet or stomach area, tell your doctor or nurse about it. You may need to cut down on the amount of salt you are using in your foods or cut out salt altogether from your diet. In addition, you may need medication to help your body get rid of the excess fluids.

Is the tingling in my fingers a result of my chemotherapy?

It may be, because some chemotherapy drugs affect the cells of the peripheral nervous system. You may feel some numbness, burning, and tingling in your hands and feet. They may feel weak or lethargic. You may have problems with walking, picking up objects, and keeping your balance. Your muscles may feel weak, tired or sore. Sometimes the nerves in other parts of your body are affected and you may feel pain in your jaw or stomach, lose some of your hearing, or become constipated. You should discuss any of these symptoms with your doctor. Many times, these effects are only temporary. However, sometimes they can signal serious problems.

Are skin rashes common during chemotherapy?

You may have some minor skin problems while you are on the drugs, including itching, peeling, dryness, redness, and acne. Most of these are easily taken care of. Use cornstarch like a dusting power to ease the itching. Take quick showers or sponge baths and apply cream and lotion to your moist skin to help prevent dryness. Do not use cologne, perfume or aftershave lotion that contains alcohol. Keeping your face clean and dry and using over-the-counter medicated creams can help your acne. Make sure you tell your nurse and doctor right away if you have sudden itching, a rash or hives, if you begin wheezing or have any trouble breathing.

Do patients sometimes suffer from irritation where the drug is being injected?

This may happen. If it is a rash that is a reaction from the drug, it normally disappears in thirty to ninety minutes. However, it may be caused by the drug leaking out at the site of the injection, which can produce serious, permanent tissue damage. If you feel any burning or pain when you are getting drugs intravenously, report it immediately to the person giving the drugs. Cold compresses and pain medication may be used to help alleviate the discomfort.

Is it unusual for dark circles to form on my fingernails?

Some drugs cause darkening of the beds of your fingernails. This is a harmless side effect and will usually disappear when the drug is stopped. You may also find that your nails become brittle or cracked or develop vertical lines or bands. Try strengthening your nails with the remedies sold for this. Protect them by wearing gloves when washing dishes, gardening or doing other work around the house. If they get worse, be sure to tell your nurse or doctor.

Do veins ever get darker when a person is on chemotherapy drugs?

Some drugs can irritate your veins and some discoloration may develop along the pathway. It may look as if someone has marked it with a felt-tipped pen. The darker your skin, the darker the vein becomes. Exposure to the sun makes the veins look even more prominent. Don't be alarmed. The coloring usually fades on its own a few months after treatment is finished.

Will I be more sensitive to the sun during my treatment?

Some drugs can increase the effects of the sun on your skin. Check with your doctor or nurse. You may need to be careful when going outside, even if you are just taking a walk. Wear a hat and use sunblock lotion. Be extremely careful if you go to the beach, being sure to wear a sunscreen with a protection factor of 15. The doctor may advise that you stay out of the sun or that you use a product to block out the sun's rays entirely.

What is meant by radiation recall?

This is a side effect that you may get if you have had radiation treatments before your chemotherapy. The skin where you had your radiation treatments may get patchy and red—anywhere from light to very bright in color—and you may have an itchy or burning sensation. A few people get blisters or wet, oozing areas of skin that peels. If you have radiation recall, clean the affected skin gently using mild soap and lukewarm water. Use cool, wet compresses to soothe the itching and burning. Tell your doctor or nurse about these reactions.

Are cancer patients on chemotherapy at a higher risk for getting shingles?

Shingles (or herpes zoster) is a painful viral infection of certain nerves that causes a skin rash along the course of the affected nerve. People with lymphoma are more susceptible to shingles. Others who are receiving chemotherapy drugs that suppress the immune system are also at a higher risk.

Is there anyone who can give me help with my hair, makeup and nails while I am undergoing chemotherapy?

There is a nationwide program, called Look Good . . . Feel Better, that has been developed by the Cosmetic, Toiletry, and Fragrance Association in cooperation with the American Cancer Society (ACS) and the National Cosmetology Association. It helps women deal with the changes in their appearances that may result from chemotherapy or radiation treatments or from the illness itself, such as loss of hair, eyebrows and lashes, changes in skin tone and texture or brittleness of nails. Cosmetologists give practical, one-on-one advice on appearance changes, including specific recommendations for skin care, hairstyles, wigs and accessories, eyebrow and eye makeup, and nail care, taking into consideration the changes you may have in your skin and nails. You can learn how to put on scarves and turbans and the different styles of wigs that are available. The American Cancer Society, along with cancer centers and hospitals around the country, runs the program locally, with members of the National Cosmetology Association offering their services on a voluntary basis to help women with cancer learn the beauty techniques. Look Good . . . Feel Better is also looking into developing programs for children and for men. Your local ACS unit, listed in the white pages of the telephone directory, can provide more information about this program. Or you can call 1-800-395-LOOK to find programs located near you.

SEXUAL SIDE EFFECTS

Will being on chemotherapy affect my sexual relations?

Chemotherapy may, but does not always, affect sexual organs and functioning in both men and women. The side effects depend on the drugs that are being used, as well as your age and your general health. In general, men and women on chemotherapy may have less desire for sex than usual. This may be due to the physical effects of the drugs, feeling unattractive due to hair and weight loss, or other side effects. In addition, several drugs used alone may cause infertility and sterility. Combinations of drugs appear to prolong infertility. Drugs that are used to manage side effects of the treatment can also alter your sexual functions.

Female Sexual Side Effects

Are irregular menstrual periods a side effect of chemotherapy?

Some drugs can affect the ovaries, reducing the amount of hormones they produce. Your menstrual cycle may come earlier or later or may last longer than usual. Sometimes it stops temporarily or altogether while you are on chemotherapy.

Will I have hot flashes as a result of this side effect?

You may have the symptoms of menopause—hot flashes, the itching, burning, or dryness of the tissues of your vagina. These symptoms may be much more intense than those that accompany naturally occurring menopause.

What can I do about the vaginal dryness?

You usually can relieve the dryness by using a water-based vaginal lubricant. There are many on the market, such as Astroglide, K-Y Jelly, Lubrin or Condom Mate, Ortho Personal Lubricant, Replens, Surgilube, Today Personal Lubricant. Some are lubricating vaginal suppositories (Lubrin, Condom Mate). Replens is used three times a week to help make intercourse more comfortable and may help prevent yeast infections. Vaseline is **not** recommended because it is greasy, rather than water-based, and can increase the chance of infection. You also should have your doctor check your estrogen level, which gives information on how well your ovaries are functioning and whether the dryness is due to a physical change in your vagina. You may be prescribed estrogen replacement treatment (unless your cancer is hormone dependent).

Am I more at risk for vaginal infections?

The changes in the tissues can make you more likely to get vaginal infections. You should consider wearing cotton underwear and pantyhose with a ventilated cotton lining. Do not wear tight pants or shorts. The doctor may also prescribe a vaginal cream or suppository to reduce the chance of infection. If you have any symptoms of infections—itching, burning or redness—check with your doctor so the problem can be diagnosed and proper treatment begun.

Can I get pregnant while I am on chemotherapy?

It may be possible for you to get pregnant while on chemotherapy, but it is not advisable because some drugs may cause birth defects. Prevention is important because even if your period stops, it is possible for you to conceive. If you are of childbearing age, you need to use birth control throughout the treatment. Once treatment is completed, menstrual periods may return and conception and normal pregnancy may be possible. If you are of childbearing age, it is important to discuss the subject of birth control and childbearing thoroughly with your doctor.

If I am pregnant before I start my chemotherapy, can I still have the baby?

If you are pregnant, it may be possible to put off starting the chemotherapy until after the baby is born. If you need the chemotherapy before then, the doctor will usually wait until after the twelfth week of pregnancy. Sometimes, however, you may need to consider terminating the pregnancy. There is more information on pregnancy and cancer in Chapter 11, "Breast Cancer."

Will a woman become infertile as a result of the treatment?

Sometimes the drug will cause damage to the ovaries that may result in infertility, making a woman unable to become pregnant. This may be a temporary condition or it may be permanent, depending on the type of drug given, the dose used and the woman's age.

Male Sexual Side Effects
What are the effects of chemotherapy on the male sex organs?

Often men who are undergoing chemotherapy have fewer sperm cells. The sperm may also have some abnormalities. These sometimes result in infertility, affecting a man's ability to father a child, either temporarily or permanently. This, of course, does not mean that erection or intercourse is affected. Production of sperm may return to normal when chemotherapy is completed, although in some cases, men have become permanently sterile. Since the effect of chemotherapy on the sperm and unborn child is not really fully known, it is advisable to use birth control during this period.

Can sperm be stored for future use?

For men desiring children, freezing or storing sperm for future use prior to chemotherapy treatments may be an option. This alternative needs to be discussed with the medical team before treatment.

Will I have sexual side effects from hormonal treatment?

Men taking estrogens sometimes get enlarged breasts and decreased sexual desires. Women taking androgens may find that their voices deepen, hair growth increases and sexual desire increases. Women who are menopausal may have bleeding. These changes usually disappear when you stop taking the drugs.

Do people on chemotherapy have personality changes?

This is not a common side effect of most of the drugs. However, chemotherapy brings major changes into a person's life and causes people to feel fearful, anxious, angry or depressed at some times during their treatments. These are perfectly normal feelings that can be dealt with, many times, by talking with friends and family members, by attending support groups made up of people going through the same kind of experiences, or by discussing them with your health care team, your clergy or a social worker.

How expensive is chemotherapy?

The costs vary depending on the drugs being used, how often they are given and in what doses, whether you get them at home, in an office or in a hospital. The cost of the visit, the tests involved and the charge to administer the drug must be added to the cost of the drug itself.

Will my insurance cover chemotherapy?

Most health insurance policies, including Medicare Part B (that helps pay for doctors' bills and many other medical services), cover at least part of the cost of many of the drugs. You need to discuss this subject with the health care team at the place where you are getting your treatment. There is more information on insurance in Chapter 24, "Living with Cancer."

LESS COMMON CHEMOTHERAPY DRUGS

Drug	Use	Side Effects
Altretamine (Hexalen, hexamethylmelamine). Given as capsule.	Ovarian cancer.	Nausea and vomiting (may worsen with continued treatment—taking drug with food at bedtime may help), fever, chills and sore throat, confusion, hallucinations, diarrhea, cramps, bloody urine, skin rash, hair loss, weight loss, loss of feeling in fingers, difficulty walking and moving, depression, second cancers (leukemia).
Amifostine (Ethyol, ethiofos, ethanethiol, WR-2721, gammaphos, NSC-296961). Given IV.	Investigational. Reduces side effects of radiation and alkylating agents.	Nausea and vomiting (may be prevented by taking antinausea medicine), drowsiness, sneezing, muscle and stomach cramps, flushing of face.
Amsacrine (AMSA, *m*-AMSA, acridinylanisidide, NSC-249992). Given IV.	Investigational. Leukemia, lymphoma, melanoma, colon and breast cancer.	Orange urine, nausea and vomiting, fever, chills and sore throat, mouth sores, seizures, headaches, dizziness, heart and liver problems, anemia, pain at injection site, skin rash.
Azacitidine (5-Azacytidine, ladakamycin, NSC-102806). Given IV.	Investigational. Leukemia, melanoma, colon and rectal cancers.	Nausea and vomiting, diarrhea, fever, chills and sore throat, anemia, hair loss, liver damage, drowsiness and sluggishness, confusion, muscle weakness, restlessness, sleeplessness, tiredness, skin rash, mouth sores.
Buthionine sulfoxime (BSO, buthionine sulfoximine, NSC-326231). Given IV	Investigational. Given before alkylating agents to enhance tumor-killing capacity.	Unknown.

(continued)

LESS COMMON CHEMOTHERAPY DRUGS (cont.)

DRUG	USE	SIDE EFFECTS
Chlorodeoxyadenosine (2-Chloro-2-deoxyadenosine, 2-CdA, Leustatin, NSC-105014). Given IV.	Leukemia and cutaneous T-cell lymphoma.	Fever, chills and sore throat, nausea and vomiting, tiredness, mild anemia, skin rash at injection site, headache, weakness when walking or moving.
CPT-11 (Irinotecan, camptothecin-11). Given IV.	Investigational. Leukemia, lymphoma, cancers of the lung, cervix, colon and ovary.	Nausea and vomiting, fever, chills and sore throat, diarrhea (may begin after second and third dose; can be severe and unpredictable), stomach cramps, mouth sores, constipation, hair loss, skin rash, shortness of breath, difficulty or pain in breathing, increased eye tears and saliva.
Dexamethasone (Decadron, Hexadrol, DXM). Given as tablets, ointment, syrup, inhaler, and IV.	Brain cancer, brain metastases, breast cancer, leukemia, myeloma and lymphoma.	Nausea and vomiting, loss of or increased appetite, weight gain, aggravation of peptic ulcers, skin rash or dryness, growth of facial hair, acne, poor wound healing, irregular or lack of menstrual periods, sleeplessness, headache, dizziness, depression, muscle weakness, swelling of arms and legs, cataracts, aggravation of or bringing on of diabetes, back pain, infections.
Dexrazoxane (ADR-529, ICRF-187, Zinecard, NSC-169780). Given as IV.	Investigational. Protective to heart.	Mild nausea and vomiting, loss of appetite, mouth sores, hair loss, tiredness, fever, chills and sore throat, seizures, shortness of breath.
Docetaxcel (Taxotere RP 56976, NSC-628503). Given IV.	Cancer of ovary, breast, lung.	Mouth sores, nausea and vomiting, diarrhea, taste changes, hair loss, skin rash, tiredness.
Edatrexate (10-EDAM, 10-ethyl-10-deaza-aminopterin, NSC-626715). Given as IV	Investigational. Cancers of lung, head and neck.	Mouth sores, diarrhea, nausea and vomiting, skin rash, mild hair loss, tiredness.

Drug	Use	Side Effects
Epirubicin (4'-Epidoxorubicin, 4'-epiadriamycin, NSC-256942). Given as IV.	Investigational. Leukemia, lymphoma, sarcomas, cancers of the breast, ovary, colon, rectum, pancreas, head and neck, and lung.	Hair loss, nausea and vomiting (usually can be prevented with antinausea medicine), red urine, fever, chills and sore throat, tiredness, headache, loss of appetite, darkening of nails and skin creases, redness of skin, redness around site of injection, hives, mouth sores, diarrhea.
Idarubicin (Idamycin, 4-demethoxy-daunorubicin, NSC-256439). Given IV.	Leukemia.	Nausea and vomiting (can be prevented with antinausea medicine), diarrhea, fever, chills and sore throat, red urine, hair loss, heart and liver problems, mouth sores.
PALA (Sparfosate sodium, PALA disodium, phosphonacetyl-L-aspartic acid, NSC-224131). Given IV.	Investigational. Given with 5-FU in treating cancers of the colon, rectum and breast.	Mild nausea and vomiting, diarrhea, mouth sores, anemia, skin rash (chest, face, back and skin creases), may reactivate skin reactions from past radiation, sluggishness, tiredness, sleeplessness, eye problems, fever, chills and sore throat.
Pamidronate (Aredia pamidronate disodium, APD). Given IV.	Used to treat high levels of calcium in blood due to cancer; bone metastases, Paget's disease.	Nausea and vomiting, anemia, stomach pain, loss of appetite, general pain, bone pain, tiredness, fever, chills and sore throat, burning at place drug was injected, sleeplessness, vision problems, heart palpitations.

(continued)

LESS COMMON CHEMOTHERAPY DRUGS *(cont.)*

DRUG	USE	SIDE EFFECTS
Pentostatin (2'-Deoxycoformycin, dCF, Nipent, Covidarabine, VP/vadaribine, NSC-218321). Given IV.	Leukemia, lymphoma.	Infections, fever, chills and sore throat, anemia, skin rash and dry skin, nausea and vomiting, mouth sores, diarrhea, loss of appetite, taste changes, muscle pain, headache, tiredness, sleeplessness, confusion, sluggishness, slurred speech, depression, seizures, coma, cough, shortness of breath.
Pipobroman (Vercyte, NSC-25154). Given as tablet.	Chronic granulocytic leukemia, polycythemi a vera.	Greater risk for infections, bleeding, nausea, vomiting, abdominal cramps, diarrhea, skin rash.
Piroxantrone (Oxantrazole hydrochloride, NSC-349174). Given IV.	Investigational. Being studied in a variety of cancers.	Infections, mild nausea and vomiting, mouth sores, loss of appetite, constipation, diarrhea, hair loss, heart problems, burning at injection site, tiredness.
Prednimustine (Sterecyt, Mostarinia, Leo 1031, NSC-134087). Given as a tablet.	Investigational. Leukemia, non-Hodgkin's lymphoma, cancers of ovary, breast and prostate.	Greater risk for infection, bleeding, mild nausea and vomiting, diarrhea, confusion, light-headedness, fever, swelling, hives.
Suramin (Antrypol, Bayer 205, Germanin, Moranyl, Naganol, Fourneau 309, NSC-34936). Given IV.	Investigational. Being studied in prostate and other cancers.	Nausea, vomiting, salty or metallic taste in mouth, anemia, constipation, skin rash, blood in urine, weakness in muscles of face, eye problems (increased tears, blurred vision), fever, chills and sore throat.
Taxotere (Docetaxel RP 56976, NSC-122819). Given by IV.	Investigational. Cancer of the ovary, breast, lung.	Mouth sores, nausea and vomiting, diarrhea, taste changes, hair loss, skin rash, tiredness.

Drug	Use	Side Effects
Topotecan (Hycamptamine, NSC-609699). Given IV.	Investigational. Being studied in a variety of cancers.	Anemia, greater risk for infections, nausea and vomiting, diarrhea, hair loss, headache, dizziness, light-headedness, fever, chills and sore throat, weight loss, general tiredness, blood in urine, loss of appetite, constipation, stomach pain, mouth sores, skin rash, dry skin, acne, fever blisters.
Toremifene (FC-1157a, toremifene citrate, toremifenum). Given as a tablet.	Investigational. Being studied in breast and a variety of other cancers.	Nausea and vomiting, stomach pain, loss of or increased appetite, diarrhea, constipation, dry eyes, cataracts, dizziness, vertigo, tiredness, lack of energy, headache, sleeplessness, hot flashes, sweating, vaginal discharge or bleeding.
Tretinoin (all *trans*-retinoic acid, tRNA, NSC-122758). Given as a capsule.	Leukemia.	Bleeding, anemia, headache, high fever, difficulty breathing, eye problems (dryness, blurred vision, night blindness), dry skin, skin rash and peeling, thinning of hair, loss of appetite, nausea and vomiting, tiredness, lack of energy, bone and muscle pain, stuffy nose, abnormalities in fetus.

(continued)

LESS COMMON CHEMOTHERAPY DRUGS (cont.)

Drug	Use	Side Effects
Trimetrexate (TMQ, TMTX, NSC-352122). Given IV.	Investigational. Lung and head and neck cancer.	Fever, shaking chills and sore throat, lack of energy, anemia, mouth sores, skin rash, partial hair loss, nausea and vomiting, loss of appetite, diarrhea, may reactivate skin reactions from past radiation.
Uracil Mustard (Uramustine, NSC-34462). Given as tablet.	Leukemias, lymphomas, and cancer of ovary.	Greater risk for infection, bleeding, anemia, nausea, vomiting, lack of appetite, diarrhea, loss of hair, skin rash, nervousness, irritability, depression, confusion, lack of menstrual periods. If you are sensitive to aspirin, may develop reactions, including bronchial asthma.
Vinorelbine (Navelbine, vinorelbine tartrate, 5'noranhydro-vinblastine, NVB). Given IV or as a capsule.	Investigational. Breast and lung cancer.	Anemia, greater risk for infection, mild nausea and vomiting with IV, severe with capsule; hair loss, chest pain, difficulty breathing, tenderness over length of vein where drug injected, tiredness, constipation, pain in jaw or tumor.

chapter 9

New Advances and Investigational Trials

Many new, exciting ideas are being tried in the cancer field. They span a whole variety of scientific advances—new substances that might prevent cancer, new methods for seeking out cancerous cells for diagnosis, new treatments and new ways of using old treatments, and genetic markers that help identify risk. Clinical trials continue to be the link between research and progress. Before you have any treatment, it is useful to check to see if there is a clinical trial for your type and stage of disease. If you are interested in joining a clinical trial, talk with your doctor, or call the Cancer Information Service and ask specifically for information on clinical trials.

Many of the most promising breakthroughs are happening in the field of molecular medicine—a science whose name was hardly in any vocabulary a few years ago. Views from this window of molecular research have dramatically changed the ways scientists think about diseases. Some of the terminology is unfamiliar. Some of the techniques are complicated and hard to understand. But this is where all the exciting new research is happening. This is where brilliant scientific minds are using high-tech instruments to find the future treatments and cures.

WHAT YOU NEED TO KNOW ABOUT NEW ADVANCES AND INVESTIGATIONAL TRIALS

- The most exciting advances are taking place in the new and growing area of molecular science that is transforming the theory and practice of medicine. You may already have heard about new specialists called molecular biologists and epidemiologists, molecular oncologists, and molecular geneticists.
- One of the newest developments involves using biological substances to trigger the body's own defense against cancer. Scientists are finding hundreds of substances that boost, direct, or restore many of the normal defenses in the body. You will hear many different descriptions, such as colony stimulating factors, tumor necrosis factor, interleukins, interferons, cytokines, and gene therapy.
- Genes responsible for illnesses, even those that have complicated genetic patterns, are being found at a dizzying rate, transforming the way that cancer is detected and diagnosed and also predicting who is at risk for developing certain cancers. These genetic tendencies are opening a new, exciting field of exploration. However, they also present many difficult decisions for families in the future.
- Tests, using molecular biology, are making the study of the disease a new art. A wide range of sophisticated molecular tools—from electron microscopes to flow cytometry (using laser instruments to analyze cells)—allows scientists to study normal and abnormal cells.
- Pathologists can be more precise and more sensitive in answering the questions of whether the tumor is malignant, how far it has spread and how much the tumor has shrunk.
- Some tests, using advanced biochemical techniques, can look for genetic changes and molecular markers that characterize particular tumor cells.
- New treatments, involving surgery, treatments with radiation, drugs, hormones, or biological agents, often used in combination with molecular approaches and computerized delivery systems, are being tested in clinical trials.
- As in the past, the clinical trial remains the critical link be-

tween researchers with microscopes and test tubes and the transfer of new techniques to patients. Each clinical trial is designed to answer a set of research questions. You need to fit into the guidelines for a trial—usually a certain type and stage of cancer and certain health status—to be eligible to take part.

- The basis for the new treatment is often the standard treatment—that is, the state-of-the-art treatment now being used. Most new treatments are designed on the basis of what has worked in the past and how it can be improved upon.

- More than fifty prevention trials are under way, scientifically studying how various substances, such as vitamins, minerals, hormones or drugs prevent cancer from ever starting or stop or reverse its development.

- Some 15,000 people each year are choosing to undergo bone marrow procedures, such as peripheral stem cell or bone marrow support, to allow the use of high-dose chemotherapy or radiation therapy treatments for their cancers. These investigational treatments sometimes use the patient's own marrow or stem cells. Other times donor marrow is the best option.

- Gene therapy could redefine the practice of medicine in the next century. It may well turn out to be a main tool to be used in treating many illnesses like cancer, as well as the more than 4,000 known genetic disorders.

PARTICIPATING IN A TREATMENT CLINICAL TRIAL

New cancer treatments, be they biologic therapy, gene therapy or new combinations of chemotherapy, radiation and surgery, start in the basic research laboratories with careful studies in test tubes and on animals. This research points out the new methods most likely to succeed, and how they can be used safely and effectively. If the investigational treatment shows promise of being better than the standard one, it is tested in a patient study, called a clinical trial. The trial helps find out if a promising new treatment is safe and effective for patients. During a trial more and more information is gained about a new treatment, its risks and how well it may or may not work. Most investigational (or experimental) drugs or agents being used are available only through doctors and scientists working closely with the National Cancer Institute or pharmaceutical companies, under strict U.S. Food and Drug Administration regulations. These regulations govern the use of investigational agents. If your physician is using a Phase II drug, for instance, it means it has already gone through extensive evaluation to determine its safe dosage.

QUESTIONS TO ASK BEFORE PARTICIPATING IN A TREATMENT CLINICAL TRIAL

- What is the purpose of the clinical trial?
- What are the possible benefits?
- Who is sponsoring it? (NCI? A major cancer center? A pharmaceutical firm?)
- Why do the doctors who designed the study believe that the treatment being studied may be better than the one now being used?
- Why may it not be any better than the standard treatment?
- Who will be giving the treatment?
- How long will I be in the study?
- What kinds of tests are involved? Are they in addition to the tests that would normally be done? Will I have to pay for them?
- What will the treatment consist of? How does it differ from the standard treatment?
- Will I be hospitalized?
- What are the possible side effects or risks of the new treatment? How do they compare with the standard treatment?
- What are my other choices?
- How does the treatment I would receive in this study compare with the other choices in terms of possible outcomes, side effects, time involved, cost to me and quality of life?
- What will happen in my case if I don't have this treatment?
- What will happen in my case if I do have it?
- How could the study affect my daily life?
- Can I stop my participation at any time? What happens if I do?
- Will I have to pay for the treatment? Does the study provide any of it free of charge?
- Will my overall charges be more than if I received standard treatment? Will insurance routinely pay for them? How often have you been successful in getting all costs reimbursed by insurance for this treatment?

- Does the study include long-term follow-up care? How often will that be and what will it consist of?

What does the word *protocol* mean?

Protocol is the term used to describe the treatment program. It is the outline or plan for use of an investigational procedure or treatment. A protocol gives the rationale for the study, and its goals. If drugs or radiation are involved, it describes the type, method of administration, dose and duration. In addition, the protocol gives the criteria for participation.

What does the term *randomization* mean?

Randomization refers to the manner of choosing people who have similar traits, such as type and extent of disease, by chance (randomly) to be placed into groups that are comparing different treatments. The groups are considered comparable. Results of the different treatment used in different groups can be compared, because irrelevant factors or preferences do not influence the distribution of people. Neither the doctor nor the persons receiving the treatment can choose the group to which they are assigned. Randomization is important because bias can alter the results of the trial.

What is meant by an experimental drug?

The words *investigational* and *experimental* are used when the new anticancer drugs are in the research stages. There are stringent guidelines that govern drug development. The Food and Drug Administration (FDA) is the agency that regulates the introduction and clinical testing of the new drugs. While the National Cancer Institute, along with drug companies, may be involved in conducting the tests, they are not regulatory agencies. The regulations governing the introduction and clinical testing of new drugs have been established and are administered by the FDA. These regulations require that certain standards of safety and effectiveness be met and that a carefully planned clinical study be undertaken.

Why should I consider participating in a cancer treatment clinical trial?

There are many reasons for participating:

- The studies offer the most sophisticated, up-to-date, high-quality cancer care available as a new treatment is tested.
- You will be carefully monitored throughout the trial.

- There are safeguards built into the trial to protect you. For example, a special review board looks at the study to see that it is well designed and that potential risks to patients are reasonable in relation to the potential benefits.
- You usually have more tests and will be monitored more frequently.
- Exploring all the options for treatment helps you feel more in control and more a part of a vital decision affecting your life.
- If a new treatment is successful, you would be the first to benefit.
- You are actively trying to help yourself and future cancer patients.

What are the disadvantages in my being treated through a clinical trial?

You need to think carefully about the downside to make sure you are making the right decision.

- Being part of a clinical trial means you may not receive the new treatment. Some people will be in the group that receives standard care for comparison to the new approach. You will be randomly assigned to receive the new or the standard treatment. You need to remember that the standard care means the best treatment generally available. However, some people are uncomfortable with the fact that they may not receive the new treatment.
- The new treatment may not be more effective than the standard one. It may produce the same results. Occasionally it may have results that are not as good as the standard one.
- You may have some side effects or some risks from the new treatment that have not been anticipated.
- The additional tests and monitoring may not be covered by your insurance.
- Some treatments may not be covered by your insurance. You need to be sure to discuss costs because they vary from study to study. What is covered by whom also varies.

What might disqualify me from participating in a clinical treatment trial?

Each study enrolls patients with certain types and stages of cancer and certain health conditions. There may not be a trial that is being done currently for your type and stage of cancer. You may not be eligible for the particular phase of the trial that is being conducted. You may have had previous treatment or a medical condition that precludes you from participating. The trial may not be done in your part of the country. You may be eligible for different phases of trials depending on your general condition and the type and stage of your cancer.

What are the different phases of clinical trials?

Clinical trials are carried out in three phases, each designed to find out certain information. Each new phase of a clinical trial depends on and builds on the information from an earlier phase.

- **Phase I** studies search for the best way to give a new treatment and how much of it can be given safely. The research treatment has been well tested in laboratory and animal studies but it is not known how patients will react to it. Harmful side effects are carefully watched. Since there may be significant risks, Phase I studies are offered only to patients whose cancer has spread and who would not be helped by standard treatments. The treatments may produce some effects and may help some people.
- **Phase II** studies determine the effect of a research treatment on various types of cancer.
- **Phase III** studies compare the new treatment with standard treatment to see which is more effective. Often researchers use standard treatment as the base to design the new treatment.

How am I protected if I participate in a clinical trial?

Any well-run clinical trial is carefully reviewed for medical ethics, patient safety and scientific merit by the research institution. In addition, most clinical research is federally regulated or federally funded (at least in part), with built-in safeguards to protect patients. (One can manufacture a drug and use it within the same state without federal regulation or manufacture and give the drug outside the U.S.) Your safeguards include regular review of the protocol (the study plan) and review of the progress of each study by researchers at other places. Federally supported or federally funded and federally regulated clinical trials (and in most major medical centers, all clinical trials) must first be approved by an Institutional Review Board located at the institution where the study is to take place. This board is designed to protect patients and is made up of scientists, doctors, clergy and other people from the local community. It reviews each study to see that it is well designed with safeguards for patients and that the risks are reasonable in relation to the potential benefits. The federally supported or regulated studies also go through reviews by a government agency, such as the National Cancer Institute, which sponsors and monitors many trials around the country.

Is the quality of life ever measured in treatment clinical trials?

There are several trials that have added measurements of quality of life issues, such as depression, self-esteem, social support, and religious involvement, to the trial. Most of the quality of life research is being conducted by nurses, either within the clinical trial itself or in separate studies. Questions that are being answered include: Must the patient make significant lifestyle changes because of the treatment? Is the patient anxious or depressed? Is the patient able to maintain relationships with family and friends?

What is informed consent?

Informed consent, which is required in federally conducted, funded or regulated studies as well as by many state laws, is the formal process by which you learn about and understand the purpose and aspects of a clinical trial and then agree to participate. The nature of the trial is explained by the doctors and nurses who are involved in it. You need to make sure you understand what is involved in participating in your specific trial. You will be given an informed consent form that defines the potential benefits and risks. Read it and consider it carefully. Ask any questions you may have. Then, if you agree to take part, you can sign the form. Of course, you can also refuse.

Can I leave a trial at any time?

Signing a consent form does not bind you to the study. You can still choose to leave the study at any time. Your rights as an individual do not change because you are a patient in a clinical trial. You may choose to take part or not, and you can always change your mind later, even after you enter a trial. You may also refuse to take part in any aspect of the research. If you have any questions, be sure to ask your doctors. If you are not satisfied with the answers, you may consider leaving the study. If you decide to leave, it will not be held against you. You can freely discuss possible other care and treatments with your health care team.

How can I find out about the clinical treatment trials being done in my kind of cancer?

There are many ways to find out your treatment choices. Talk with your doctors. Get a second opinion from other cancer specialists. Go to or call a comprehensive cancer center if there is one in your area. Call the Cancer Information Service (1-800-4-CANCER) and ask the information specialists the questions you have about the treatment being offered. Request a PDQ search for clinical trials that pertain to your type and stage of cancer.

What is a PDQ?

PDQ is a helpful data-based treatment information system supported by the National Cancer Institute. PDQ offers state-of-the-art treatment statements, compiled and updated monthly by panels of the country's leading cancer specialists, giving the range of effective treatment options that represent the best available therapy for a specific type or stage of cancer. PDQ also gives the latest information on clinical treatment trials being offered around the country for each type and stage of cancer. It is a ready reference, with over 1,000 active trials, that is updated monthly by a review board composed of cancer specialists.

What do I need to know in order to have a PDQ search of clinical trials for my kind of cancer?

If you call the Cancer Information Service and request a PDQ search, you will be asked a series of questions to determine the information needed to complete the search for you:

- Whether or not you are currently receiving treatment. If you are already being treated, a search of potential clinical trials is not appropriate.
- Whether you are interested in participating in a clinical trial.
- Whether you are able or willing to travel to a participating center and how far you are willing to travel for treatment.
- The primary site of your cancer, the stage, and if possible cell type and grade; for breast cancer patients, hormonal and menopausal status.
- The site of metastases, if any.
- What previous treatments you have had, type of treatment, when and where, including names of drugs previously received and when.
- Major medical conditions that might preclude participation.

Can I be treated at the Clinical Center at the National Institutes of Health?

The National Institutes of Health, the federal government's agency for medical research, has a medical research center and hospital—the Warren Grant Magnuson Clinical Center located in Bethesda, Maryland, just outside of Washington, D.C. The hospital portion of the Clinical Center, with room for 540 patients, is especially designed for medical research. The number of beds available for a particular project and the length of the waiting list of qualified patients are important in determining whether and when you can be admitted. Research on a particular disease may allow only one or two patients to be studied at any given time.

How are patients selected for treatment at the Clinical Center?

You can be treated at the Clinical Center only if your case fits into a research project. Each project is designed to answer scientific questions and has specific medical eligibility requirements. For this reason you must be referred by your own doctor, who can supply the Clinical Center with the needed medical information, such as your diagnosis and details of your medical history. If your doctor feels that you might benefit by participating in a cancer research study at NIH, the doctor should call the National Cancer Institute's public inquiries office at 301-496-5593 or write to the Clinical Director, National Cancer Institute, Building 10, Room 12N214, Bethesda, MD 20892.

How will I know if I have been accepted as a patient at the Clinical Center?

If the scientists at the Center determine you are eligible, your doctor will be notified. Occasionally it may be necessary for you to be seen at the Clinical Center for a preliminary interview and study of your case. The Clinical Center provides nursing and medical care without charge for patients who are being studied in clinical research programs. However, the Center generally cannot pay transportation costs.

What is the Office of Alternative Medicine at the National Institutes of Health?

This office was established in 1992, to find practical treatments that may be of use to physicians—even if the way those treatments work is not understood for years. It has begun to fund research in areas such as acupuncture, biofeedback, hypnosis, music therapy, massage therapy, yoga and prayer, as they relate to many different diseases including cancer. It is giving an opportunity to demonstrate scientific validity to those who are practicing alternative medicine.

BONE MARROW TRANSPLANTS AND PERIPHERAL STEM CELL SUPPORT

People throughout the world—some 15,000 people each year—are choosing to undergo bone marrow procedures, such as peripheral stem cell or bone marrow support, to allow the use of high-dose chemotherapy or radiation therapy treatments for their cancers. Sometimes the patient's own marrow or stem cells are used. Other times donor marrow is the best option. Using peripheral stem cells instead of bone marrow is making the process easier and sometimes less costly.

WHAT YOU NEED TO KNOW ABOUT BONE MARROW TRANSPLANTS AND PERIPHERAL STEM CELL SUPPORT

- Bone marrow transplants date back to the mid 1950s. They were developed as a potential therapy for fatal blood diseases such as leukemia and aplastic anemia. Healthy bone marrow from a donor, usually a family member (called an allogeneic transplant), is transplanted into a patient whose diseased cells have been wiped out by radiation and chemotherapy.
- Bone marrow is the soft, spongelike material that is found in the cavities of your bones. The chief function of bone marrow is to produce the three types of cells found in the blood—red blood cells, white blood cells and platelets. Chemotherapy and radiation therapy, when given at very high doses, destroy the bone marrow and the body's ability to produce new blood cells.
- Autologous transplants, using the patient's own bone marrow, became possible in the 1970s, when the technique of freezing the marrow while the patient was given radiation and chemotherapy, thawing it and returning it to the patient was perfected.
- In the early 1990s, it became possible to replace blood cells by using a special type of cell that circulates in the blood vessels, called a peripheral stem cell. Peripheral stem cells, taken from the patient's own blood, began to be used to support patients undergoing high-dose chemotherapy, mak-

ing the process simpler and less expensive. Unlike bone marrow, which requires the patient to undergo general anesthesia to remove it, peripheral stem cells are easier to get. The process is similar to donating blood.

- Today, bone marrow and peripheral stem cell support are used to regenerate the bone marrow so that it can begin dividing and producing blood cells after high-dose treatments are given for treatment of cancers such as Hodgkin's disease, non-Hodgkin's lymphoma and high-risk breast cancer. Sometimes there is a concern that cancerous cells may be in the bone marrow that is removed. Procedures have been developed to kill remaining cancer cells.

- Since bone marrow and stem cell support are investigational treatments in some diseases, it is important to have these procedures done in major medical centers, where you can participate in a clinical trial. There are many hospitals performing bone marrow transplants and peripheral stem cell support. It is essential that you ask how many of the procedures have been done in the institution where you are planning to have your transplant and how many have been done for your kind of cancer. The American Society of Clinical Oncologists has established minimum standards for bone marrow transplant programs that include a requirement that the facility conduct at least ten transplants a year.

- A specially trained support team, including nurses, pharmacists, social workers and other support staff, is also needed for bone marrow transplants. This team must be able to recognize and resolve complications that might arise.

QUESTIONS TO ASK YOUR DOCTOR ABOUT BONE MARROW TRANSPLANTS AND PERIPHERAL STEM CELL SUPPORT

- Am I a candidate for peripheral stem cell support or for bone marrow transplantation?
- What kind of bone marrow transplant will you do? Will you be using donated marrow?
- Is this the best treatment for my condition? Why?
- Is this treatment part of a clinical trial? If not, why not?
- How many of these procedures have been done in this hospital? How many for my kind of cancer? What was the success rate?
- Can you put me in touch with other people who have had this procedure?
- What are the risks and possible side effects? Can I die from the procedure?

- With my condition, what are my chances of being cured?
- If you will be using donated marrow, what are the chances that the donated material will not grow in me?
- If this procedure is done, will I need other treatment?
- What is the cost of the treatment and how does it compare with the cost of other possible therapy?
- Will my insurance pay for this treatment? Can you help me with dealing with my insurance company? Is there any other financial help available? Will I need to make a payment before this treatment can be started?
- How long will I have to stay in the hospital? Can any of it be done on an outpatient basis?
- Will I have to be treated far from home?
- What kind of support team is available? Do you have a support group for patients?
- Can friends and family visit me in the hospital? If so, are there special places for my family to stay while I'm in the hospital?
- How long will I be treated as an outpatient?
- How long will I be out of work?
- What changes in my normal activities will be required?
- How soon after the transplant will I be able to resume normal activity?
- What kind of complications may occur?
- After the transplant, how often will I need medical checkups?

Why is peripheral stem cell or bone marrow support being used in cancer treatment?

Although neither of these procedures is considered treatment itself, both are being done to allow you to receive very high doses of radiation or chemotherapy. The treatment doses that are given are so high that they severely damage the bone marrow or might even destroy it. The damaged marrow needs to be replaced with healthy marrow to allow you to produce new cells so you have the ability to fight off infections, to clot blood and to transport oxygen.

What kind of hospital should I go to if I am going to have a bone marrow transplant or peripheral stem cell support?

You must be sure that you are being treated at a major medical center that specializes in the kind of bone marrow transplant you will be having for your specific kind of cancer or that has done stem cell support for your kind of cancer. The doctor should be experienced in this specialized treatment, supported by a trained team. You will need to be at a center that has access to the blood products that may be needed if you have complications. Moreover, since for most cancers these are investigational treatments, it is important that you be at an institution that is carrying out clinical trials. The number of treatment centers that perform these procedures has grown considerably in recent years, but it is important to ask enough questions to make sure you are making the right choice.

TYPES OF TRANSPLANTS	
TYPE	**DESCRIPTION**
Peripheral stem cell support Uses your own stem cells, whose growth is stimulated by growth factors	Least complex of three procedures. Shorter hospital stay; some institutions beginning to perform on outpatient basis. Less risky than other two procedures. Less expensive than other two procedures.
Autologous bone marrow transplant Uses your own marrow	Complex procedure. Risky procedure with many complications but fewer than allogeneic transplant. Hospital stay approximately one month. Less expensive than allogeneic transplant.
Allogeneic bone marrow transplant Uses bone marrow from another person—brother, sister, parent, or an unrelated donor	Most complex of three procedures. You need to find a donor who can match at least three markers (antigens) found on your white blood cells. Donor will need to be in hospital day of transplant. This transplant carries risk that your body may reject the foreign marrow (called graft-versus-host disease—GVHD). Many complications may result. Most risky of three procedures. Hospital stay ranges from one to two months, followed by outpatient care. Most expensive of three procedures.

PERIPHERAL STEM CELL SUPPORT

What is meant by peripheral stem cell support?
Peripheral stem cells are cells that circulate in your blood vessels rather than in your bone marrow. Researchers are exploring the

use of these cells to restore the normal formation and development of blood cells rather than using a bone marrow transplant. A process, called apheresis, uses a machine to separate your blood components. The components that are not needed are returned to your body. Usually growth factors, proteins that stimulate the production and growth of blood cells, are given before the stem cells are returned to the patient.

Is the end result the same for autologous bone marrow transplant and peripheral stem cell support?

The end result of both stem cell and autologous bone marrow transplants is the same—your bone marrow function recovers. However, the early results from several major centers suggest that recovery after the stem cell treatment is faster than after bone marrow infusion. This more rapid recovery reduces side effects, such as serious infections, and the need for blood and platelet transfusions. In addition, stem cell support does not usually mean a long hospital stay. Rather, you can be cared for at home during most of the process. The theory is the same but the stem cell procedure is less complex, has fewer side effects and is less costly. The rapid recovery after stem cell "rescue" makes it possible that some patients can be treated with multiple courses of high-dose chemotherapy.

Where do the stem cells or bone marrow to be used come from?

The stem cells come from the patient. There are three sources for the bone marrow—your own marrow (autologous transplant), your twin's marrow (syngeneic), or another person's marrow (allogeneic transplant). In an allogeneic transplant the marrow usually comes from your brother, sister, parent, or sometimes from an unrelated donor.

How are the stem cells produced?

Usually you are injected with a substance, called a growth factor, to stimulate the bone marrow to produce greater numbers of stem cells than the body usually produces. As these stem cells are released by the bone marrow into the bloodstream, they can be collected by a process called apheresis.

How is apheresis done?

It is usually done in a blood bank of a hospital. To collect the stem cells, your blood is withdrawn. You will be connected to a cell separator for about two to four hours for each of four or five collections. Sometimes these collections will be separated by several days, to allow your body to produce more cells in between the withdrawals.

What kind of growth factors are given?

Growth factors, also called cytokines, are routinely used to stimulate the bone marrow to begin dividing. Two types—granulocyte macrophage colony-stimulating factor (GM-CSF) or granulocyte colony-stimulating factor (G-CSF)—are generally used. In stem cell support, they may be given before and during the gathering of the stem cells.

Will I have any side effects during the process of collecting these stem cells?

You may experience some tingling, chilling sensations or light-headedness during the procedure, similar to those felt when a person is giving blood.

What happens to the blood that is taken out?

The blood is separated and the red blood cells, platelets and plasma are returned to you. Once collected, the cells are purified and frozen for storage, while you get your high-dose chemotherapy or whole body radiation treatments. This also may be done in an out-patient setting. If you have severe complications, you may be admitted to a hospital until they are under control. When the treatments are completed, the stem cells are reinjected into your system.

How are the peripheral stem cells then transplanted back into my body?

The cells are thawed and reinjected into your system through your veins. This procedure can take up to two hours and may be done in a hospital or in an outpatient facility. Sometimes patients complain that their rooms smell like garlic or that they experience a garlic taste in their mouths. This is due to the solution used to freeze the stem cells.

What kinds of complications might I have while the cells are being reinjected?

You may have shortness of breath, or problems with your liver or your heart requiring hospitalization. However, some patients may not need to stay in the hospital because they may have few side effects and may recover more quickly.

What are the long-term effects of peripheral stem cell transplants?

Effects are not yet known since the procedure is relatively new. Both the advantages and disadvantages of this transplant method and the long-term side effects are presently being studied in major centers around the country. In addition, improved techniques for collecting and storing the stem cells, and for adding growth factors to restore disease-free marrow function will be tested in the future. Further research will determine the optimal use of this treatment.

DIFFERENCES BETWEEN PERIPHERAL STEM CELL AND AUTOLOGOUS BONE MARROW SUPPORT

ITEM	PERIPHERAL STEM CELL	AUTOLOGOUS BONE MARROW
Hospitalization	up to 10 days	21 days
Time for white blood cells to reach greater than 500	10 days	20–25 days
Time for platelets to recover to 20,000	16 days	20–25 days
Transfusion of red blood cells needed	6 units	40 units
Transfusion of platelets needed	6 units	Up to 100 units
Estimated cost	$50,000–$85,000	$80,000–$135,000

BONE MARROW TRANSPLANTS

What are the different kinds of bone marrow transplants?

There are basically two kinds of bone marrow transplants—autologous, which uses your own marrow, and allogeneic, which uses marrow from another person, such as your brother, sister, parent or an unrelated donor. A third type, syngeneic, uses the marrow from an identical twin. The most complex of the bone marrow transplants is the autologous transplant.

What kinds of cancers are treated with bone marrow transplants?

Bone marrow transplantation is considered a standard treatment option for some patients with relapsed Hodgkin's disease, non-Hodgkin's lymphoma, and neuroblastoma—where it has been shown to cure patients. It is being evaluated as a treatment for patients with breast cancer, leukemia, germ cell tumors, ovarian cancer, non-seminoma testicular cancers, certain childhood cancers and some primary brain tumors in adults and children. It is also being studied in the treatment of Ewing's and other sarcomas, melanoma, metastatic cancer, and cancers that do not respond to treatment or cannot be removed by surgery. In addition, several noncancerous disorders, including aplastic anemia, severe combined immunodeficiency disease and thalassemia, are also being treated with bone marrow transplants. Preliminary investigations are under way to evaluate the usefulness of transplantation for some people who are HIV positive.

What steps are involved in bone marrow transplantation?
It depends upon the institution where you are going to have the transplant and what kind of transplant you are going to be having. However, there are usually five steps you need to go through: evaluation, pretreatment and supportive care, the transplant itself, engraftment, and convalescence, both in and out of the hospital.

STEPS IN BONE MARROW TRANSPLANT

STEP	ESTIMATED TIME INVOLVED
Evaluation, including donor identification (if needed)	4 weeks
Pretreatment	2–10 days
Transplant	Several hours
Engraftment process	14–30 days
Inpatient care	1–2 months after transplant
Outpatient care	1–3 months after hospitalization

How can I use my own bone marrow for support?
If you are having an autologous bone marrow transplant, you serve as your own donor. Usually, your bone marrow is removed, or harvested, as the health professionals say, when you are in remission or when no cancer cells can be found when looking at your cells under a microscope. The purpose of removing your bone marrow is to collect enough stem cells—cells from which blood cells develop—for the transplant. The stem cells will produce the new red blood cells, white blood cells and platelets that you need.

How will I be evaluated?

The doctor carefully examines you and your history to make sure that the transplant is the best treatment. The doctor will discuss the complications and risks with you. You and your family, along with the doctor, will look at all the factors, especially your condition, outlook and what other treatments might be available, before making the decision to go ahead with the transplant.

What will happen to me during the pretreatment phase?

You will have several days of tests and other procedures. You will probably have a catheter inserted into one of the large veins in your chest. It will be used to withdraw blood samples as well as to give you blood, drugs, and nutrition. In addition, the catheter will be used in transplanting the new marrow. The catheter will probably remain in place for several months.

Will I also be given chemotherapy during this pre-treatment phase?

Yes. Before you can have a transplant, the cancer cells must be killed. You will receive intensive chemotherapy. Some patients will also get radiation treatment. If you have leukemia, you may receive whole body radiation. These high-dose treatments will destroy your healthy marrow as well as the cancer cells. You will be given medicines to help manage and lessen the side effects of the high-dose chemotherapy and the radiation therapy. The pretreatment phase usually lasts from two to ten days, depending upon the procedures being used.

What side effects should I expect during this time?

You might experience nausea, vomiting, mouth sores, diarrhea, lowered blood counts, loss of appetite and loss of your hair. There may also be the possibility of damage to vital organs. Since your bone marrow is being destroyed, your body will be unable to defend itself against infection for a time.

What kind of supportive care will I get during the pretreatment phase?

Usually you must stay in a hospital room, where it is easier to keep the environment as free from infectious agents as possible. You will be given antibiotics to help prevent infections. In addition, you will need periodic blood transfusions because the chemotherapy and radiation will damage parts of the bone marrow that produce red blood cells and platelets. If you are unable to eat, you will be given nutrition through the catheter.

Will I feel very tired?

Yes, you probably will. Bone marrow transplants take a great deal of energy, not only for you but also for your family. You may get tired from the treatment itself, which is long and severe. You may also get tired from not knowing what the final results will be. In addition, your family may need to travel a long distance to the treatment center or need to live away from home for an extended period of time. This adds pressure on both you and your family.

How is the actual transplant of the bone marrow done?

Soon after the chemotherapy and radiation treatments are finished, you will receive bone marrow through the catheter. You might hear the health professionals calling this the transplant or the rescue process. The new marrow will travel through your blood to your bone marrow, where it will begin to make new red and white blood cells and platelets. This is called engraftment. It will take from 14 to 30 days for this to happen. Your doctor will take blood tests or remove a small amount of marrow to make sure it is growing and that the cancer has not returned.

How is the process of donating bone marrow different if I am the donor myself?

If you are having an autologous transplant and thus are the donor yourself, your bone marrow may be treated to remove malignant cells. Your bone marrow cells may be combined with a preservative to keep the cells alive when they are frozen and stored in a liquid nitrogen freezer until the day they will be transplanted. The marrow may also be purged with anticancer drugs, or other methods may be used to remove any cancer cells before it is frozen.

If I am having an allogeneic transplant, how will the donor be matched with me?

The matching of bone marrow is a very complicated process. It is based on markers found on the white blood cells. Scientists look at six markers, called human leukocyte antigens or HLA, to judge whether there can be a good match between you and the donor. These antigens are proteins that play a critical role in protecting the body from disease. Each person's antigens are a combination inherited from the mother and father. Related donors, such as brothers and sisters, have a 35 to 40 percent chance of being a match. The chances among unrelated donors are much lower—estimates range from one in a thousand to one in a million, depending on the frequency of your tissue type in the general population. Special blood tests show whether any of these antigens are shared by you and the other person. Most institutions require a match on at least three antigens. The more matching antigens you have, the fewer the complications will be.

Who can help me find a bone marrow donor?

There are several resources to help find donors. However, although the number of donors increases constantly, there is still a possibility that you may not find a donor with enough matching antigens. The National Marrow Donor Program was created to help you find a suitable donor. It receives requests for bone marrow donors from transplant centers throughout the United States, searches its computer file for a match, coordinates additional testing of donors, helps with transplantation arrangements and collects and analyzes data. Local American Red Cross chapters may also be helpful in locating bone marrow donors. See Chapter 26, ''Where to Get Help,'' for further information.

What does the donor have to do during the transplant?

Donors for allogeneic or syngeneic transplants usually go into the hospital the day before or the day of the transplant. Depending on the hospital, donors will get either local anesthesia to deaden the area of the body where the marrow will be removed, or general anesthesia to put them to sleep. The process to extract the marrow takes about forty-five minutes and must be done in an operating room under sterile conditions. The marrow is usually taken from the hip bones. The doctor makes six to ten punctures with a large needle and, using a series of smaller needles, draws about one to two pints of fluid, containing marrow, out of the donor's bones. The marrow is then strained to remove blood and bone fragments and put into the patient (the recipient) within two to four hours. Because there may be some blood loss, donors usually store two units of their own blood beforehand, to be used as needed during or after the procedure.

Does the donor have any side effects from giving the marrow?

There may be some soreness around the puncture sites for a few days. Within a few weeks, the donated marrow will have been replaced by the donor's system. Most people are back to their regular routines within a day or two, although some may take a little longer. In some rare instances, there may be infection around the incision site.

How long do I need to stay in the hospital after the transplant has taken place?

Most people stay in the hospital, in a protective isolation room, for a month or two after the transplant has taken place. Usually, you will be able to go home when your neutrophil count, a subtype of your white blood cells, is greater than 500 for at least two consecutive days. In addition, your general condition, your red blood cell and platelet counts—and whether or not you have infections—are all taken into consideration in making this decision.

Why do I need to stay in the hospital so long?

You will need to be monitored to make sure that the new bone marrow is growing. You will also be checked regularly for infections. If you had an allogeneic transplant you will be watched carefully for acute graft-versus-host disease so that you can be treated if any problems develop. You will also be given high-calorie, highly nutritious feedings through an intravenous line. In addition, you will be taught how to care for yourself at home, learning such things as how to take care of your catheter, which will be left in place for three or four months after the transplant.

What side effects need to be considered?

There are many side effects. The extent of them will vary from one person to another and will depend upon what kind of bone marrow transplantation you have. Some, such as hair loss, are temporary. Others, such as infections and graft-versus-host disease (GVHD—a side effect of an allogeneic transplant), can be serious, and sometimes fatal. You may have bleeding in the nose, mouth, under the skin or in the gastrointestinal tract. You may also have some liver damage. The period of highest risk is between fourteen and thirty days after your transplant has taken place, while your body begins to manufacture new red and white blood cells and platelets.

What kind of infections are common during this recovery period?

You may get viral, bacterial or fungal infections. For instance, herpes simplex, herpes zoster and cytomegalovirus are frequent causes of infections. Pneumonia is another common complication. You may have inflammation in your mouth and intestinal tract, called mucositis. You can be treated with antibiotics or antiviral and antifungal therapies. You may also be given antibiotics to prevent infection.

What is graft-versus-host disease?

When you have a bone marrow transplant, your immune system is replaced. If you are getting donor marrow, the new marrow, particularly its T-cells, identifies your system as foreign. It may launch an attack against you, just as whatever remains of your original immune system may reject the marrow graft. This is called graft-versus-host disease or GVHD.

Who gets GVHD?

It happens to people who have allogeneic transplants. If you are older, you are more likely to develop GVHD than if you are younger. If you have more matching antigens with your donor, you are less likely to develop GVHD. In addition, if your donor is of the same sex as you are, you are less likely to develop GVHD than if your donor is of the opposite sex. Nearly half of the people develop symptoms of GVHD soon after the transplant, some as soon as nine days after the procedure. When it happens soon after, it is called acute GVHD. When it develops later, it is called chronic GVHD.

What are the symptoms of GVHD?

If you have acute GVHD, you may have skin rashes, jaundice, liver disease or diarrhea. They may be mild or they may be severe. If you have chronic GVHD, you may have temporary darkening of the skin and hardening and thickening of the patches of skin and the layers of tissues under it. You may also have bacterial infections and weight loss. GVHD affects the liver, the skin and the gastrointestinal tract—you can have it in all three sites. Corticosteroids and other drugs are used for treatment.

Can anything be done to prevent GVHD?

Yes. Since the T lymphocytes are the major cause of the immune attack, drugs that help suppress them are given to patients routinely after transplantation. Also under study is the use of a procedure called T-cell depletion. Monoclonal antibodies or other processes are used to destroy T lymphocytes in donated marrow before it is given to the patient.

Are there any benefits to developing GVHD?

Many studies have shown that mild GVHD is actually beneficial over the long term because it kills tumor cells. People with leukemia and lymphoma who develop mild GVHD are less likely to have a relapse than are those who never have the reaction.

How often will I need to come back to the hospital after my bone marrow transplant?

It depends on your condition. You will probably need to be seen several times in the first few weeks. For the next several months, you will need to visit the health care team every two to four weeks. The doctor will want to check your catheter. Your blood counts will be checked to see if you need to have platelet and blood transfusions. If you have had an allogeneic transplant, your doctor will also look for symptoms of liver complications, infections and chronic graft-versus-host disease, which may appear as early as three or four months after the transplant. The doctor will also need to check to see that the cancer has not returned. After the first six months, your schedule of checkups will change, probably to every six months. Most of your checkups will probably include a bone marrow biopsy.

How can the doctor tell if the bone marrow transplant is failing?

There are several signs. If the graft is being rejected by your body, the donor's cells do not grow and your own cells may not begin growing again. If you have leukemia, your leukemia cells may return to your bone marrow.

How long will it take for me to get back to feeling like my normal self?

You will probably need a full year to recover fully from your transplant. You need to understand, however, that you may have to change your normal habits, to help you cope with the long-term effects of your treatment. You may feel tired, have dry eyes, skin sensitivity, and reproductive disorders. Because of changes in your liver, you may need to modify your diet. You may also need to take medication for a long time.

What are the major long-term side effects of bone marrow transplants?

Most people who have had transplants feel their overall health is good and that the benefits of the transplant outweigh the side effects. There may be several major long-term side effects. They include infertility, cataracts (especially for persons who have had allogeneic transplants) and second cancers. Persons who have had transplants complain most often about muscle spasms, leg cramps, numbness of extremities, eye problems and infertility. Slow return of energy and memory loss are also frequent complaints.

Will the transplant affect my sexual ability?

It depends on your age, and the dose and length of treatment you have as part of the transplant procedure. If you receive whole body radiation as part of your transplant procedure, you (both men and women) will most likely become sterile—that is, unable to produce a child. However, you will probably still have the desire and will be able to be active sexually. Men who undergo chemotherapy for bone marrow transplants commonly become infertile. You may wish to discuss sperm banking before you begin the transplant procedure. Many women who receive chemotherapy alone as part of the transplant procedure will have irregular periods, which usually will return to normal within three to twenty-eight months after the transplant. If you are a woman, are over 26 years old, and have both chemotherapy and whole body radiation, you will probably develop early menopause because your ovaries will stop producing certain hormones. You may be given hormone replacement therapy. However, if you have had breast cancer, hormone replacement therapy is not appropriate for you.

How often do transplant patients get cataracts?

Cataracts are a common long-term side effect among allogeneic bone marrow transplant patients who have single-dose total body radiation, with about 75 percent of patients getting cataracts some three to six years later. If you had total body radiation in several small doses, your risk is reduced to 25 percent.

Do many patients who have transplants get secondary cancers?

It is not yet clear, because bone marrow transplants have been done for a relatively short period of time. However, there is concern that the high-dose chemotherapy, radiation therapy and other factors related to the procedure could cause other cancers. The risk varies and depends on your age, general health, menopausal status, drug dose and previous treatment.

How much do bone marrow transplants cost?

Allogeneic transplants are the most expensive, costing from $150,000 to $300,000. At most institutions autologous transplants cost about half as much. Insurance coverage varies depending upon many factors. In most hospitals, you will need to have the funds to cover the costs before the transplant procedure is started.

What are the bone marrow transplant clinical trials being done in conjunction with Blue Cross and Blue Shield?

The National Cancer Institute is sponsoring four national multicenter breast cancer trials that are designed to enroll 1,500 women. The trials are comparing the benefits and risks of high-dose chemotherapy with autologous bone marrow transplant support to those of conventional chemotherapy for treating localized breast cancer at high risk of recurrence, or metastatic breast cancer. The Blue

Cross and Blue Shield Association is helping fund a substantial portion of the patient care costs for Blue Cross and Blue Shield members who are randomized to the high-dose chemotherapy–bone marrow transplant arm of the trials. Call the Cancer Information Service (1-800-4-CANCER) for further information.

Is it normal to worry about relapse?

Yes, it is normal. Unfortunately, some people do have relapses, most from their original tumors, although some persons may also develop other cancers from the chemotherapy and radiation. It is possible for some patients to get a second transplant, although it may involve a different regimen, without whole body radiation. New immunologic agents, such as interleukin-2, interferon and ricin are being evaluated for use in decreasing the risk of relapse.

DIAGNOSIS

New high-technology imaging techniques have replaced exploratory surgery in the diagnosis of cancer for some patients. Magnetic resonance imaging can be used to detect hidden tumors by mapping the variations of the various atoms in the body on a computer screen. Computerized tomography, a painless procedure, uses cross-x-rays to examine parts of the body, producing cross-sectional pictures. Positron emission tomography (PET), which produces three-dimensional images of the body's metabolic and chemical activity, is being used in diagnosing brain cancer.

Some of the advances in the diagnosis of cancer:

- Viewing the inside of the body through a thin, flexible fiberoptic instrument, called an endoscope, that can be equipped with a light, a video camera, and electronic instruments and can be inserted to obtain tissue and remove small growths. One of the most rapidly advancing fields in medicine, this microchip technology lets the doctor see clear details inside organs that once could be viewed only by operating. It allows the doctor to take out small amounts of tissue for biopsy, to determine diagnosis, to stage tumors and to decide whether or not an operation is needed.
- Adding high-resolution video technology to this fiberoptic equipment allows the entire operation team to observe the endoscopic procedures, permitting surgeons to perform more complex procedures.
- Exploring new techniques to improve the quality of mammo-

grams and developing new technology to detect and distinguish different kinds of breast tumors. Digital mammography, which uses computers to increase the ability to view breast tissue that is more dense; telemammography, which transmits images electronically; and stereotactic needle biopsies, for lumps that cannot be felt, are among some techniques that are being researched.

- Using thin hollow needles guided by x-rays to perform biopsies. Called a skinny or thin needle aspiration biopsy they allow access to both superficial and deep areas of the body without causing tissue damage. They can be used with great precision to reach tissues in the deepest recesses of the body, such as the liver, pancreas and prostate and lymph nodes in the pelvis. A syringe attached to the needle allows cells to be withdrawn. These biopsies are playing an increasingly important role in diagnosis, in reducing a patient's discomfort and in cutting costs by eliminating major surgery and hospital stays.

- Using new scanning devices, such as PET scanners (positron emission tomography), which show the body in motion to detect cancer and monitor the course of the disease. Using radioactive isotopes injected into the blood, this nuclear equipment looks at the changes in the metabolism of the tissues that might indicate cancer.

- Measuring the amount of DNA in cells, with a laser-powered instrument with a computer system, to evaluate the risk of the recurrence of some cancers, including breast, prostate and bladder cancer. Called flow cytometry, the procedure is performed on cancer cells that have been removed from a patient. It can suggest whether some patients would benefit from less aggressive treatment or detect whether the person is resistant to certain drugs.

- Using radio-labeled monoclonal antibodies to detect tumors undetectable by present technology and to pinpoint the spread of metastatic tumors. The antibodies collect wherever the cancer has spread and pass through the body if no cancer is present.

- Differentiating between cysts and solid masses using ultrasound equipment.

- Researching the use of sensitive molecular techniques to distinguish between malignant and benign disease.

- Finding means of identifying gene alterations or rearrangement that might predict whether a tumor will be aggressive or if it has metastasized.

TUMOR MARKERS

What are tumor markers?

A tumor marker is a general medical term for the substance that is found in higher amounts than normal in the blood, other body fluids or tissues of people who have cancer. There are several different kinds of tumor markers presently being used in the cancer field. Some, like the p53 gene, pinpoint people with an inherited trait who may be at a higher risk for developing cancers. Others, such as the PSA test for prostate cancer and the CA 125 test for ovarian cancer, are used in diagnosing disease, to monitor patients during treatment and to look for recurrence. Most tumor markers cannot be used alone in diagnosing cancer. For instance, when adults have a higher than normal amount of carcinoembryonic antigen (CEA) in their blood it may indicate that cancer of the colon or rectum may be present. However, since this protein is also found in the blood of people who do not have cancer, such as smokers, it cannot be used as a definite diagnostic tool. Many tumor markers presently are being researched in clinical trials.

What is a genetic screening test?

That is a test to determine whether a person has an inherited gene, like the p53 gene, that predisposes a person to some kind of cancer. It is now believed that people are born with weak spots in their genetic makeup that may make them more susceptible to cancer.

What is Lynch syndrome 2?

Lynch syndrome 2, sometimes known as the hereditary nonpolypotic colonic cancer, type 2 or the family syndrome of Lynch, is one of the cancer family syndromes. It is used to describe a family with two or more generations of cancer of the colon and endometrium, and sometimes ovary and breast, that have been diagnosed at an early age with many persons in the family having multiple primary cancers. Lynch 1 is the term used for a family that has many members with colon cancers without polyposis or other cancers.

What is the Li-Fraumeni cancer family syndrome?

The Li-Fraumeni cancer syndrome, also called SBLA syndrome, describes a family that has three or more members who have one or more cancers and are at risk for developing sarcomas; breast, bone and brain tumors; lung, laryngeal cancer and leukemia; and adrenal cortical neoplasia. It is believed that changes in one gene, p53, may account for the Li-Fraumeni syndrome.

What will someone do when an inherited tendency is found?

The family members will need to be tested and counseled. For some kinds of cancer, people who are found to inherit a trait will be able to take preventive action. For instance, a test that detects mutant proteins in people with an inherited gene for familial adenomatous polyposis (a rare condition in which the lining of the colon sprouts hundreds of tiny wartlike polyps, which left untreated almost always leads to colon cancer) has been developed. High-risk families can be tested to see if they have inherited the gene. Those who have might choose to have more frequent exams to find new polyps. They may decide to have preventive surgery. They may, in the future, be encouraged to enter trials to test chemo-preventive agents that might prevent colon cancer. There are, however, many ethical questions that need to be looked at in this newly emerging field.

Who can counsel families who are found to have a genetic tendency?

Some of the major medical centers have genetic counselors who have expertise in discussing the issues with families who have this tendency. If you need this kind of counseling, be sure to seek out the experts in this emerging field.

What are some of the ethical issues around genetic screening tests?

There are many, including privacy, freedom of choice for testing, family relationships, insurability, availability of widespread screening, and its economic impact.

TREATMENTS

Is research being done on ways to turn cancer cells back into normal cells?

This is called differentiation research and it is being conducted in several areas of the country. In laboratory experiments, scientists have successfully used chemical agents to halt the continuous reproduction of cancer cells. The cells do not become normal—that is, they do not perform all of the activities of regular cells. However, they are no longer immature cancerous cells, and rather than continuously replicating themselves, they eventually die as normal cells would. Researchers also have found that some of the agents used to make the cells "mature" can increase the efficiency of anticancer drugs and radiation and may be useful in treating advanced disease. This promising research is in early stages and undergoing investigational trials both in the United States and Europe.

TUMOR MARKERS THAT MAY INDICATE CANCER

Test	How May Be Used in Cancer
Alpha-fetoprotein (AFP)	Higher levels may indicate cancer of the testicles, liver, stomach, pancreas, lung or ovary. May be used to monitor treatment and recurrent disease. Level also higher in cirrhosis, hepatitis, and toxic liver injury.
Beta2-Micro-globulin	Investigational use. Higher levels may indicate multiple myeloma. Used in staging and determining extent of disease.
BRCA 1	Investigational use. Alteration of this region on chromosome 17q may indicate predisposition for breast and ovarian cancers.
c-erbB-2 (HER-2/neu)	Investigational use. Higher levels may indicate early recurrence and shorter survival in cancers of the breast, ovary and stomach. May be used in future to diagnose breast cancer.
Calcitonin	Used in diagnosis of cancer of thyroid. Higher levels also may indicate cancer of the breast, liver, lung, and kidney.
Cancer Antigen 15-3 (CA15-3)	Investigational use. May be used to monitor response to breast cancer treatment or to determine metastatic breast cancer.
Cancer Antigen 19-9 (CA 19-9)	Investigational use. May be used to differentiate between benign and malignant disease in cancer of the pancreas, stomach and colon. May also be used with other procedures such as CEA to monitor cancer patients.
Cancer Antigen 50 (CA-50), Cancer Antigen 195 (CA-195)	Investigational use. Higher levels may indicate cancer of the pancreas, colon and rectum.
Cancer Antigen 125 (CA-125) Protein found in blood	Higher levels of this protein found in women with ovarian cancer. Used to assess prognosis, to monitor treatment and to determine recurrence in ovarian cancer. Also found in women with endometriosis, pelvic inflammatory disease and peritonitis.

Carcino-embryonic Antigen (CEA)	High levels may indicate cancer of colon and recurrence of cancer of breast, lung, prostate, pancreas, stomach, colon and rectum. May be found in higher levels in smokers, people with lung and bowel diseases and others who do not have cancer.
Cytokeratins	Investigational use. May be used to detect lung, bladder and cervical cancers.
Epidermal Growth Factor Receptor (EGF-R)	Investigational use. Higher levels may indicate cancers of breast, bladder, head and neck, lung and kidney.
Estrogen or Progesterone Receptor (ER) or (PR)	Used to determine whether breast cancer will respond to hormone treatment and whether person is at increased risk for recurrence.
Human chorionic gonadotrophin (HCB)	Higher levels may indicate choriocarcinoma, gestational trophoblastic tumors, breast and testicular cancers. Used in detection and in monitoring treatment. Higher levels also found in pregnant women and among people taking certain medications.
Human Papilloma Virus (HPV)	More than 70 similar viruses that tend to cause warts. Strains number 16 and 18 associated with cervical cancer.
Interleukin-2 Receptor (IL-2 Receptor)	Higher levels may indicate adult T-cell leukemia, hairy cell leukemia and other tumors. Used in monitoring treatment.
Ki-67	Investigational use. Monoclonal antibody. May be used to determine prognosis in non-Hodgkin's lymphoma and breast cancer.
Lipid-associated Sialic Acid (LASA-P)	Investigational use. Higher levels may indicate cancers of the breast, stomach, lung, colon, rectum, leukemia, lymphoma, Hodgkin's disease, or melanoma. Used with other tumor markers.
MLH 1 MSH 2	Investigational use. Defects in these genes, part of the cells' molecular repair may cause colon carcer.
MTS 1 (p16)	Investigational use. Inherited gene located on chromosome 9 that may predispose persons to melanoma.
myc	Investigational use. Family of oncogenes (c-myc, N-myc, L-myc). Seen in cancers of the breast, lung, stomach, colon, and in leukemia and neuroblastoma. (continued)

TUMOR MARKERS THAT MAY INDICATE CANCER (cont.)

Test	How May Be Used In Cancer
p53 gene p16 gene	Investigational use. Alteration of a gene, p53, located on chromosome 17p, or p16 gene, located on chromosome 9, may indicate predisposition for many cancers including colon, lung, breast, bladder, liver, leukemias, or melanoma.
Philadelphia chromosome (Ph[1])	Abnormal chromosome that indicates chronic myelogenous leukemia. Used in determining treatment and prognosis.
Prostate Specific Antigen (PSA)	Higher level may indicate prostate cancer. Used in combination with other tests to detect prostate cancer. Useful in monitoring for recurrence. Also higher in men with prostatitis, or nodular prostatic hyperplasia.
Prostatic Acid Phosphatase (PAP)	Cancer cells from prostate that have spread excrete greater amounts of this enzyme. Also higher in other prostate diseases. Not a definitive test to detect prostate cancer. Should not be performed for 48 hours after prostate exam, prostate massage, enemas, colonoscopies or other physical stimulation of the prostate.
ras	Investigational use. Family of oncogenes (N-ras, H-ras, K-ras). Have been detected in cancers of the bladder, lung, colon, rectum, breast, and in some leukemias.
Squamous cell carcinoma antigen (SCC)	Investigational use. Higher levels may indicate cancer of the uterus, cervix, and head and neck. May be used to detect advanced disease.
Tumor-associated glycoprotein 71 (TAG 72)	Investigational use. Higher levels may indicate cancers of the colon, rectum, stomach, ovary or breast.

NEW SURGICAL TECHNIQUES

Are there new techniques being used in surgery?

There are several new tools and methods that make surgery easier. Among them:

- The loop electrosurgical excision procedure (LEEP) that uses an electrified wire loop to increase the accuracy of detecting hidden cancers and stemming sexually transmitted disease. The low-cost treatment can be performed in young women who have an abnormal Pap smear in which precancerous cells are found.
- Stereotactic surgery, using computer-assisted techniques to allow the surgeon to remove deep or difficult-to-reach tumors.
- Laser surgery, using a carbon dioxide, argon or Nd:YAG (neodymium:yttrium-aluminum-garnet) laser to remove colon polyps and tumors blocking the esophagus and colon, to treat abnormal tissue and early cancer of the cervix, vagina and vulva or the head and neck, the respiratory system, small tumors on the vocal cords and breast cancer. Lasers are also being used to shrink brain tumors.

NEW RADIATION TECHNIQUES

Are there any new advances in treating people with radiation?

There are several areas of research, including:

- Linking a radiosensitizer, a substance or a procedure that makes cancer cells more sensitive to the radiation treatment. Some chemotherapy drugs are being used, making tumor cells that were previously resistant to radiation more susceptible.
- Attaching radioactive isotopes in the laboratory to antibodies produced from cells taken from a patient's tumor. The antibodies, reinjected into the patient and carrying the radioactive isotopes, travel through the bloodstream to the tumor, where the antibody-carrying isotopes attach to the tumor and kill the cells. This treatment, called radio-labeled antibody therapy, is being tested in Hodgkin's disease, non-Hodgkin's lymphoma, lung and liver cancer.
- Using particle radiation, such as fast neutrons, protons, helium ions, deutrons, heavy ions (carbon, neon, argon) and

negative pi-mesons, to give greater doses or distribute doses with less harm to surrounding tissues than the substances now being used. Studies include use in sarcomas, gliomas, melanomas, cancer of the sinuses, salivary gland, lung, prostate, and head and neck cancer.

- Using new computerized technologies, such as specialized computer-driven radiation-producing machines, on-line imaging devices and 3-D treatment designs, to give more accurate and larger doses without increasing side effects, to monitor automated treatments and assure treatment quality have recently been introduced for patient use in several centers that allow 3-D treatment designs that give the radiation dose more accurately to the boundaries of the tumor. Called CD-CRT, it allows more radiation to be given to the tumor.

- Giving a large single dose of radiation directly to the tumor during an operation with minimum effects to nearby normal tissue. Called intraoperative radiation, this is being tested with cancers of the breast, colon, rectum, stomach, brain and gynecologic organs.

- Trying new ways to get the most tumor kill with the least damage to normal cells by changing the schedules, such as giving smaller daily doses of radiation more frequently—often twice a day (called hyperfractionation) or the regular dose of radiation in a shorter time (accelerated fractionation).

- Using radioprotectors, chemical compounds that protect normal cells against short-term radiation damage, allowing the normal cells to repair themselves while the tumor cells are still being treated and permitting higher doses of radiation than would normally be safe for the surrounding tissues.

- Using high-energy photons to destroy minute regions of the brain with minimal damage to surrounding tissues. Called stereotactic radiosurgery, it allows patients to arrive early the day of the treatment, undergo radiosurgery that is focused on the site, and go home the next day.

New Chemotherapy Treatments

What new methods are being used in chemotherapy treatment?

There are several new methods under investigation in clinical trials for different kinds of cancers. Among them are:

- Using more intensive drug treatments, in sequence, for shorter periods of time to make sure that full doses of each drug are given as quickly as possible, and adding growth factors to help overcome the side effects of the more intense doses.

- Linking chemotherapy drugs or other toxins to antibodies (such as monoclonal antibodies) or other agents that are able to find their way to specific cells, delivering a higher dose of cancer-killing substances directly to the tumors while sparing healthy tissues.
- Giving drugs directly to a limited area of the body, such as the liver, to prolong the time that the tumor is exposed to the chemotherapy, while doing little damage to normal tissues. Adding an agent that causes the blood to slow down, making the cancer cells more vulnerable to the drugs.
- Finding drugs that can overcome the resistance sometimes developed by cancer cells to chemotherapy agents. Chemosensitizers are being tested that may reverse resistance in some patients.
- Giving drugs at carefully selected times of day, based on the rhythmic biologic cycle that takes place in people, using portable pumps to deliver single or several drugs. This area of research, called circadian chemotherapy, is testing whether some anticancer drugs may be more effective if given during certain parts of the circadian cycle.
- Giving chemotherapy to shrink the cancer and then removing it with surgery. Called neoadjuvant chemotherapy, it is being tested in several types of cancer. In addition, there are several new chemotherapy agents that are in Phase I trials or will soon be entering those trials.

What clinical studies are being conducted using angiogenesis?

There is considerable research in the field of blood vessel formation (angiogenesis), looking at the level of oxygen found in tumors to help identify those people whose cancers are more likely to recur and those who might benefit from more aggressive treatment. The trials are studying both sides of the issue—how to get more oxygen into tumors to enhance the effect of treatment and how to use drugs (angiogenesis inhibitors) to choke off the oxygen supply to tumors, thus starving them.

HYPERTHERMIA

Is hyperthermia being used in treatment?

Heat therapy (hyperthermia) is a potential treatment that has been studied for many years and continues to be investigated in Phase I trials, either alone or with radiation and chemotherapy. Scientists think that exposing tissue to high temperatures may shrink tumors by damaging cells or depriving them of substances they need to live. Local (applying heat to a small area such as a tumor), regional (heating an organ or a limb) and whole body hyperthermia are being studied.

How is the area to be treated heated?

External and internal heating devices can be used. For local hyperthermia, the area may be heated externally with high-frequency waves. Or it may be heated internally with a sterile probe, such as thin, heated wires or hollow tubes filled with warm water, implanted microwave antennae, radiofrequency electrodes, or laser implants that emit very high frequency sound waves. In regional hyperthermia, magnets and devices that produce high energy are placed over the region to be heated or the area is treated with perfusion—the patient's blood is removed, heated and then pumped into the region that is to be heated internally. Whole body heating uses warm-water blankets, hot wax, inductive coils (like those in electric blankets) or thermal chambers. There are a number of clinical trials of this treatment method being conducted.

Photodynamic Therapy

What is photodynamic therapy?

Photodynamic therapy, also known as phototherapy, photochemotherapy or photoradiation therapy, uses three elements: a light-sensitizing drug, light (usually from a laser) and oxygen. The drug is a photosensitizing substance that makes cells more sensitive to light. The substance is injected into the body and is absorbed by all cells. The agent remains in or around tumor cells for a longer time than it does in normal tissue. When the treated cancer cells are exposed to a light (usually red) from a laser, the light is absorbed by the photosensitizing agent. This light absorption causes a chemical reaction that destroys the tumor cells. The light exposure must be carefully timed to coincide with the period when most of the agent has left healthy cells but still remains in cancer cells. Advancements in photosensitizers, fiberoptic probes and two new types of lasers (argon-pumped dye and pulsed gold vapor) have created a new interest in photodynamic therapy because they have enabled doctors to use the treatment on tissue that was once unable to be reached by the treatment.

What are the advantages and disadvantages of photodynamic therapy?

There are several advantages. Cancer cells can be selectively destroyed while most normal cells are spared, the damaging effect of the photosensitizing agent occurs only when the substance is exposed to light and the side effects are relatively mild. A disadvantage is that the laser light cannot pass through more than about one-third of an inch of tissue (one centimeter).

What kind of cancer has been treated with photodynamic therapy?

This treatment has been used in an investigational manner in basal and squamous cell skin cancers, malignant and ocular melanomas, cutaneous T-cell lymphoma, gynecological cancers and cancers of the lung, bladder, esophagus, stomach, and head and neck.

Are there any side effects from photodynamic therapy?

The most common side effect is skin sensitivity for four or more weeks. Exposure to sunlight can produce a severe sunburn. Other side effects may include some pain in the treatment area, a skin reaction similar to a mild sunburn, nausea, vomiting, chills, hives, metallic taste, eye sensitivity to light, and mild liver problems.

Must patients take any precautions when being treated with photodynamic therapy?

The substance remains active for about four to six weeks after the injection. You need to protect yourself from direct and indirect sunlight. When outdoors, nontransparent clothing that covers the body from head to toe must be worn, including a wide-brimmed hat, gloves, socks and shoes. The eyes must also be protected with sunglasses that have a 100 percent ultraviolet block to prevent eye injury. Other substances are being tested to lessen these side effects.

ENHANCING THE IMMUNE SYSTEM WITH BIOLOGICAL RESPONSE MODIFIERS

One of the newest developments in cancer involves using biologicals to trigger the body's own defenses against cancer. Scientists are finding hundreds of substances that boost, direct, or restore many of the normal defenses of the body. Many of them occur naturally in the body while others are made in the laboratory. Many are still years away from being used for ordinary medical practice. Doctors are just beginning to experiment with ways of combining various biologicals with each other and with standard treatments for more effective use. It is believed that cancer cells probably are present at some time in everyone, but that the immune system is usually able to stop the cells before they have a chance to become cancers. The latest methods for preventing, diagnosing and treating cancer, now in clinical trials across the country, are known as biological therapies.

What substances are used in the biological area?

The substances are called biological response modifiers and include monoclonal antibodies, tumor growth factors, colony-stimulating factors, interleukins and gene therapy.

What are monoclonal antibodies?

A monoclonal antibody is a substance that can find and attach to a specific protein on cancer cells. Monoclonal antibodies are produced in the body in small quantities. However, they can be produced in a laboratory in great quantity and designed to hone in on target cancer cells. They have potential in the prevention, detection and treatment of cancer.

How can monoclonal antibodies be used in treating cancer?

They can potentially be used to attack and damage, or destroy, cancer cells. They may be used to deliver anticancer drugs, toxins or radiation directly to specific cancer cells, thereby increasing the attack on those cells while causing less damage to normal healthy cells. There are several trials using different monoclonal antibodies for several kinds of cancer, including leukemia, lymphomas, melanoma, cancers of the colon, rectum, ovary, pancreas, and prostate.

What are radio-labeled monoclonal antibodies?

They are monoclonal antibodies that have been made radioactive and can be used to detect minute cancer that has spread in the body. After being injected into the bloodstream, the radio-labeled antibodies attach to cancer cells in the body and can be detected by special sensing devices. Investigations using radio-labeled monoclonal antibodies in the detection of many different cancers are ongoing.

What are some of the agents linked to the monoclonal antibodies?

The agents include radioisotopes, plant and bacterial toxins, chemotherapy drugs and biologic agents. One of the toxins, ricin, is being tested in clinical trials for leukemia, lymphoma, melanoma, and cancers of the colon, rectum, lung and breast.

What are tumor growth factors?

Tumor growth factors, which are also called cytokines, colony-stimulating factors or hematopoietic growth factors, are naturally occurring substances that stimulate the bone marrow to produce white and red blood cells and platelets.

How are tumor growth factors used for in treating cancer?

Investigations are under way in many areas:

- To produce more red blood cells and lessen bleeding problems, enabling patients to tolerate larger doses of chemotherapy.
- To boost white blood cells that fight infection, allowing greater amounts of chemotherapy to be given.
- To enhance chemotherapy drugs, increasing their effectiveness.
- To separate cancer cells from bone marrow that has been removed from a patient.
- To enhance wound healing.

What different tumor growth factors are being investigated?

There are several types that are being used:

- Sargramostim to stimulate the growth of early bone marrow cells. Also called granulocyte-macrophage CSF, GM-CSF, Leukine, Prokine or Leukomax.
- Filgrastim to stimulate the growth of granulocytes. Also called G-CSF or Neupogen.
- M-CSF to stimulate the growth of macrophages.
- Erythropoietin to stimulate the production of red blood cells. Also called Epogen.
- Interleukins to stimulate the growth of bone marrow cells, the production of eosinophil, and of platelets. Also called IL-1 or hematopoietin-1, IL-3 or multi-CSF, IL-5 or eosinophil CSF, IL-6 or thrombopoietin.
- Pixy that combines the elements of both GM-CSF and IL-3.
- GF beta to promote tissue repair.

How are growth factors given to patients?

Growth factors are usually given either intravenously or subcutaneously (under the skin). Sometimes patients are able to give it to themselves, after instruction by a nurse.

What is interferon?

Interferon, discovered in 1975, is a cytokine, a protein that helps to regulate the immune system. Interferons used in cancer treatment are made naturally by the body when cells are stimulated by an agent such as a virus, or produced synthetically in a laboratory by putting some interferons into bacteria and cultivating a large quantity of them.

Are there different kinds of interferons?

There are three groups of interferons: alpha, beta and gamma. It appears that alpha and beta interferons are made by virtually all white blood cells. Gamma interferon is made only by T-cells (a type of white blood cell processed in the thymus gland) and large granulocytes (a white blood cell made in the bone marrow). Gamma interferon is more powerful in its effect on the immune system than alpha or beta interferon.

Is interferon used alone in cancer treatment?

Interferon seems to be more effective when it is used with chemotherapy drugs, such as 5-fluorouracil or other biological agents such as tumor necrosis factor and other interferons.

What is interleukin?

Interleukin is a group of natural, hormonelike substances that are made in the body by lymphocytes, a type of white blood cell. Interleukins are a type of cytokine that carry signals between the blood-forming cells that are part of the immune system. There are several interleukins, each distinguished by a different number—Interleukin-1 (IL-1) to Interleukin-12 (IL-12).

How do the different interleukins work?

Each of the interleukins performs different duties:

- IL-1 triggers a wide range of processes involved in inflammation, activates T-cells and stimulates bone marrow growth. Also called hematopoietin-1.
- IL-2 stimulates the growth and activities of a wide range of cells including several types that can kill cancer cells, such as LAK cells (lymphokine-activated killer cells), TIL cells (tumor-infiltrating lymphocytes) and CTL (cytotoxic T-lymphocytes). Also called Proleukin.
- IL-3 stimulates the growth of precursor bone marrow cells, young cells that have the potential to grow into mature blood cells. Also called multi-colony-stimulating factor or Multi-CSF.
- IL-4 enhances the growth of B-cells, the production of antibodies, and stimulates the production of other immune system cells. Also called B-cell stimulatory factor-1 or BSF-1.
- IL-5 stimulates the growth of blood cells that kill bacteria. Also called eosinophil colony-stimulating factor or eosinophil CSF.
- IL-6 stimulates the growth of B-cells. Also called B-cell stimulatory factor 2, BSF-2, or interferon beta-2.
- IL-7 stimulates the expansion of immature lymphoid cells,

induces production of IL-2, and is active in the growth of T-cells.

- IL-10 is believed to promote growth of both B- and T-cells, and it acts with IL-7, IL-2 and IL-4 on thymocytes.
- IL-12 stimulates the proliferation of natural-killer and T-cells and triggers a surge of gamma interferon from both cell types.

What are LAK cells?

LAK, or lymphokine-activated killer cells, are being used in investigational trials. IL-2 injected into the body can stimulate the production of lymphocytes, which can be taken from the patient's blood and exposed to more IL-2, which causes them to reproduce at a faster rate than normal. These stimulated cells, known as LAK cells, are then returned to the patient's bloodstream, where they have the potential to destroy cancer cells.

What are TIL cells?

TIL, or tumor-infiltrating lymphocytes, are a type of white blood cell that can invade or infiltrate growing tumors and kill cancer cells while sparing normal cells. TIL can be produced in a laboratory, using IL-2 to treat cancer cells from the patient's tumor. As the number of TIL cells expands, the cancer cells decrease. The tumor-infiltrating lymphocytes are returned to the patient along with more IL-2. This is an investigational treatment.

What are CTL cells?

CTL stands for cytotoxic T-lymphocytes, a type of white blood cell also known as killer cells. They can attack and destroy cancer cells.

What is tumor necrosis factor?

Tumor necrosis factor, produced by specialized white blood cells called macrophages in response to infection, is a substance that occurs naturally in the body in small amounts. It can kill cancer cells, as well as damage the blood vessels of a tumor, preventing nutrients and oxygen from reaching it. Tumor necrosis factor is being used in combination with chemotherapy drugs and other biologic response modifiers.

How is BCG used?

BCG, or bacillus Calmette-Guerin, is being used in patients with metastatic colorectal or kidney cancer or melanoma. The patients receive injections of BCG and antibodies, produced from cells taken from a patient's tumor, followed by IL-2 to stimulate their immune system.

USES AND SIDE EFFECTS OF COMMON BIOLOGICAL RESPONSE MODIFIERS

NAME	USE	SIDE EFFECTS
Bacillus Calmette-Guerin (BCG, TheraCys, TICE BCG). Intravascularly, into skin, intralesional, intrapleural.	Urinary tract cancer, melanoma, and other cancers.	Small red area that scales and dries leaving small pink or bluish scar after 3 months (if given on skin), skin rash, increased urination, pain during urination, blood in urine, fever, chills, tiredness, sluggishness, mild nausea and vomiting, loss of appetite, diarrhea.
Filgrastim (G-CSF, Neupogen). Given IV or injected under skin.	Decreasing infection for bone marrow transplants, stem cell support and other high dose treatments.	Bone pain in lower back, pelvis or chest, fluid retention, swelling at injection site, flare in psoriasis, tiredness, mild headache, chest tightness. Rarer are skin rash, mild hair loss, nausea and vomiting, diarrhea, loss of appetite, flushing.
Interferon alpha n1 (Wellferon). Investigational. Interferon alpha n2a, 2b (Roferon, Intron A). Hairy cell leukemia, Kaposi's sarcoma of AIDS. Interferon alpha-2c (Berofor). Investigational. Given subcutaneously, topically and IV.	Hairy cell leukemia, Kaposi's sarcoma of AIDS, multiple myeloma, leukemia, lymphoma, melanoma, and cancers of the bladder, colon-rectum, and kidney, as well as condyloma and hepatitis.	Fever, chills and sweats (usually occur in 1 to 2 hours; last less than 18 hours), tiredness, lack of energy, loss of appetite, change in taste, pain in muscles, headaches, sleeplessness, depression, visual disturbances, tremor, seizures, agitation, anxiety, dizziness, mild nausea and vomiting, diarrhea, gas, constipation, mild hair loss, skin rash and dryness, burning in area where drug injected.

Agent	Uses	Side Effects
Interferon gamma 1b (Actimmune). Given intramuscularly and IV.	Infections associated with chronic granulomatous disease.	Headache, fever, chills, diarrhea, nausea and vomiting, stomach pain, loss of appetite, dizziness, confusion, disorientation, hallucinations, seizures, tiredness, night sweats, shortness of breath, heart problems.
Interleukin 2 (IL-2, Aldesleukin, Proleukin). Given IV.	Melanoma, cancer of the kidney.	Nausea and vomiting, diarrhea, fever and chills, lack of energy, irregular heartbeat, disorientation, sleeplessness, loss of memory, anemia, skin rash and dryness, hair loss, weight gain, angina, shortness of breath, cough, lung congestion, less frequent urination (begins within 24 to 48 hours, lasts 7 to 30 days), mouth sores.
Interleukin-3 (IL-3). Given IV or injected under skin.	May be used in combination with G-CSF or GM-CSF to stimulate production of platelets for patients getting high-dose chemotherapy, bone marrow transplants or stem cell support.	Fever, chills, nausea, mild bone pain, rash and swelling at injection site, headache (may need to take acetaminophen or codeine).
Levamisole (Ergamisole). Given as a tablet.	Used in combination with fluorouracil after surgery to stimulate macrophages and T-lymphocytes in colon cancer (Duke's C).	Dizziness, agitation, confusion, nausea and vomiting, diarrhea, loss of appetite, constipation, bitter taste, mouth sores, skin rash, sleeplessness, headache, tiredness, fever, chills, muscle weakness, arthritis, swelling of arms and legs, fluid retention, dizziness, blurred vision, shaking, agitation, confusion, nightmares and hallucinations, paranoia, tremors, jitters, seizures.

(continued)

USES AND SIDE EFFECTS OF COMMON BIOLOGICAL RESPONSE MODIFIERS *(cont.)*

Name	Use	Side Effects
Pixy.	May be used to increase leukocytes and platelets in patients getting high-dose chemotherapy; bone marrow transplants or stem cell support.	Fever, chills, nausea, rash and swelling at injection site, headache, flushing sensation, low or high blood pressure, nausea and vomiting, bone pain in back, pelvis or chest, fluid retention, irregular heartbeat, confusion, tiredness.
Sargramostim (GM-CSF, Leukine, Prokine, Leukomax, granulocyte-macrophage CSF). Given IV or injected under skin.	Increasing red blood cell and platelet growth for bone marrow transplants and other high-dose treatments.	Flushing sensation, low or high blood pressure, nausea and vomiting, fever, leg spasms, skin rash at injection site, bone pain in back, pelvis or chest, fluid retention, irregular heartbeat, headache, confusion, fever, chills, tiredness.
Tumor necrosis factor (rTNF-Alpha, cachectin). Given IV.	Kaposi's sarcoma, melanoma.	Tenderness and rash around area where injected, high or low blood pressure, stomach pain, loss of appetite, nausea and vomiting, diarrhea, headache, confusion, speech disorders, sleeplessness, lack of energy, hallucinations, seizures, wheezing, fever, chills, lack of energy.

GENE THERAPY

What is gene therapy?

Gene therapy takes a healthy gene and inserts it into the cells of a patient to compensate for a missing or defective one. Instead of giving a patient a drug to treat or control the symptoms of a genetic disorder, physicians attempt to correct the basic problem by altering the genetic makeup of some of the cells. Recent advances in understanding and manipulating genes have set the stage for scientists to alter genetic material to fight or prevent disease.

How does gene therapy work?

In some current clinical trials, cells from the blood or bone marrow are removed from the patient and grown in the laboratory under conditions that encourage them to multiply. The desired gene is inserted into the cells with the help of a disabled virus (called a virus vector), and the successfully altered cells are selected out, encouraged to multiply and returned to the patient's body. In other cases, liposomes (fatty particles) or disabled viruses may be used to deliver the gene directly to the cells.

When was gene therapy first used?

The first use of gene therapy was in September 1990, at the National Institutes of Health to correct a rare genetic disorder (adenosine deaminase deficiency) in a four-year-old girl from Cleveland. Her white blood cells were removed, the human ADA gene was added in a laboratory and the white blood cells with the ADA gene were then reinfused into her body. Over fifty gene therapy studies are under way.

Has gene therapy ever been used in cancer patients?

In January 1991, two patients with advanced melanoma were treated at the National Cancer Institute with gene therapy. Both are still alive and functioning. Additional melanoma patients have been added to the trial. Gene therapy is still extremely new and highly experimental. The number of approved trials is small and relatively few patients have been treated to date. It is being done only at selected major centers in the country.

Are there any cancer gene therapy trials presently being done?

A number of clinical trials are currently approved to test gene therapy in the United States and in other countries, including cancers such as melanoma, neuroblastoma and brain tumors. Scientists are working on ways to genetically alter immune cells that are naturally or deliberately targeted to cancers:

- One method being used experimentally in treating melanoma genetically alters immune cells, arms them with cancer-fighting genes and returns them to the body, where they can more forcefully attack the cancer cells.

- Another method, being used in a variety of clinical trials, genetically alters cancer cells taken from the body so that they elicit a strong immune response. These cells are returned to the body with the hope that they will act as a cancer vaccine.

- It is now also possible to inject a tumor with a gene that renders the tumor cells vulnerable to an antibiotic or other drug. Subsequent treatment with the drug should kill the cells that contain the foreign gene. It may also be possible, though a mechanism known as the bystander effect, to kill tumor cells that are not usually affected by the substance. Two trials are under way using these approaches for the treatment of brain tumors.

NEW PREVENTION TECHNIQUES

The new term in the area of prevention is *chemoprevention*. It means using drugs and other substances to prevent cancer. There are several kinds of research studies being done in this new field. Some are directed at people who have been successfully treated for one cancer and are at high risk for getting a second cancer. Others are aimed at people who have a medical condition that may lead to cancer or are at risk for getting cancer. Still others enroll healthy, disease-free people.

What are chemoprevention trials based on?
They are based on the belief that various chemoprevention agents may stop or reverse cancer development or prevent it from ever starting. These agents need to be studied scientifically over time to find out if they can indeed prevent cancer.

Does everyone on a chemoprevention trial get the agent being tested?
People who take part in the trial are separated into different groups. In some studies, the chemoprevention agent will be tested against no agent at all. That means that one group will get the agent and others will receive an identical-looking pill, called a placebo, that contains no drug at all. You will be put into one group or the other purely by chance and usually you will not be told what

group you are in. Other times, the agent will be tested against another agent. The people in each group take a different agent or a different dose of the same agent.

What kinds of agents are being tested in chemoprevention trials?

They are usually drugs that have shown through research some success in preventing a type of cancer when given in a specified dose over an extended period of time. The agent may be a vitamin, mineral, nutritional supplement, such as vitamins A or E, high-fiber materials such as wheat bran and other dietary components, or drugs that have been widely used for many years.

Are there side effects or risks in chemoprevention trials?

There may be. Some agents used in chemoprevention may cause side effects depending on what they are and how you respond to them. Every possible effort is made to identify the risks associated with the agents being used. Generally, they are not expected to cause serious side effects.

Are there any costs involved?

Each trial is different. Some are entirely cost-free to those who participate. In others, you may have to pay for some or all of the costs of the tests and examinations that are required. The trials, however, are designed so that most of the tests are considered to be part of routine medical care, so that if possible, they are costs that your insurance can pay for. The tests may be a mammogram, a Pap test, or a cholesterol test. These are examinations that healthy people are encouraged to do on a regular basis. You need to discuss the costs with the doctor or nurse before you decide whether or not you wish to participate.

QUESTIONS TO ASK BEFORE JOINING A CHEMOPREVENTION TRIAL

- What is the purpose of the trial?
- What part of the trial is experimental?
- What is my alternative choice if I do not choose to be in the trial?
- What kinds of tests are required?
- Whom do I contact with questions about the research?
- What are the potential risks and potential benefits?
- What are my responsibilities while in the trial?
- How long will the trial last?
- What costs may I expect?
- Will my records be confidential?

- How can the trial affect my daily life?
- What side effects could I expect from the agent being used?
- Do I have any further responsibilities after I have completed the study?

What are some of the chemoprevention trials that are under way?
There are several, including:

- The Breast Cancer Prevention Trial, to determine whether taking an antiestrogen drug (tamoxifen) for five years will prevent breast cancer from developing in women who are at increased risk for the disease. The study is enrolling 16,000 healthy higher-risk women, half of whom will receive tamoxifen and half of whom will receive a placebo (an inactive pill that looks like tamoxifen).
- The Prostate Cancer Prevention Trial, to evaluate whether taking the drug Proscar (finasteride) for seven years will prevent prostate cancer from developing in men. This study is enrolling 18,000 men ages 55 and older, half of whom will receive finasteride each day for seven years and half of whom will receive a placebo (an inactive pill that looks like finasteride).
- The Prostate, Lung, Colorectal and Ovarian Cancer Screening Trial, to determine whether the widespread use of certain screening tests to detect these cancers will save lives. This test will study digital rectal exam and PSA (prostate), chest x-ray (lung), flexible sigmoidoscope (colorectal) and physical exam of the ovaries, CA-125 and transvaginal ultrasound (ovary). Doctors expect to enroll 148,000 men and women between the ages of 60 and 74 at ten medical centers across the country.
- Several trials that are testing the effectiveness of vitamins and minerals in preventing cancer. Beta-carotene, the retinoic acid (chemical cousin of vitamin A), vitamin C, folic acid, selenium and calcium are among those being studied. Beta-carotene, for instance, is being studied alone or in conjunction with other agents in the prevention of cancer of the cervix, lung, skin, colon, and head and neck.
- There are some studies in the area of diet, for instance, looking at the effects of fiber on colon cancer and the effects of lowering the fat content of the diet of women who have had breast cancer.

chapter 10

Unproven Treatments

Cancer patients are frequently lured into trying unproven methods of treatment by the promise of a cure. It is important to be an informed consumer in assessing any "cures" reported in the popular press. Ask the hard questions about the unproven methods being offered, and do your own research into what is promising Use your own common sense and sound judgment—if it sounds too good to be true, it probably is.

Everyone is susceptible to the promises of a "sure cure" that is without risks or pain, using natural products with no side effects. And cancer patients and their families are no exception. The cures that are commonly offered by the proponents of unproven methods include diets, devices and drugs. This subject is a controversial one, with information that can be misleading and claims that can be difficult to interpret. Some people turn to unproven methods because they think the treatments will be easier for them to withstand. Others mistrust doctors or fear the usual treatments for the disease. Sometimes friends or family members encourage the patient to try "miracle cures." Many people are using some unproven methods along with their regular treatments. There are stringent ethical and procedural controls in place in the medical system. It seems only fair that practitioners of unproven methods should be held to the same research standards as any other scientist—that a discovery is completely and accurately described so that other researchers can independently verify and expand upon those results.

What You Need to Know About Unproven Treatments

- Usually there is little scientific evidence presented by those promoting unproven methods. Patients are encouraged to have the treatment even though there is no true evidence that it really works. There are some promoters who engage in unethical sales techniques, make misleading promises, charge high fees and neglect prudent conventional medical supervision and care. Many times the write-ups for the unproven methods use scientific words or phrases in a misleading manner.
- Some treatments that have been tested and found useless, such as Laetrile, are renamed and repackaged and continue to be sold to unsuspecting patients.
- Although some unproven methods are being prescribed by physicians, many cures are being promoted by doctors with unrecognizable degrees such as N.D. (Doctor of Naturopathy), Ph.N. (Philosopher of Naturopathy), DA BB-A (Diplomate of American Board of Bio-Analysts), and Ms.D. (Doctor of Metaphysics).
- If you are using an unproven method in combination with standard treatment, it is important to discuss it with your health care team to make sure that it does not interfere with your treatment and to review potential side effects. There may be a risk, for instance, in mixing some chemotherapy drugs with unorthodox substances.
- For many who want to explore approaches to self-care that would improve their quality of life, such as meditation, deep relaxation and hypnosis, imagery, a wholesome balanced vegetarian diet, psychological or spiritual support or the traditional Chinese medicine, there are ethical and appropriately qualified practitioners available locally at moderate cost.

Questions to Ask Before You Use Unproven Methods

- Why do I want to use this kind of treatment?
- What do I think it will accomplish?

- What evidence is there that the unproven method will work? How has it been evaluated?
- Has it been written up in a scientific journal? Why not?
- Do the practitioners of the method claim that the medical community is trying to keep their cure from the public?
- Does the treatment have a "secret formula" that only a small group of practitioners can use? Has the treatment been evaluated by an independent group of researchers?
- How long has the establishment been in operation? Is it certified by any authoritative body?
- What are the qualifications of the people who will be treating me? Have they graduated from accredited schools?
- Does it sound too good to be true?
- Have I discussed the treatment with my doctor?
- Will the doctor continue to care for me if I am using this treatment?
- Is there some way my doctor and I can come to a compromise?
- Can I continue my regular treatments and try the unproven method at the same time?
- Is there some kind of investigational or experimental treatment that would give the same or better results?
- What costs will be associated with the unproven method?
- How do these costs compare to conventional treatment?

What is the difference between investigational treatment and unproven methods?

Investigational treatments, sometimes called experimental treatments, are conducted using specific scientific methods and standards to evaluate new therapies or procedures. (These procedures are described in Chapter 9, "New Advances and Investigational Trials.") Unproven methods, sometimes called alternative treatments, cannot be proven effective, either because no studies exist or because whatever data are available have not been produced using the specific standards and methods required of scientific research. Although the standards being used for investigational treatments are complex and strict, they are put in place for the safety of the public and to make sure that any new treatment offered to patients actually works.

Is the subject of unproven methods new?

Unproven remedies for the treatment of cancer are as old as the disease itself. In 1784, the House of Burgesses of the General Assembly of Virginia, of which George Washington was a member, passed a resolution appointing a committee to make a trial of Mary Johnson's "receipt of curing cancer," consisting of garden sorrel, celandine, persimmon bark and spring water, and to report on its effect. In 1754, the committee after hearing the testimony of many witnesses who had taken the remedy report that they had been cured

STANDARDS FOR INVESTIGATIONAL TREATMENTS COMPARED TO UNPROVEN METHODS

INVESTIGATIONAL	UNPROVEN
Must have scientific evidence that treatment being used has some effectiveness against cancer.	People giving treatment usually claim it has high degree of activity against cancers that are considered incurable with no basis for the claim.
Objectives of study must be clearly stated.	Usually no study has been outlined with objectives.
Methods used to achieve objectives must be stated in protocols and in reports of results.	Usually no written protocol or standardized methods of giving drugs or medication. Even the same patient may get different doses given in different manners.
Study includes comparison groups to determine whether treatment is better than standard treatment.	No comparison groups.
Must be reviewed by human subjects committee in qualified medical institution.	No review by human subjects committee. Institution normally not certified by usual authorizing agencies.
Informed consent, including written explanation of the purpose and aspects, the potential benefits and risks of the trials, is required.	Most unproven methods are used without any explanation and without your signing a consent form.
Must be clear evidence that patients have cancer.	Many times no biopsy evidence to prove that person had cancer.
Patients randomly assigned to treatment and control groups to eliminate bias.	No control groups used.

(continued)

STANDARDS FOR INVESTIGATIONAL TREATMENTS COMPARED TO UNPROVEN METHODS *(cont.)*	
INVESTIGATIONAL	**UNPROVEN**
Response to treatment must be objectively assessed using sound, well-defined methods.	Unproven treatment being studied often used after or along with standard treatment. No way to tell which treatment caused improvement.
Results must be analyzed thoroughly enough to determine effects of treatment.	Claim that treatment works is based many times on stories of people who appear to be cured or on testimonials from people who believed they were cured by unproven method.
Other researchers using same method must be able to achieve same results.	Records often scanty, inadequate or nonexistent. No means of replicating results or even of knowing what results have been.
Results must be published in reputable scientific journals.	Results not reported in scientific journals and not reviewed by experts in field. Findings are reported directly to press.

of cancer, put the report into the minutes of the House of Burgesses and voted Mrs. Johnson a reward of £100.

Why are doctors so opposed to unproven methods?

Most of them feel that there are risks to patients using an unproven method instead of a conventional treatment. The most substantial one is the delay in getting a treatment that could offer a cure. Many standard treatments are highly successful, especially in curing cancers that are found early. If you use an unproven treatment first and then go to the standard treatment after the unproven one does not work, your cancer could be at an advanced stage. The delay could result in the loss of valuable time in receiving a treatment that could have been effective for you—and reduce your chances for curing your cancer or at least controlling it. You are spending money for treatment, usually not covered by insurance, that is not effective.

Is it difficult to get information about treatment results of un-proven methods into scientific journals?

Papers that are published in reputable medical and nursing journals require that scientifically sound methods be used to conduct the study and that objective evidence be presented so that the overall effectiveness of the treatment can be evaluated. The papers are reviewed by professionals in the same field as the study though a process called peer review. Without hard evidence, the studies, whether they are reporting on unproven methods or other treatments, do not get published. There is no lack of places to present scientific data, with over 500 high-quality medical and nursing journals and nearly 3,000 health-science journals where new medical developments are regularly communicated. In addition, there are thousands of regularly scheduled meetings of doctors and scientists at which to present well-documented scientific evidence.

Can those who provide unproven treatments get any help from the government in conducting trials of their treatments?

The Office of Alternative Medicine, established in 1992 at the National Institutes of Health, has begun to fund research in areas such as acupuncture, biofeedback, hypnosis, music therapy, massage therapy, yoga and prayer. The primary interest of the office is to find practical treatments that may be of use to physicians—even if the way those treatments work is not understood for years. This office was established to give an opportunity to those who are practicing alternative medicine to demonstrate the scientific validity of their treatments.

Is there a congressional report on unproven methods of cancer treatment?

There is a report from the U.S. Congress Office of Technology Assessment, *Unconventional Cancer Treatments,* that summarizes a four-year study of unconventional cancer treatments by the Congressional Office of Technology Assessment. It examines many of the better-known and most controversial therapies and diet regimens. The report is available from the Government Printing Office (Report OTA-H-406), Washington, D.C. 20402-9325. Produced by a panel of experts in both standard and alternative treatments, it describes those that are most common and reviews their claims.

What are antineoplastons?

Dr. Stanislow Burzynski of the Burzynski Research Institute in Houston has identified a group of peptides produced by the body,

QUESTIONABLE METHODS OF CANCER TREATMENT REVIEWED BY THE AMERICAN CANCER SOCIETY

Antineoplastons
Bio-Medical Center (Hoxsey method)
Brych, Vlastimil (Milan)
Contreras method
Dimethyl sulfoxide (DMSO)
Ecology therapy (Kelly malignancy index)
Electronic devices
Fresh cell therapy
Gerson method
Greek cancer cure (Alivizatos therapy)
Hoxsey method
Hydrogen peroxide and other "hyperoxygenation" therapies
I.A.T (Immunoaugmentative therapy)
Iscador
Kelly malignancy index
Laetrile
Livingston-Wheeler therapy
Macrobiotic diets
Harold W. Manner, Ph.D. (Metabolic therapy)
Metabolic therapy
"Psychic surgery"
Questionable cancer practices in Tijuana and other Mexican border clinics
Questionable "nutritional" therapies
Revici method
Simonton, O. Carl, M.D.

Information on these topics is available from the American Cancer Society. Call 1-800-ACS-2345.

which he calls antineoplastons. He and his colleagues claim that these peptides are produced in individuals as part of a "biochemical defense system" that inhibits cancer cell growth. According to Dr. Burzynski, "The failure and deficiency of antineoplastons will result in perpetuation of neoplastic growth and development of cancer." He restores this "cancer defense system" by giving antineoplastons to people with cancer.

Has the National Cancer Institute reviewed Dr. Burzynski's antineoplastons treatment?

The National Cancer Institute (NCI) reviewed seven cases of primary brain tumor that were treated by Dr. Burzynski with antineoplastons A10 and AS2-1. It concluded that antitumor responses had occurred. To determine whether the antitumor activity was due to treatment with antineoplastons, NCI is conducting Phase II clinical trials using antineoplastons in patients with brain tumors. The NCI explains that the decision to study the agent in clinical trials does not indicate that the agent will be useful in the treatment of cancer, only that it merits evaluation.

What is the Greek cancer cure?

Dr. Hariton-Tzannis Alivizatos was a microbiologist who used a series of serum injections to treat individuals with cancer. Before he died in 1991, Dr. Alivizatos claimed to have been curing cancer for more than a decade at his clinic in Athens, Greece. However, his findings were never published in a scientific journal, his serum was never tested by other scientists to see whether or not it did what Dr. Alivizatos claimed and he never allowed an independent review of his findings. In addition, he refused to make the contents of his serum known.

What is shark cartilage treatment?

The theory is that shark cartilage can inhibit the development of the network of blood vessels that tumors need for nourishment and to remove waste products. Scientists say that an insignificant number of sharks—one out of a million or less—get cancer. Sharks seem to resist tumors naturally. Rather than bones, the skeletons of sharks are made of pure cartilage, a hard gristly material formed from proteins and complex carbohydrates and toughened by rodlike fibers. Clinical trials are under way to determine whether shark cartilage has a role in cancer treatment.

What is laetrile?

Laetrile is a product made from apricot pits which contains a chemical called amygdalin. Promoters of laetrile, which they also called vitamin B_{17}, claim that it is a harmless, effective treatment for cancer and that it is useful in cancer prevention. However, no scientific evidence supports these claims. The National Cancer Institute tested laetrile in laboratory animals several times but found no convincing evidence that it is effective against animal cancers. However, because of widespread public use and interest in the subject, the National Cancer Institute conducted a clinical study of laetrile with cancer patients. The conclusion of the researchers who participated in the trial was that laetrile was ineffective as a treatment for cancer and did not substantially improve symptoms of the disease in the patients studied. A detailed report of the study was published in the *New England Journal of Medicine* in January 1982 (volume 306, number 4).

What is the macrobiotic diet?

The macrobiotic diet, also known as the Zen macrobiotic diet, consists mainly of cereal products, such as rice. Individuals following the diet must not eat any sugar, meat or animal products and must restrict their intake of fluids. There are many variations of the macrobiotic diet. The principle of all of the diets is to recommend that liquids, usually in the form of miso or tamari broths, be used only sparingly. Meats (including poultry), dairy products, tropical or semitropical fruits and juices, sugar, honey, or anything artificial are to be avoided. The most restrictive of these diets, not usually followed today, uses only cereals, mostly in the form of brown rice. Those who recommend the diet for cancer patients believe that cancer is a toxic blood condition that has developed because of poor eating habits.

Can the macrobiotic diet be harmful to cancer patients?

The macrobiotic diet lacks nutritional elements needed even by healthy people. It is low in many vitamins and minerals. Since milk products are excluded, getting enough calcium can be a problem. For cancer patients under treatment, there can be additional difficulties. Many are already experiencing weight loss and lack of appetite. Many have difficulty in maintaining their weight, in eating enough calories and consuming the necessary protein. It is common for cancer patients to feel full both during and after eating. Persons on the macrobiotic diet need to eat large amounts of food, mostly bulky foods, just to obtain the number of calories required by the diet. The diet does not allow vitamin and mineral supplements. The macrobiotic diet also requires a person to devote many hours in preparing the food.

What is immunoaugmentative therapy?

The Immunology Researching Centre was established in the Bahamas in 1977 by Lawrence Burton, Ph.D., a zoologist, who claims that his treatment, called immunoaugmentative therapy or IAT, is effective against cancer, multiple sclerosis and AIDS. In media interviews, Dr. Burton has described his great success in treating patients with a serum created from a combination of agents in human blood. The Food and Drug Administration has not granted permission for IAT to be given to cancer patients because there is not enough laboratory evidence of antitumor activity to warrant its use or testing in human beings. Dr. Burton also has never formally reported in the scientific literature details of his treatment methods or results of studies he conducted at the clinic. Since the research results have never been published, other scientists have not been able to evaluate his claims.

Has the National Cancer Institute evaluated Dr. Burton's treatment?

The National Cancer Institute repeatedly offered to screen Dr. Burton's materials to evaluate them for antitumor activity and to test them for purity and toxicity. Dr. Burton has neither supplied nor identified the IAT treatment materials. However, five American patients who returned to the United States from his clinic in the Bahamas gave the National Cancer Institute sealed IAT specimens. The analyses of these specimens showed they were dilutions of blood proteins with no evidence of the immunologic components described by Dr. Burton and with no evidence of biological or antitumor activity. In addition, all of the samples analyzed were contaminated with bacteria and four of them were positive for hepatitis. These results have been confirmed by subsequent analyses of more than seventy additional samples by the Centers for Disease Control and Prevention, NCI and other independent laboratories. Moreover, HIV has been found in Dr. Burton's treatment material, confirming that this material has the potential to transmit AIDS, as well as hepatitis and bacterial infection, to those who receive IAT. In 1986 the Bahamian government closed the clinic, but it was reopened several months later after Dr. Burton promised quality control and sterile conditions.

What is the Livingston-Wheeler Clinic?

Dr. Virginia Livingston-Wheeler, who died in 1990, operated the Livingston-Wheeler Clinic in San Diego, California. She believed that cancer is caused by a bacterium she called *Progenitor cyptocides*. Dr. Livingston-Wheeler's treatment involved a vaccine prepared for each patient (derived from bacteria usually cultured from the patient's urine), along with a low-carbohydrate diet, antibiotics and certain enzymes. She published reports on her bacterium beginning in the 1950s. However, other researchers have not been able to confirm the existence of the unique organism that Dr. Livingston-

Wheeler described. Cultures that she submitted to the American Type Culture Collection, a private organization that collects, grows, preserves and distributes authentic cultures of microorganisms, have been identified as *Staphylococcus epidermidis.* The California Department of Health Services Cancer Advisory Council, which includes nine cancer experts and five consumer representatives, conducted a review of the available information and concluded that there is no scientific basis for believing that the Livingston-Wheeler vaccines are safe and effective in treating cancer. As a result, in 1990, the state of California ordered the clinic to stop treating cancer patients with these vaccines, which were not approved by the FDA (Dr. Livingston-Wheeler never sought FDA approval for her vaccine).

chapter 11

Breast Cancer

Finding a lump in your breast or being told you have a suspicious mammogram is a jolting, shocking emotional experience. Today, with the new knowledge of how breast cancer behaves, there are many new options and alternatives available for women facing this diagnosis.

Despite the good news of sensitive, breast-sparing treatments, breast cancer is a disease that arouses women's fears more than any other. There is no simple blueprint for breast cancer treatment, so it is essential for women to learn all they can about the disease. While women once complained that the doctors made all the decisions about breast cancer treatment for them, today women are being given a staggering array of choices—and are finding it difficult to decide among the various treatments.

What is important for you to know if you have a breast problem is that no longer is a disfiguring operation to remove a breast the only answer. Much of the thinking about breast cancer has changed in the last few years. Scientists once thought that breast cancer first spread to nearby tissue and underarm lymph nodes before extending to other parts of the body. Therefore, doctors believed that the spread of breast cancer could be controlled with extensive surgery to remove the breast, chest muscles and underarm lymph nodes. Today scientists think that cancer cells in some cases may break away from the primary tumor in the breast and begin to metastasize even when the disease is in an early stage. Therefore, you may have additional (adjuvant) treatment recommended after your primary breast treatment. Studies have shown that adjuvant treatment, given in addition to the primary treatment in breast cancer, increases chances for long-term survival.

WHAT YOU NEED TO KNOW ABOUT BREAST CANCER

- About 80 percent of breast cancers are diagnosed in women over age 50. Men sometimes get breast cancer, but they are a small minority of cases.
- Many women have one or more risk factors for breast cancer. However, most risks are at such a low level that they only partly explain the numbers of women who have breast cancer.
- Most women have lumpy, uneven breasts that change with age, the monthly menstrual cycle, pregnancy, menopause and taking hormones, such as birth control pills.

WHO IS AT RISK FOR BREAST CANCER?

- Females.
- Over age 40, risk increases with age.
- Family history of breast cancer (mother, sister or daughter), especially if your relative's cancer developed before menopause or affected both breasts.
- Menstrual period started at early age.
- Late age of menopause.
- Never had children or late age at first live birth.
- History of cancer of the endometrium, ovary or colon.
- Higher education and socioeconomic status.
- Personal history of cancer in other breast.
- Postmenopausal obesity.

POSSIBLE RISK FACTORS:

- Estrogen replacement therapy.
- High intake of animal fat.
- Alcohol consumption.

- Mammograms are an important screening test, since they find breast cancer early before there are any symptoms.
- Early diagnosis is very important since most breast cancer found when tumors are small can be cured.
- The two treatment options for early stage breast cancer are the modified radical mastectomy and partial mastectomy (also known as breast-conserving surgery) followed by radiation therapy. A recent reanalysis of the data reaffirmed that survival rates are comparable for these two treatments.
- Adjuvant treatment, either chemotherapy or hormonal therapy, is important in breast cancer. Designed to kill any cancer cells that may have spread, it increases chances for long-term survival.

Who is most likely to get breast cancer?

Women over the age of 50 are most likely to get breast cancer. Women who have a mother, sister, daughter, grandmother or aunt who has had breast cancer and women who have already had breast cancer in one breast are also at increased risk. White women and women with higher incomes are more likely to get the disease, as are women who had their first period at an early age, have menopause at a late age, women who deliver their children later in life or who remain childless, and postmenopausal women who are overweight. There is evidence suggesting that women who eat a diet high in fat, who drink alcohol or who take estrogen replacements may have an increased risk of breast cancer.

SYMPTOMS OF BREAST CANCER

- A lump or thickening in the breast or under the arm.
- A change in the size or shape of the breast.
- Discharge from the nipple.
- A change in the color or feel of the skin of the breast or the skin around the nipple; this may be dimpling, puckering or scaliness of the skin.
- Other changes in skin color or texture, such as "orange peel" skin.
- Swelling, redness or feeling of heat in the breast.

What kind of doctor should I see if I have signs of breast cancer?

If you have a lump or notice any of the other symptoms, you should first see the doctor or nurse who normally takes care of you—your internist, family practitioner, gynecologist or nurse practitioner. Your doctor will order whatever tests are necessary to determine whether or not your symptom is actually cancer or will refer you to a specialist for further testing.

MAJOR DECISION-MAKING POINTS IN BREAST CANCER

- You find a lump or another symptom yourself or your mammogram shows a potential problem.
- Your biopsy shows you have cancer.
- You need to make a choice about the type of operation—breast-conserving surgery with radiation therapy or mastectomy.
- You need to decide whether to have reconstructive surgery after mastectomy.
- You are told you need adjuvant treatment.

What kinds of treatments are used for breast cancer?

Generally, four major kinds of treatment are recommended, alone or with one another: surgery, taking out the cancer in an operation; radiation therapy, using high-dose x-rays to kill the cancer cells; chemotherapy, using drugs to kill cancer cells; and hormone therapy, using hormones to stop the cells from growing. Biological therapy, using your body's immune system to fight cancer, bone marrow transplants and peripheral stem cell support are being studied as treatments for breast cancer. It is important for you to be a part of this decision-making process since in many cases more than one kind of treatment will be available for your stage of disease.

RISKS AND CAUSES

How does the breast function?

Your breast is a very complicated organ. It is made up of glands (or lobules) that make milk, channels (ducts) that connect glands to the nipple, fibrous connective tissue and fat. The breast is made up of fifteen to twenty sections called lobes, each with many smaller lobules. Your muscles lie underneath the breast and cover your ribs. Each month, before and during menstruation, changes, such as swelling, tenderness, pain and even lumps, may occur in your breasts.

Do most women have "lumpy" breasts?

Women's breasts come in all sizes and shapes. Most women's breasts are lumpy and uneven, especially in women under 35 years old. Sometimes, especially right before a menstrual period, they feel swollen and tender. Women's breasts also change because of age, pregnancy, menopause, or taking birth control pills or other hormones. By doing a breast self-exam every month, you will learn what is normal for your breasts and will be more likely to notice when something feels different.

If I have lumpy breasts, am I at a higher risk to get breast cancer?

At one time, doctors used to refer to women with lumpy breasts as having fibrocystic disease or benign breast disease or fibrocystic changes. They believed that these women were at a higher risk for developing breast cancer. Doctors now find that 70 percent of the women with such changes who have been biopsied have little increased risk of developing cancer. Of the remaining group, about 5 percent are diagnosed with atypical hyperplasia, with both excessive cell growth (hyperplasia) and cells that are not normal (atypia). These women have a moderately increased risk of getting breast cancer. The other 25 percent show signs only of excessive cell growth, called hyperplasia, and have a slightly increased risk of having breast cancer. Women with intraductal papilloma and sclerosing adenosis are included in this last group.

What is my personal risk of getting breast cancer?

One woman in eight will develop breast cancer in her lifetime—this is the average lifetime risk assuming you live to age 85. Your risk is different at different times in your life. If you are between the ages of 35 and 45, your risk is one in 100. If you are 50 to 60 years old, your risk is roughly one in 50.

Do women with inverted nipples have a greater chance of developing breast cancer?

No, not if this is your normal condition. Inverted nipples are subject to infection if not kept clean and dry, but there does not seem to be a relationship between inverted nipples and breast cancer. However, if your nipple is normally erect and retracts—or if you see dimpling or puckering in your breast—you should see the doctor to have it checked.

lymph nodes
and fat
under armpit
(axilla)

chest muscle

mammary lobes

nipple

milk ducts

fat body
of breast

chest muscle

Breast

What causes breast cancer?

Scientists do not know what causes breast cancer and cannot explain why one person gets the disease while another does not. Breast cancer also does not spread from one person to another, and cannot be caught from another person.

Can blows or injuries to the breast cause breast cancer?

No, bumping, bruising or touching the breast does not cause breast cancer. Such injuries often draw attention to a lump in the breast, even though the lump is not a result of the injury.

Is breast cancer inherited?

A small proportion may be. If your mother, grandmother, aunts or sisters had breast cancer before menopause, especially if it occurred with another related cancer, such as cancer of the ovary, or if it was in both breasts, you are more likely to develop the disease than women with no family history of the disease. If you are at higher risk, you should be checked regularly by a doctor who specializes in breast diseases. You may also wish to see a genetic counselor.

What is the Li-Fraumeni syndrome?

This is a rare, inherited cancer syndrome found by scientists in 1990. It is due to an alteration of a gene, called p53, that ordinarily controls normal cell growth. If this gene is damaged, cancer may occur. If you have this syndrome in your family, you inherit a predisposition for certain cancers, including breast cancer. There are also other genes under study that might influence cancer risk. However, more work must be done to identify the crucial genes and to characterize them before scientists can gain an understanding of an inherited predisposition for breast cancer in families. For more information, see Chapter 9, "New Advances and Investigational Trials."

What is preventive mastectomy?

Preventive mastectomy—sometimes referred to by the doctor as a prophylactic mastectomy—is the removal of one or both breasts to reduce the risk of cancer. Some women who have a very high risk for cancer choose this alternative, such as a woman who has had several biopsies or has close relatives who have had breast cancer before menopause. Some women who have had cancer in one breast and have many lumps in the other breast or women who have had several surgical biopsies on one breast, all of which have been noncancerous, may also decide to have this operation.

Are there reasons against having a preventive mastectomy?

There is some controversy about the advisability of this procedure, even for high-risk women. You should know that in most women who have had this operation, no cancer has been found in the breasts that have been removed. In addition, some breast tissue is left behind when a mastectomy is done, so there is no guarantee that you will be free of cancer. Most doctors will recommend that you perform monthly breast examination and have checkups every three months instead of having this operation. If you are considering a preventive mastectomy, you should discuss the procedure, reconstructive surgery, possible complications and follow-up care with your doctor and a plastic surgeon. You may want to get a second opinion and you would be wise to request a consultation with a genetic counseling service affiliated with a university medical school. Furthermore, you may wish to talk with someone who has had a preventive mastectomy before you make this decision. You need to study the pros and cons carefully before you decide.

Can breast feeding cause or prevent breast cancer?

For many years, it was thought that nursing helped to immunize women against breast cancer. Later studies seemed to indicate that women who nursed were more prone to cancer. The most recent analysis found that the longer mothers breastfeed and the younger they begin, the more they lower their risk of getting cancer before menopause.

Do birth control pills cause breast cancer?

Several studies have been conducted on this subject, with conflicting results. Some studies show an increased risk of developing breast cancer among women under age 45 who used the birth control pills for long or short periods of time at a relatively young age, generally before age 25, or before their first full-term pregnancy. Others showed that women who have not had children, women who used certain high progesterone combinations of birth control pills and women with a family history of breast cancer were at increased risk. It is not known whether the differences found in the studies are due to chance, to differences in the types of birth control pills or to some undetected factor. While the relationship between birth control pills and breast cancer is still under study, if you have used the pills for a long time, began use at an early age, have a family or personal history of breast cancer or a personal history of benign breast disease, you should discuss the use of birth control pills with your doctor.

Does estrogen replacement therapy cause breast cancer?

The association between hormonal replacement therapy, either estrogen or a combination of estrogen and progestin, is not clear. There is a controversy in the medical profession about whether the benefits of estrogen replacement, such as reduction in cardiovascular disease and osteoporosis, outweigh the risks. A study, carried out by the National Cancer Institute, of premenopausal women who had taken estrogen for twenty years or more showed a 50 percent increase in risk of developing breast cancer compared with women who had not taken it. A number of other studies support this association. A Swedish study of over 23,000 women who had used replacement hormones, both estrogen and estrogen-progestin combinations, showed they had about a 10 percent higher incidence of breast cancer than expected. Additional studies are underway to further study estrogen replacement therapy, its benefits and its risks. Women who have had breast cancer are usually advised not to take replacement therapy. You should discuss the question of hormone replacement therapy, along with how long you should use it, with your doctor.

Does diet play a role in breast cancer?

Research findings, especially of large population groups, indicate that diet may be a possible factor in breast cancer, but at this time these epidemiologic studies have not yet been supported by stronger case control studies. However, in areas of the world where breast cancer is common, diets are high in fat and animal protein. Americans, for instance, consume three times as much fat and more animal protein than the Japanese, and have proportionately more breast cancer. When Japanese women move to the United States, their rate of breast cancer begins to rise and continues in each generation until the rate approaches that of American women. In addition, postmenopausal women who are overweight have an increased risk of developing breast cancer. The National Cancer Institute and the American Cancer Society both recommend cutting total fat intake to less than 30 percent of calories. There are research studies under way to determine whether reducing the amount of fat eaten by women at high risk for breast cancer will affect the number of breast cancer cases.

Does drinking alcohol cause breast cancer?

There are some studies that suggest that women who drink alcohol may have a slightly higher risk for breast cancer, although the evidence is weak. The risk seems to go up with the amount of alcohol consumed.

If I have lobular cancer in situ, am I at higher risk for getting cancer in the other breast?

If you have lobular cancer in situ, you are at higher risk for getting an invasive cancer in both breasts.

Do men ever get breast cancer?

Yes. However, it is uncommon, with only 1,000 new cases diagnosed each year as compared to 181,000 new cases for women. The data on this rare cancer are limited but it seems to have similar risk factors as does female breast cancer. Most occur in middle age or older, with the most common kind being infiltrating ductal carcinoma. Male breast cancers are usually found in a more advanced stage than are female breast cancers. The majority of cases are estrogen receptor positive. Men also can develop Paget's disease and inflammatory carcinoma.

What are the symptoms of male breast cancer?

A painless lump, usually discovered by the man himself, is by far the most common first symptom. Nipple discharge, nipple retraction and a lump under the arm are also symptoms commonly seen in male breast cancer. Diagnosis and staging are the same as for women.

Is breast cancer in men treated differently from that in women?

The treatments are similar to those used for women: surgery, radiation and chemotherapy, depending on the stage of disease, because male breast cancer shares a similar natural history with female breast cancer. Modified radical mastectomy is the usual surgery, since saving the breast is not an issue in males. However, lumpectomy, with removal of some lymph nodes under the arm, can be done if the patient is unable to undergo extensive surgery. Metastatic breast cancer involves hormonal treatment, with tamoxifen, or the removal of hormone-producing organs.

What is the Breast Cancer Prevention Trial?

This study, being run in the United States and Canada, will determine whether taking an antiestrogen drug (tamoxifen) for five years will prevent breast cancer from developing in women who are at increased risk for the disease. The study is enrolling 16,000 healthy higher-risk women, half of whom will receive tamoxifen and half of whom will receive a placebo (an inactive pill that looks like tamoxifen). Women who are 60 years of age or older or younger women who have a combination of other risk factors are eligible for the trial. If you wish to learn more about this trial, call the Cancer Information Service (1-800-4-CANCER).

MAMMOGRAMS, BREAST EXAMS AND BREAST SELF-EXAMINATION

How often should I check my breasts for cancer?

There are some general guidelines. First, you should do breast self-examination every month, starting with your teenage years. Second, you should have the basic screening exams—a breast exam by a doctor or a nurse and a mammogram. Both are necessary. Third, if you have had breast cancer, or if your mother or sister has had breast cancer, you need to be under the care of a doctor who specializes in breast cancer, with your screening schedule tailored to your specific needs.

At what age should I start having a mammogram and a breast exam by a doctor or nurse?

Both the American Cancer Society and the National Cancer Institute agree that after the age of 50, you should have a breast exam by a physician or nurse and a mammogram every year. However, there is some controversy as to when to begin these tests. The American Cancer Society recommends that you start these two screening tests at age 40 and have them every one to two years between the ages of 40 and 49. The National Cancer Institute does not recommend for or against screening women age 40–49 but suggests you discuss mammograms with your doctor.

Where in the breast does most cancer develop?

About half of all breast cancers develop in the upper outer portion of the breast, the part of the breast closest to the underarm. The second most common site is the area beneath the nipple. Breast cancer is more often found in the left than in the right breast.

Are there standards for mammography facilities?

As a result of the 1992 Mammography Quality Standards Act passed by Congress, all medical facilities that perform and interpret mammography tests must be certified by the Food and Drug Administration (FDA). Under these regulations mammography facilities must be certified by an accrediting body approved by the FDA and comply with the following:

- The personnel who perform mammography and physicians who interpret the mammograms must be certified or licensed and have adequate training and experience.

SIZE OF BREAST TUMORS FOUND BY MAMMOGRAPHY AND SELF–EXAM

MAMMOGRAM

⅛ inch
found by regular
mammogram

¼ inch
found by first
mammogram

SELF-EXAM

½ inch
found by women who do
regular breast self–exam

1 inch
found by women who do
occasional breast
self–exam

1½ inches
found by women untrained
in breast self–exam

- All certified facilities must be inspected annually by federal inspectors or state inspectors working under contract to the FDA.
- Equipment must be specifically designated for mammography and monitored closely to ensure proper radiation levels.
- Facilities must set up quality assurance programs to ensure that mammograms are as clear as possible and that positive results are followed up properly.
- Mammography and other patient records must be retained for five years.

How much radiation will I receive when I get my mammogram?

The federal government has set standards that limit the amount of radiation used in mammograms—one-tenth of a rad per two views for one breast. The machines in most facilities deliver a lower dose than this. However, the amount needed depends on several factors. For instance, if your breasts are dense, they may require a higher dose to get a clear image. You need to be sure that you are in an institution that has good equipment, good technology and expert technicians. These will assure quality mammograms with the lowest possible doses of radiation.

Does it hurt to have a mammogram done?

When you have a mammogram, your breast must be compressed between two flat plates in order to get a good picture. While most women feel uncomfortable while this is being done, it lasts only for a few seconds. It is a good idea to schedule your mammogram after your menstrual period, when your breasts are less likely to be as tender. Those few women for whom mammography is very painful should discuss the problem with the technologist and the radiologist before the mammogram is done.

What preparations are necessary before having my mammogram?

On the day of the examination, you may be asked not to use any deodorant, perfume, powders, ointment or preparation of any sort in the underarm area or on your breasts. Also, it is more convenient to wear a blouse or sweater with a skirt or slacks, since you will be asked to undress to the waist for the examination.

What is digital mammography?

Digital mammography, a technique that is still being studied, records x-ray images in computer code instead of placing them on film. Using computer software, the radiologist enhances subtle variations in the image, making tumors easier to spot. Digital mammograms also can be sent electronically (called telemammography), allowing consultation with experts. It is expected that, in the future, digital mammography may help improve mammograms, especially for those with dense breast tissue.

What is contour mammography?

Contour mammography is done with a special type of equipment that makes the exam more comfortable, photographs more breast tissue and uses lower doses of radiation.

What does a mammogram show?

Mammograms are x-rays of the breast. You will usually have two taken of each of your breasts, one from above and one from a side angle. A mammogram can show a lump as early as two years before it can be felt. The lump that cannot be felt is usually smaller than one than can be felt. Also, if it is cancer, it usually has not spread and is usually curable. It is also important to do a monthly breast self-examination, and have a doctor or a nurse examine your breasts each year, because some changes, including lumps that can be felt, **may not** show up on a mammogram.

Are mammograms difficult to interpret?

The radiologist looks for unusual shadows, clusters of white specks, distortions, special patterns of tissue density, any mass and its shape, and the differences between the images of the two breasts. The radiologist must have experience in interpreting these different areas, which can be difficult, depending on the size, shape and density of your breasts. For instance, mammograms of younger women are more difficult to interpret because their tissue is more dense. As you grow older, your breasts become less dense. It is important that your mammogram is "read" by a radiologist who is an expert in this field.

Will the radiologist compare my mammograms from year to year?

It is essential for the radiologist to be able to compare earlier mammograms with new ones, in order to evaluate the areas that look suspicious. If you change the place where you have your mammograms taken or you move, be sure to ask your radiologist for your films so they can be put on file. They are an important part of your health record that cannot be replaced.

Should I have a mammogram if I have had a breast implant?

If you have had a breast implant after you have had surgery for breast cancer, you should check with your doctor to find out whether you need to have a mammogram on that side. If you have had implants for other reasons, you should talk with the professionals at the facility to make sure that they are experienced in doing mammography in women with implants. There are special techniques which must be used, both in taking the x-rays and in reading them.

What special mammography techniques need to be used if I have had a silicone implant?

First of all, silicone implants are extremely dense on x-rays, so they can block the view of the tissues that are behind them. The breast needs to be positioned in certain ways in order to detect any abnormal areas. Secondly, the technician needs to take special care to avoid rupturing the implant when compressing the breasts. Lastly, reading these mammograms is more difficult. You must be sure that the radiologist has had experience in interpreting mammograms in implant patients. Unless it is done properly, the screening may be inadequate and cancers missed.

How much does a screening mammogram cost?

It depends on where you live and the facility you are using. Most mammograms used for screening cost between $100 and $150. Remember that high cost does not always mean high quality. Many insurance companies cover all or part of the cost of screening mammograms. For women 65 and older, Medicare will pay for a part of this cost once every two years.

WHEN YOU FIND A SYMPTOM OR THERE IS A PROBLEM ON YOUR MAMMOGRAM

What should I do if I find a lump in my breast?

First of all, examine your other breast to see if it feels the same. If it does, what you are feeling is probably a normal part of your breast. You should make sure, however, that you mention it to your doctor. If the lump does not go away after your period, see your doctor. If you are past menopause and you find a new lump or a thickening in your breast, you should see your doctor. Most often, the problems are not breast cancer, but only a doctor can tell for sure.

QUESTIONS TO ASK YOUR DOCTOR IF YOU HAVE A SUSPICIOUS LUMP IN YOUR BREAST

- What does the lump feel like?
- What do you think it is?
- Will I need to get a mammogram? What will it show?
- Who gets the report of my mammogram? How long will it be before you let me know the results?
- What other tests should I have? How will these tests be done? Where will I go to get these tests? Will these tests have any side effects?
- How long will it take to get the results of each of these tests? What will they show?

What is a cyst?

A cyst is a sac filled with fluid. It can be as tiny as a pinhead or as big as an egg. Sometimes a cyst appears and disappears practically overnight. Cysts are caused by a buildup of tissue related to the changes that normally take place in the breast during each menstrual cycle. They are usually found in both breasts. Cysts tend to get larger toward the end of the menstrual cycle and shrink or disappear after it. These changes may be exaggerated if the menstrual cycle becomes irregular, particularly if there is a long time between periods. You are more likely to develop cysts as you approach menopause. If you take estrogen after menopause you may also develop cysts. Cysts are rarely cancerous.

Can a doctor tell the difference between cancer and cysts by feeling them?

Sometimes. Cysts feel different from cancerous lumps. A large cyst near the surface of the breast feels smooth, slightly squishy and may be somewhat movable. Cancers are usually harder and more irregular in shape and tend to be more fixed. If the cyst is deep in the breast, it cannot be felt but may be found through a mammogram. One way to determine whether or not it is a cyst or cancer is to do needle aspiration.

Will ultrasound be used if I have a cyst?

Ultrasound is most useful in telling the difference between solid masses and cysts, especially in younger women whose breasts are very dense. It may also be used for pregnant women or a woman who has been recently nursing whose breasts are extremely dense. The doctor may order an ultrasound if your cyst does not disappear when the fluid is taken out (aspirated). Some cysts are very small or have thick walls or may have thick fluid that does not flow through the needle. Ultrasound does not, however, show microcalcifications or identify very small cancers, so it is not used for general screening.

If the doctor finds a solid tumor on the ultrasound does it mean I have breast cancer?

No. Sometimes the doctor will find a benign tumor in the breast—that is one that does not have any cancer cells in it. These tumors, called fibroadenomas, are harmless growths. They are not usually found in women who have had menopause, unless they are taking estrogen. However, the only way to know whether the solid tumor has cancer cells in it is to have a biopsy.

Are there other lumps in the breast that are not cancer?

Yes, there are several other conditions that you might hear the doctor talk about, such as fat necrosis, sclerosing adenosis, intraductal papilloma, mastitis, and mammary duct ectasia. Some of these conditions, such as fat necrosis, sclerosing adenosis and intraductal papilloma, will require a biopsy to make sure the lumps are not cancerous.

Are most breast lumps cancerous?

No, they are not. With all the information on breast cancer that has been written in the past few years, it is important for you to know that chances that a lump in your breast is **not** cancer are really excellent. In fact, eight out of ten lumps are found to be benign. However, it also is important to know that lumps found in postmenopausal women are more likely to be cancerous than those found in women who are still menstruating. Remember that about 80 percent of breast cancers are diagnosed in women over the age of 50.

What if my mammogram does not show the lump I can feel in my breast?

If you have a lump that does not go away, it needs to be tested further and biopsied, even if it **does not** show on the mammogram. About 10 percent of mammograms do not show lumps even when they are there. These are called "false-negative" results.

A lump should not be ignored just because it cannot be seen on a mammogram. About 10 percent of mammograms do not show lumps even when they are there.

Is discharge from the nipples of the breast a cause for alarm?

It is wise to call any discharge from the nipples to the attention of your doctor. If the discharge is pink or bloody or comes on suddenly and is from only one breast, you need to have a doctor look at it immediately to determine its cause. Some young women may have a slight clear or yellowish nipple discharge at the time of menstruation. This is not unusual and should not cause alarm but should be mentioned to the doctor. Breast discharges may occur prior to menopause when other changes are taking place in the body and should be checked by the doctor to determine if there is a problem. Some of the fluid can be put on a slide and analyzed.

Are any new tests being used to detect and diagnose breast cancer?

There are some studies being done to look at the use of new technologies in this area but they are not a standard part of testing at the present time. Positron emission tomography (PET), magnetic resonance imaging (MRI), and laser scans, along with ultrasound and CT scans, all seem to have some potential when added to mammography for diagnosing breast cancer. PET, for instance, may be useful as a problem-solving tool to detect tumors in women whose screening mammograms do not reveal them. MRI can show tumors in breasts that are dense or may tell the difference between fibrocystic disease and cancer. They may also play a role in detecting cancers in women who have silicone implants. Laser beams along with

---

TESTS THAT MAY BE USED TO DIAGNOSE BREAST CANCER

- Complete history and physical exam.
- Careful inspection of breasts and lymph node areas.
- Mammography.
- Ultrasound.
- Aspiration biopsy to remove fluid from cyst.
- Fine needle aspiration for cytology.
- Needle biopsy.
- Stereotactic biopsy.
- Mammographic localization with biopsy.
- Excisional or incisional biopsy.
- Chest x-rays and blood tests.
- Estrogen and progesterone receptor tests.
- MRI or CT scan.

a camera to record the image are also being used. Ultrasound can often show whether a lump is solid or filled with fluid. CT scans sometimes locate tumors that are hard to find. However, since these tests are more expensive than mammography—PET, for instance, costs about $1,500 per test—they cannot be used for mass screening, but may become useful tests for diagnosing the disease.

Are thermography, transillumination, microwaves, lasers or monoclonal antibodies being used to diagnose breast cancer?

Although research has been done with thermography, transillumination, microwaves, lasers and monoclonal antibodies, none has been shown to be useful, either in screening or in diagnosing breast cancer.

What is meant by the term *calcifications*?

Calcifications, often called microcalcifications, are tiny specks of calcium in the breast. When these specks form a certain pattern it is called a cluster. A cluster signifies to a doctor that the tissues surrounding the calcium specks may be cancerous. If the pattern is not clear, the doctor may advise you to have another mammogram in three to six months. If the pattern of calcifications looks suspicious to the doctor, you will have a biopsy. About half of the cancers detected by mammography are seen as these clusters on the mammogram.

What will the doctor do if he has any doubts about my lump or suspicious cluster of cells?

If the doctor has any doubts, further studies will be suggested. These may include more mammograms, or one of several procedures to determine whether or not the lump is cancer. Remind yourself again that eight times out of ten it usually turns out that the lump is **not** malignant.

What is a diagnostic mammogram?

This is a mammogram done when you have specific symptoms, such as a lump or a thickening, or when an irregularity is found on your screening mammogram. The technician will take different views, from different angles. The area in question may be magnified to allow the doctor to see the details more clearly so that an accurate diagnosis can be made.

Can the mammogram tell whether or not cancer is present?

Mammograms indicate to a trained doctor a suspicion that cancer may or may not be present. They can be used by surgeons to locate the site of the tumor and to check if there are additional tumors in the breast. However, they should not be used alone to definitely tell whether there is cancer in the breast. Only the pathologist, looking at cells under a microscope, can tell whether they are cancerous. In addition, even a negative mammogram **does not** guarantee that there is no cancer in the breast.

WHAT HAPPENS WHEN A PROBLEM IS FOUND ON A MAMMOGRAM OR THERE IS A BREAST SYMPTOM	
Problem is compared with a prior mammogram	This is why it is important to make sure your mammograms are kept on file and sent to your new doctor when you change doctors.
Additional mammograms or tests done	The doctor may order another mammogram or different views. Ultrasound may be done to see if lump is solid or filled with fluid.
Stereotactic fine needle biopsy or needle core biopsy done	These types of biopsies are used to take fluid out of cyst or to take cells out of breast, after numbing breast. Usually used if the doctor suspects that a problem may be present. May be followed by excisional or incisional biopsy.
Excisional or incisional biopsy done	If the doctor is highly suspicious that a problem is present, an excisional or incisional biopsy may be done immediately rather than the stereotactic fine needle or core biopsy.
Second opinion consultation	Many women, unless their diagnosis was made in a center that has multidisciplinary opinions, decide they wish to get a second opinion at this time.

What kind of examination will the doctor do if I have symptoms?

The doctor will ask about your health and medical history and will do a physical examination. In addition, the doctor will carefully feel the lump and tissue around it (called palpation by the medical community). If you have had a recent mammogram, it will be compared with ones done in the past. A new mammogram or additional views may be needed. Sometimes a doctor will order an ultrasound, also called a sonogram, which can show whether the lump is filled with fluid or is solid. Lumps that are filled with fluid are usually not cancer. Depending on the results of these tests, you may need to have a biopsy done.

What happens after either the doctor or I find a breast lump?

There are numbers of ways in which your case can proceed. This is an important decision point. You must prepare yourself to make a decision about how you want to proceed if, after the examination, the doctor suggests there is a possibility that the lump may be cancer. You need to decide, for example, whether you wish to have a second opinion on the kind of treatment you will have.

Is a second opinion important in breast cancer?

In our view, a second opinion is important in cancer because it is such a complex disease. In breast cancer, there are many options and differences of opinion. Unless you are at a comprehensive breast center or a medical center where you are getting a multidisciplinary consultation, a second opinion would probably be useful for you to help you think through your choices.

What does a multidisciplinary consultation consist of?

You will be seen by a team of specialists, usually at the same time or at least during the same visit. The team will include a surgeon, radiation oncologist and a medical oncologist. You should be told by the team what treatment would be best, in its opinion, for your kind of breast cancer. Some women use this team for a second opinion only, while others wish to use it for their entire treatment. Sometimes the team may also include other members, such as a diagnostic radiologist, plastic surgeon, pathologist, oncology nurse and a social worker.

HOW BIOPSIES ARE DONE

QUESTIONS TO ASK YOUR DOCTOR BEFORE YOU HAVE A BIOPSY

- What type of biopsy will I have? Exactly what will you be doing?
- How long will the biopsy take? Will I be awake? Will it hurt?
- Where will you do the biopsy? Will I be able to drive myself home after I have it done?
- How much tissue will be taken out? Will the biopsy leave a scar? Will it change the shape of my breast?
- How soon will I know the results of the biopsy?
- Will you be arranging for estrogen and progesterone tests?

How will the doctor determine whether or not the growth is breast cancer?

The only certain way to tell whether any growth is cancerous is for the doctor to do a biopsy—removing all or part of the lump and sending it to the laboratory to be analyzed. You may have one of several kinds of biopsies: needle, incisional, excisional, stereotactic, and needle localization.

What is needle aspiration?

The doctor uses a long thin needle to draw out any fluid that may be present in the lump. Once the fluid is gone, the cyst collapses. If the lump is solid, the doctor may remove some cells with the needle and send them to the laboratory for further testing. Needle aspiration, also called aspiration or fine needle aspiration, is usually done in the office and is relatively painless.

What is needle localization?

If the doctor sees a definite area of change on your mammogram which cannot be felt manually, a surgical biopsy may be necessary. The area that is to be removed must be pinpointed and marked by the radiologist before the surgeon can perform the biopsy. This procedure is called needle localization or mammographic localization with biopsy.

How is needle localization done?

Using your mammogram as a guide, a needle is placed in the breast with its tip at the abnormal spot. The wire is placed through the needle. The needle is removed, leaving the wire in place. The top of the wire may be taped to your breast so that it won't move. This part of the procedure is usually done in the radiology department. You then will be brought to wherever the surgery will be done.

How big is the wire?

The wire is about the size of a strand of hair, with a tiny hook at the tip holding it in place in the breast. During the biopsy, this wire guides the surgeon, who will cut along the wire and follow it inside your breast to the suspicious area which cannot be seen with the naked eye. The surgeon will remove the area along with the marker wire.

Is needle localization painful?

Not usually. Before placing the needle, the doctor numbs your skin with a painkiller. The skin of the breast is sensitive to pain but the tissue inside the breast is not. Many women say the insertion of the

TYPES OF PROCEDURES TO DETERMINE IF A LUMP OR SUSPICIOUS CLUSTER IS CANCER

TYPE	DESCRIPTION
Fine needle aspiration	Uses fine-gauge needle to take fluid out of cyst or to take cells out of lump. Usually done in doctor's office or outpatient area of hospital. No scar. May be followed by excisional or incisional biopsy.
Core needle biopsy	Uses larger needle with special cutting edge to take a core of tissue out of breast. Uses local anesthesia. Not used for very small lumps. Usually done in doctor's office or outpatient area of hospital. Usually no scar.
Needle localization; may also be called **localization biopsy** or **mammographic localization with biopsy**	Two-part procedure. Fine needle containing a wire is put into breast so that tip rests in area of change seen on mammogram. Second mammogram confirms needle is in right place. Surgeon takes out lump or cluster in area where wire is. Fine needle portion done in radiology department, with surgery in operating room with local anesthesia. Scar depends upon amount of tissue taken out.
Stereotactic biopsy or **stereotactic localization biopsy**	Patient may be sitting up or lying on table with hole in it to allow breast to hang down. Computer plans exact position for needle. Either fluid or cells can be taken from lump. Local anesthesia may be needed. No scar.
Incisional	Takes out part of the lump to be examined by a pathologist. Uses local or general anesthesia. Usually done in outpatient department of hospital. Operation lasts less than one hour, followed by an hour or two in the recovery room. Small scar. Since the advent of fine needle and core biopsy, rarely used for breast cancer.
Excisional	Takes out the entire lump or the suspicious area. Used for lumps that are small. Uses local or general anesthesia. Usually done in the outpatient department of a hospital or a surgical center. Operation lasts less than one hour, followed by an hour or two in the recovery room. May change the shape of your breast, depending on size of lump, where located and how much additional tissue is removed. Scar depends on type of surgery done.

needle is painless. Others find it rather uncomfortable You may feel some tugging if the needle needs to be moved into a different position.

What is a stereotactic biopsy?

The stereotactic biopsy, sometimes called a stereotactic needle-guided biopsy, is a new procedure used when something is found on the mammogram that cannot be felt. It can be used to tell whether the cells are benign or malignant, without leaving a scar. It takes place in the radiology department. You may be sitting up. Or you may be lying on an examining table that has an opening in the front end, so that the breast hangs downward. You will be given local anesthesia to numb your breast. The radiologist will use imaging equipment to position the needle. Both aspiration and core biopsy samples can be taken. If a surgical biopsy is needed, a small hook wire is inserted into the area where the samples are taken.

When is an excisional biopsy recommended?

There are several circumstances when a doctor may want to do an excisional biopsy, including: if the ultrasound shows the lump to be solid, if the results of the other procedures are not definitive enough to allow the doctor to make a diagnosis, or if the doctor, when looking at the mammogram, becomes highly suspicious that the problem is cancer.

What kind of doctor will perform a breast biopsy?

The biopsy will be done by a surgeon. You need to be sure that the surgeon is skilled in performing breast biopsies.

What should I expect as side effects from a biopsy?

It depends on what kind of biopsy is done. In general, however, you can except that you might have some mild pain that can be relieved by pain medicine, that you may need to wear a soft bra for 24 hours for support, that you might not be able to use your arm on the side of the biopsy for a few days, and that the area where the biopsy was done will be tender for a while. You may also have some bruising and an indentation in your breast where the biopsy was done. However, within a month or two it should fill in, unless you have additional surgery at the same site. If you have had stitches, they will probably be taken out in a week.

Will I have to go to the hospital for the excisional biopsy?

It depends on your doctor and the kind of procedure being done. It is usually done on an outpatient basis, either in a surgical center or in a hospital. It is usually done with local anesthesia and you will go home the same day.

Is the biopsy ever done as part of the operation for breast removal?

There are some doctors and some women who prefer to do the biopsy as part of the mastectomy. If it is done in this manner, it is known as a one-step procedure. If the biopsy is done separately, it is known as a two-step procedure.

Is there an advantage to having a two-step procedure rather than a one-step procedure?

There are some differences between the two procedures that you need to be aware of. Approximately 80 percent of the women who have a suspicious lump biopsied will not have cancer. The two-step procedure allows you to have the biopsy, go home and find out the results. If it turns out to be cancer, you will have time to have needed additional tests done. You will be able to have hormonal testing. If you wish, you will be able to get another opinion on what kind of treatment you should have. You will have time to make arrangements at work and at home for your recovery period and time to prepare yourself emotionally for your surgery. In addition, the doctor will be able to read both the frozen-section biopsy and the regular biopsy.

Are there any women for whom the one-step procedure makes sense?

Some women and some doctors prefer the one-step procedure. If you have already decided on your choice of treatment if cancer is found, a one-step procedure may be the right choice for you. It means that you will have only one surgery. You will not have to wait between knowing you have cancer and having the final operation. On the other hand, you will not have the ability to get a second opinion or to have additional tests done. The doctor will use a frozen-section biopsy. There are pros and cons for each choice that you need to investigate before you choose one over the other. This is the kind of decision you need to think about yourself and discuss with your doctor and your family.

What is the difference between a frozen-section biopsy and a regular biopsy?

The main difference is in how much the pathologist can tell about the nature and type of cancer. A full discussion of the two kinds of biopsies is in Chapter 4, ''How Cancers Are Diagnosed.''

If the doctor has found that I have breast cancer, what other tests need to be performed?

If the pathologist looking at your breast cells under the microscope determines they are cancerous, several other tests may be called for. There may be hormonal receptor tests, called estrogen and progesterone receptor tests, done in a special laboratory to show whether the cancer is sensitive to hormones. The doctor usually orders x-rays of the lungs and blood tests. A bone scan may be done. Since breast cancer tends to spread to the lungs, liver, or bones, these tests may be required to find out whether the cancer has spread. The additional testing is important to help the doctor recommend what kind of treatment should be done.

What is an estrogen receptor test and how is it done?

This is a test to measure for protein on a cell to which estrogen will attach. Preparations for the test must be done before the tumor is removed, because it must be tested immediately after its removal from the breast. The doctor sends a sample of the tumor (about one gram) to the laboratory where the measurement is done. If chemotherapy is being planned to shrink the tumor before the operation, the test should be done before chemotherapy treatments are started, since chemotherapy may alter its accuracy.

What is a progesterone receptor test?

It is similar to the estrogen receptor test, but it measures the progesterone receptors.

Why are estrogen and progesterone receptor tests important?

They are a means of predicting whether the cancer was dependent on hormones for growth and whether or not you will respond to hormonal treatment. Scientists believe that changing the normal hormonal environment may affect cancers, such as those in the breast, which may depend on the presence of hormones for their growth. If the tests are positive, the doctor may treat you with hormonal drugs, or, in rare cases, may remove one of your hormone-secreting organs (such as the ovaries, adrenal glands, or pituitary gland). Women who are estrogen-receptor-positive have a 50 to 60 percent chance of responding to hormonal therapy. If you are both estrogen and progesterone-receptor-positive, you have nearly an 80 percent chance of responding to this kind of treatment.

Do most women with breast cancer have positive estrogen receptors?

Yes. Studies show that about two-thirds of all breast cancers are estrogen-receptor-positive (ER+). In addition, about two-thirds of

ER+ cancers are also progesterone-receptor-positive (PR+). Generally women who are past menopause are more likely to be estrogen-receptor-positive, while premenopausal women are more likely to be estrogen-receptor negative (ER−).

Is there more than one type of breast cancer?

There are at least fifteen different varieties. However, over 80 percent of breast cancer starts in the ducts—and is called ductal carcinoma. The next most common (about 12 percent) starts in the lobules and is called lobular carcinoma. The remaining start in the surrounding tissue.

What is meant by the term *infiltrating* or *invasive*?

Infiltrating—sometimes the word *invasive* is used instead of *infiltrating*—means that the cancer has grown outside of the duct or lobule where it started, into the surrounding tissue. You can have infiltrating (or invasive) ductal cancer or infiltrating (or invasive) lobular cancer.

What is inflammatory breast cancer?

This is an uncommon type of breast cancer which often spreads rapidly to other parts of the body. The breast is warm, red and swollen. You may feel a lump in your breast, an enlargement or thickness, discharge from or a pulling back of your nipple or a pain in your breast or nipple. Ridges may appear on the skin, or the breast skin may display a pitted appearance known as *peau d'orange*. Generally, this type of breast cancer is treated with all three types of treatment—chemotherapy, surgery and radiation therapy. Sometimes, the chemotherapy is given first, followed by mastectomy and radiation therapy. The order of the treatment varies.

What is Paget's disease?

Paget's disease is a form of breast cancer that involves the nipple. The tumor is in the ducts under the nipple. The tumor cells grow through the ducts onto the nipple's surface.

Are there any other types of breast cancer?

There are some other cell types of ductal cancer—comedo, medullary, mucinous (colloid), papillary, scirrhous, and tubular. In addition cystosarcoma phyllodes is a rare type of breast cancer.

What is meant by lymph node involvement?

The doctor checks to see whether or not the cancer which started in the breast has spread to the lymph nodes under the arm. The treatment used for breast cancer which has spread to the lymph nodes is different from treatment for localized breast cancer that has not yet begun to spread.

UNDERSTANDING BREAST CANCER OPERATIONS

Probably the most difficult decision is the kind of operation you will have for your breast cancer. You will have several choices. Different doctors use different terms for the same operation, which makes it very confusing. We have described them, using the terms as they are most commonly referred to today. **However, you need to be sure you ask your doctor to explain exactly what is going to be done, how much tissue will be removed and what your breast will look like after the operation.**

QUESTIONS TO ASK YOURSELF BEFORE DECIDING ON A BREAST OPERATION

- How important is it for me to save my breasts?
- Is the tumor of a size and in a position that makes it possible to save my breasts?
- Am I willing to have breast-conserving surgery followed by six weeks of radiation treatment?
- Do I want to get another opinion?
- If I have the breast removed, do I want to have immediate reconstruction?

What choices do I have for surgery?
You may have one of several operations:

- Partial mastectomy—sometimes called breast-conserving surgery, lumpectomy, excisional biopsy, or segmental mastectomy—removes the tumor, and usually some tissue around it.
- Simple mastectomy, sometimes called total mastectomy, which removes the breast.
- Lymph node dissection, which takes out the lymph nodes underneath your arm (usually done in combination with a partial and simple mastectomy).
- Modified radical mastectomy, which removes the breast and lymph nodes.

A radical mastectomy, sometimes called the Halsted radical mastectomy, is rarely performed today.

What is the most common operation for breast cancer?

Today, the most common operation for breast cancer is the modified radical mastectomy, despite studies that have shown that this operation and the breast-conserving surgery followed by radiation therapy are equal in terms of survival. The second most common operation today is the partial or segmental mastectomy (breast-conserving surgery), followed by radiation therapy. This surgery takes out the cancer, some of the breast tissue around it, the lining over the chest muscle and lymph nodes under the arm. This operation is then followed by radiation treatment.

Many women assume that if they have a mastectomy, it means that the doctor will get all of the cancer out of the body. However, scientists now believe that cancer cells may break away from the primary tumor and spread to other parts of the body even when the disease is at an early stage. If the doctor tells you that you can have an operation for breast cancer that can save your breast, a mastectomy will not increase your chances of being cured.

What factors determine whether or not I can have an operation which saves my breast?

If the microcalcifications in your breast are not extensive, or if your tumor is less than four centimeters in diameter and can be totally taken out, you will probably be able to have this kind of operation. Most of the time, breast-conserving surgery is done only for early (Stage I and Stage II) breast cancer. If you have more than one primary tumor in your breast, or if you have extensive microcalcifications on your mammogram, you probably will not be able to have this kind of operation. The doctor will also have to take into account several other factors, such as the size of your breast, the technique used to do the biopsy, the amount of breast tissue that will be taken out along with the tumor and whether or not you are willing to have radiation therapy after the surgery.

What is involved in having breast-conserving surgery?

The doctor will take out the entire tumor along with some of the normal tissue surrounding it, and the lymph nodes under the arm. After two to four weeks of recovery, external radiation will be deliv-

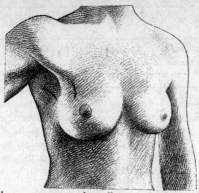

lumpectomy with axillary node dissection

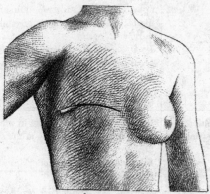

simple mastectomy

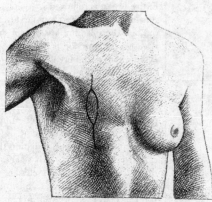

radical mastectomy with skin graft

Examples of breast operation scars

TYPES OF OPERATIONS

TYPE	DESCRIPTION
Partial mastectomy; also called **breast-conserving surgery**, **lumpectomy**, or **wide excision**	The lump in your breast is taken out, along with some of the normal breast tissue around it, to get clear margins. This is followed by radiation therapy to the part of the breast that remains. Survival rates are the same as with the modified radical mastectomy when cancer is treated in its early stages. *Advantages:* If you are large-breasted, most of your breast is preserved. You have a better appearance than with a modified radical mastectomy. There is little possibility of loss of muscle strength. *Disadvantages:* If you have small or medium-size breasts, you will have a noticeable change in your breast shape. You must undergo radiation treatments. If lymph nodes are not taken out, cancer may spread undetected.
Lymph node dissection; also called **axillary lymph node dissection**	Lymph nodes are taken out in the hollow of your armpit. Usually done at the same time as breast operation. *Advantages:* Doctor can check to see if there is cancer in nodes. *Disadvantages:* You have a risk of developing lymphedema.
Total or simple mastectomy	Entire breast is removed. *Advantages:* Your chest muscles are not taken out and there is little loss of arm strength. Breast reconstruction is easier. *Disadvantages:* The breast is removed. This operation is not a common one today.
Modified radical mastectomy	Entire breast, lining over chest muscles and lymph nodes under arm taken out. Usually only the smaller of the two chest muscles taken out. Survival rates are the same as with the partial mastectomy plus radiation therapy when cancer is treated in its early stages. *Advantages:* Your chest muscles are not taken out. You can have breast reconstruction and you can plan it before your operation. *Disadvantages:* Your breast is removed. You have a risk of developing lymphedema.

ered to the entire breast. For some patients, a boost of radiation to the area where the tumor was found will also be needed.

Will my breast look different after I have breast-conserving surgery?
Yes, it will. How different it will look depends upon the size of your breasts and amount of tissue that has been taken out.

Is the breast-conserving surgery done more often in one part of the country than another?
Data from the national data base of the American College of Surgeons and the American Cancer Society show there are great variances in whether you will have breast-conserving surgery (a partial mastectomy) or a modified radical mastectomy depending upon what part of the country you live in. The women who live in New England are most apt to have partial mastectomies (53 percent) while those who live in the eastern south-central region of the country are least likely to have partial mastectomies (18 percent). Moreover, smaller hospitals are less likely to be doing partial mastectomies. These data show that the regional differences are similar to those comparing the use of modified radical mastectomies versus radical mastectomies in the 1970s.

What are the reasons for choosing a modified radical mastectomy instead of breast-conserving surgery?
There are several reasons why you might decide to have a modified radical mastectomy rather than breast-conserving surgery.

- If you have many microcalcifications in different parts of your breast, or if you have tumors in more than one area of your breast.
- If too great a proportion of your breast must be removed either because the tumor is large or your breast is very small.
- If you have a schedule that would not allow you to have radiation therapy every day for five or six weeks; or if suitable medical facilities for radiation treatments are too far away or require extended travel time.
- If you have a prior history of high-dose radiation to the breast area.
- If the tumor is directly beneath the nipple and the surgery would require taking out all or part of the nipple areola complex.
- If you are in your first or second trimester of pregnancy, you would not be able to have breast conservation because you could not have the radiation therapy. (Women in their third

trimester might be able to have the breast-conserving surgery, with the radiation treatments done after delivery.)

In addition, there are some women who believe that taking out the breast means that the cancer is all gone and choose to have a mastectomy for that reason. You need to remember that if the doctor tells you that you could have breast-conserving surgery, a mastectomy will not increase your chances of being cured.

QUESTIONS TO ASK YOUR DOCTOR IF THE BIOPSY SHOWS BREAST CANCER

- How big is the tumor? Where is it in my breast?
- What kind of breast cancer do I have? Is it invasive?
- What do the estrogen and progesterone receptor tests show?
- What other laboratory tests were done on the tumor tissue and what did they show?
- What other tests will need to be done before we decide on the treatment?
- What kind of operation do you recommend? Am I a candidate for breast-conserving surgery?
- Is there another type I should consider?
- What are the pros and cons for each one?
- Will you take out some lymph nodes under my arm? How many? Why? What are the risks and side effects of doing this?
- What will my breast look like after the operation? How much tissue will be taken out? Where will the scar be? How big will it be?
- How will we decide on the operation? How long can I take to make this decision?
- Where can I go for another opinion?

How long can I wait to have my operation for breast cancer?

Most doctors agree that you can delay two to three weeks without any problem. Studies have shown that a short delay between biopsy and treatment will not affect the spread of disease or reduce the chances for successful treatment. Many women want time to think and to get a second opinion on treatment, looking at all the alternatives. For these women, getting all of the necessary information about the extent of the cancer is well worth the time it takes. On the other hand, if you are the kind of person who wants to have it done and over with and feel comfortable with your choice, you should proceed with your treatment.

Are lasers ever used in operating for breast cancer?

Some doctors do use a laser instead of the traditional scalpel in both mastectomy and lesser surgery, feeling that they reduce pain and the length of the hospital stay, but there is no widespread agreement that it has any advantage.

STAGES OF AND TREATMENTS FOR BREAST CANCER

How will the doctor decide on what treatments will be used for my breast cancer?

There are many factors that your doctor will consider in making these decisions, such as the size and location of your tumor, cell type of your cancer, the stage of your disease, size of your breast, your age and menopausal status, and your overall health. In addition, estrogen and progesterone receptor levels, tumor grade (nuclear and histologic), the doctor's experience, and your personal preference will have a role in making these decisions.

Why does the doctor want to find out the stage of my breast cancer?

The most important factor in making the decision about the right treatment for your cancer is to understand the stage of your disease. The stage is based on the size of the tumor and whether the cancer has spread to other organs.

What is meant by tumor grade?

Grading takes into account the structure of the cells and their growth patterns. Histologic grade refers to how much the tumor cells resemble normal cells (called differentiation). The lower the grade, the more the tumor cells resemble normal cells. (Differentiation is discussed in Chapter 3, "What Is Cancer?") Nuclear grade refers to the rate at which the cancer cells in the tumor are dividing to form more cells (called proliferation). Cancer cells that divide more often are faster growing and more aggressive than those that divide less often. The nuclear grade is determined by the percentage of cells that are dividing. Again, the lower the grade the more normal.

What does flow cytometry measure?

Flow cytometry, an instrument with a computer system, measures several features of cells. It can evaluate the amount of DNA, deter-

STAGES OF BREAST CANCER

STAGE	DESCRIPTION
In situ (TIS, N0, M0)	Very early cancer is found in only a few layers of cells. It has not spread to nearby tissues.
Stage I (T1, N0, M0)	Cancer is no bigger than about 1 inch across (2 centimeters) and has not spread outside the breast.
Stage II (T0–3, N0–1, M0)	Cancer is no bigger than about 1 inch across (2 centimeters) but has spread to lymph nodes under arm (axillary lymph nodes); **or** cancer is between 1 and 2 inches across (2 to 5 centimeters). It may or may not have spread to lymph nodes under the arm; **or** cancer is bigger than 2 inches across (5 centimeters) but has not spread to lymph nodes under arm.
Stage IIIA (T0–3, N1–2, M0)	Cancer is less than 2 inches across (5 centimeters) and has spread to lymph nodes under the arm which have grown into each other or into other structures and are attached to them; **or** cancer is bigger than 2 inches across (5 centimeters) and has spread to lymph nodes under arm.
Stage IIIB (T4, any N, MO or any T, N3, M0)	Cancer has spread to tissues near the breast (chest wall, including the ribs and the muscles in the chest); **or** cancer has spread to lymph nodes near collarbone.
Stage IV (any T, any N, M1)	Cancer has spread to other organs of body, most often the bones, lungs, liver or brain.
Inflammatory breast cancer	Rare breast cancer. Breast has red appearance and warmth. Skin may show signs of ridges and wheals or may have pitted appearance. Tends to spread quickly.
Recurrent	Means cancer has come back after it has been treated. May come back in breast, in muscles of chest (chest wall) or in another part of body.

HISTOLOGIC AND NUCLEAR GRADES OF BREAST CANCER

GRADE NUMBER	HISTOLOGIC	NUCLEAR
Grade 1	Well-differentiated cellular features and growth patterns	Cells have low proliferation capacity with well-differentiated tumor nuclei
Grade 2	Intermediate changes in cellular features and growth patterns	Cells have intermediate proliferation capacity with intermediate changes in tumor nuclei
Grade 3	Poorly differentiated cellular features and growth patterns	Cells have high proliferation capacity with poorly differentiated tumor nuclei
Grade 4	Undifferentiated	(No nuclear grade 4)

mining whether tumor cells have too many or too few pairs of chromosomes. If the cells have the expected amount, they are known as diploid tumors. If they have too much or too little DNA, they are known as aneuploid. In addition, flow cytometry can also measure the growth rate of the tumor—the percentage of cells that are dividing at any one time and producing new cancer cells, called the S-phase fraction. Diploid tumors and those with a low S-phase fraction are considered less aggressive. This information is important in deciding treatment, especially for women with breast cancer in whom no cancer was found in the lymph nodes.

Are there any other indicators that doctors use to tell whether a patient will do well with breast cancer treatment?

There is an array of other new "markers" being studied. They include cathepsin-D, NM23, epidermal growth factor, and the c-*erb*B-2 (HER-2-neu) oncogene. These and other markers can tell doctors such things as how fast the cells are growing and how likely the cancer is to spread or recur. Most of the markers are still being studied and refined. They are discussed further in Chapter 9, "New Advances and Investigational Trials."

What is breast cancer in situ?

Breast cancer *in situ* is cancer found at its earliest stage, confined to the place where it started. There are two types: intraductal carci-

TREATMENT CHOICES FOR BREAST CANCER

STAGE	TREATMENT
In situ	*If you have ductal cancer:* Total mastectomy or excisional biopsy followed by radiation therapy. *Clinical trials:* Surgery to remove the cancer followed by radiation therapy. *If you have lobular carcinoma in situ:* Biopsy to take out the cancer, followed by regular mammograms and checkups; **or** total mastectomy on one or both breasts. Lymph nodes under the arm may be taken out. *Clinical trials:* For patients who have not had a mastectomy, use of taxomifen to prevent cancer from recurring.
Stage I	Partial mastectomy followed by radiation therapy; or total mastectomy; or modified radical mastectomy. Lymph nodes under the arm may be removed. Chemotherapy or hormonal therapy may also be given. *Clinical trials:* New chemotherapy drugs, combinations of drugs and new ways of giving chemotherapy.
Stage II	Partial mastectomy and removal of lymph nodes under the arm, followed by radiation therapy; **or** modified radical mastectomy; **or** total mastectomy. Chemotherapy or hormonal therapy may be given following any of the above treatments. In some cases radiation therapy may be given to the chest following mastectomy to reduce the risk of recurrence. Radical mastectomy is used only in special situations. *Clinical trials:* New chemotherapy drugs, combinations of drugs, new ways of giving chemotherapy, elimination of chemotherapy or hormonal therapy for certain patients or breast preservation.
Stage IIIA	Modified radical mastectomy. Some lymph nodes under the arm may be taken out; **or** radical mastectomy. Chemotherapy, sometimes with hormonal drugs, is given after surgery. Radiation therapy may be given before or after surgery. *Clinical trials:* New chemotherapy and hormonal drugs, combinations of drugs, new ways of giving chemotherapy and breast preservation.

(continued)

TREATMENT CHOICES FOR BREAST CANCER *(cont.)*

STAGE	TREATMENT
Stage IIIB	Biopsy, followed by radiation therapy to the breast and lymph nodes. Additional external or implant radiation therapy or mastectomy may follow the radiation therapy. Chemotherapy or hormonal therapy may be given before or after surgery and radiation therapy. *Clinical trials:* New chemotherapy drugs and biological therapy, new combinations of drugs and new ways of giving chemotherapy.
Stage IV	Biopsy followed by radiation therapy or mastectomy. Hormonal therapy or chemotherapy. *Clinical trials:* New chemotherapy and hormonal drugs and new combinations of drugs or biologic agents.
Inflammatory breast cancer	Combination of chemotherapy, hormonal therapy and radiation therapy. Surgery to remove the breast. Treatment is usually similar to that for Stage IIIB or IV breast cancer.
Recurrent	*If it has come back in only one place:* Surgery or radiation therapy. *If it has come back in more than one place:* Chemotherapy or hormonal therapy; **or** radiation therapy to help relieve pain due to the spread of cancer to bones and other places. *Clinical trials:* New chemotherapy drugs, new hormonal drugs, biological therapy or bone marrow transplants.

noma *in situ* and lobular carcinoma *in situ*. With the increasing numbers of women being screened with mammography, more breast cancers are being found at this early stage.

How is lobular carcinoma in situ treated?

Many doctors feel that rather than being a premalignant tumor, lobular carcinoma in situ is a marker for invasive cancer at some later time—since about a quarter of the women who have it will develop invasive cancer of the breast within twenty-five years. There are differing opinions on how to treat this cancer. Some doctors believe there should be no treatment, with careful follow-up by physical examination and mammography (usually every three months), so long as the person understands her particular risk for developing invasive cancer and the possibility of metastasis. Others feel a mastectomy of either one or both breasts should be the treatment of choice. There are clinical trials for women who choose to have local excision followed by tamoxifen therapy to help prevent development of invasive cancer.

Will I have to have treatments after the operation?

There are many factors that your doctor will consider in making this decision. They are discussed later in this chapter under the heading "Adjuvant Treatment."

HAVING THE OPERATION

Will I need to bank my blood for my operation?

Most breast cancer operations (except for some of the flap operations done in reconstruction) do not need blood transfusions. However, it is a question you need to ask your doctor. If your doctor thinks you will need blood transfusions during your operation, it would be wise to make plans to bank your own blood.

What should I expect the operation to be like?

It depends on what operation you are having, where you are having it and what that hospital's procedures are like. You may be asked to go to the hospital prior to your surgery in order to have the routine tests done, such as chest x-rays and blood work. On the day of the operation, you will probably be given medications to make you relax. Then you will be taken to the operating room, where electrocardiogram sensors will be attached to your arms and legs to check your heart rate during surgery. You will be put to sleep. After you are asleep, a tube will be placed in your throat to carry air to your lungs. Your operation should take about two to four hours, depending on what is being done. You will be awakened in the recovery room.

QUESTIONS TO ASK YOUR DOCTOR BEFORE YOUR BREAST OPERATION

- How long will the operation take?
- How should I expect to feel after my operation?
- Will I need blood transfusions during the operation and should I bank my own blood before going to the hospital?
- What will the scar look like? Please show me where it will be.

- Will I be in pain? What will you do for my pain?
- How long will I be in the hospital?
- Will I need special care at home after surgery?
- When can I get back to my regular routine? Will I have to take any special precautions?
- What kind of exercises should I do?
- If I decide to have breast reconstruction, can it be done as part of this operation?
- If I decide not to have reconstruction, what other choices will I have?

How long will I be in the recovery room?

You will probably spend an hour or so in the recovery room. Don't be surprised if your mouth feels dry and you feel drowsy and a little nauseated—these are common side effects of the anesthesia. There will, in all likelihood, be tubes in the area of your operation to drain away fluid, an IV (intravenous) tube in your arm so you can get liquid nourishment, wires taped to your chest to measure your heartbeat, and bandages on the area of the operation.

Will I stay in the hospital?

In most places, you will stay for one or two days, although some hospitals and surgical centers will let you go home the same day. If you stay in the hospital, what happens when you go back to your room depends on the type of surgery you have had and the practices in that hospital. Usually, the nurse will be in often to take your temperature, pulse, and blood pressure. The area where you have been operated on will also be checked. You will be asked to turn, cough and breathe deeply to keep your lungs clear, and to move your legs and feet to improve your blood circulation. By the next day, you will probably get up out of bed, with help, and walk around. You will soon start eating solid foods and be able to take a sponge bath. In most hospitals, you will go home after one or two days, usually with the drains that are taking fluid out of the underarm area still in place.

Will I feel any pain?

You will probably feel some pain in the area of the operation. You may also feel some numbness, tingling, or pain in your chest, shoulder area, upper arm or armpit. If you are in pain, do not hesitate to ask for medication to relieve it.

How will I take care of the area where the operation was done?

You usually will be taught how to clean the area and put on a new dressing. In addition, you need to take special care of the armpit where lymph nodes were taken out. You will also be taught how to take care of the drains that are in that area (and how to measure and record the volume of drainage), if they are not removed before you go home. You will need to be gentle with the site of your operation. Gently pat it dry, rather than rubbing. It is important for you to protect the area of your operation from any friction or bumps until it is completely healed—that will take anywhere from five to seven weeks. You can use lanolin cream or cocoa butter to keep the scar from drying and shrinking. Cornstarch can be used to lessen itching or friction from your clothes.

When will the stitches be taken out?

The stitches are usually taken out seven to ten days after the operation.

When can I take a bath or a shower?

You can usually take a sponge bath or a tub bath a few days after the operation as long as you make certain that the areas of the drain and incision stay dry. You will not be able to shower until after the stitches and drains are taken out.

What problems might I have after the operation?

You may have swelling in your arm, infection around the area of your operation, weakness in your upper body, a tired feeling, or shoulder pain.

Why do I need to exercise after my operation?

You need to exercise for several reasons. Exercises can help you regain motion and strength in your shoulder and your arm. They can also help decrease the stiffness and the pain in your neck and your back. If you have had the lymph nodes taken out under your arm, there are certain kinds of exercises you will need to do to help prevent or reduce lymphedema—a swelling of your arm and hand due to buildup of fluid.

When can I begin to do exercises after my operation?

You can usually begin carefully planned exercises as early as 24 hours after surgery. You need to discuss with your nurse and your doctor what exercises you can do and when you can begin to do them. Here are a few simple ones that you may be able to do within a day after surgery. Be sure that you do these only to the point of pulling or pain. Do not push yourself.

- **Breathing exercises.** Practice deep breathing. Lying on your back, breathe in deeply, expanding your lower chest as much as possible. Then let the air out and relax. Concentrate on relaxing while letting the air out. Do this three or four times, breathing in deeply and relaxing.
- **Hand stretches.** Flex your fingers. Rotate your wrist in a circle. Touch your fingers to your shoulder and, holding them there, lift your bent arm straight out.
- **Shoulder and head rotations.** Raise your shoulders and rotate them to the front. Now rotate them to the back. Try going from back to front in a circular motion. Slowly rotate your head in a circular direction, then move it from left to right, then move it from front to back. This helps to loosen your neck, back, chest, and shoulder muscles.
- Use your elbow and hand as much as you can for normal activities.

When can I do more active exercising?

Usually you can begin doing more active exercises after the stitches and drains have been taken out. Again, you need to talk with your nurse and doctor about your exercises. The Reach to Recovery volunteer from the American Cancer Society may also give you exercise information. Here are some suggested exercises to try. Start gradually and work up to doing each exercise five times a day, then increasing until you do a maximum of twenty times per day per exercise. If you get tired, be sure to rest before continuing.

- Stand up straight, feet apart, with toes six to twelve inches from and facing the wall. Bend your elbows and place your palms against the wall at shoulder level. Work both hands up the wall parallel to each other until the incision pulls or pain occurs. Mark the spot so that you can check your progress. Work your hands down to shoulder level. Move your feet and body closer to the wall if it is more comfortable. Rest and repeat.
- Stand straight, feet apart. Place your hand on your hip of the side that was not operated on for balance. Bend the elbow of your arm on the operated side, placing the back of your hand on the small of your back. Gradually work your hand up your back until your fingers reach the opposite shoulder blade. Slowly lower your arm. Rest and repeat.
- Lying in bed, clasp your hands behind your head and push your elbows into the mattress.

Will I do different exercises depending on the operation?

If you have breast reconstruction immediately after your mastectomy, you will need special exercises. Be sure to ask your doctor and nurse to give you specific instructions tailored to your own situation.

Is there any special care I should take of my arm where I had the lymph node dissection?

Yes. You should elevate that arm, resting it on a pillow or on the back of a sofa (your elbow should be level with your heart) for 30 to 45 minutes every two hours for the first two to three weeks and then two to three times a day for an additional six weeks. For the first eight weeks, you should limit the use of this arm to 30 minutes at any one task. When you are sleeping your forearm should be higher than your elbow and your elbow higher than or level with your heart. If you sleep on your side, be sure you sleep on the side away from the surgery.

How long will it take before I get the full motion and strength back to my arm and shoulder?

It could be two or three months, depending on the kind of treatment you have had. The stiffness and tightness felt in the tissues of the chest and armpit after surgery or radiation therapy will come and go for a while. It is important to concentrate on activities that involve your shoulder on the side of the surgery, doing the stretching exercises slowly and smoothly. Continue to work at exercising at least three times a day, gradually improving your motion, until the feeling of tightness is no longer a problem. Over time, the numbness under your arm will decrease, but total feeling may not return for a long time.

How will I know when I have my normal shoulder motion back?

You will know that you have normal shoulder motion when you can do the same things with your arm on the side of the operation as you can on the nonoperated side.

Will all the pain, numbness and tingling sensations ever disappear?

Yes, they most likely will. However, some women continue to have symptoms up to a year after the operation. Some say that when they touch under their armpit, they have pain radiating from under the arm to the waist. Some describe the sensations as heaviness or a feeling of "pins and needles" and skin sensitivity. Others say that the sensations change from time to time. Some women who have had a mastectomy feel pain in the breast that was removed. Doctors and nurses are not sure why this "phantom pain" occurs, but it does exist. It is not imaginary. As with other operations, the symptoms are affected by the weather. If you have unusual sensations, discuss them with your doctor.

Will I have trouble sleeping?

Some women do have trouble sleeping, for a time, on the side of the operation. Others say that they cannot wear their prosthesis to bed because the elastic in the bra is too tight. (You can get a "sleeping bra" which is much softer and more comfortable to wear.) Some women describe the feeling as like being in a cast, saying it is difficult to sleep because it is hard to find a comfortable position. Others talk about the difficulty of lying flat on their backs because of the pulling sensation. Yet others experience very little difficulty with this problem.

Will I be able to shave under the arm where I have had the lymph node dissection?

You should probably refrain from shaving and from using deodorants for two to four weeks. You need to ask the doctor and nurse when you can start using strong deodorants or depilatory creams and when you can shave under the affected arm.

How long will it be before I can return to my regular activities?

You will probably find that two or three weeks after your operation you will be doing many of the things you have always done. After six weeks, you probably will be able to go back to all your normal activities. However, listen to your own body. When you get tired, make sure to rest. Be careful not to overdo. This is a time to be good to yourself.

Is swimming a good exercise for me?

Yes, swimming, aerobics and dance exercises are all good for you, but should not be started until about six weeks after your operation. Many communities offer swimming, exercise and dance classes specifically for breast cancer patients. You need to discuss with your doctor and nurse how soon after your surgery you will be able to resume these activities.

Will I be able to play tennis or golf?

Yes, but you should check with your doctor as to when you can take up these active sports again.

Will I have a swollen arm after my operation?

Removing the lymph nodes under the arm interrupts the flow of lymph fluid. In some women, the buildup of this fluid in the arm and hand causes them to swell. This swelling is referred to by health professionals as lymphedema. The swelling might occur shortly after your operation or many years later. If it occurs shortly after your operation, it is more likely to come and go. If it happens many years later, it is more likely to be a permanent condition. If you have radiation to the area under your arm after your operation, had an infection or are greatly overweight, you are more likely to get lymphedema. If you notice that your arm is beginning to swell, get in touch with your doctor or nurse as soon as possible.

What causes lymphedema?

The lymph channels are one of three channels in the body that move fluids. Two of the channels, veins and arteries, move blood. The lymph channels, a series of cells that line up to form channels, move clear fluids. The surgery interrupts or destroys the paths that are used to drain the fluid. What is not clear is why two women who have identical surgery have different side effects—with one getting lymphedema and the other one not getting it.

Does this swelling mean that cancer has come back?

Normally, this swelling does not mean that your cancer has come back. Rather, it is a side effect that some women experience after surgery for breast cancer. Be sure to contact your doctor at any sign of swelling or infection in your arm.

Will exercise help my lymphedema?

It might. General physical activity is essential for improved circulation. It is good for you to move around and use your swollen limb. Swimming, walking and biking are particularly good exercises. But exercise when it is cool since heat and humidity can aggravate lymphedema.

What can be done for the swelling?

Your doctor will check to see if you have an infection. If so, you will need to take medicine to control the infection. If not, there are several steps you can take:

- Consult with a physical therapist.
- You can elevate your arm to help reduce the swelling.
- You may need to wear an elastic sleeve or use an elastic cuff to improve the circulation of the lymph fluid.
- You may need to use an air-driven pump that pushes the fluid out of your arm, along with a compression garment that prevents the fluid from returning.

- Most insurance companies cover the cost of both sleeves and pump. The American Cancer Society sometimes has a pump that can be borrowed.

Although all of these may help control the swelling, they will not cure it. When you stop using them, the swelling usually will return.

Why can't the doctor put a needle in and drain the fluid out?

It is not possible to do this because the fluid is within the tissues. What you need to do is to move the fluid from the affected area, past the obstruction and back into the system to get rid of it.

Are there any new treatments for lymphedema?

A type of massage, called manual lymph drainage, which has been used in Europe for many years, is now also being used in the United States. A therapist, using her hands like a milking device, milks the fluid out of the affected limb. Sometimes the limb is then bandaged overnight until the next massage session. When the limb is close to normal, a made-to-measure elastic support garment is used. In the research stages are microsurgery, to reconnect the damaged lymph channels, cold laser, to promote the production of new channels, freeing up the existing ones, and drug treatment.

What is the National Lymphedema Network?

The National Lymphedema Network provides information about lymphedema and locations of centers in the country for its treatment. See Chapter 26, "Where to Get Help," for additional information.

Will I be more susceptible to infections after my operation?

It is more difficult for your body to fight infection after lymph nodes have been taken out. You will need to protect your arm and hand on the side of your operation from any kind of injury for the rest of your life. If you get an infection, you should call the doctor immediately. You should also be careful about any cuts, scratches, insect bites or other injuries you get on your arm and hand on that side of your body.

What will I need to do to take special care of my affected arm ?

There are several lifelong precautions you will need to take:

- Don't carry suitcases or a briefcase with that arm.
- Do not wear tight-fitting or elasticized cuffs, tight sleeves or

tight jewelry, such as rings, wristwatches or bracelets, on that side.

- Whenever possible, avoid injections, vaccinations and drawing of blood from the affected arm.
- Wear loose rubber gloves when washing dishes. Do not expose the hand or arm to excessive temperatures.
- Keep the affected side covered when you are out in the sun. Use sunscreen and avoid sunburn.
- Avoid insect bites and stings by using protective insect repellent.
- Pamper your arm by carrying your purse or packages on the other side. Don't push heavy furniture with the arm.
- Wash cuts promptly, treat them with antibacterial medication and cover them with sterile dressing. Change the dressing and check them often for redness, soreness or other signs of infection.
- Avoid burns while cooking or smoking.
- Wear a thimble when sewing to avoid pinpricks.
- Wear gloves or mitts when gardening and working with sharp objects or hot objects. Use a mitt when taking hot dishes out of the oven.
- Use an electric razor to avoid cutting this area. Underarm shaving may be a problem for a while because of the lack of mobility or numbness, so take great care.
- Never pick or cut cuticles or hangnails. Use cream cuticle remover for nail care. Apply lanolin hand cream to hand and arm several times a day.
- Though you should be cautious, it is also important to use your arm normally. Don't favor it or keep it dependent.
- If you do notice pain, swelling, or redness on your scar or arm, with or without fever being present, call your doctor.

Why do I have pain in my neck and back?

When your breast is removed, your weight may shift and be out of balance, particularly if you have large breasts. This can cause you to have some pain in your neck and back.

Why do I feel numbness and tingling in my arm?

Sometimes during the operation, some nerves may be injured or cut. You may feel some numbness and tingling in your arms, shoulder, underarm and chest, especially in the first few weeks after your surgery. Most likely, the numbness and tingling will go away over time, but the total feeling may not return for a long time and some numbness may be permanent.

HAVING RADIATION TREATMENT AFTER BREAST-CONSERVING SURGERY

Is it possible to have breast-conserving surgery without having radiation therapy?

It is not recommended, since studies have shown that at least 40 percent of women who have only the breast-conserving surgery are most likely to have a local recurrence in the breast.

QUESTIONS TO ASK ABOUT RADIATION WITH BREAST-CONSERVING SURGERY

- When will the treatments begin? How long will each treatment take? When will the treatments end?
- Who will be responsible for my radiation treatments? Who will be giving them? Where will they be done?
- What kind of short-term and long-term side effects will I have? What are the risks of this treatment?
- Will I have to spend any time in the hospital as part of these treatments? How long?
- Can I continue my normal lifestyle during treatments? Is there anything special I can do to take care of myself during these treatments? Should someone come with me to the treatments?
- Will my breast change in appearance after treatment? How?
- Will the costs of the treatment be covered by my health insurance?
- How often will I have to have checkups and tests after my treatment is finished?

If I have breast-conserving surgery, what kind of radiation treatment is used?

High-energy x-rays are aimed at your breast and sometimes at nearby areas that still contain some lymph nodes, such as under the arm (if only a sample of lymph nodes was taken during surgery), above the collarbone, and along the breastbone. The goal is to destroy any cancer cells that may still remain in the breast and surrounding areas. The high-energy x-rays are delivered by a linear accelerator or cobalt machine. You may get treatment in four areas: different sides of your breast, around your collarbone, in the center of your chest and under your arm.

How is the radiation treatment done?

After you have had your operation and you have recovered from it—usually two to four weeks after the operation—you will start on radiation treatment. You will lie on your back, usually with your hand under your head, under a machine that will beam the x-rays.

How often will I go for my radiation treatments?

You will usually go for five days each week, for about five weeks. Each treatment takes about 20 to 25 minutes. Only a few minutes of this time are for the treatment; most of the time is spent putting you in the proper position. Many people continue with work or their regular activities during the treatment period. (There are more details about radiation treatment and its side effects in Chapter 7, "Radiation Treatment.")

How is the boost done?

One to two weeks after the radiation treatment has been completed, most women receive a concentrated booster dose of radiation to the area where the breast lump was located. The boost is usually done with external radiation. If you have the external radiation boost, you will have daily visits for five days using a linear accelerator machine.

Will my breast feel firmer after radiation treatment?

Your breast, after being treated with radiation, may be different. It may feel firmer. It may be larger because of the buildup of fluid. Or it may be smaller because of tissue changes. Some women say that the skin of their treated breast is more sensitive after treatment, while other women say it is less sensitive. You may find you have itchy, red, or dry skin. If your skin blisters, be sure to report it to the doctor and nurse. If you have the booster with external beam radiation, you may notice an increase in skin redness at the site of the treatment.

Are there any other side effects from the radiation treatments?

Other side effects depend upon where the radiation is given and how much is used. Many women find their breasts are sore or tender. They report feeling tired. (There are more details about radiation therapy and its side effects in Chapter 7, "Radiation Treatment.")

How many women have local recurrences after their breast-conserving surgery and radiation therapy treatment for their Stage I and II breast cancers?

About 20 to 40 percent of women choosing this treatment have local recurrences, so it is important that you have careful follow-up. If you should have a recurrence, you can have a mastectomy to control the local disease. If you are under 35 years old, you have a greater risk of local recurrence so you must be carefully followed.

ADJUVANT TREATMENT

What is meant by adjuvant treatment?

An adjuvant treatment is one that is being used in addition to a primary form of treatment.

Why is adjuvant treatment important in breast cancer?

Adjuvant treatment is one that is used in addition to the primary form of treatment. It is an important part of the treatment for breast cancer, based on studies that have changed the thinking on how breast cancer spreads. Scientists once thought that breast cancer first spread to nearby tissue and underarm lymph nodes before extending to other parts of the body. Therefore, doctors believed that the spread of breast cancer could be controlled with extensive surgery to remove the breast, chest muscles and underarm lymph nodes. However, scientists now believe that cancer cells may break away from the primary tumor in the breast and begin to metastasize even when the disease is in an early stage. The adjuvant treatment is designed to kill any cancer cells that may have spread. Studies have shown that adjuvant treatment, given in addition to the primary treatment in breast cancer, increases chances for long-term survival.

What kind of adjuvant treatment is used for breast cancer?

Usually chemotherapy or hormones are used because they can affect cancer cells throughout the body (called systemic treatment). In some cases, such as before or after a mastectomy, radiation therapy might be used as an adjuvant treatment to kill breast cancer cells that have spread to nearby parts of the body, such as the chest wall.

What factors determine the kind of adjuvant treatment I am given?

The kind of adjuvant treatment you will be given depends on the stage of your disease, your general health, and other prognostic factors. These factors include whether or not you have lymph node involvement, the size and grade of your tumor, whether you have undergone menopause, and whether your tumor is positive or negative for estrogen or progesterone receptors. In addition, the doctor may look at the rate at which the cells in your tumor are dividing, sometimes referred to as nuclear grading. In some medical centers, testing for other markers will also be done.

Do these factors affect my chance of recovery from my breast cancer?

These factors are used by the doctor to plan your treatment. Some of them also tell your doctor how well you might do on different kinds of treatment. For instance, if your breast cancer has not spread to the lymph nodes under the arm (called node-negative), you are less likely to have a recurrence of breast cancer than those women who do have cancer in their lymph nodes. If you have a smaller tumor, you have a better chance of recovery than those who have a large tumor. If your breast cancer is hormone-receptor-positive your tumor tends to grow less aggressively and you are more likely to respond to hormone therapy. A low histologic or nuclear grade (Grade 1) is more favorable than a higher one (Grade 3).

When will my adjuvant treatment begin and how long will it last?

Your adjuvant treatment usually begins between four and twelve weeks after surgery. If you are having chemotherapy treatment, it usually lasts for three to six months, with a cycle of treatment followed by a recovery period, then another cycle of treatment and so on. You will get the drugs either by mouth or by injection into your blood vessel, usually in a doctor's office or in the outpatient area of a hospital. If you are having hormonal treatment, you will take two tamoxifen pills a day, for a period of at least two years. Most doctors in this country are giving this treatment for five years, since the ideal length of treatment is still under study.

QUESTIONS TO ASK YOUR MEDICAL ONCOLOGIST BEFORE STARTING CHEMOTHERAPY OR HORMONE TREATMENT

- Why do I need this treatment?
- Are there any other treatments for my stage of disease?
- Why have you chosen the one you are recommending?
- What are the benefits and risks of each of the treatments?
- If I need hormone treatment, would drugs be better for me?

- What regimen of drugs will I be taking?
- Are there any other regimens you considered?
- What side effects will I have?
- How long would I have to stay on them?
- How will it affect my normal lifestyle?
- Are there any clinical trials I should consider for my stage of disease?

What kind of adjuvant treatment will I have if I am node-positive?

- If you are node-positive and are premenopausal, you will probably have chemotherapy.
- If you are node-positive and are postmenopausal, you will probably get hormonal treatment.

Studies that have been done to date show that adjuvant treatment with both tamoxifen and chemotherapy for node-positive women appears to be more beneficial for postmenopausal women than for premenopausal women.

Will I have adjuvant treatment if I am node-negative?

This is a very complex issue, since between 60 to 70 percent of node-negative women with breast cancer can be cured with primary treatment alone. However, these statistics mean that in about a third of the node-negative women, breast cancer does recur—and there is nothing at the present time that tells the doctor exactly whether you will be one of the women who will have a recurrence and thus would benefit from adjuvant therapy. You and your doctor must weigh the possible benefits against the possible risks, looking at the prognostic factors, your age and general health and your treatment preference.

Are there any guidelines for making these choices for node-negative women with breast cancer?

There are some:

- If you are estrogen-receptor-positive and have a fairly small tumor, you will probably receive hormonal therapy (probably tamoxifen), whether you are pre- or postmenopausal. The side effects are relatively few for most women, so doctors generally agree that the possible benefits outweigh the risks.
- If you are estrogen-receptor-positive and have a large tumor, you may receive chemotherapy if you are premenopausal,

tamoxifen alone if you are postmenopausal, or a combination of the two treatments.
- If you are estrogen-receptor-negative, you will probably receive chemotherapy, whether you are pre- or postmenopausal.

What is hormonal treatment?

Hormonal treatment is used to keep the cancer cells from getting the hormones they need to grow. You may need to take drugs to change the way your hormones work. Another type of hormonal treatment is the removal of your ovaries, which are organs that produce hormones.

What hormone drug is usually used?

Tamoxifen is the drug most commonly used for hormone treatment. Taken in pill form, tamoxifen (its trade name is Nolvadex) blocks your body's use of estrogen, but does not stop your own estrogen production. It has been used for almost twenty years to treat patients with advanced breast cancer. More recently, it has been used as an adjuvant therapy following primary treatment for early stage breast cancer. In addition, the National Cancer Institute is sponsoring a large clinical trial to determine whether tamoxifen can prevent breast cancer in women who have an increased risk of developing the disease.

Are there other beneficial effects of tamoxifen?

Yes. While tamoxifen acts against the effects of estrogen in breast tissue, it acts like estrogen in other body systems. If you take tamoxifen, you may share many of the beneficial effects of menopausal estrogen replacement therapy, such as a lowering of blood cholesterol and a slowing of bone loss.

What are the side effects of tamoxifen?

The side effects are not usually severe and not all women experience them. You may have nausea and vomiting, dizziness, headaches and fatigue. You also may have hot flashes, vaginal bleeding, dryness or irritation. Your periods may become irregular, but they usually will not stop completely. You will not go into menopause or become infertile. If you are premenopausal, you may become more fertile, so you should use some type of birth control while taking tamoxifen (do not take oral contraceptives because they may change the effects of tamoxifen). If you do become pregnant, you should not take tamoxifen during pregnancy or while breast feeding.

If I take tamoxifen, will I begin my menopause?

No. Tamoxifen does not cause women to begin menopause, although it can cause some symptoms that occur during menopause. Your ovaries should continue to act normally and produce female hormones in the same or slightly increased amounts.

Are there any side effects of taking tamoxifen over a long period of time?

This is an issue that is still being studied. A few women who have taken very high doses of tamoxifen have reported vision and other eye problems. A few have developed blood clots, particularly if they were also having chemotherapy while taking the tamoxifen. In one trial, depression was reported by about 1 percent of the postmenopausal women using tamoxifen as adjuvant therapy. In addition, some studies have suggested that women taking tamoxifen have an increased risk of developing cancer of the endometrium, about two or three times higher than women in the general population (an increase similar to that associated with single-agent estrogen replacement therapy in postmenopausal women).

Is it possible to treat Stage II or Stage III breast cancer with only tamoxifen instead of having an operation plus adjuvant treatment?

If you take only tamoxifen, you have a very high risk of having a local recurrence. This choice is only for women who cannot have a mastectomy or breast-conserving surgery plus radiation therapy because of their age or other complications that make an operation impossible.

Is RU-486 being used to treat breast cancer?

RU-486, the abortion pill, is being tested in clinical trials in France and Canada in the treatment of metastatic breast cancer. The French study is enrolling women who are resistant to tamoxifen treatment, while the Canadians are studying women who are not known to be resistant to tamoxifen. There are currently no studies being conducted in the United States using RU-486.

What are the side effects of having my ovaries taken out?

If you have your ovaries removed as a hormonal treatment for breast cancer, you will no longer be able to have children. This is referred to as surgical menopause and, if you are premenopausal, the side effects will probably be more sudden and intense than those of people who have natural menopause. You may have hot flashes and dryness or irritation of your vagina among many other possible symptoms.

What chemotherapy drugs are used as adjuvant breast cancer treatment?

Adjuvant chemotherapy involves a combination of anticancer drugs, usually using one of three combinations—CMF (cyclophosphamide, methotrexate and fluorouracil), CAF (cyclophosphamide, Adriamycin and fluorouracil), or CA (cyclophosphamide and Adriamycin).

Will I have menopause due to my chemotherapy treatments?

Some of the drugs used as adjuvant treatment for breast cancer can damage your ovaries. If you are premenopausal and your ovaries stop producing hormones, you may have symptoms of menopause, such as hot flashes and dryness of your vagina. Your periods may become irregular or may stop completely. You may become infertile and no longer be able to have children. If you are over the age of 35, some of these side effects, such as infertility, may be permanent. (There is more information on side effects in Chapter 8, "Chemotherapy.")

Are there any other side effects if my ovaries stop producing hormones?

Having your ovaries suddenly stop producing hormones means the symptoms will be exaggerated. You may feel less sexual desire, have soreness and dryness in your vulva or vagina, burning in the vagina during intercourse or light spotting after intercourse. You may have persistent hot flashes and sweats. You should use a water-soluble lubricant during vaginal intercourse. You might try avoiding highly seasoned foods, caffeine and alcohol to minimize your hot flashes. In addition, you may want to consult a specialist to help treat your symptoms, such as a gynecologic-endocrinologist, who has knowledge of menopause and nonestrogen replacement therapies.

Will I lose my hair as a result of the chemotherapy treatments?

It depends on the regimen you will be on. If you are on CAF (cyclophosphamide, Adriamycin and fluorouracil), you will probably lose your hair soon after you begin the treatments. Only about 10 to 15 percent of the women on CMF (cyclophosphamide, methotrexate and fluorouracil) lose all of their hair. Thinning is more common.

Will I gain weight as a result of my chemotherapy?

Weight gain can be due to treatment for women who are on prednisone or oral cyclophosphamide. Other women do gain weight, but research indicates that weight gain is due to eating more calories rather than to the treatment itself. The women who gained the weight reported feeling more unhappy, more worried and more distressed about their appearance than those women with breast cancer who did not gain weight while on treatment. If you are having problems with weight gain, you may need to get help from a dietitian.

What kinds of new treatments are being studied for breast cancer?

There are studies on many new kinds of treatments for all stages of breast cancer. They include new treatment methods, new doses and treatment schedules and new ways of combining treatment. In addition, work is under way with various anticancer drugs and drug combinations as well as several types of hormone treatment and new ways of combining chemotherapy with hormone treatment and radiation therapy. Biological therapy—treatment with substances that boost the immune system's response to cancer—is also being studied in clinical trials. New approaches such as bone marrow transplants, peripheral stem cell support and colony-stimulating factors are also being researched.

How is peripheral stem cell support being used for breast cancer patients?

In some institutions, you can get high-dose chemotherapy with peripheral stem cell support for some stages of breast cancer. Stem cells in your blood are removed, purified and frozen. The high-dose chemotherapy is given and then your stem cells are given back to help your bone marrow recover and to produce healthy blood cells. This treatment is being studied in clinical trials. Call the Cancer Information Service to find centers where this is being done. You will find more information on this procedure in Chapter 9, "New Advances and Investigational Trials."

How are bone marrow transplants being used for breast cancer?

Like peripheral stem cell support, bone marrow transplants also allow high-dose chemotherapy to be given. Because these high doses can destroy your bone marrow, marrow is taken from your bones before this treatment is started. The marrow taken out is treated to remove malignant cells, and frozen. You are given the high doses of chemotherapy, sometimes followed by radiation therapy, to treat your cancer. Your marrow that was taken out is thawed and given to you through a needle in your vein. You will find more details about bone marrow transplants in Chapter 9, "New Advances and Investigational Trials."

Will I be eligible for clinical trials using bone marrow transplantation?

There are several clinical trials available in the country. The National Cancer Institute is running four clinical trials for two general groups of breast cancer patients—women with Stage II and IIIA breast cancer with ten or more positive lymph nodes and women with Stage IV breast cancer. The trials are evaluating the effectiveness of high-dose chemotherapy with autologous bone marrow transplant support, comparing the benefits and risks of this treatment to those of conventional chemotherapy. The Blue Cross and Blue Shield Association, and the Federal Employee Program, are supporting the clinical trials by helping to fund a substantial portion of the patient care costs of Blue Cross and Blue Shield members who participate in the clinical trials and receive their treatment at a contracting hospital. If you want to be part of this clinical trial, you need to make sure you have your bone marrow transplant in a hospital that is participating. Call the Cancer Information Service at 1-800-4-CANCER to get information on this and other clinical trials.

How expensive are bone marrow transplants for breast cancer patients?

Bone marrow transplantation is an expensive procedure, because it is very labor intensive and includes many tests, services, laboratory work and medicine. Depending on the length of recuperation and whether peripheral stem cell or bone marrow support is used, your bill can range from $50,000 to over $300,000.

BUYING A PROSTHESIS

If I have had a mastectomy, are there medical reasons why I should wear a prosthesis?

There are reasons why you should wear a prosthesis—a form to replace the missing breast. The weight of the remaining breast, particularly if you have medium-to-large breasts, can cause shoulder, neck and back pain. You may find that your posture will change, with the affected shoulder rising, if you do not have a prosthesis. The larger the remaining breast, the more vital the need, not only for appearance but also for the weight. In many cases, a well-fitted prosthetic device means the difference between a prompt, cheerful, total recovery and long-term personal distress.

What does a prosthesis look like?

Usually it is flesh-colored. The prostheses are sized to match the remaining breast both in shape and weight. Normally they are shaped like a teardrop. The flat side goes against the wall of the chest and the tail end goes toward the armpit. Some companies make reversible ones that can be used on either side.

Does a prosthesis feel cold against the chest?

It depends on the type of prosthesis, what it is made of and how it is supposed to be worn. Many of them feel a little cold when they are first put on. After they have been worn for a few minutes, they warm to body temperature.

When should I be fitted a breast prosthesis?

Most doctors will tell you to wait until the scar is fully healed before you get fitted for a breast prosthesis. Most patients can begin using a full prosthesis a month or six weeks after surgery. However, soft forms can be worn from the very beginning. For instance, at the very beginning you can use simple clean padding in your brassiere. The Reach to Recovery volunteer who visits you may provide you with a temporary Dacron-filled prosthesis to wear while the wound is healing and the area is tender and swollen. Some patients tell us they use items such as cotton balls, lamb's wool, handkerchiefs, sanitary napkins, shoulder pads or padded bras during the period between their operation and being fitted for a prosthesis. You should check with your doctor before you start wearing the permanent prosthesis.

How can I be sure I find the right prosthesis?

First of all, you should not shop for the prosthesis by yourself. It is much better if an involved person, such as your sister, mother, husband, or a good friend, goes along with you. Second, you should make sure you try on several different kinds and models so that you can be sure the one you finally buy is what you really want. There are several dozen different breast forms on the market. You should try on several to compare the way they feel and look.

What should I be looking for in a prosthesis?

The breast form should feel comfortable, have a natural contour and consistency, and should remain in place when you stretch, bend or reach. A properly weighted form provides the balance your body needs for correct posture and anchors your bra, preventing it from riding up. There are some forms that are designed with adhesive skin supports, and include an optional nipple, that you can wear without a bra. It is important to pay close attention to how the prosthesis feels and how it fits—the form should match your other breast when seen from the side, the bottom and the front. Your clothes should fit the way they did before you had your operation. The form may feel too heavy at first, but will feel natural in time. Take your time in choosing a form. Remember you will be wearing it every day for a long time to come.

What are the different kinds of prostheses available?

There are several different kinds of breast forms made by several companies. Generally they fall into these classifications:

- **Silicone:** Form made of silicone skin or polyurethane and filled with silicone gel or glycerine or fluid. Very soft and flexible with the look, feel and weight of the natural breast. Some have different forms for left and right breasts, with side wings. Depending on manufacturer, made to be worn on the skin, with or without regular bra or bra with pocket. Adjusts to body temperature; may need to be warmed before using. Some can leak if fingernail or pin pricks them. May be worn for swimming. Also available in customized model using pre-operative impression. Silicone-filled prostheses range in cost from $75 to $300; silicone gel from $150 to $450, with customized forms costing up to $1,400.

- **Organic:** Made of cotton or other organic material. Filling is organic fiber, with glass beads or other weights cushioned into the form. Made in left and right breast forms. Warms quickly and remains at room temperature. Some can be worn directly on skin. Odorless. May be worn for swimming. Cost ranges from $60 to $200.

- **Foam:** Lightweight, they are molded polyurethane foam or foam chips; weights can be added. Spongy feeling. May get stiff and yellow with wear. Good for leisure wear or swimming (need waterproof cover). Especially useful with lounging bra for postoperative period, although some like them for general wear. Cost ranges from $30 to $175.

- **Temporary:** Lightweight and long-wearing. Soft pads with tricot filling. Can also be cotton with cotton filling. Good for sleepwear and postoperative wear. Cost ranges from $5 to $50.

Where do I go to buy a prosthesis?

There are several places: corset shops, surgical supply houses, foundation departments of some large department stores, and some special outlets. Some American Cancer Society offices offer a variety of forms that a woman can examine (they are not for sale) in a noncommercial setting. The Reach to Recovery volunteer or the American Cancer Society office can give you material describing the various forms, their manufacturers and a list of suggested outlets available. Most of the outlets have fitters who can help you. The large mail-order houses also have prostheses available.

What should I wear when I shop for the prosthesis?
You should bring along some figure-revealing clothes to see how natural the form will look—a sweater or one of your more revealing dresses. If you want to use your own bras, make sure you bring them along so they can be altered if needed.

Can I make my own prosthesis?
Some people do make their own prostheses. Some of the materials put out by the American Cancer Society have instructions for making your own breast forms and night bras. Some small-breasted women or women who have had both breasts removed find that they can use homemade forms. However, in many cases, the homemade forms are too lightweight and tend to ride up. Again, you must be careful because you can end up with posture changes and discomfort in your shoulders or back if you wear a prosthesis which isn't the proper weight for you.

What is a special mastectomy bra?
It is a bra with a built-in pocket to hold the form in place. It also has extra material under the arm and above the breast. The form is placed in the pocket of the bra, which holds it in place. You can bend, stretch, or stoop without jarring it out of place. Some patients have complained that special mastectomy bras do not fit properly or that they are cumbersome and unattractive. Many patients have altered their own bras by adding pockets, and still others have had seamstresses make pockets for their regular bras. In some stores, fitters will sew pockets into your bras to hold the prosthesis. Some companies make mastectomy bras that are individually fitted.

What kinds of covers are available for the form?
Some of the forms, both lightweight and heavy ones, have nylon or cloth covers. The covers are made of washable, fast-drying materials. The cover allows the forms to be pinned directly into regular brassieres for occasional use instead of in the specially made pocket. Some women prefer to wear the covers on the forms at all times. They like the way they feel. The tricot covers, especially, are easy to wash out and dry.

Can I get a breast form with a nipple?

Some forms are made with nipples. Nipples also are sold separately and can be easily attached either to the prosthesis, or directly to the skin. Some women who have had breast reconstruction without the nipple also use these separate nipples.

Can I get a form in a dark skin color?

Some forms are made in both light and dark skin colors.

Can I wear my prosthesis all the time?

Many women do wear their prostheses around the clock. Some women start by wearing it a few hours a day and gradually increasing the number of hours of wear. Wearing the form to bed at night may help prevent a stiff neck and shoulder problems. Waterbeds also have been recommended by some, since they provide support and conform to the body.

Are there any cosmetics to cover the scars I have after surgery?

There is a special brand of cosmetics, Covermark, which is designed to blend into one's individual skin color. The cosmetics are waterproof and when carefully applied are particularly useful for swimming. Available from Lydia O'Leary (One Anderson Avenue, Moonachie, NJ 07074) and in many drug and department stores.

Is there anything I can do about the tightness of the elastic in my bra?

Notion stores and girdle and corset shops sell bra extenders that can be used to make a bra more comfortable. They also sell shoulder-strap pads which some women use to relieve discomfort on the shoulder-strap area.

Can I have a prosthesis custom-made?

There are a few manufacturers who custom-make prostheses. The American Cancer Society can give you an up-to-date listing.

Will my insurance cover a prosthesis?

It depends on your insurance plan. Some health insurance (and Medicare) covers part or all the cost of the first prosthesis. A replacement form is not usually covered. The doctor should write the prescription for the form and for mastectomy bras. When you are buying them, ask that the term *surgical* be written on the bill. You should also write "surgical" on your check. Breast forms, mastectomy bras and even bra alterations may be tax deductible when medically prescribed. Be sure to read your insurance policy, because some say you must buy the form within a specific period of time and buy a certain type. If you are planning to have reconstruction, ask your insurance company whether they will also pay for a prosthesis and mastectomy bras. Some women have found that submitting a claim for a prosthesis and mastectomy bras makes them ineligible for payment for subsequent reconstruction. You also need to keep all your receipts, since most prostheses are covered by warranty.

Can I do anything about the perspiration under my prosthesis during the summertime?

You can buy a thin sheepskin pad, which you wear facing your body, behind the form, to absorb perspiration. Some women find using facial tissue under the form during the summer will also do the trick.

Is anyone making special bathing suits for women with mastectomies?

Many of the major bathing suit companies make special bathing suits for mastectomy patients. You can usually get them through the same source where you got your prosthesis or in large department stores. Your local unit of the American Cancer Society can usually supply you with a list of available styles.

BREAST RECONSTRUCTION

If I plan to have breast reconstruction when should I see the plastic surgeon?

If there is a possibility that you want to have breast reconstruction after your mastectomy, it would be useful for you to see a plastic surgeon before you have your mastectomy operation. The reconstruction can be done at the same time as your mastectomy or at some future time. If it is done after the mastectomy, you will have to wait three to six months.

QUESTIONS TO ASK YOUR PLASTIC SURGEON BEFORE YOU HAVE BREAST RECONSTRUCTION

- What are the different choices of reconstructive surgery? What type do you think is best for me? Why?
- Should I have the reconstruction at the time of my mastectomy or should I wait until later? How much later

can I have it done? If I need to have chemotherapy, should I wait until I have finished that treatment?

- What are the advantages and disadvantages of having reconstruction at the time of my mastectomy? Of waiting to have it until later?
- What are the side effects and risks that I should consider?
- Will you be using tissue expanders? A saline-filled implant? Can you use my own tissue?
- Will you explain how the surgery will be done? What kind of anesthesia will you use?
- What will I look like after the surgery? What kind of scars will I have and where will they be?
- What will my new breast look like? Will it match my other breast? Will it change over time? Will I have to have anything done to my other breast?
- Can I have my nipple reconstructed? How will it be done?
- What is your experience with this operation?
- Do you have any before-and-after pictures you can show me?
- May I talk with someone who has had the operation?
- How many operations will I have to have? Will I need to be in the hospital each time? For how long? How long will I need for recovery?
- Will I be in much pain? For how long?
- Will I need to wear a special bra after my operation?
- How much will it cost? Will my insurance cover any part of it?
- What can be done if the surgery is not successful?

Can I have breast reconstruction at the same time I have my mastectomy?

That is certainly a possibility, depending upon what stage and type of breast cancer you have and your general health. Generally, if you have breast cancer in situ or Stage I and II infiltrating cancer, reconstruction may be done if you are having a mastectomy as your treatment. You should ask your surgeon for a consultation with a plastic surgeon before the mastectomy. The plastic surgeon will identify whether you are a candidate for immediate reconstruction or whether you would be better off waiting. If you don't have immediate reconstruction, you will probably have to wait three to six months until your scar has healed. If you are having chemotherapy or radiation treatments, most doctors prefer to wait some one to three months after completing them. In addition, most doctors wait another three months between the operation to create the breast and the construction of the nipple. If you smoke, the doctor will ask you to stop smoking in order to ensure an adequate blood supply.

Are there advantages to my having the reconstruction at the same time as my mastectomy?

Having the reconstruction at the same time may make you feel better psychologically, make you feel attractive and may help with your sexual life. It means, however, that your doctors must cooperate with each other, including scheduling the operating room for two operations instead of one. You will be in surgery and under anesthesia for a longer time and you may have additional complications from having two surgeries. It is important to be sure that the plastic surgeon has had experience in performing immediate reconstruction. There is no evidence of harmful effects—that is, having the two operations at the same time does not interfere with or delay adjuvant treatment and does not interfere with the management of recurrent disease. However, many doctors still prefer to do the reconstruction as a separate operation.

Will my breast look like it did before the mastectomy?

You should not expect that it will. The new breast will probably look more flattened than tapered. It may be firmer than your natural breast and it may not match it exactly. There is a limit to the size of the constructed breast, based on what the skin can support. Sometimes, women choose to have the remaining breast reduced (or in some cases augmented) to more closely match the new reconstructed breast. However, under clothing, you can probably not notice the difference between the two. Most women are pleased with the results of the reconstruction. Although the new breast will not be a perfect replica of the old one, most women who have the reconstructive surgery can wear a normal bra or a bikini. You need to talk to the plastic surgeon about your expectations. Ask to see before-and-after pictures of women who have had this surgery. If your expectations are not realistic, you may be better off not having the reconstruction.

How can I know before the surgery if I will have a good result?

It is difficult to know, but there are some factors that will give you and your doctors some clues. They include your overall health, your chest structure and body shape, how your body heals, the effects of other breast surgery you have had, the skill of your plastic surgeon and the type of reconstruction operation you will be having.

Will I have scars as a result of the reconstruction?

You will have some scars, but the doctor will try to hide them as much as possible. The scars will depend upon the kind and extent of the surgery you will be having. When you talk with your plastic surgeon, ask where the scars will be, how long they will be, and what they might look like. Like most scars, they will fade in time, but probably they will never disappear completely. If you have darker skin, the scars usually look more prominent.

What is involved in breast reconstruction?

Breast reconstruction usually means one or more operations, even when you have it done at the same time as the mastectomy. You may have an implant (tissue expansion or simple breast reconstruction) or use your own tissue. If you are going to use your own tissue, there are three operations that can be done—latissimus dorsi reconstruction, transverse rectus abdominus muscle flap and free flap reconstruction. Having a nipple reconstructed or decreasing the size of the other breast means additional surgery.

Why has the doctor asked me to stop smoking?

Cigarette smoking can narrow your blood vessels, reduce blood flow to the tissues, and impair healing. Because it can seriously affect the results of the reconstruction, the plastic surgeon usually will insist that you not smoke for at least three weeks before your surgery and for several months after it.

What is expansion reconstructive surgery?

This is the most common reconstructive surgical approach. It can be done using one of several types of expanders. The expander, with a valve attached to it, is implanted behind the chest wall muscles, using the lines of the mastectomy incision. After a few weeks, when the wound has healed, you will return to the doctor's office every week or two, where sterile saline (salt water) is injected into the valve until the expander is slightly larger than the desired final size. The filled expander is left in place for several months to stretch the breast tissue. The surgeon operates again, taking out the expander and inserting a permanent breast implant. This process results in a more natural, supple contour to the reconstructed breast. The entire process takes from four to six months to complete.

What does a simple breast reconstruction entail?

If it is done after you have had a mastectomy, the surgeon makes a small incision along the lower part of the breast area near the mastectomy scar (or the mastectomy incision may be used) and

OPERATION CHOICES FOR BREAST RECONSTRUCTION

DESCRIPTION	COMMENTS
Expander Can be of several types. Empty silicone sack or double envelope with silicone layer and empty sack implanted under skin and muscle, gradually filled with saline (saltwater) solution through a valve over a period of weeks, stretching skin. Local or general anesthesia. Inpatient or outpatient. Surgery takes 1 to 2 hours.	Most common type of reconstruction. Provides greatest flexibility in breast size. Requires additional office visits (15 to 30 minutes) to add saltwater solution to stretch skin. May be uncomfortable for some women. Can have problems with valve. Another operation often needed to convert expander to permanent implant.
Implant, also called **fixed-volume implant** Sack, filled with silicone gel or saline fluid, implanted under skin and chest muscle. General or local anesthesia used. Can be outpatient or inpatient. Surgery takes 1 to 2 hours. Short recovery time. Low rate of complications.	Implants filled with silicone gel can be used only if a woman is enrolled in a clinical trial. Saline filled have silicone layer or envelope that contains filling.
Latissimus flap, also called **back flap** Muscle, called latissimus dorsi, and eye-shaped wedge of skin moved from back to chest wall and sewn in place, leaving tissue attached to original blood supply. Inpatient with general anesthesia. Surgery takes 2 to 4 hours.	May need blood transfusion. Major surgery that can be painful. Need to stay in hospital 3 to 6 days. Scar left on back or side. May have drain in for several weeks. May have fluid buildup in back area. May have slight bulge under arm that will shrink in time.
TRAM flap (transverse rectus abdominus myocutaneous), also called **tummy tuck.** Fat, skin and muscle taken from stomach area and moved up to form breast. Tissue usually remains connected to abdominal blood supply, although in some cases microsurgery used. Inpatient, with general anesthesia. Surgery takes 3 to 5 hours.	May need blood transfusion. Major surgery that can be painful. Hospital stay of several days. Recovery period may take several weeks, including inability of patient to stand straight for days or even weeks. Healing problems may occur, including thick tissue on flap. Scar in abdominal area. *(continued)*

OPERATION CHOICES FOR BREAST RECONSTRUCTION *(cont.)*

DESCRIPTION	COMMENTS
Microsurgery, also called **free flap** Muscle and fat from other parts of body, such as buttock or thigh, are cut free from blood supply, moved to breast and reattached to breast blood supply by microsurgery. Inpatient with general anesthesia. Surgery takes 3 to 8 hours.	May need blood transfusion. Most complex of all operations for reconstruction. Needs surgeon with great expertise in procedure. Hospital stay of several days. Scar in buttock or thigh. May have serious complications. Longer recovery period.
Nipple Can be made from existing skin, pinched and tacked to make nipple, or created from tissue from other nipple or groin and attached to breast mound.	Areola reconstruction may also be done. May need tattoo to match color of other breast. If created from other nipple or groin, that area will feel tender for about 2 weeks.

puts the implant into a pocket created under the chest muscle. Different types of implants can be used—saline, silicone gel or double lumen implants. A drain may be put in to take away the fluid that may accumulate during the first few days, and the incision is closed. The operation takes about one to two hours and is usually done under general anesthesia.

What is capsular contracture?

Capsular contracture is the term used by health professionals to describe the hard scar the body forms around an implant, resulting in a hard breast. The newer implants have textured surfaces that help reduce the chances of scar formation. These textured surfaces also seem to produce a softer breast.

What is latissimus dorsi reconstruction?

This operation is used when chest muscles have been removed and where there is too little skin to hold and cover an implant. The surgeon transfers skin, muscle and other tissue from the back to the mastectomy site. To create a new muscle on the front of the chest, a broad flat muscle on the back, below the shoulder blade—called the latissimus dorsi—is used. An implant is then placed under the new chest muscle. Drains may be put in and kept in place for several days after the surgery to remove fluid. This operation takes three to four hours. You will probably stay in the hospital for several days. You will have a scar on your back as well as on your chest.

What is transverse rectus abdominus muscle flap?

This operation is sometimes called the "tummy tuck." The surgeon transfers one of the two abdominal muscles (the rectus abdominus) to the breast along with skin and fat from the abdomen. This flap of muscle, skin and fat is shaped into the contour of a breast. If there is enough abdominal tissue available, no implant is needed. Transferring tissue in this way also results in tightening of the stomach, thus the use of the term *tummy tuck*. This operation usually offers you a better cosmetic result. However, it is considerably more complicated and you will be in the operating room a longer time. You will have a horizontal scar across the lower abdomen plus the scar on your chest.

What is free flap reconstruction?

This is one of the newest operations for breast reconstruction. You need two teams of surgeons, using microsurgical techniques. The first team removes the flap and the second prepares the blood vessels. A portion of the skin and fat is taken from your buttocks or lower abdomen and grafted onto the mastectomy site. The success of this surgery depends on the tissues getting enough nourishment from the blood vessels after the operation and the experience of the surgeon doing this procedure.

How is the nipple reconstructed?

The nipple is usually constructed by shifting a layer of skin and fat on the reconstructed breast to the place where the nipple and areola (the circle of darker skin that surrounds the nipple) will be formed. It can also be reconstructed by using tissue from the nipple of your opposite breast or tissue from other areas, such as your upper inner thigh. A prosthetic nipple that can be attached directly to the skin is available in stores that sell prostheses.

Is tattooing a procedure in nipple reconstruction?

Tattooing may be used to match the color for the area of the areola. If it is done, a local anesthetic is often used. The pigment is placed directly onto the skin, using a tattooing device that has been dipped into the pigment. The new tattoo often looks darker than the selected color at first and fades in time.

CHOICES

Can I have an operation on my opposite breast if it is larger than my reconstructed breast?

The surgeon can reduce the size of your remaining breast so that it will more nearly match the new breast. This operation may be done at the time of reconstruction or as a second operation. The operation to reduce the size of the remaining breast is called reduction mammoplasty.

What is the difference between the different kinds of implants?

The saline implant is a silicone rubber envelope filled, during surgery, with sterile salt water. The silicone implant is a silicone rubber envelope filled with soft silicone gel that feels like thick jelly. The envelope may have either a textured or a smooth surface. The double lumen implant has two silicone rubber envelopes, one inside the other; one filled with silicone gel and the other filled during surgery with a small amount of saline water which allows the surgeon to adjust the size.

What are the health risks of these implants?

All of the implants have some health risks associated with them and the Food and Drug Administration (FDA) is looking at both types. There are several possible side effects. You may find some hardening of the scar tissue that normally forms around the implant. This can sometimes cause you to have pain, hardening of the breast or changes in the appearance of your breast. Calcium deposits can also form in surrounding tissue, which also can cause you pain and hardening of the breast. The saline implant is more likely to rupture, so you need to be careful not to hit it, for instance, if you play sports. The silicone implant can rupture, too, allowing the gel filling to be released into surrounding tissue. In addition, tiny amounts of silicone might leak or "sweat" through the silicone gel implant, even if it does not rupture.

What are the risks if the silicone gel is released in my body?

The FDA is restricting the use of silicone gel implants to special situations, while studies are being carried out to assess the extent of the health risks. There are some possible risks that if silicone gel escapes from the implant it may reach distant parts of the body. It has been suggested that even very small amounts could cause certain autoimmune (connective tissue) diseases, such as lupus, scleroderma and rheumatoid arthritis in some women. Although some doctors have reported that a few patients have developed arthritis-like diseases after receiving breast implants, it is not clear whether women with implants are more likely to develop these conditions than those without implants. There are also questions as to whether the silicone can increase the risk of cancer, find its way into breast milk, or pose a risk to unborn babies. The studies presently under way are designed to answer these questions.

What are the symptoms of the autoimmune-like diseases caused by leaking silicone gel?

The symptoms include pain or swelling of joints; tightness, redness or swelling of the skin; swollen glands or lymph nodes; unusual or unexplained fatigue; swelling of the hands and feet; and unusual hair loss. You might have a combination of these symptoms. But you need to remember that these immune-related disorders are relatively rare.

Do the silicone implants cause cancer?

At the present time, there is no evidence that the silicone-gel-filled implants cause cancer in humans. Two reported studies have shown no increased risk for breast cancer. Other studies are presently under way.

Is the silicone envelope that is on all the implants dangerous?

This also is not known, and cannot be totally ruled out, even for the saline-filled implants.

How long does an implant last?

This can vary from woman to woman. Some implants last for many years in some women. In others they have to be replaced more frequently. The exact length of time an implant lasts cannot be guaranteed at this time.

Is a saline-filled implant safer than a silicone-gel-filled implant?

It probably is but this issue is not completely settled at this time. The Food and Drug Administration has asked the manufacturers of the saline-filled implants to submit safety and effectiveness information on them, especially since saline-filled implants use a silicone rubber envelope, whose long-term safety is unproven. However, leakage or rupture of a saline implant would result in release of salt water. Since salt water is not foreign to your body, it is assumed that it would not present the risks that are associated with the gel.

Where would the salt water in the saline implant go?

The salt water would be absorbed in your body within a few hours. The implant would be deflated quickly and would need to be removed surgically.

If I wish to have a silicone-gel-filled implant for my reconstruction will I be able to do that?

You probably will. The Federal Drug Administration (FDA) has issued guidelines which limit the use of these implants to reconstruction and have imposed a moratorium on the use of silicone-gel-filled implants for breast enlargement. You can have a silicone-gel-filled implant only if you are enrolled in a clinical scientific study through the surgeon who is doing your reconstruction. Under these guidelines, if you have had breast cancer, you may still, if you wish, choose to have immediate or delayed reconstruction, using silicone-gel-filled implants, so long as you are participating in the clinical trial.

How can I enroll in a study?

You first need to contact the doctor you choose to do the implant surgery. The doctor then makes the necessary arrangements with the implant manufacturer. The doctor will need to certify that you qualify medically for the implant. You will need to sign a special informed consent form, certifying that you have been told about the risks of the implant. You will be enrolled in a registry so that you can be notified in the future, if needed, about new information on implants. (You can get additional information by contacting the FDA Breast Implant Information Service at 1-800-532-4440.)

What complications might I have from the surgery for breast reconstruction?

You must remember that there is always the possibility of complications from any surgery, even with the best surgeon. You might have an infection at the breast site, or large areas of the skin might die. Part or all of a transferred muscle may fail to survive. If you have had an implant and these complications happen, the implant may need to be removed temporarily and then replaced. You should not expect that the reconstruction will restore the sensation lost through your mastectomy. Make sure you discuss the possible complications with your plastic surgeon before the operation, realizing that, as with any type of plastic surgery, it is difficult to predict the overall results.

Will I have to do anything to my breast after reconstruction?

If you have had an implant, you will be taught how to massage it after the operation and how to exercise the muscles surrounding your implant. It will take a few months for the skin and muscle to stretch and for the reconstructed breast to take on a natural appearance.

How long is the recovery period after reconstruction?

It depends on what operation and how much surgery you have had. You will generally have a large bulky dressing and a drain, and will probably need pain medicine for the first couple of days. You may have more pain and discomfort from this operation than from the mastectomy, especially if you are having reconstruction that involves the movement of muscle and tissue from other parts of the body. Most women are able to resume normal activities in two to three weeks, although it is usually several more weeks before they can do strenuous exercise.

Should I be doing breast self-examination if I have a breast implant?

Yes, you should be doing monthly breast self-examination so you will be familiar with how your breasts feel normally and would be able to detect any complications that are due to your implant. It is particularly important for you to pay attention to changes in the firmness, size or shape of your breast. You should also be attentive to pain, tenderness or color changes in the breast area or any discharge or unusual sensation around the nipple. You should report these changes promptly to your doctor. In addition, you need to pay attention to the other breast. If you are not sure how to do breast self-examination, ask your doctor to teach you.

Will I need to have mammograms on my reconstructed breast?

Most doctors feel there is no need to have a screening mammogram of the side with the mastectomy and reconstruction since there is no breast tissue remaining on the reconstructed side.

If I have surgery to reduce my other breast, will I need special views when I have a mammogram?

If you have had breast reduction surgery, you need to tell the technician and the radiologist before the mammogram is done. Usually the scar tissue that is seen in the reduced breast does not present a problem in reading the mammogram. If an implant was placed in the other breast at the time of the reduction surgery, you need to have special views taken.

Can I have breast reconstruction if I had my mastectomy ten years ago?

There are women who have had successful reconstructions twenty years after their mastectomies. The fact that you had a mastectomy many years ago does not disqualify you as a candidate for the operation, nor does your age.

Can I have breast reconstruction after I have had radiation treatments?

It depends on many factors. However, radiation-damaged skin, grafted, thin, or tight skin or the absence of chest muscles are not the obstacles to breast reconstruction that they once were.

How much does breast reconstruction cost?

The operations are expensive and cost depends upon the extent of the surgery as well as other factors. The surgeon's fee can run from $2,500 to over $10,000, with hospital costs ranging from $3,000 upward. Many private insurance plans now cover postmastectomy surgery, but coverage varies greatly. Some cover only the hospital costs, while others will also pay part or all of the plastic surgeon's cost. Be sure you know the cost and what your policy will cover before deciding on the operation.

GETTING SUPPORT

What is Reach to Recovery?

This is a volunteer program sponsored by the American Cancer Society. It is based on the idea that those people who have been through breast surgery and have experienced the pain, anxiety, and convalescence are able to help others who are going through the same experiences. Trained volunteers offer emotional support and furnish information, including a kit with a realistically written manual of information and exercise materials. For women who have had a mastectomy, a temporary breast form and bra may be supplied. Call the local office of the American Cancer Society.

What is Look Good . . . Feel Better?

Look Good . . . Feel Better is a nationwide program that has been developed by the Cosmetic, Toiletry, and Fragrance Association in cooperation with the American Cancer Society (ACS) and the National Cosmetology Association. It helps women deal with the changes in their appearances that may result from chemotherapy or radiation treatments or from the illness itself, such as loss of hair, eyebrows and lashes, changes in skin tone and texture or brittleness of nails. Cosmetologists give practical, one-on-one advice on appearance changes, including specific recommendations for skin care, hairstyles, wigs and accessories, eyebrow and eye makeup and nail care, taking into consideration the changes you may have in your skin and nails. You can learn how to put on scarves and turbans and the different styles of wigs that are available. The American Cancer Society, along with cancer centers and hospitals around the country, runs the program locally with members of the National Cosmetology Association offering their services on a voluntary basis to help women with cancer learn beauty techniques. Look Good ... Feel Better is also looking into developing programs for children and for men. Your local ACS unit, listed in the white pages of the telephone directory, can provide more information about this program. Or you can call 1-800-395-LOOK to find programs located near you.

Would it be useful for me to go to a support group?

Joining a support group can help you discuss your feelings with others who have shared your experience. A study, conducted in California with women who have metastatic breast cancer, concluded that group therapy may help patients adapt to their disease and possibly prolong survival. Your nurse, social worker, your local American Cancer Society, or the Cancer Information Service (1-800-4-CANCER) can put you in touch with a group in your area.

Why am I afraid to let my partner get near me since my operation?

This happens to some after breast surgery. You may worry about the scar hurting or you may be afraid of letting your partner see your new body. Sexual relations can be resumed as soon as you feel ready. The body's ability to heal is quite rapid. Intimacy can help to make you feel better psychologically. A small, soft pillow to protect the scar may be helpful at first. You may need to experiment to find comfortable positions that do not put pressure on the area where you had surgery. Be honest with your partner. Explain your fears and enlist your partner's help. Your partner may also be nervous and scared.

Why it is that since my mastectomy I seem to be having difficulties with my partner—having sex less often and not enjoying it as much?

Several studies have shown that some, but certainly not all, women who have had breast surgery may be faced with a problem involving their sexuality. There seem to be several parts to it, depending upon what kind of surgery you have had:

- You may be afraid of showing your scars to your partner.
- You may be afraid of having your partner see you with only one breast, or with a breast that is not as perfect as before.
- You may feel you will never be the same person sexually as you were before.

- Your partner may be afraid of causing you pain.
- Your partner may be upset with the change in your body.
- Your emotional problems may be more involved than having the breast operation.

For some, the loss is so great they cannot overcome it alone. If you are having a problem of this kind, it is important for you to get some professional help.

Are there any other activities that will make me feel better about myself?

Physical exercise, such as tennis, swimming, dance classes or exercise classes, can help to improve your feelings about yourself. Your sense of grace and balance can be enhanced through dance-exercise classes. Yoga has been recommended as a way of achieving a sense of wholeness about the body. Many persons have taken up such challenging new activities as skiing. Others have returned to college and found a whole new sense of self-worth. Creative activities, such as music, painting, sewing, needlepoint and writing, are excellent fields to explore to help strengthen your self-image. In addition, you may want to explore the possibility of breast reconstruction if you have not already done so.

Is there anything a family member or friend can do to help someone who has gone through a breast cancer experience?

- Many women find that talking about their experience and how they feel about it is very helpful.
- A partner who tells you that you are still loved and needed will help you get through the difficult days and make you feel worthwhile.
- Friends and family members who are willing to talk and who are not afraid to bring up the subject make it easier for conversation to begin.
- Nurses who encourage the patient to look at the site of the operation and who listen to what you have to say are helpful.
- People who are willing to go with you to buy your prosthesis or wig are helpful.

Is it normal for me to feel depressed after a few weeks, when earlier I felt like I was facing the facts honestly and well?

Much of your reaction, it has been found, depends upon the expectations you have and how you approached the operation. It is not unusual to have emotional distress. It may be a feeling of panic. Some cry. Others say they don't feel like eating. Some cannot sleep or concentrate. Still others cannot talk about their cancer to anyone. Many women have a "why did this have to happen to me" feeling. These are normal kinds of feelings for breast cancer patients. Some people reach this stage directly after the operation, others not until a month or several months have gone by. Just understand that these are normal reactions to having a cancer diagnosis and to the feeling of helplessness about it. Above all, don't feel that you are strange because you have these feelings. It is normal to have them. Find someone to talk to—either a family member, a good friend, a support group, the Cancer Information Service, the American Cancer Society, a social worker, a nurse, doctor or cleric.

Do younger women have more difficulty coping with breast cancer?

It seems that they do. Younger women seem to be more likely to be depressed, angry, and resentful, have more sexual problems and more fears about recurrence than do older women with breast cancer.

What can I do to help my children cope with my situation?

Children react in different ways and are influenced by their age and stage of development. Some are angry because you are ill. Others are frightened or worried. Some wonder whether or not they have caused your illness. It is better to tell them what is going on, because even young children know when something is happening. It's a good idea to tell your children the truth as simply and positively as possible. Ask for their questions and answer them honestly, but be careful not to burden them with any more information than is necessary. There is more information on helping your family cope with your illness in Chapter 24, "Living with Cancer."

PREGNANCY AND BREAST CANCER

Can a woman who has had breast cancer safely have a baby?

This is becoming a more common question, since about a quarter of all breast cancer patients will develop their disease during their childbearing years. There have been several studies assessing the possible effects of pregnancy on breast cancer patients. A summary of those studies shows that pregnancy after breast cancer treatment has no effect on recurrence or on survival rates. This appears to be true regardless of the number of pregnancies, the time between treatment and the pregnancy, lymph node status, or the stage of the initial breast cancer.

Should I get pregnant while I am getting my treatment?

You should not get pregnant while you are still undergoing treatment. Therefore, it is important to practice family planning while you are being treated.

How long should I wait after my treatment before I become pregnant?

Many doctors suggest that you wait a minimum of one year. The most important consideration is your overall risk for recurrent cancer based on your initial stage of disease. If, for instance, you have node-negative disease, there is no scientific evidence that you need to wait more than a year before attempting to get pregnant. You need to consider the time you need to get back to your normal activities before you decide to get pregnant. You and your partner should discuss the risks involved with your doctor. A consultation with a genetic counselor may also be useful. Of course, the decision of whether or when to attempt to become pregnant is one that only you can make.

Where can I find support during my pregnancy?

This is a difficult issue. Many times family members will not be supportive of your decision to become pregnant. You may have additional concerns, especially about your breasts, since they become fuller than normal during pregnancy. It is useful to find professionals who can be supportive during this time. You may need to go back to the health professional team that took care of you during your cancer treatment. You might also ask for help from an oncology nurse or social worker at a cancer center, or a genetic counselor. If they cannot help you themselves, they can suggest others who can.

Will I be able to breast-feed my baby and will it be safe for the baby?

Some women find that they can breast-feed from the other breast. Most women do not produce milk from a breast that has been radiated. If you plan to breast-feed, you need to know that breast-feeding has not been shown to increase the risk of breast cancer in the infant.

How is breast cancer detected during pregnancy?

It is usually a painless lump which has been felt by the doctor or the woman herself. Mammograms in pregnant women are difficult to read because of the increased water density of the breast.

What is the outlook for women who discover breast cancer during pregnancy?

About 7 percent of women who develop breast cancer happen to be pregnant at the time of the diagnosis. The outlook for a pregnant woman is just as favorable as that for nonpregnant women of the same age with a similar stage of disease—provided that the cancer is diagnosed and treated promptly.

What kind of doctor should be taking care of me if I am diagnosed with breast cancer during my pregnancy?

It is important that you have a multidisciplinary group of doctors taking care of you, including your obstetrician, an experienced breast surgeon and a medical oncologist. In addition, it may be necessary for a radiation oncologist to be involved.

How will a biopsy be done if the doctor finds a suspicious lump in my breast while I am pregnant?

As with nonpregnant women, a prompt biopsy is essential to establish a diagnosis of breast cancer. Breast biopsy under local anesthesia is safe any time during pregnancy.

Should I have a bone scan?

This is also a difficult decision to make. Under most circumstances, a bone scan will not be done because of the danger to the fetus from radiation exposure. However, if there is other evidence that suggests to your doctor that you may have bone metastases, there are some ways of doing a bone scan with decreased radiation exposure to the fetus.

Will estrogen and progesterone receptor tests be done?

It is not clear whether estrogen and progesterone receptor tests taken during pregnancy are as valid a predictor on which to base treatment as they are in nonpregnant breast cancer patients, since very few studies have been done on this question.

Should I terminate my pregnancy if breast cancer is detected?

The types of biologic changes that occur during pregnancy—high output of hormones like estrogen and prolactin—are known to favor breast tumor growth. However, there have been several small studies that show that having an abortion does not change the course of your breast cancer, nor does it improve your survival rates. Breast cancer has never been known to spread across the placenta to the fetus.

Will I be able to have a healthy baby?

Breast cancer does not seem to affect the developing fetus.

Can I have an operation for breast cancer while I am pregnant?

Most doctors will recommend mastectomy during the first six or seven months of your pregnancy. Later in your pregnancy, lesser surgery may be recommended, with your radiation treatment delayed until after your delivery. Radiation poses hazards to the baby and its use is discouraged during pregnancy.

Will I have general anesthesia for my operation?

You probably will, particularly if you are having a mastectomy. Studies have found that it is safe for you to have general anesthesia after your first trimester, so long as the usual precautions are taken to compensate for the normal changes that occur to your body functions during pregnancy.

Will I be able to have chemotherapy treatment while I am pregnant?

Chemotherapy is hazardous to the development of the baby during the first three months. Therefore, chemotherapy should be avoided at that time, if possible. If this is not feasible, then your doctor needs to decide whether treatment can be safely postponed until the second trimester or later. Studies show that single and combination chemotherapy can be given during the second and third trimesters with a very low risk of fetal damage, although other side effects such as premature labor may be a risk. However, many doctors feel that chemotherapy should be delayed until after delivery. Your doctor may also recommend an early induced delivery or a cesarean delivery. You and your doctor need to discuss the advantages and disadvantages of each choice.

What if advanced local disease or metastatic breast cancer is discovered early in my pregnancy?

Advanced local disease or metastatic breast cancer in nonpregnant women is usually treated with both chemotherapy and radiation therapy. As a pregnant woman, you will need to think about whether or not you wish to end the pregnancy in order to begin the treatment. Although there is no evidence that termination of the pregnancy improves the outcome for breast cancer patients, it does permit standard aggressive treatment to be given for advanced disease.

Can I breast-feed if I am taking chemotherapy?

Probably not. This is another question you need to discuss with your doctors. Systemic chemotherapy drugs may reach significant levels in your milk, especially if you are being treated with cyclophosphamide or methotrexate or some hormonal drugs. In addition, if you are scheduled to have breast surgery after you deliver, it is safer if you have not been breast-feeding.

Is there any special care that a pregnant woman needs during treatment?

There are several issues that are especially important for pregnant women with cancer:

- You may need to increase the amount of food you eat so that you can maintain the appropriate weight gain during your pregnancy.
- If you are receiving chemotherapy, there are several other potential problems:
  —if nausea and vomiting are potential side effects, you may need to take antinausea medicine. Your doctor will need to determine which medicines are appropriate to control it.
   —you need to make sure you are getting good dental care and oral hygiene to prevent oral infections.
  —you will need to pay greater attention to constipation, since this is a problem associated with both pregnancy and some chemotherapeutic drugs.
  —if infection or hemorrhage are potential side effects, you will need to be especially careful and watchful.

Will my delivery be specially timed if I am taking chemotherapy?

The doctor will plan your delivery so that your blood counts are not dangerously low, thus putting you at risk. Following delivery, the doctor will reassess your treatment, particularly if it was planned to avoid risks to the fetus.

FOLLOW-UP AFTER BREAST CANCER

How often will I need to return for checkups following breast cancer?

Your doctor will tailor-make a follow-up schedule for you. Generally, the doctor will ask you to come back every three months for the first year and then every six months. After five years, you will probably have yearly visits. You will probably have a bone scan and a chest x-ray yearly; blood tests at every visit and a mammogram every year.

Why are these checkups important?

You need to make sure you have the checkups to see whether or not your cancer has reappeared (or recurred, as the medical community says). Even when a tumor in the breast appears to have been completely removed or destroyed, the disease sometimes returns because undetected cancer cells have remained in the area after treatment or because the disease had already spread before treatment. Most of the recurrences, about 60 percent, happen within the first three years after your first treatment. Another 20 percent happens within the next two years, with 20 percent happening in the later years. It is important that you continue to be checked by the doctor on a regular schedule.

QUESTIONS TO ASK YOUR DOCTOR ABOUT FOLLOW-UP EXAMS

- How often will I need to be checked and who will I go to for checkups? What kind of tests will be done then?
- Who will be in charge of my follow-up care? Will I have to go to more than one doctor?
- What kinds of tests will I need? Can they be done at the same time as my visit with you?
- Will I need a mammogram on the other breast?
- Should I be doing breast self-exam? Can you show me what to look for?
- What symptoms should I be checking between examinations with you?
- Are there any specific symptoms or problems I should report to you?

What kind of doctor will be doing the follow-up exams?

This is an issue that you need to discuss with the team of doctors who have treated you. In the first few years after treatment, you will probably have to see more than one doctor. The surgeon will want to check you. If you have had breast reconstruction, the plastic surgeon will also want to see you. If you have had radiation treatment and chemotherapy, the radiation oncologist and the medical oncologist will need to be included in your follow-up. It is most useful if you can have an agreement among the team as to who is your lead doctor, how you can alternate visits (so you don't have to see two doctors in the same week), and how the results of the tests will be shared and discussed among the different specialties.

Is there anything special I should look for between these checkups?

Call your doctor if you have the following problems: pain in your breast, shoulder, hip, lower back or pelvis; changes in your breast or in your scar such as lumps, thickenings, redness or swelling; loss of weight or appetite; a persistent hoarseness or cough; nausea, vomiting, diarrhea or heartburn that lasts for several days; changes in your menstrual cycle or flow; dizziness, blurred vision, severe or frequent headaches or trouble walking; or digestive problems that seem unusual or that do not go away. Remember that these symptoms can be caused by many other things, such as the flu, a common cold, menopause or arthritis. They are not sure signs that the cancer has returned, but you need to report them to your doctor so that an accurate diagnosis can be made.

Why should I do a monthly breast self-exam?

Monthly breast self-examination is particularly important after you have had breast cancer because you have a greater chance of getting cancer in the other breast. Doing breast exams after you have had cancer is different—you need to learn what is normal for you now. Ask your doctor or nurse to help you learn what to expect and how to perform the examination. If you have had a breast removed, you need to understand the scar area and what to look for. If you have had breast reconstruction, you need to feel carefully around the implant and under your arm. If you have had radiation, you need to understand the different feeling of the breast tissue itself. What you will be looking for is any change that you need to bring to your doctor's attention.

RECURRENCE

What is meant by a local recurrence?

A local recurrence is when the cancer returns only in the breast area. If the disease returns in another part of the body, it is called metastatic breast cancer or distant disease.

Where is breast cancer most likely to spread?

The lungs, bone and liver are the areas where breast cancer is most likely to spread. Other sites include the kidneys, ovaries, pituitary gland, adrenal glands and thyroid gland.

Can breast cancer that comes back be treated?

Breast cancer that recurs locally can often be treated and, in some instances, can be cured. However, if it comes back in another part of the body, it usually cannot be cured, although many women have lived for many years following their recurrence.

What will my treatment choices be?

Your choice of treatment depends on your hormone receptor levels at the time of your recurrence, the kind of treatment you had before and your response to that treatment, the length of time from first treatment to when the cancer came back, whether your recurrence is local or widespread, whether you still have menstrual periods and other factors. The treatments may be radiation, surgery, chemotherapy or hormones. You should consider going into one of the ongoing clinical trials testing newly developed chemotherapy and biologic agents, bone marrow transplants, or peripheral stem cell support in Phase II studies. (Call the Cancer Information Service to get information on these studies.) There is more information on clinical trials in Chapter 9, "New Advances and Investigational Trials."

Will I have pain with recurrent breast cancer?

It depends on where it recurs. If you have pain, there are several treatments that can be used. You may be given pain medication or you may be given radiation therapy if the pain is due to bone metastases. One recent development for treating pain from bone metastases is Strontium-89 (Metastron) which is given on an outpatient basis in a single intravenous injection and provides relief which usually lasts an average of six months. More information on Strontium-89 can be found in Chapter 25, "When Cancers Recur or Metastasize." Further detailed information on pain is in Chapter 24, "Living with Cancer."

What are the experiences of other cancer patients in dealing with recurrence?

We have been told by many people who have had cancer that recurrence is their greatest fear. When recurrence does happen, most people deal with it in much the same way as they did their first bout with the disease. However, many feel more upset about their recurrence than they were with their original diagnosis. This may be because many are sicker, or feel they have less support from their families. Some also feel angry about their treatment choices. Some think that because the cancer has come back they are going to die. Some women say that they find it hard to talk about recurrence with their spouses and family members, but are able to talk about it with people outside of their families. There is more information on this subject in Chapter 25, "When Cancers Recur or Metastasize."

Is there any information on what recurrence means to the spouse and family of the patient?

Recurrence is very difficult on the families of patients. Some feel angry and fearful. Others talk about the injustice of the recurrence and express feelings of grief, as well as concern with coping and with the impact that this event has on the family.

Is it usual to feel that your doctor thinks you have more family support than you have?

Many patients have noted this fact. They feel that their doctors and nurses assumed they had adequate support from their families and that they were coping better than they actually were. They also felt that their doctors presumed they had more knowledge about the disease than they actually had.

If I have had breast cancer, am I at higher risk for getting other kinds of cancer?

Women who have had breast cancer are at higher risk for getting cancers of the endometrium, ovary and colon. You are also at higher risk for getting cancer in the other breast.

If I have had radiation therapy, am I at an even higher risk for developing a new cancer in the opposite breast?

Having breast cancer in the first breast puts you at higher risk for developing it in the opposite breast, compared to women without the disease. Radiation treatment for breast cancer—which can cure breast cancer—adds a little, but not very much to that risk. A study by the National Cancer Institute showed that fewer than 3 percent of the second primary breast cancers that occurred in women diagnosed with breast cancer between 1935 and 1982 could be attributed to radiation therapy administered five years or more previously. The small increased risk of cancer in the opposite breast due to radiation therapy occurred only in women who were treated when they were under 45 years of age. If you are under 45 years of age and having radiation treatment, talk to the radiation oncologist about what steps will be taken to minimize radiation exposure of the opposite breast during treatment.

chapter 12

Prostate and Other Male Cancers

> Prostate is often mispronounced as "prostrate"—with the addition of an *r* in the last syllable. The correct pronunciation is "prostate," without the *r* in the second syllable.

The longer a man lives, the greater his chance of developing prostate cancer. Autopsies show that nearly every man over the age of 80 has some evidence of prostate cancer. Many of these men have lived with these cancers and never known they existed. Not all prostate problems turn out to be cancer. About eight out of ten times, the problems can be traced to other causes. Symptoms of prostate cancer are often the same as those caused by the enlargement or inflammation of the gland. Three out of four men over age 50 have some symptoms of an enlarged prostate, which in most cases is not due to cancer.

While survival is the most important factor in determining treatment, there are many other considerations for men facing treatment of disease in this sensitive area. For example, sexual function and urinary function are major concerns following treatment. It is important for any man facing treatment to assess each treatment and its side effects before making a decision. With new techniques available for detection and treatment, men have more choices than ever before—which can result in making the decisions more difficult to make than ever before. Gathering information and talking with doctors from different disciplines may help you in making your decision.

What You Need to Know About Prostate Cancer

- Prostate problems don't always mean prostate cancer.
- Most men have at least one bout of prostatitis (inflammation of the prostate) in their lifetimes.
- Acute prostatitis is characterized by an abrupt onset of fever, pain at the base of the penis, and painful urination.
- Chronic prostatitis is characterized by low-grade, recurring infections that cause discomfort.
- The prostate also becomes enlarged as the result of hormonal changes associated with aging. This condition is known as Benign Prostatic Hypertrophy, or BPH. By the age of 60, prostate enlargement is found in almost all men. When this happens, it narrows the passageway for urine flow, causing a variety of symptoms, such as difficulty in starting the flow of urine, decreased force of the urinary stream, dribbling of urine and increased frequency of urination. This blockage of the urine can lead to serious infections of the urinary tract.
- Proscar (finasteride is the generic name) is a new drug being used to treat symptoms of enlarged prostate glands. Clinical studies show the drug offers some symptom relief for enlarged prostate glands in about one of three men though it may take at least 6 to 12 months before relief is achieved. Continuing studies are under way to determine if the drug can prevent prostate cancer from developing.
- Prostate cancer is usually first detected through a digital rectal examination the doctor performs as part of a physical examination. Most men should have a digital rectal exam each year after age 40.
- About 30 percent of men over 60 have prostate cancer. Only about 1 percent of prostate cancers occur in men under 50.
- Prostate cancer, which is less common than BPH, may require treatment depending on the stage of the disease, the age of the patient, and a full understanding of the treatment options available. No treatment for prostate cancer is totally free of the possibility of some sexual or incontinence prob-

lems. It is important that treatment be discussed with, and undertaken by, a skilled, experienced urologist.

WHO IS AT RISK FOR PROSTATE CANCER?

Age	Risk increases with age, especially after age 55.
Race	Black men in parts of the U.S. have the highest incidence of prostate cancer.
Genetics	Increased risk if first-degree relative has had prostate cancer.
Diet	High fat intake suspected.
Occupation	Working with cadmium, zinc, rubber, dewaxing process in oil refining indicated in studies.
Other	Obesity and previous bouts with sexually transmitted diseases.

How often should a man be checked to see if there are signs of prostate cancer?

A digital rectal examination should be performed every year on all males over the age of 40. Those in high-risk groups, such as African Americans, or where family members have a history of prostate cancer, are advised to begin the yearly testing earlier. The American Cancer Society is also recommending that a PSA test (a test which detects prostate-specific antigen, a protein produced by prostate cells) be performed yearly on men 50 years of age and over. The National Cancer Institute's early detection guidelines do not include routine PSA screening for men without symptoms.

What are some of the issues involved in the controversy in using the PSA test as an early detection tool?

A number of issues and a number of "unknowns" are involved. Like all medical tests, PSA is not foolproof. It can indicate a cancer when none exists. However, the American Cancer Society believes that PSA can increase the ability to find early, localized prostate cancer with further testing. According to the National Cancer Institute, much remains unknown about the interpretation of PSA levels, the test's ability to discriminate cancer from benign prostate conditions and the best course of action following a finding of elevated PSA, especially in younger men. Since in some cases men with suspicious PSAs will receive treatment that may cause impotence and incontinence, the concern is that PSA screening may result in treatments without any benefit and with unnecessary side effect.

SYMPTOMS OF PROSTATE CANCER

Small prostate cancers often do not cause any symptoms. When symptoms do occur, they may include:

- Frequent urination, especially at night.
- Trouble starting or holding back urinating.
- A weak or interrupted urine flow.
- Pain or burning during urination.
- Blood in the urine.
- Continuing pain in lower back, pelvis or upper thighs.

What kind of doctor is best for treating prostate problems?

A urologist, a doctor who specializes in treating diseases of the genitourinary system, is best qualified to determine whether symptoms are caused by prostate cancer, BPH, or some other condition such as an infection.

QUESTIONS TO ASK IF THE DOCTOR THINKS YOU HAVE PROSTATE CANCER

- What sort of lump did you feel on the prostate?
- Is the prostate enlarged or is there a definite nodule or ridge?
- Where was it located?
- Were the PSA (prostatic-specific antigen) test results elevated?
- What was the PSA reading?
- How high was my PSA level above normal?
- Will you be rechecking the extent of the tumor with an ultrasound probe?
- Will the biopsy be done with an ultrasound probe?

Who usually gets cancer of the prostate?

The risk of developing cancer of the prostate increases with age. Cancer of the prostate usually occurs in men over 55 years of age. The incidence varies from country to country. Black American males have the highest incidence. Japanese-American men have the lowest. Statistics show that men with relatives who have had prostate cancer are more than three times as likely to develop the disease. There is some evidence that workers who have been exposed to cadmium, zinc, rubber or the dewaxing process of oil refining may be at higher risk for prostate cancer. Those who have had past bouts with sexually transmitted diseases are also at increased risk.

What causes prostate cancer?

It is believed that changes in the sex hormones have an influence on prostate cancer. Hormones are required for the normal growth and development of the prostate and men who have been castrated almost never develop prostate cancer. Prostate cancer can be induced in mice by prolonged administration of testosterone. Testosterone levels are higher in patients with prostate cancer than in those with other prostate problems. However, doctors cannot explain why one person gets prostate cancer and another does not. The effects of diet are being studied. Some evidence suggests that a diet high in fat increases the risk of prostate cancer, but this link has not been proven. Other studies point to an increased risk to workers exposed to the metal cadmium during welding, electroplating or making batteries. Rubber industry workers also appear to develop prostate cancer more often than is normal. Studies are also being conducted to determine whether benign prostatic hyperplasia or a sexually transmitted virus increases the risk for prostate cancer.

Is it true that men who have had vasectomies are more likely to develop prostate cancer?

There have been some studies that appear to point to the possibility that men who have had vasectomies may be at greater risk for prostate cancer as well as other studies that questioned these findings. An expert committee convened by the National Institutes of Health has found that the association, at most, is a small one. Further studies are needed to determine whether or not vasectomy is associated with prostate cancer in any way. In the meantime, screening for prostate cancer should not be any different for men who have had a vasectomy than for those who have not.

What does the prostate look like?

The prostate gland is about the size of a walnut. It is located below the bladder and in front of the rectum. It is a male sex gland, part of a man's reproductive system. Its only known function is its

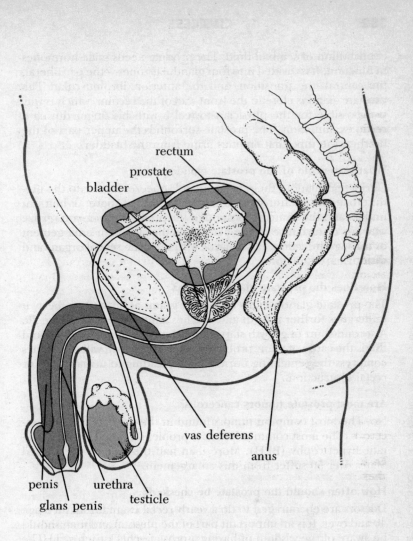

Male reproductive organs
(Illustration by Dolores Bego)

contribution of seminal fluid. The prostate needs male hormones to function. It is divided into four glandular zones—the peripheral, the central, the transition, and the anterior fibromuscular. The prostate gland is close to the front wall of the rectum, which is why it is possible for the physician to feel it with his finger during a rectal examination. The prostate surrounds the upper part of the urethra, the tube that empties urine from the bladder.

What is the role of the prostate gland?

During ejaculation, the prostate gland squeezes fluid into the urethra to aid in the transport and nourishment of sperm. When you understand the strategic location of the prostate gland, you realize why any disturbance to the gland, whether through enlargement or through infection, raises havoc with the male sexual organs and with urinary functions.

How does the prostate gland develop?

The prostate gland weighs only a few grams at birth. At puberty it undergoes further growth and reaches adult size by about age 20. A second spurt of growth starts in most men at about age 50—and this is the cause of many problems, since the growth will sometimes compress the remaining normal gland, leading to urinary and/or rectal obstruction.

Are most prostate tumors cancerous?

No. The most common tumors found in the prostate are not cancerous. The most common prostate problem is called benign prostatic hypertrophy (BPH). More than half the men in the United States over 50 suffer from this enlargement.

How often should the prostate be checked?

Doctors are encouraged to do a yearly rectal exam for all men age 40 and over. It is an important part of the physical and men should be aware of the wisdom of having a prostate check each year. The doctor can do this examination in a very few minutes. Some doctors also will do a PSA test. As discussed above, the use of the PSA as a screening test is still under study. It is wise to talk with your doctor about prostate cancer, the symptoms to watch for and an appropriate schedule for checkup. The doctor's advice will be based on your age, your medical history and other factors.

How is the digital rectal exam done?

The doctor is able to feel the prostate gland with a rubber-gloved finger inserted through the anus. A cancerous lump feels firm, like a marble, in what is normally a fleshy gland. Though not the most dignified of examinations, the checking of the prostate gland so that any abnormality can be detected early is an important part of any physical. The doctor will ask you to either bend from the hips with elbows on the examining table or on your knees. Some doctors prefer to have the buttocks elevated in the knee-chest position. In either case, the doctor will ask you to "bear down" as he inserts his finger. It is normal to experience sensations of having to urinate or defecate during the examination.

Is the PSA test a substitute for the digital rectal exam?

No. Many men wish they could skip the digital rectal exam and just have what seems to be the simpler blood tests. However, used alone, the PSA test does not diagnose prostate cancer. It is important to have the digital rectal exam because it gives the doctor the chance to feel whether or not there are lumps on the part of the prostate that can be felt.

What are the symptoms of cancer of the prostate?

Symptoms which should not be ignored include a weak or interrupted flow of urine, inability to urinate or difficulty in starting urination, need to urinate frequently (especially at night), blood in the urine, urine flow that is not easily stopped, painful or burning urination and continuing pain in the back, pelvis or hips. These symptoms are often the same symptoms that indicate other prostatic problems, but they are symptoms which should be checked by the doctor, who can detect the difference between a cancerous and noncancerous enlargement of the prostate. **Be aware, however, that early prostate cancer often does not cause any symptoms, which is why regular digital exams are recommended.**

What tests are usually recommended when the doctor finds a problem with the prostate?

Any abnormality which the doctor feels when doing a digital rectal exam will make it necessary for other tests to be ordered. Usually the doctor will try to determine what is causing the lump, and whether it is a benign or a cancerous lump. Blood tests such as the PSA (and sometimes PAP) and urine studies will usually be ordered. The doctor may order other tests such as bone scans and chest films, kidney-function tests, intravenous pyelogram and lymphography to determine the extent of disease. A biopsy is the final definitive test.

What does the PAP test measure?

The Prostate Acid Phosphatase (PAP) test measures a protein produced by prostate cells. An elevated PAP suggests that the cancer may have spread beyond the prostate capsule.

What does the PSA test tell the doctor?

The PSA (Prostate-Specific Antigen) is a protein measured in the blood which is produced by normal and malignant prostate cells. The PSA test alone is not a definitive test and must be used with other indicators to determine diagnosis. The PSA readings can range from zero to the hundreds. Establishing a normal range for the PSA value has been difficult—cancer has been discovered in patients with ranges from 0.2 to over 150. An abnormally high PSA level may suggest cancer of the prostate. Progressive elevation of the PSA over a period of time is of particular concern. To further complicate the picture, the rise in PSA is sometimes seen in men who do not have cancer, and occasionally it is not detectable in men who do have cancer of the prostate. Nonetheless, the PSA does serve as an indicator, and when it is found to be beyond the normal range, further testing must be done to determine if the cause is cancer.

Important note: PSA blood tests should be done <u>before</u> cystoscopy or needle biopsy, because these procedures may <u>raise the PSA levels.</u> The PSA level may not return to normal for several weeks. The digital exam by itself does not significantly increase serum PSA, but cystoscopy and needle biopsy may.

What are considered to be normal PSA levels?

Researchers are continuing to study this question. It appears that normal levels may differ according to age. Recent studies suggest the following age-specific PSA levels:

- Age 71–80: 6.5 ng/ml
- Age 61–70: 4.5 ng/ml
- Age 51–60: 3.5 ng/ml
- Age 41–50: 2.5 ng/ml

In addition, an annual rise in PSA level of about 0.04 ng/ml in men over age 60 is not considered abnormal. These continuing studies will suggest changes both in the guidelines and in follow-up practices.

What happens if the doctor finds I have an elevated PSA?

In most cases, the doctor will want to do further testing to determine why the reading is high. An elevated PSA does not always indicate that cancer is present. Thirty-six percent of patients with nonmalignant tumors have a moderately elevated PSA. The presence of cancer can sometimes be confirmed by the removal of a small piece of prostate tissue for microscopic examination. In the past, a finger-guided needle biopsy was used or a surgical procedure was required. Most doctors will obtain a needle biopsy with ultrasound probes.

How is an ultrasound-guided needle biopsy done?

The probe is placed in the rectum and bounces high-frequency sound waves into the prostate. The different densities between normal prostate tissue and cancer show up as shadows on the ultrasound image. The ultrasound probes are often able to discover cancerous tissue that is missed by a digital examination. The biopsy is then done using the ultrasound to guide the probe. Ultrasound images allow the surgeon to guide a spring-loaded device that fires a needle through the wall of the rectum into the prostate to capture bits of possibly cancerous tissue. The needle is withdrawn so the sample can be analyzed.

Does it hurt to have an ultrasound-directed biopsy?

The device fires the needle so rapidly that it is virtually painless. Some 5 to 10 percent of patients feel a little ache when the gun is fired. There is no anesthesia or catheter and you can usually return home when the procedure is completed.

What other techniques are used to determine if there is cancer?

A CT scan of the abdomen and pelvis may be ordered. The doctor may also order urine tests and may look into the urethra and bladder through a thin, lighted tube called a cystoscope.

Does cancer of the prostate sometimes spread?

Cancer cells can break away from the original tumor in the prostate and spread through the bloodstream and lymphatic system and form tumors in other parts of the body. When cancer of the prostate spreads outside the prostate itself, it often shows up in nearby lymph nodes or lymph glands. Prostate cancer can also spread to the bones, liver, bladder, and other organs. When cancer spreads from the prostate to other parts of the body, often to the bone, the disease is called metastatic prostate cancer rather than bone cancer, liver cancer, etc. To determine if there are other signs of cancer, the doctor may order a CT or CAT scan, to check for abnormally enlarged lymph nodes, or an MRI, to check the prostate and nearby lymph nodes. A bone scan may be ordered to check the bones since increased turnover may be a sign of spreading cancer, although it can also be the result of other bone problems. A chest x-ray will probably also be done to check the status of the lungs.

Can the doctor tell from a biopsy whether my cancer is likely to be the type that spreads?

Prostate cancer shows a wide variation in terms of how likely it is to spread. If the cancer cells closely resemble normal microscopic prostate cells, the tumor is usually considered to be "low grade." If the cancer cells invade neighboring tissue structures such as nerves or blood vessels, the tumor is designated as "high grade" to indicate a more aggressive form of prostate cancer. What is most difficult about prostate cancer is that many tumors remain small and never cause any problems, but some break away from the prostate and appear in the bones. However, researchers say they do not know for certain which will spread and which can be ignored—thus posing a difficult dilemma for patients and doctors.

QUESTIONS TO ASK YOUR DOCTOR BEFORE DECIDING ON PROSTATE CANCER TREATMENT

- What type of treatment do you suggest?
- Why do you feel this treatment is better for me than other possible treatments?
- Are there other treatments that will achieve the same results?
- Is it possible for me to have no treatment at this time, but to have you follow me closely to see if there are future changes?
- What are the benefits and drawbacks of each kind of treatment?
- What are the drawbacks to having radiation instead of surgery or surgery instead of radiation?
- Is internal radiation a possibility for my condition?
- Will radiation be prescribed following surgery?
- How often do you do this type of surgery or radiation?
- Can I have radiation (either internal or external) and later, if it doesn't work, have surgery to remove the prostate? Is it worth the risk?
- How extensive will the surgery or radiation be?

- Where will the scar be?
- Is cryosurgery a possibility?
- How will the treatment affect my sex life?
- Can you do nerve-sparing surgery so that I will not be impotent? How successful has this surgery been in your patients to date?
- If I lose my ability to function sexually, what are my alternatives?
- Will treatment make me incontinent? How long will incontinence continue? Will incontinence be permanent? Will exercises help me alleviate incontinence?
- Will you be doing extensive lymph node dissection to check for cancer spread? Why? What are the side effects in your experience?
- What restrictions will there be on my activities after treatment?
- When can I return to normal activities after this treatment?

If the cancer of the prostate is discovered in a very early stage should I risk the side effects of surgery or radiation or should I wait and see if the cancer progresses?

Unfortunately, there are not, at this time, foolproof guidelines, although many doctors feel it is safest to have radiation or surgery to remove the prostate. Research presently in progress assesses the benefits of various treatments. Treatment is not a guarantee against metastatic cancer, but seeks to reduce the risk, though by an uncertain amount. If cancer is discovered in the very early stages, one choice, with a full understanding of the risks, may be to wait and watch. These thoughts may be helpful:

- Age makes a difference. If over age 70 to 75, waiting and having frequent checkups is a possible treatment option.
- If the cancer appears to be low-grade in appearance when viewed under the microscope and clearly confined to the prostate, you may be advised to wait and watch. (One population-based study has shown excellent survival without any treatment in patients with well or moderately well-differentiated tumors clinically confined to the prostate, irrespective of age.)
- If the cancer is too small to be felt with a digital rectal exam, you may want to proceed slowly.

Important note: In any of these cases, if no treatment is immediately recommended, it is important that you have frequent, regular digital examinations, PAP and PSA testing and ultrasound follow-up to detect any changes as soon as they occur.

What type of cancer are most prostate cancers?

Over 95 percent of prostate cancers that are found in the prostate gland are adenocarcinomas that vary in appearance and differentiation. The remainder are usually squamous cell or sarcomas. Most adenocarcinomas are found in the posterior lobe and are usually multifocal.

What are the stages of prostate cancer?

Prostate cancers are staged from A to D. The results of all the testing will help the doctor decide which stage best describes a patient's cancer.

What is the Gleason score?

The Gleason score is a method used by doctors to determine how close to normal the cells look when the tissue is examined under the microscope. Scores from 1 to 4 indicate that the tumor is well differentiated, 5 to 7 indicate that it is moderately differentiated and 8 to 10 indicate that it is poorly differentiated. The term *differentiated* is used to describe how closely tumor cells resemble their normal counterparts. Tumor cells are described as well differentiated when they look much like normal cells of the same type and are able to carry out some functions of normal cells. Poorly differentiated and undifferentiated tumor cells are disorganized and abnormal-looking. As a general rule, the more undifferentiated the cells look under the microscope, the more active they are likely to be. The greater the difference in the appearance of the cell from what is normal, the higher the number that is assigned on the Gleason scale. (More information about cell differentiation may be found in Chapter 3, "What Is Cancer?")

TREATMENT CHOICES

What are the common treatments for prostate cancer?

Three kinds of treatment are commonly used for prostate cancer:

1. Surgery (removing the cancer).
2. Radiation (using high-dose x-rays to kill cancer).

3. Hormone therapy (using hormones to stop cancer cells from growing).

In addition, cryosurgery, radiation implants, and different ways of giving radiation treatment are being studied as treatment options. Treatment will depend on your medical history, age and stage of disease. Before deciding upon a treatment, it is important to know precisely what the diagnosis is and to understand what risks, side effects and benefits there are concerning each suggested treat-

STAGES OF PROSTATE CANCER	
STAGE	**DESCRIPTION**
Stage A	Cancer confined to the prostate. It cannot be felt and there are no symptoms. Found through ultrasound or accidentally when surgery is done for other reasons. In Stage A1, cancer cells are found only in one area of the prostate and are well-differentiated. In Stage A-2, cancer cells may be moderately or poorly differentiated or are found in many areas of the prostate.
Stage B	Cancer can be felt during rectal exam. Cancer cells found only in prostate gland. In Stage B1, a single tumor is found on one lobe of the prostate. In Stage B2, there is more extensive involvement of one lobe or involvement of both lobes.
Stage C	Cancer cells have spread outside the covering (capsule) of the prostate to the tissues surrounding it. Seminal vesicles may have cancer in them.
Stage D	Cancer cells have spread to lymph nodes or to organs and tissues far away from prostate. Stage D1 means that cancer cells have spread to the lymph nodes near the prostate. Stage D2 means cancer cells have spread to lymph nodes far from the prostate and to other parts of the body, such as the bone, liver or lungs. Stage D1 involves regional lymph nodes only; Stage D2 involves distant lymph nodes or metastases in other parts of the body; Stage D3 indicates prostate cancer patients who have relapsed after adequate endocrine therapy.
Recurrent	Cancer has come back after it has been treated. It may come back in the prostate or in another part of the body.

ment. It is also important for you to confront the very personal factors and feelings that involve the possible sexual and urinary side effects before you make your decision.

Does age make a difference in deciding what kind of treatment option to choose for prostate cancer?

Since prostate cancer is slow-growing, many doctors feel that a 70- to 75-year-old man diagnosed with an early stage of prostate cancer should probably opt for the least invasive treatment. Radiation might be recommended rather than surgery, since it has fewer side effects. In younger or more active men, the decision is less clear. In younger men, surgery to remove the entire prostate may be recommended as insurance against future spread. You should be aware that there is a great deal of controversy about what treatment is best. Studies are incomplete as to how the effectiveness of each of the treatments compare in long-term results.

How curable is cancer of the prostate?

Cancer of the prostate may be cured when it is localized and frequently responds to treatment for long periods of time even when it has spread beyond the prostate.

What is the role of testosterone in prostate cancer?

The normal prostate is dependent upon circulating androgens, principally testosterone, to function. Prostate cancer is also dependent on the male sex hormone testosterone, which can stimulate its growth. That is the reason why hormone therapy that counters the production of testosterone is sometimes prescribed to curb the cancer.

PROSTATECTOMY

What is a prostatectomy?

A prostatectomy is the surgical removal of all or part of the prostate. A radical or total prostatectomy is the removal of the entire prostate. Removing the prostate always results in infertility because the gland is essential for a man to father a child. However, the prostate itself does not affect potency, the ability to have an erection and sustain it during sexual intercourse. Potency relies on normal hormone production, an intact supply of blood to the penis and clusters of microscopic nerves close to the prostate gland. However, depending on the location of the cancer, the surgeon performing the prostatectomy may have to cut the nerves that control erection. Additionally, the skill of the physician has a great deal to do with his ability to perform the operation so that incontinence and impo-

TREATMENT CHOICES FOR PROSTATE CANCER

STAGE	TREATMENT
Stage A1	Careful observation without further immediate treatment in selected patients. Younger patients may consider treatment as for Stage A2.
Stage A2	• External beam radiation (If transurethral resection done, delay 4–6 weeks.) **or** • Radical prostatectomy, may be followed by radiation therapy; **or** • Careful observation without immediate treatment. *Clinical trials:* Interstitial implantation of radioisotopes with pelvic lymphadenectomy; cryosurgery or external beam radiation with new techniques.
Stage B	• Radical prostatectomy, may be followed by radiation therapy; **or** • External beam radiation; **or** • Careful observation without immediate treatment. *Clinical trials:* Interstitial implantation of radioisotopes with pelvic lymphadenectomy, external beam radiation using new techniques, cryosurgery, neutrons or protons.
Stage C	• External beam radiation (If transurethral resection done, delay 4–6 weeks.) **or** • Radical prostatectomy, usually with pelvic lymphadenectomy plus postoperative radiation if capsular penetration or seminal vesicle invasion or if PSA level is elevated 3 weeks after surgery. • Careful observation without immediate treatment. NOTE: If control of urinary symptoms is needed, radiation therapy, transurethral resection of prostate or hormonal manipulation, through either orchiectomy, LHRH agonists or estrogen may be indicated. *Clinical trials:* Interstitial implantation with ultrasound or alternate forms of radiation or ultrasound-guided percutaneous cryosurgery.
Stage D	• Hormonal manipulation through orchiectomy, leuprolide, leuprolide plus flutamide or estrogens. • External beam radiation for selected D1 patients. • Radiation therapy for palliative results. • Transurethral resection to relieve urinary symptoms. • Observation without immediate treatment. *Clinical trials:* Mixed beam radiation, radical prostatectomy plus orchiectomy, chemotherapy or antiandrogens.
Recurrent	• Depends on previous treatment, site of recurrence. Radiation for local recurrence; in selected patients, prostatectomy for recurrence following radiation therapy, hormonal therapy. Radiation for bone pain.

tence can be avoided whenever possible. According to the National
Cancer Institute, among men over 65 years of age, 63 percent who
have had their prostates removed surgically are incontinent and
60 to 90 percent are impotent following surgery. It is important
to question the doctor carefully about experience and the results
achieved with patients, since studies show that results can differ
from doctor to doctor.

Are there different kinds of prostatectomy operations?

A prostatectomy is done in one of two ways. In retropubic prostatectomy, the prostate and nearby lymph nodes are removed through
an incision in the abdomen. In perineal prostatectomy, an incision
is made between the scrotum and the anus to remove the prostate.
Nearby lymph nodes sometimes are removed through a separate
incision in the abdomen. It is important to ask your doctor which
of these is planned.

QUESTIONS TO ASK YOUR DOCTOR ABOUT PROSTATE SURGERY

- What kind of operation will you be doing? Will you do
  nerve-sparing surgery? Where will the scar be?
- How long will I be in the hospital? Is a nurse needed?
- How long will the catheter be needed? Are bladder spasms
  to be expected?
- How long can I expect my urine to look cloudy?
- When will the stitches be removed?
- How long will the dribbling and feeling of urgency to
  urinate continue?
- How long can I expect to be incontinent?
- Are there exercises I can do to strengthen the muscles that
  control urination?
- When can I start driving a car, using stairs, lifting, walking,
  playing tennis or other active sports again?
- Will I be impotent? Will this be temporary or permanent?
- What sort of limitations will the operation put on my
  sexual activity?
- How much does my own psychological state play in
  determining my sexual future?
- What can be done if I am impotent?

If a man has undergone surgery for a benign disease of the prostate,
does this mean he can no longer have prostate cancer?

No. Most operations performed for prostate problems other than
cancer do not remove the entire prostate. Unless a man has under-

gone a total prostatectomy, he should understand that it is still possible for him to develop prostate cancer. Remaining prostatic tissue should be examined as part of every annual examination.

Is it possible to have a prostatectomy and not lose the ability to have an erection?

Impotence—being unable to have an erection—is the most common long-lasting side effect of prostate cancer treatment. A nerve-sparing procedure to retain erection was developed in 1982 by Patrick Walsh, M.D., of Johns Hopkins University. Many surgeons now use this procedure, which, when done by experts in the field, preserves potency in 50 to 70 percent of patients. About 75 percent of patients can have the special procedure. The other 25 percent need more extensive surgery. It is wise to ask your surgeon about the procedure so that the doctor understands your concerns. Most surgeons are doing the nerve-sparing procedure as long as it does not compromise the cancer treatment—something which sometimes cannot be determined until the surgery is being performed. The return to potency may take as long as two years after surgery. If nerves that preserve potency must be removed, then you must face the fact of sexual impotence. This is a question which you should discuss with your partner and with your doctor beforehand. Whatever the outcome, it is helpful to be open about your concerns and discuss them with your partner.

Is incontinence to be expected following a prostatectomy?

Many men are shocked to discover that the operation causes them to lose their ability to control urine after surgery. They are embarrassed to discover that they must use incontinence pads to control dribbling. Very often, incontinence will lessen as the healing continues. A small percentage of men who undergo radical prostatectomy will have total loss of bladder control. Many more have occasional dribbling during coughing or exertion. Incontinence can sometimes be overcome through the strengthening of muscles with simple exercise. Urinary sphincter implants are also possible to help control incontinence.

Will I be sterile after a total prostatectomy?

Since the prostate gland produces most of the fluid released at the time of sexual intercourse and climax, patients are sterile—unable to father a child—following this operation.

Questions to Ask Yourself

- **Have I checked fully with the doctor about all my options and the risks involved?**

- Am I prepared to accept the fact that treatment to remove my prostate may leave me incontinent, impotent or both?
- Do I want to get another opinion before proceeding with the treatment this doctor recommends?
- Do I want to get a second opinion from a surgeon if I originally saw a radiation oncologist or see a radiation oncologist if I saw a surgeon?

Why is pelvic lymph node dissection done and is it important?

Pelvic lymph node dissection is done to determine if the cancer has spread to the lymph nodes, since prostate cancer spreads by way of the blood vessels and lymph system. Physicians do not agree about how extensive dissection of the lymph nodes needs to be, though most physicians are using "modified" dissection. Side effects associated with this type of procedure include wound infection and blood clots. Discuss your concerns with your physician to see how aggressive the plan is for removing lymph nodes when operating. This question should be asked if you are having a prostatectomy as well as when implant radiation is being planned.

What preparation needs to be done before prostate surgery?

Preparation is similar to that for most abdominal surgery. Daily enemas and laxatives may be given. You will be shown how to deep-breathe and how to cough and turn properly to minimize postoperative complications. It is important for you to let doctors and nurses know about any other health issues, such as hypertension, heart disease, diabetes or lung problems, as well as any drugs that you are presently taking.

Are blood transfusions needed during prostate operations?

Whether or not transfusions are needed will depend upon the surgery being done. Many people bank their own blood to use during the operation and plans must be made in advance with your doctor.

Why is the catheter needed during and after surgery?

The catheter helps maintain urine outflow. Care must be taken to prevent accidental removal, so try to refrain from pulling on the catheter. Premature removal can interfere with recovery.

How long does the catheter remain in place?

Depending on the patient's progress, the catheter usually remains in place for two to three weeks after radical prostatectomy. Following removal, there may be some dribbling and urgency to urinate for several weeks. For most individuals, this condition gradually improves as muscles heal and strengthen.

Are bladder spasms common after prostatectomy surgery?
Bladder spasms may occur after prostatectomy. These spasms have a rapid onset and usually subside in a few minutes. They can be quite painful. Sometimes these spasms can be caused by the obstruction of the catheter due to kinked tubing, mucus plugs or blood clots. In some cases antispasmodic drugs are prescribed.

Is it normal for my urine to be cloudy?
Your urine may be cloudy for several weeks after surgery. It will clear up as the wound heals.

Is there anything I can do to help strengthen muscles so I will not be incontinent?
Your doctor may suggest that you do corrective exercises, known as Kegel exercises, designed to strengthen your perineal muscles. Here are a few suggestions that may be helpful:

- Empty your bladder. Try to relax yourself completely. Tense your muscles by pressing your buttocks together. Hold this position and count to ten. Relax and count to ten. Do this exercise for ten minutes each time, three times a day. At the beginning, you may not be able to hold the position for the count of ten or you may tire before you have completed the entire set. If so, stop exercising and go back to it later.
- When starting to void, shut off the stream for a few seconds, then start voiding again. Do this exercise each time you urinate to improve urinary control.
- Remember to urinate as soon as you feel the need. Do not wait.
- It may take several weeks or months of daily exercise before you notice a difference.

Following a prostatectomy, is radiation sometimes recommended?
In some cases, for example, when the surgery finds that the cancer has spread beyond the prostate capsule or into the seminal vesicles, or when the PSA level remains elevated three weeks after surgery, postoperative radiation may be prescribed.

RADIATION THERAPY

What kinds of radiation therapy are used for prostate cancer?
Two kinds of radiation treatments are possible. Most common is external radiation given with an x-ray machine. Doctors are also

presently reexamining the use of internal or implant radiation therapy. Sometimes both internal and external radiation are used.

How effective are radiation and radiation implants in treating prostate cancer?

Both kinds of radiation therapy are being used to treat some prostate cancers and the success rates indicate that these treatments are as effective as radical surgery, depending upon the spread of the disease. Since it is estimated that potency is maintained in 50 to 60 percent of patients following external beam radiation, this is a consideration, particularly in men who are still sexually active. About 85 percent of men who have had radiation implants with iodine-125 maintain potency, but since radiation implants tend to be done in younger men, age may play a role in this difference. It is important that you discuss this question with your doctor before undergoing treatment.

QUESTIONS TO ASK YOUR DOCTOR ABOUT RADIATION THERAPY

- What type of radiation will I be getting?
- Do I have a choice of having external radiation or internal implant radiation?
- Which has proved to be best in my type of case?
- Does radiation have less of a chance of controlling my cancer than other treatments?
- What side effects will there be? Will I be incontinent? Will I have erection problems? Will I be impotent?
- Who will be responsible for my radiation treatments?
- Can I continue to carry on normal activities while I am in treatment?
- How long will each treatment take?
- Do I have to worry about making anyone else radioactive?
- If I have problems with my radiation treatments should I discuss them with you? If not, who should I discuss them with?

External Radiation
What is involved with external radiation therapy?

The patient goes to the outpatient department of the hospital for a period of time—usually five days a week for five to seven weeks. With a machine, the rays are aimed at the tumor and the area around it. At the end of treatment, an extra "boost" of radiation is often given to a smaller area of the pelvis where most of the tumor is found.

What kinds of side effects can be expected from external radiation therapy?

Many men who have radiation therapy are able to continue their normal routines, although during the last weeks of therapy, many complain of feeling very tired. Some find that there are skin reactions as well as diarrhea, bleeding, difficult urination, abdominal cramping, rectal soreness, hemorrhoids and cystitis. Some men find that they have some temporary pain upon ejaculation and there may be a permanent decrease in semen volume.

What can be done about cystitis caused by radiation?

Cystitis, the inflammation of the urinary bladder that causes pain on urination, usually occurs during the first few weeks of therapy. The patient should try to drink at least 2 quarts of fluid each day. The doctor may also prescribe antispasmodics and analgesics to help alleviate some of the symptoms.

Why would I have rectal soreness as the result of radiation?

Rectal soreness (referred to as proctitis) can be the result of radiation damage to the surface of the intestinal tract. A low-residue diet will help to allow healing. Some doctors will suggest the use of steroid enemas or suppositories to help alleviate symptoms. Antidiarrhea medication is sometimes prescribed.

What do I do about skin reactions due to radiation?

Skin reactions commonly occur several weeks after radiation is begun. The irradiated area should be kept clean and dry. Direct sun exposure should be avoided and the skin should not be exposed to extreme heat or cold. Commercial skin creams or lotions should be avoided because some contain metal bases, which can cause further burning. Some water-based lotions, such as Aquaphor, may be used with approval of the radiologist. (More information on radiation treatment and side effects can be found in Chapter 7.)

What are the long-term side effects of external radiation therapy?

There is a chance, with external beam radiation, that serious injury to the bowel and bladder may result. For this reason, it is essential that your radiation treatment be done by a qualified radiation oncologist who understands sophisticated radiation techniques, such as the use of linear accelerators and careful simulation and treatment planning. For those who have had a transurethral resection of the prostate (TURP), there will probably be delay of radiation for four to six weeks after the surgery.

Will I become incontinent as a result of external radiation therapy?

Although you may have some difficulty in urination, including pain and increased frequency, incontinence is not usually a major side effect of external radiation. Acute, temporary reactions may occur, but chronic problems or late reactions are unusual.

How does radiation affect erections?

Radiation can affect erections by damaging the arteries that carry blood to the penis. As the radiated area heals, internal tissues may become scarred. The walls of the arteries may lose their elasticity so they can no longer expand enough to let blood speed in and create a firm erection. So it is possible that although potency is preserved, it may diminish over time.

Internal Radiation (Interstitial Implantation)
What is interstitial implantation?

Interstitial implanation, usually called internal radiation, and sometimes referred to as brachytherapy, is being evaluated again as a treatment for prostate cancer. It involves the implantation of a radioactive substance directly into the prostate. The procedure was used extensively at one time, being done with freehand implantation with I-125 seeds. However, the results were not completely satisfactory, so new evaluation studies are in progress to test suitable radioactive sources and ultrasound imaging to help achieve more satisfactory results.

How is internal radiation done?

The patient is admitted to the hospital for abdominal surgery. The doctor implants radioactive materials directly into the tumor. Radioactive iodine implantation (I-125), palladium (^{103}PD) and interstitial radioactive gold (198 Au) are most commonly used. The procedure and results are presently under clinical evaluation. Doctors feel that the use of ultrasound imaging techniques for guiding implantation directly to the cancer is a big step forward in perfecting this technique. Be sure to ask about the extent of lymph node dissection (pelvic lymphadenectomy), if your treatment plan includes internal radiation therapy. (There is more information about radiation treatments in Chapter 7, "Radiation Treatment.")

Is cryosurgery being used in treating prostate cancer?

Cryosurgery is being studied as a treatment for prostate cancer. This procedure uses liquid nitrogen or carbon dioxide to destroy tissue by freezing. The substance is placed in a hollow metal probe that is inserted into the tumor or applied to its surface. The treatment is a surgical procedure and takes two to three hours under general or spinal anesthesia. (More information about cryosurgery can be found in Chapter 5, "Treatment.")

SEXUAL PROBLEMS FOLLOWING TREATMENT

When treatment makes the patient impotent, is there any way that he can regain sexual functioning?

If the nerves were not removed during surgery, sexual function may return—though it may take a considerable period of time, often as long as a year or more, before it returns to normal. For those where function is no longer possible, there are other alternatives. A number of prostheses have been invented which can be implanted so that normal sex can be resumed. However, most experts suggest that it is important to wait at least six months to a year to see if function will return before deciding upon implant surgery. You may want to discuss your sexual concerns with an oncology clinical nurse specialist, a sex therapist or sex counselor.

Why do I still have problems having an erection even though the doctor says my prostate surgery or radiation therapy was successful?

There are many reasons for a man to lose his ability to have an erection. It happens to everyone at times—even to those who don't have cancer. Emotional stress—worry about cancer, depression, being tired, trying too hard, worry, alcohol—all can result in erection problems. Any signs of an erection give you proof that your body is cooperating, but the psyche is so sensitive that it may take quite a long time for you to feel certain enough of your masculinity for you to resume normal intercourse. A number of men report that they had their first orgasm after cancer treatment while asleep, during a sexual dream. If you have such an experience, it is proof that you can achieve erection, since sleep erections are not affected by psychological factors. Perhaps this is a good time for you to experiment with other pleasuring techniques. If the doctor says there is no physical reason for the problem, perhaps the cause is psychological, due to pressure you yourself feel about getting an erection. The pace of sexual adjustment after treatment often depends upon your feelings about yourself. An appointment with a sex therapist or a self-help book on sexuality may help you to gain a better understanding of the problem.

What methods are used to allow men who have had surgery or radiation that has resulted in impotence to have intercourse?

There are a number of nonsurgical and surgical approaches now available.

What are the nonsurgical approaches?

There are external, noninvasive systems which use vacuum devices that are quite effective. One such device is worn like a condom but is made of a semirigid material. The sheath is put on and a vacuum is applied to draw the penis out to fill it. The device is left in place for intercourse. Another device requires putting the penis in a vacuum which draws blood into the organ. When an adequate erection has been produced, it can be maintained by putting a constricting band around the base of the penis. The disadvantage of this method is the loss of spontaneity involved in making preparations since three to five minutes are required to produce an erection. In addition, because the rigidity of a normal erection depends on the engorgement of internal tissue, and since only the part of the penile shaft beyond the constricting ring is engorged, the result is a less firm erection.

Is there an injection available that helps produce erections?

There is a medication, papaverine, that produces erections in many men when it is injected with a needle into the side of the penis. Some urologists are teaching men how to administer papaverine to themselves.

How do surgically implanted devices work?

There are a number of different prosthetic designs which can help a man to achieve a controlled erection. Some are simple malleable, semi-rigid rods that are implanted inside the penis. Newer types of inflatable penile prostheses operate hydraulically to make the penis hard or soft. A plastic reservoir about the size of a tangerine is implanted inside the body beneath muscles near the bladder. The implanted reservoir serves as a permanent storehouse for water. The reservoir is connected by two thin plastic tubes to a hydraulic pump planted in the scrotal sac, which in turn is attached to two hollow cylinders, much like balloons, that are implanted in the penis. To achieve an erection, the small pump is gently squeezed. This releases the salt water which fills the reservoir, which flows down into the cylinders and causes the erection. The fluid returns to the reservoir when a release valve implanted inside the scrotum is pressed.

Does the body sometimes reject these implants?

Prophylactic antibiotics are used and most times the implants are successful. Only about 1 percent of implants are rejected or create infections. In those cases the prosthesis is removed and the infection is treated. Many times the prosthesis can be reimplanted.

How long does penile implant surgery take?

Implant surgery takes from about thirty minutes to two hours. Many patients spend two to five days recuperating in the hospital. Full recovery requires four to six weeks. The usual complications of surgery are possible—infection, bleeding, abnormal scarring do sometimes occur. On the whole, complication rates are low. Although no mechanical device is a perfect replacement, most men who have had the surgery say they are satisfied with the implant results.

Dealing with Urinary Problems

Once I am past the initial recovery period will I still have to deal with dribbling of urine?

Unfortunately, for some men it may take some time following treatment before the muscles are strengthened enough to control urination. However, if you do the daily corrective exercises described in this chapter, the problem should lessen and in many cases will eventually disappear.

Are there any devices to cope with long-term urinary problems following prostate surgery?

There are devices that are similar to the penile implant that are sometimes used to solve the problems of urine control. A reservoir is implanted which is controlled by a small pump implanted in the scrotum. A cuff is implanted around the urethra. When the cuff relaxes as the control pump is squeezed, the urine gathered in the bladder is released. The cuff closes on its own in about two minutes. The system automatically repressurizes until the man feels the need to urinate again.

Can the same patient have prostheses for both impotence and incontinence?

It is possible for the same patient to have two prostheses implanted—one to restore potency and the other to control incontinence.

Hormonal Treatment

What is the role of hormonal treatment in prostate cancer?

Hormonal treatments—both through surgical removal and with hormone drugs—are usually used when it is found that prostate cancer has spread or when it returns, or in some cases when it is localized but in an advanced stage. For years, scientists have known that prostate cancer cells depend on male sex hormones, known as androgens, for their growth. The purpose of hormone therapy is to lower levels of testosterone, upon which prostate tumors thrive. Hormone therapy is used to treat prostate cancer that has spread, because it is systemic therapy—which means that it can affect cancer cells throughout the body. The treatment may be given before or after the prostatectomy or the radiation therapy.

What are the different types of hormonal treatments used for prostate cancer that has spread?

A number of different therapies are available. These include:

- Estrogen.
- Luteinizing hormone-releasing hormone agonist.
- Antiandrogen.
- Orchiectomy (removal of testicles).

How does estrogen therapy work?

Estrogen therapy is a hormonal approach which relies on the administration of estrogen, a female hormone that reduces or eliminates the body's production of testosterone. Diethylstilbestrol (DES) is sometimes prescribed. There are side effects to this treatment, such as breast enlargement or tenderness, nausea, vomiting and loss of libido and impotence. This form of treatment is not appropriate for men who have a history of heart disease or embolism.

What are luteinizing hormone-releasing hormone agonists, often referred to as LHRH?

LHRH suppresses testicular androgen, which is linked to tumor growth. This hormone is the normal brain hormone that controls the secretion of luteinizing hormone, the hormone that is responsible for increasing the secretion of male hormones by the testes. The natural hormone LHRH is secreted by the brain in minute amounts and successive pulses of the hormone are released approximately once every ninety minutes. When first discovered, it was hoped that LHRH would be useful for increasing fertility and gonadal functions. Unexpectedly, when copied in the laboratory and made 100 to 300 times more potent than the natural hormone, it was found that it had the opposite effect. Therefore, LHRH is now being used to inhibit testicular functions. Several forms being made in the laboratory are being used, including the leuprolides (Lupron and Depo Lupron) and goserelin (Zoladex). LHRH has shown in some studies to be equivalent to orchiectomy or DES. This treatment can be expensive and can cause loss of potency. Use of these drugs can also result in a "flaring" of problems—such as increased bone pain when first taken. The addition of antiandrogen helps block tumor flare in the first few weeks or months of treatment, after which it is often discontinued.

Are there side effects to hormonal drug treatments?

Studies have shown that hot flashes, loss of libido, and cardiovascular side effects can occur with hormonal drug treatments.

What is flutamide?

Flutamide (Eulexin) is a synthetic nonsteroidal antiandrogen approved for use in the United States. Flutamide causes adrenal androgen suppression (as opposed to testicular androgen suppressed by LHRH). Side effects are minimal and generally are limited to mild diarrhea and breast enlargement. (Usually radiation is given to the breasts before treatment is started to alleviate this side effect.) This drug has been used alone as well as in combination with LHRH or immunotherapy in an attempt to suppress tumor growth in prostate cancer. In many cases, when the drug is used alone, sexual potency can be preserved. Results of the effectiveness of this treatment are still to be determined.

When is an orchiectomy used for prostate cancer?

Orchiectomy, the removal of the testicles, has been used for many years to control prostate cancers that have spread or when prostate cancer recurs. The spread can often be controlled by removing the testicles—man's natural source of the male sex hormone. Removal of both testicles is called a bilateral orchiectomy. This procedure, which is considered a low-risk operation, eliminates the major source of testosterone. Without these hormones, the growth of prostate cancer cells slows down. Though this procedure is still being used, studies show that drug therapy may be as effective.

Are chemotherapy or biological therapy being used?

Chemotherapy and biological therapy for advanced prostate cancer are being tested in various types of clinical trials. Some of the anticancer drugs being tested include Suramin, lovastatin, strontium, CPT-11, topotecan, taxol, taxotere, didemnin B, retinoids 4 HPR and all-trans retinoic acid, and interferon.

What can be done to treat painful bone metastases caused by prostate cancer?

For those with painful bone metastases, hormonal therapy is the mainstay of treatment. If the metastatic cancer is confined to one area, external beam radiation may be used. Where there are more widespread problems, investigation is under way with bone-seeking radioisotopes and radioactive monoclonal antibodies. Strontium-89, sometimes referred to as Metastron, is an injectable form of radiation that is sometimes used for treatment of painful bone metastases. One injection can give relief for up to six months. Additional information about Strontium-89 can be found in Chapter 25, "When Cancers Recur or Metastasize."

Is Proscar being used for prostate cancer?

Proscar (finasteride), which was developed for the treatment of benign prostatic hypertrophy, is being investigated for preventing prostate cancer. This drug blocks the action of an enzyme involved in androgen (male hormone) metabolism. Because androgens stimulate prostate growth, including cancer, researchers believe finasteride may prevent cancer from developing. The Prostate Cancer Prevention Trial, which will enroll 18,000 men, has been started by the National Cancer Institute to assess the drug's effect on the development of prostate cancer.

Are there support groups for men with prostate cancer?

Groups for men with prostate cancer are springing up all over the country. They offer newly diagnosed patients and those who have undergone treatment a chance to get information about different treatment options, prognosis and posttreatment follow-up in a relaxed atmosphere. Us Too and Man to Man are two support groups for prostate cancer patients with chapters around the country. There are also support groups for the partners of patients. For information about support groups in your area, you can contact the Cancer Information Service, the American Cancer Society or the American Urological Association. (Also see Chapter 26, "Where to Get Help," for more information.)

What kind of follow-up is needed for prostate cancer?

During the first year, checkups should be scheduled every three months; the second to fifth year every six months; and thereafter, every twelve months. Blood and urine tests will be done at each checkup, acid and alkaline phosphatase and PSA tests will be done every six months for the first five years. The PSA test has been found to be a sensitive test for the detection of recurrence.

CANCER OF THE TESTICLE

WHAT YOU NEED TO KNOW ABOUT TESTICULAR CANCER

- It occurs mostly in younger men, aged 25 to 35.
- It is highly treatable, usually curable.
- If localized, both fertility and sexual potency can usually be maintained.

Discovering you have testicular cancer is devastating and frightening—especially since it usually occurs at the prime of a young man's life. Cancer of the testicle is one of the most common cancers in white males between 15 and 35 years of age. Men with undescended testicles are at greater risk for developing testicular cancer. It most commonly occurs in only one testicle. Though it was once considered to be incurable, the many advances in treatment make this a highly curable form of cancer, especially when discovered in an early stage.

SYMPTOMS OF TESTICULAR CANCER

- Lump in either testicle.
- Painless enlargement of testicle.
- Dull ache in lower abdomen or groin.
- Heaviness in scrotum.
- Sudden collection of fluid in scrotum.
- Dragging feeling in scrotum.
- Tenderness or enlargement of breasts.

Do I need a special kind of doctor for treatment?

Since this is an unusual type of cancer, the patient with suspected testicular cancer would be well advised to seek out a urologist who specializes in testicular cancer in one of the large medical centers. Close cooperation among surgical oncologist, radiation oncologist

and medical oncologist will help ensure the most successful outcome.

QUESTIONS TO ASK YOUR DOCTOR BEFORE DECIDING ON TESTICULAR CANCER TREATMENT

- **Are you planning to do a needle or simple biopsy?** *(If the answer is yes, get a second opinion before allowing the procedure.)*
- **Will only one testicle be removed?**
- **Is the tumor confined to one testicle?**
- **What is the cell type—seminoma or nonseminoma?**
- **Will this operation make me sterile?**
- **As insurance, will you make arrangements for sperm banking in case I become sterile?**
- **Will my sex life change?**
- **Are you planning any follow-up treatment?**

What are the testes and how do they function?

The testes are egg-shaped glands situated in the scrotum. They produce spermatozoa. The sperm is collected at the back of the testicles in a maze of coiled tubes called the epididymis. It then travels up toward the seminal vesicles and prostate through a long tube known as the vas deferens.

Who is most likely to get testicular cancer?

Most testicular cancers are found in young men. It is more common in white men than in blacks. Many cancers of the testicle appear to have some relation to undescended testicles. Damage to testicular tissue from viral infections which may appear at the same time as mumps may increase the risk of testicular cancer, but this has not been confirmed. Low birth weight (below five pounds) seems to increase the risk of testicular cancer. Sons of women with a history of unusual bleeding or spotting during pregnancy, those who used sedatives, alcohol or were exposed to x-rays while pregnant may be at higher risk. It is not contagious.

Are men with undescended testicles at greater risk for testicular cancer?

Testicular cancer is most often found in young men who have unde-
scended testicles. In the male fetus, the testes are formed near the kidneys and, in normal development, descend to the scrotum shortly after birth. If they never make this descent or descend after the age of 6, the chances of having testicular cancer are three to fourteen times more than in men with normally developed testicles.

Surgery is sometimes done before the age of 6 to place the testicle in the appropriate place in the scrotum. However, the risk, even when this is done, appears to be greater in men who were born with undescended testicles.

Is testicular cancer a common type of cancer?

Testicular cancer accounts for only 1 to 2 percent of cancer in American men. The peak age is 20 to 40, then it declines until age 60, when there is a slight increase. It is more common among white men than blacks. Scandinavian men have the highest incidence. In Denmark it accounts for 6.7 percent of all cancers. Asian and African countries have the lowest rate.

How is testicular cancer usually discovered?

Most are discovered accidentally by the patient. Most are found on the sides of the testicle, but some appear on the front. Young men should get into the habit of practicing a simple exam known as TSE or testicular self-exam. It is easily accomplished and should be done each month, during or soon after a warm bath or shower. While standing, the man gently rolls one testicle between his thumb and fingers, checking for lumps, swelling or other changes. The process is repeated for the other testicle. Any hard, firm or fixed area should be checked by a physician.

What are the symptoms of testicular cancer?

Painless enlargement of the testicle is the most common symptom. The first sign might also be a small, hard lump, about the size of a pea, which is painless when touched. There may be a dull ache in the lower abdomen and groin, or a heaviness in the scrotum. Some men complain of a dragging sensation. The breasts may feel tender or be enlarged. In some rare cases there may be a painful mass which can indicate bleeding within the testicle.

How is cancer of the testicle diagnosed?

Ultrasound will usually be used to evaluate the tumor. After ruling out infection and other diseases that can mimic testicular cancer through careful physical examination and medical tests, the standard procedure for a suspicious lump in the scrotum is surgical removal of the entire affected testicle, done through an incision in the groin. The operation is performed to establish the diagnosis, as well as to remove the tumor.

Are tumor markers used in diagnosing, staging and monitoring cancer of the testicle?

Germ cell tumors produce marker proteins that are being tested for use in diagnosis, staging and monitoring cancer of the testicle. (See Chapter 9, "New Advances and Investigational Trials.")

TESTS THAT MAY BE USED FOR DIAGNOSING AND STAGING TESTICULAR CANCER

- Testicular ultrasound (to help distinguish between epididymitis and tumor).
- CT scans of abdomen and pelvis.
- Orchiectomy, after determining that the mass is not caused by infection or other underlying problem, to remove the entire testicle for biopsy. The surgery constitutes the diagnostic step and the first phase of treatment.

Important: Biopsy of the testicle prior to removal of the affected testicle is not recommended. A second opinion should be sought.

- Intravenous pyelogram.
- Blood tests to help in proper planning for treatment.
- Surgery may be recommended to remove lymph nodes.

Why isn't a biopsy of the lump done without removing the whole testicle?

If the problem is cancer—and most tumors in the testicles are cancerous—cutting through the outer layer of the testicle may cause the disease to spread locally. If the doctor suggests a simple biopsy, you should seek another opinion before surgery.

What are the implications of having a testicle removed?

Many men assume that the removal of the testicle will affect their ability to have sexual intercourse or make them sterile. A man with one healthy testicle can still have a normal erection and produce sperm. A prosthesis which has the weight, shape and texture of a normal testicle can be inserted surgically to restore normal appearance. If part of the scrotal skin must be removed, it may be more difficult to restore the scrotum to a normal appearance.

Is it a good idea to bank sperm when you have testicular cancer?

You will want to ask your doctor if this is necessary or advisable. Recent studies have shown that the majority of men with testicular cancer recover fertility, although this might take two to three years after treatment has been completed. Some men with testicular cancer have impaired sperm production and could be ineligible for sperm banking.

STAGES OF TESTICULAR CANCER	
STAGE	**DESCRIPTION**
Stage I	Cancer found only in testicle.
Stage II	Cancer found in lymph nodes in abdomen (often in region of the kidney) as well as in testicle.
Stage III	Cancer spread beyond lymph nodes in abdomen to other parts of body such as lungs or liver. (Nonbulky Stage III means metastases are limited to lymph nodes and lungs with no mass larger than 2 cm. in diameter. Bulky Stage III indicates 5 cm. and more extensive spread.)
Recurrent	Cancer has returned after being treated—either in the testicles or in another part of body.

What are the differences between seminoma and nonseminoma cancer of the testicles?

There are many different kinds of testicular cancer, but they are generally placed in two broad categories of germ cell tumors: seminoma and nonseminoma. Seminomas account for 40 percent of all testicular germ cell tumors. Nonseminomas are actually a group of cancers which include choriocarcinoma, embryonal carcinoma, teratoma and yolk sac tumors. Each of these two major types of testicular cancer grows and spreads differently and each is treated differently. It is important to find out the extent or stage of the disease so that proper treatment can be planned.

What does lymph node dissection do?

This operation, referred to as lymphadenectomy, is sometimes done to determine if the cancer has spread so that the disease can be treated properly. Since cancer of the testicle spreads first to the retroperitoneal lymph nodes (the nodes deep in the abdomen below the diaphragm), this surgery may also help control the disease by taking out any nodes which are involved. You should understand that this diagnostic procedure, since it removes many nerves necessary for erection and ejaculation, may alter sexual ability and function. Statistics show that 90 percent of men who had undergone this surgery had a reduction in or total loss of ejaculation.

TREATMENT CHOICES FOR TESTICULAR CANCER

STAGE	TREATMENT
Stage I: Seminoma	Removal of testicle (radical inguinal orchiectomy) followed by external beam radiation to lymph nodes in abdomen. *Clinical trials*: Radical inguinal orchiectomy with close follow-up.
Stage I: Nonseminoma	Removal of testicle (radical inguinal orchiectomy) and removal of lymph nodes in abdomen (lymph node dissection). Monthly blood tests and chest x-rays first year and every 2 months second year. Chemotherapy at any signs of recurrence; **or** if CT scan and tumor markers are negative, removal of testicle without lymph node dissection with monthly checkups first 2 years and close follow-up beyond.
Stage II: Seminoma	*If tumor is nonbulky:* Removal of testicle followed by external beam radiation to lymph nodes in abdomen. *If tumor is bulky:* Removal of testicle followed by external beam radiation to lymph nodes in abdomen and pelvis; **or** removal of testicle followed by chemotherapy.
Stage II: Nonseminoma	Removal of testicle and lymph nodes in abdomen (lymph node dissection). Chemotherapy may be given following surgery. If cancer remains following chemotherapy, further surgery may be needed. High-dose chemotherapy with bone marrow transplant. *Clinical trials:* Chemotherapy instead of lymph node dissection.
Stage III: Seminoma	Removal of testicle followed by multidrug chemotherapy. *Clinical trials:* Other chemotherapy protocols.
Stage III: Nonseminoma	Chemotherapy followed by surgery to determine if any cancer cells are still left. Further chemotherapy if cancer cells remain; **or** high-dose chemotherapy with bone marrow transplant. *Clinical trials:* New chemotherapy drugs.
Recurrent	Chemotherapy with or without bone marrow transplant. *Clinical trials:* New chemotherapy drugs.

Some patients may recover their ability to ejaculate as a result of the healing of nerve tissue or regeneration of nerve fibers.

How often should I see a doctor for checkups after being treated for cancer of the testicles?

Generally, patients are checked and have blood tests to measure their tumor marker levels every month for the first two years after treatment. Regular x-rays or scans may be ordered. After that, checkups may be needed just once or twice a year. Testicular cancer seldom recurs after a patient has been free of the disease for three years. Follow-up may vary for different types and stages of testicular cancer.

CANCER OF THE PENIS

This is a very rare cancer that sometimes occurs at the tip of the penis and is almost exclusively found in uncircumcised males between the ages of 50 and 70. It is usually of squamous cell origin. When diagnosed early, it is highly curable. Sometimes cancers from the bladder, prostate, lung, pancreas, kidney, testicle or ureter can spread to the penis. Since it is an unusual and rare type of cancer, it should be treated by an oncologist at a large medical center who has expertise in this type of cancer.

What are the symptoms of penile cancer?

A pimple or sore on the penis, a small nodule, white thickened patches, a raised, velvety patch, a wart or ulcer, especially one that is painless, can all be symptoms. In addition, bleeding associated with erection or intercourse, persistent abnormal erection without sexual desire, foul-smelling discharge, or a lump in the groin should all be carefully investigated.

STAGES OF PENILE CANCER	
STAGE	**DESCRIPTION**
Stage I	Limited to glans and foreskin.
Stage II	Found in deeper tissue of glans and spread to shaft of penis. Not spread to lymph nodes.
Stage III	Found in penis and lymph nodes in groin.
Stage IV	Found throughout penis and lymph nodes in groin and/or spread to other parts of the body.

What is the usual treatment for cancer of the penis?

The usual treatment is surgery. Approximately 90 percent of patients with cancer of the penis, if it is found in the early stages, will be cured through the surgical removal of the tumor. If the cancer has spread to the groin, nodes in the groin usually will be removed. Radiation therapy and chemotherapy are also sometimes used in these cases.

\	
TREATMENT CHOICES FOR PENILE CANCER	
STAGE	**TREATMENT**
Stage I	*If limited to foreskin*: Wide local excision and circumcision. If *in situ or Bowen's disease*: Fluorouracil cream; **or** microsurgery. *If infiltrating tumors of glans*: Penectomy; **or** internal or external radiation; **or** microsurgery. *Clinical trials*: Laser therapy.
Stage II	Partial, total or radical penectomy; **or** radiation therapy followed by penectomy. *Clinical trials:* Laser treatment or removal of lymph nodes following penectomy.
Stage III	Penectomy and removal of lymph nodes on both sides of groin and/or radiation treatment. *Clinical trials:* Chemotherapy.
Stage IV	Surgery; **or** radiation. *Clinical trials:* Chemotherapy plus surgery or radiation therapy.
Recurrent	Radiation or surgery. *Clinical trials:* Chemotherapy or biological therapy.

How is surgery performed?

There are different types of surgery used for operating on cancers of the penis. Any one of these methods may be used:

- Wide local excision, removing the cancer and some normal tissue on either side.
- Microsurgery, removing the cancer and as little normal tissue as possible.
- Radiation.

- Laser surgery, using a narrow beam of light to remove cancer cells.
- Circumcision, removing the foreskin.
- Partial penectomy, removing part of the penis.
- Total penectomy, removing the entire penis.
- Lymph nodes may also be removed during surgery or at another time.

Will I have sexual problems as a result of surgery on the penis?
If only part of the penis has been removed, you may still be able to achieve erection and have the ability to perform penile-vaginal intercourse to the point of ejaculation.

Are prosthetic devices available?
There are several kinds of penile prostheses. Your doctor can advise you where to get information.

What is the treatment for a metastatic tumor that appears on the penis?
Usually if the tumor has metastasized from another part of the body, the doctor will remove the tumor surgically and use radiation to help relieve any pain or side effects.

What kind of follow-up is necessary for cancer of the penis?
The doctor will teach you how to check yourself to detect any changes in the penis area, and this self-examination should be done monthly. The first year, checkups will usually be scheduled every three months, the second year, every six months and yearly thereafter. Urine and blood stool tests will be done at each visit; chest x-rays every six months for the first year, then yearly; and CBC, IVP and CT scan of the pelvis yearly.

chapter 13

Lung Cancer

We've all heard about lung cancer and about its relationship to smoking. It is estimated that about 80 percent of all lung cancers could be eliminated if everyone stopped smoking tomorrow. But if you already have lung cancer, that discussion really has no bearing on your reality. What you need to know now is how to deal with the fact that you have lung cancer.

There are an expanding number of choices available for treatment of lung cancer. Although in the last ten years, the overall pulmonary cancer cure rate has nearly doubled, most lung cancers are discovered in an advanced stage because there is presently no effective screening test to find these cancers early. The many-pronged effort continues with surgical, medical and radiation oncologists as well as pathologists, molecular biologists and immunologists attempting to answer the very basic questions of how to treat and cure lung cancer.

WHAT YOU NEED TO KNOW ABOUT LUNG CANCER

- Symptoms of lung cancer are elusive. Many of them are not painful or distinctive—and they vary depending on where the cancer is located and on its growth pattern.

- A cough is the most common symptom of lung cancer. It occurs when a tumor irritates the lining of the airways or blocks passage of air.
- Many lung cancers are discovered during routine annual checkups, when doctors perform chest x-rays on people who smoke.
- Most lung cancers are in an advanced stage when they are found.
- Not all lung cancers are alike and different types are treated differently.
- Small cell lung cancer is usually found in people who smoke. It is usually treated with chemotherapy.
- There are three main kinds of nonsmall cell lung cancer—squamous cell (or epidermoid), adenocarcinoma and large cell. These are usually treated with surgery, radiation or chemotherapy.
- Lung cancer is the most common cause of cancer death in

WHO IS MOST LIKELY TO GET LUNG CANCER?

- Men and women who smoke. The risk is 10 times greater for men who smoke and 5 times greater for women who smoke.
- Smokers who have bullous emphysema.
- People between 50 and 75 years of age, more often from 65 to 75 than from 50 to 64.
- People whose lungs have been scarred due to past lung infections and those with chronic pulmonary disease.
- Asbestos workers, especially those who also smoke.
- Persons exposed to radon.
- Uranium and hard rock miners and those who work with coal tars, petroleum, chromates, nickel, arsenic and mustard gas.
- Persons who live in polluted urban areas or have been exposed to secondhand smoke.
- People with certain genetic factors or hereditary conditions that may predispose some to cancer. A slight increase has been seen in the incidence of lung cancer among siblings and children of those with lung cancer.
- People who are deficient in vitamin A.

men, claiming more lives than the next four most common cancers combined.

- In women, lung cancer has replaced breast cancer as the prime cause of cancer death.
- The longer a person has smoked, the more cigarettes smoked per day, the greater the length, tar content and depth of inhalation, the greater the risk.
- The incidence of lung cancer decreases when smoking is stopped, and after fifteen years the risk of lung cancer is the same as for nonsmokers.
- Studies show that a diet low in vitamin A makes smokers more susceptible to lung cancer.
- Lung cancers are very difficult to cure because they are usually found when they are in an advanced stage.
- Patients who have had lung cancer are at risk for developing a second primary lung cancer.
- Lung cancer is regarded as one of the most preventable cancers, because of its strong link with cigarette smoking.

What causes lung cancer?

Scientific research indicates that most lung cancers (more than 80 percent) are caused by smoking. A small proportion of lung cancer patients have never smoked, but have lung cancer due to other causes. People who have been exposed for many years to smoking, or irritating substances in the air, including secondhand smoke and pollution, are more likely to have lung cancer than people who have breathed unpolluted air all their lives. It is also possible that the tendency to get lung cancer may be inherited. Clinical studies suggest that blood relatives of lung cancer patients are more likely to have lung cancer than people who do not have a family history.

Can the damage from smoking be undone?

Once a person stops smoking, the body can clean the lungs and protect them from further damage as well as decrease the risk for lung cancer. It takes a significant amount of time for the lungs to get rid of tars and other substances and a number of years, some researchers say about fifteen years, depending on how long the person has smoked, to reduce the risk of cancer to the level of someone who has never smoked. However, the lungs are able to repair themselves and physicians report that they start to "pink up" and recover shortly after smoking is stopped.

Is marijuana smoking harmful to the lungs?

There is some evidence that marijuana may have the same harmful effects as cigarette smoke. Since marijuana cigarettes contain much more tar than do tobacco cigarettes, they may be more harmful. Marijuana smokers inhale very deeply and hold the smoke for a

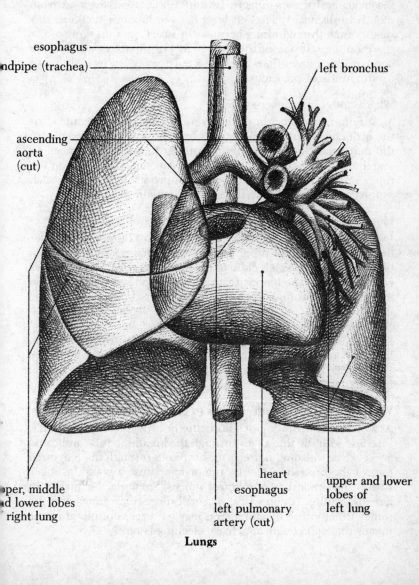

esophagus

ndpipe (trachea)

left bronchus

ascending
aorta
(cut)

upper, middle
d lower lobes
right lung

heart
esophagus

left pulmonary
artery (cut)

upper and lower
lobes of
left lung

Lungs

long time in their lungs and smoke the cigarette down to the very end, where tar concentrations are the highest.

What do the lungs look like?

The lungs are two spongy, pinkish-gray organs that take up much of the room inside the chest. They enfold the other organs of the chest such as the heart, the large blood vessels entering and leaving the heart and the esophagus (the tube which carries food from mouth to stomach). The left lung has two lobes or sections. It is smaller than the right lung because the heart takes up some of the space on the left side of the chest. The right lung has three lobes and is a little bigger than the left one. Tubes called bronchi make up the inside of the lungs.

Where does lung cancer start?

Most lung cancers begin in the bronchi (the larger air tubes) or the bronchioles (the smaller tubes branching off the bronchi) in the moist mucous layer of the breathing tubes. Some cancer researchers believe that twenty or more years may pass between the time someone is first exposed to a cancer-producing substance such as tobacco smoke and the time cancer actually develops.

How does lung cancer spread?

Lung cancer usually begins as a tiny spot, most often on the inner lining of a bronchial tube. Because lungs have a rich supply of blood and lymph vessels close to the lining, it is easy for the cancer cells to get into the bloodstream or the lymph system and spread to other parts of the body.

Where does lung cancer usually spread?

Lung cancer most commonly spreads, or metastasizes, to the brain, liver and bone, although it may spread to any organ of the body (see Chapter 25, ''When Cancers Recur or Metastasize,'' for additional information).

What happens when cancer starts to grow in the lung?

As a tumor on the lining of a bronchus or bronchiole grows, it may interfere with the flow of air through the breathing tube and cause a wheeze or whistling noise as the air passes through the narrowed part of the bronchus. Or the tumor may cause a cough as it obstructs the upward movement of mucus. Sometimes it makes an already existing cough worse or small ulcers may appear on the tumor which cause bleeding. You may see streaks of blood in the mucus that you cough up. Heavy bleeding is rare.

If the cancer has spread outside the lung, what symptoms am I likely to have?

Sometimes fluid accumulates in the lining outside the lungs, causing fluid to collect in the pleural cavity. This can cause chest pain and make it hard to breathe. A tumor growing between the two lungs may press on the esophagus and make it hard to swallow. It may affect the nerves that go to the voice box and make you hoarse. When it grows in one of the smallest bronchial tubes, it may grow to the size of a golf ball without having any effects that you will notice and it may not be discovered for many years unless an x-ray is taken.

SYMPTOMS OF LUNG CANCER

- Symptoms often depend on the location of the tumor.
- Cough is the most common symptom. Any change in a smoker's cough is a significant symptom not to be ignored.
- Wheezing.
- Constant chest pain.
- Shortness of breath during routine, everyday activities that have not caused breathing difficulty in the past. (Don't worry about the shortness of breath that develops after rapidly running up several flights of stairs, since even the healthiest person will feel short of breath under those conditions.)
- Spitting up sputum, even a small amount, especially in the early morning.
- Flecks or streaks of blood, coughed up or in the sputum (may look rusty rather than red).
- Hoarseness.
- Fever.
- Neck enlargement.
- Repeated pneumonia or bronchitis.
- Weight loss.
- Clubbing of the fingers.
- Arm and shoulder pain.

In what type of lung cancer is arm and shoulder pain a symptom?

One type of lung cancer, known as a superior sulcus tumor, is sometimes incorrectly diagnosed as cervical arthritis or bursitis because of arm and shoulder pain symptoms. The tumor is located in the upper part of the chest and usually extends into the adjoining ribs and spine, producing shoulder and arm pain, sometimes extending to the forearm and the fourth and fifth fingers. An x-ray of the chest, with special attention to the superior sulcus area, helps to diagnose this tumor.

Are lung tumors ever benign?
Benign tumors (adenomas) do occur, but they are rare. Prior to surgery they are difficult to distinguish from cancerous tumors and therefore are treated in the same manner.

TESTS THAT MAY BE USED TO DIAGNOSE LUNG CANCER

- Sputum cytology (studying the mucus for signs of cancer).
- Chest x-rays.
- CT scan.
- Spirometry (measures breathing efficiency of lungs).
- Bronchoscopy exam (to look into breathing passages).
- Ultrasound (sonogram).
- Needle aspiration (to remove cells that are hard to reach with bronchoscope).
- Mediastinoscopy (surgery to check for diagnosis).
- Thoracentesis (to check fluid from pleura).
- Pulmonary function tests.
- For small cell lung cancers, a bone marrow biopsy may be done.
- Thoracotomy.

NOTE: Not all of the tests are done on all patients. However, it is important to have thorough testing and staging before any treatment is started. There is more detailed information on these tests in Chapter 4, "How Cancers Are Diagnosed."

What kind of doctor should be treating me if I have lung cancer?
Usually your internist or general physician will refer you to a specialist. Specialists who treat lung cancer include thoracic surgeons, radiation oncologists, and medical oncologists. Before any treatment is begun, a review of the biopsy should be done by an experienced lung cancer pathologist at a major medical center.

QUESTIONS TO ASK YOUR DOCTOR ABOUT LUNG CANCER TREATMENT

- What kind of lung cancer do I have?
- Is it small cell or nonsmall cell lung cancer?

- Has the cancer spread outside the lung?
- What is the stage of the disease?
- What are my treatment choices?
- Is surgery a choice for me?
- Can radiation be used before surgery to reduce the size of the tumor?
- Is laser surgery or cryosurgery an option?
- Will the remaining lung work well enough so that I can be active after the operation?
- Is the operation considered a risk?
- In my condition, will anesthesia be a problem?
- How long will the operation last?
- How will I feel after the operation?
- How long must I stay in the hospital?
- Would you suggest that I get involved in a clinical trial?
- If I am not operated on, what other treatment do you suggest?
- Will I need radiation therapy?
- Will chemotherapy be used?
- What are the risks and side effects of each treatment?
- What will treatment cost?
- What kinds of follow-up tests will I have after treatment?

Is a biopsy always necessary?

A biopsy is essential because it gives the pathologist a specimen to study so the cell type and the degree of malignancy can be identified.

Why is it important to have my biopsy reviewed?

It is important, before allowing any treatment to begin, to make certain that your diagnosis is correct. Some cases of small cell lung cancer, which respond well to chemotherapy, can be confused on microscopic examination with nonsmall cell carcinoma.

Why is staging so important?

Staging plays a critical role in the selection of treatment, so careful initial evaluation to define the location and extent of your cancer is critical. Staging depends on the combination of clinical examination, x-rays and laboratory information, and an understanding of the pathology—determined by the biopsy of lymph nodes, bronchoscopy, and any surgical biopsy procedures. The doctor will try to determine as accurately as possible through thorough testing the full extent of your cancer and whether it has started to spread.

What are the different categories of lung cancers?

Lung cancers fall into two broad categories—nonsmall cell lung cancer and small cell lung cancer. Nonsmall cell lung cancer is more common than small cell lung cancer. There are three main kinds of nonsmall cell lung cancer, each named for the type of cells in the tumor. In all, there are more than a dozen different kinds of lung cancers. How your lung cancer is treated and how successful the treatment is depend partly on the cell type.

What are the different kinds of nonsmall cell cancers?

The three main kinds are:

1. **Squamous cell,** also called **epidermoid.** It is most common in men, begins in the bronchi and usually does not spread as quickly as other types of lung cancer. This is the most common type found in men and most often occurs in the major bronchi.
2. **Adenocarcinoma** is the most common type in women and in people who have never smoked. It usually begins along the outer edges of the lungs and under the lining of the bronchi.
3. **Large cell lung cancers** are a group of cancers with large, abnormal-looking cells. These tumors usually begin along the outer edges of the lungs.

What is mesothelioma?

Mesothelioma is a relatively rare cancer that affects the membrane lining the chest cavity or the membrane lining the abdominal cavity. The most common first symptoms are shortness of breath, pain in the wall of the chest which is aggravated by deep breathing, or abdominal pain which may vary from vague discomfort to severe spasms. There is believed to be a connection between asbestos exposure and mesothelioma. Treatments for malignant mesothelioma include surgery, radiation, chemotherapy and intraoperative photodynamic therapy.

NOTE: Although most tumors of mesothelial tissue are malignant, benign tumors can occur, usually in the pleura. They may grow to be quite large, but surgery is usually curative for the benign tumors.

What are some of the more uncommon types of lung cancers?

Some of the more unusual types include carcinoid and mucoepidermoid. Carcinoid tumors are low-grade malignant tumors often found in young patients and are considered to have an excellent long-term prognosis. Mucoepidermoid tumors have varying grades of severity.

Are there clinical trials for lung cancer?

Because lung cancer is so hard to control, many researchers are studying ways to make treatment more effective. Clinical trials are available for all stages of lung cancer. These trials are designed to find out whether the new approach is both safe and effective and to answer scientific questions. Some trials involve treatments to shrink or destroy the primary tumor. In others, scientists are testing ways to prevent lung cancer from coming back in the chest or spreading to other parts of the body after the primary tumor has been treated. Still others involve treatments to slow or stop the spread of lung cancer. (See Chapter 9, ''New Advances and Investigational Trials,'' for more information on how you can get involved in a clinical trial.)

Are all kinds of lung cancer treated the same way?

No. There are different treatments depending on the cell type, the extent of the disease, and the way the disease responds to treatment. Surgery, radiation therapy and chemotherapy are all used. Surgery is done when it is likely that all of the tumor can be removed. Radiation is used to damage cancer cells and stop them from growing and dividing. Chemotherapy is used, especially in small cell lung cancer, which spreads quickly, to try to kill cancer cells not only in the lung but in other parts of the body.

What is small cell cancer and why is it treated differently?

Small cell cancer, sometimes called oat cell cancer, is a fast-growing, fast-spreading variety of lung cancer. It has usually spread beyond the lung when it is found. Even when it is found only in the lung, because of its ability to spread quickly, it is usually treated with chemotherapy to which it is responsive, so that all cancer cells, no matter where they are, are treated. In many cases, treatment also includes radiation therapy, to shrink or destroy the primary tumor in the lung or tumors found elsewhere in the body.

What is prophylactic cranial irradiation (PCI)?

This is radiation that may be given to the brain of small cell lung cancer patients to prevent tumors from forming in the brain, even though no cancer is found there. Usually, this treatment is reserved for patients whose lung tumor has responded well to other treatment.

When is surgery usually used in treating lung cancer?

Surgery is used in treating nonsmall cell lung cancers and, in very selected instances, for small cell lung cancers when there is a good chance that the tumor is confined to only one lung. The affected part, or possibly the whole lung, may be removed. If the cancer has spread to the lymph nodes in or near the affected lung, the surgeon still may be able to remove all of the cancer. Sometimes it is possible for the surgeon to remove a cancer that has grown outward from the lung into a small part of the chest wall. The operation will include the removal of the lung and the cancerous tissue on the chest wall.

What is a segmental or wedge resection?

This operation removes only a small part of the lung.

What is a lobectomy?

A lobectomy is the removal of an entire lobe of the lung.

What is a pneumonectomy?

A pneumonectomy is the removal of an entire lung.

When is surgery *not* used in treating lung cancer?

Surgery will not be used when the cancer has spread to the other lung. The reason for that is that there would not be enough lung capacity left for breathing if both lungs were removed. Surgery is usually not possible for a tumor that has grown from the lung into organs in the chest, such as the heart, esophagus, trachea or large blood vessels. Also, surgery cannot cure lung cancer that has spread to the lymph nodes in the neck, or to other organs such as the liver, kidneys or brain (see Chapter 25, "When Cancers Recur or Metastasize"). Surgery is seldom recommended for small cell lung cancer because it is faster growing and often not as confined as nonsmall cell lung cancer.

Does the surgeon sometimes operate and not remove the lung?

If the surgeon finds that the cancer has spread too far to remove it all, or is in an area where removal is impossible, the lung may be left untouched and the operation ended. Radiation and chemotherapy will be used to help shrink the tumor growth.

Will the surgeon sometimes remove the lung even though the cancer cannot be totally removed?

This is the surgeon's judgment call—and this is the reason why you want to have the most experienced and knowledgeable doctor you can find. If, for example, the tumor is causing serious bleeding and you are coughing up blood or if there is an infection with abscess formation, it may be necessary to remove the lung. Radiation with or without chemotherapy may then be used to help reduce the remaining cancer.

How do I breathe during a lung operation?

Special equipment is used to assist you in breathing. Your other lung continues to function while the surgeon is working on the diseased lung.

After a lung is removed, what happens to the space that's left in the chest?

Like an empty closet, space left after surgery manages to get filled up. Body fluid and scar tissue help to fill the void. Structures from the opposite side may shift toward the side of the operation. The other lung usually expands. Until this happens, there may be a feeling of one-sidedness or emptiness on the side of the operation. During your recovery period you will be encouraged to lie on the unoperated side so that the operated lung can heal unrestricted.

Where are the incisions made for a lung operation?

Usually they are made beneath and behind the shoulder blade, paralleling the ribs. They are visible when the back is exposed.

How long do most lung cancer operations take to perform?

Approximately two to five hours.

When can I get out of bed?

You will probably be up in 24 hours or more, depending upon the extent of the operation and your physical condition.

Will it be painful to lift my arms or take a deep breath?

For a week or so after lung surgery, you may find it painful. Your nurse or doctor will instruct you in breathing deeply. You will be encouraged to breathe each time to the point of pain. Amazingly enough, the pain on breathing will go away more quickly if you breathe deeply than if you try to prevent the lung pain by shallow breathing.

Can I breathe and live normally if I have a lung removed?

You can breathe and live normally after the removal of one or two lobes of the lung, except that there might be restrictions placed on doing strenuous physical exercise. If your entire lung is removed, you may tend to get short of breath when you exert yourself. However, at rest, you will breathe normally.

What if I decide I don't want my lung removed?

If your general health is good and the cancer is confined to one lobe or one lung, the doctor will probably recommend removal of the entire tumor. If all the cancer is removed, statistics show there is an excellent chance for recovery and you would be wise to follow that recommendation. Don't make this kind of decision without talking it through with your physician. Explain your concerns and reservations and let the doctor give you the rationale for why the

TYPES OF SURGERY USED IN LUNG CANCER

Type	Description
Thoracotomy	Exploratory chest operation, used as diagnostic tool. Major surgery. Allows examination of lung and surrounding areas. If tumor is found to be operable, may be combined with one of procedures below.
Segmentectomy or wedge resection	Removal of small portion of lung.
Limited pulmonary resection	Any surgery that is less than the removal of the entire lobe of the lung.
Lobectomy	Removal of entire lobe of one lung.
Bilobectomy	Removal of two of the right lung's three lobes.
Pneumonectomy	Removal of entire lung.
Sleeve pneumonectomy	Removal of entire lung as well as lower trachea. Airway is reconstructed.
Extended resection	When part of chest wall, left atrium, and diaphragm are removed. Reconstruction usually done with prosthetic material.
Sternotomy	Midline splitting of sternum, sometimes used so doctor can see both sides of chest to locate undetected cancer; possible removal of small portion of each lung.
Mediastinotomy or Mediastinoscopy	Surgical procedure to allow doctor to check whether lung cancer has spread to lymph nodes behind breastbone.

surgery is necessary. This is not a decision to be made lightly or without being fully informed of the risks involved in postponing or rejecting surgery.

When is radiation used to treat nonsmall cell lung cancers?

Traditionally, radiation has been used for two purposes—as an effective treatment for nonsmall cell cancer that is inoperable but localized or to reduce pain or obstruction in cases where a cancer is not operable, since radiation can be concentrated in small areas rather than acting throughout the body as chemotherapy does. Doctors may use radiation therapy following surgery or to treat patients whose cancer has spread from the lung to other parts of the body. Some radiation treatments may be given in two slightly smaller doses in one day to allow a higher daily dose to be delivered in smaller, but more frequent, dosages. The use of neutron or particle beam radiation is also sometimes used in lung cancer. There is more information on radiation in Chapter 7, "Radiation Treatment."

When is chemotherapy used to treat patients with lung cancer?

Chemotherapy is the treatment of choice for small cell lung cancer which is not controllable with surgery. Sometimes chemotherapy is given in combination with radiation therapy or before or after surgery, especially for patients with nonsmall cell cancers that are localized but need to be shrunk in order to be surgically removed. It may also be used for some nonsmall cell lung cancers in persons who are not candidates for surgery or radiation therapy. There is more information on chemotherapy in Chapter 8, "Chemotherapy."

Is the laser used in treating lung cancer?

The laser is sometimes used in treating lung cancer, but it is important that it be done by someone with special technical expertise and knowledge of laser therapy. In some cases of Stage IIIA nonsmall cell superior sulcus lung cancers with little or no node involvement that have not metastasized, endobronchial laser therapy is sometimes used. Laser is also sometimes used to treat tumors that are blocking a breathing tube when radiation is not effective.

Is photodynamic therapy used in treating lung cancer?

This form of treatment is used only for small, early cancers that are inoperable due to medical reasons or for small, multiple lung cancers. This treatment does not eradicate tumors that extend

TREATMENT CHOICES FOR NONSMALL CELL LUNG CANCER

STAGE	TREATMENT
Occult: Cancer cells in sputum, no tumor found in lung	Testing done to try to find site of cancer. Surgery to remove it.
Stage 0: Also called carcinoma in situ, found in local area, in a few layers of cells; has not grown through top lining	Surgery to cure; or photodynamic therapy used internally.
Stage I: Only in lung; normal tissue surrounds it	Surgery; or if not operable, radiation. *Clinical trials:* Chemotherapy following surgery; or chemoprevention therapy; or endoscopic photodynamic therapy.
Stage II: Spread to nearby lymph nodes	Surgery to remove tumor and lymph nodes; or radiation, if patient cannot be operated; or surgery and radiation, adjuvant chemotherapy.
Stage III-A: Spread to chest wall or diaphragm near lung; or spread to lymph nodes in mediastinum; or to lymph nodes on other side of chest or in neck, but is operable	*Small primary tumor:* Surgery; or surgery and radiation; or radiation; or chemotherapy combined with other therapy. *Superior sulcus tumor:* Radiation and surgery; or radiation alone; or surgery alone; or chemotherapy combined with other treatment; or laser therapy and/or brachytherapy. *Chest wall tumor:* Surgery; or surgery and radiation; or radiation alone; or chemotherapy combined with other treatment.
Stage III-B: Same as above but is found to be inoperable	Radiation; or chemotherapy plus radiation; or chemotherapy plus radiation followed by surgery; or chemotherapy alone; or cryotherapy plus radiation.
Stage IV: Spread to other parts of body	Radiation; or chemotherapy; or chemotherapy and radiation; or treatment such as laser therapy and/or brachytherapy to control obstructions and other problems.
Recurrent: Returns after previous treatment	Radiation therapy and/or chemotherapy, laser therapy or internal radiation.

TREATMENT CHOICES FOR SMALL CELL LUNG CANCER

STAGE	TREATMENT
Limited stage: Found in one lung and nearby lymph nodes	Combination chemotherapy and radiation to chest with or without radiation to brain (prophylactic cranial irradiation); **or** chemotherapy with or without cranial irradiation; **or** surgery followed by chemotherapy with or without cranial irradiation. *Clinical trials*: New drugs, surgery or radiation in addition to chemotherapy, new radiation schedules.
Extensive stage: Spread outside lung to other tissues in chest or other parts of body	Chemotherapy with or without radiation to brain; **or** chemotherapy and radiation to chest with or without radiation to brain; **or** radiation to parts of body where cancer has spread, such as bone or spine; **or** *Clinical trials:* New drugs and new ways of giving all of above treatments.
Recurrent: Returns after previous treatment.	Radiation; **or** laser therapy and/or brachytherapy to reduce discomfort; **or** *Clinical trials:* New drugs.

through the bronchial wall or have metastasized to regional lymph nodes.

Is endobronchial brachytherapy used in treating lung cancers?

This technique, which is sometimes used to eliminate bronchial obstruction, places a small plastic catheter in the involved bronchus, into which a radiation source is inserted directly into the center of the cancer. It can be used for patients who have recurrent lung cancer and have previously received external radiation.

Is cryotherapy used in treating lung cancer?

Cryotherapy may sometimes be used in treating inoperable non-small cell lung cancers.

TREATMENT CHOICES FOR MALIGNANT MESOTHELIOMA

STAGE	TREATMENT
Localized (Stage I): Only in lining of chest or abdomen	If in only one place in chest or abdomen, surgery to ensure wide disease-free margins; **or** if in larger part of the lining, surgery to remove lining and tissue near it, with or without radiation; **or** external radiation; **or** surgery to remove sections of pleura, lung, part of diaphragm and part of lining around heart; **or** *Clinical trials:* Surgery followed by intrapleural chemotherapy; **or** photodynamic therapy during surgery; **or** surgery, radiation and chemotherapy.
Advanced (Stages II, III and IV): Spread beyond lining to other parts of chest or abdomen	Draining of fluid in chest or abdomen with drugs put into chest or abdomen to prevent further fluid buildup; **or** surgery to relieve symptoms; **or** radiation to relieve symptoms; **or** chemotherapy. *Clinical trials:* Multimodalities, intraperitoneal chemotherapy.
Recurrent: Cancer returned either in lining of chest or abdomen or in another part of body, after previous treatment.	Depends on many factors, including where cancer returned. *Clinical trials:* Biologicals, chemotherapy and other approaches.

Will I need special treatment if I have chronic bronchitis or emphysema as well as lung cancer?

Many patients with lung cancer also have other lung problems. These conditions, along with the cancer, may make you more susceptible to lung infections. Your total condition will be assessed before treatment is started. The assessment will take into consideration whether your preexisting condition prevents you from having surgery and whether it is possible for you to have radiation treatment. If you have one of these conditions, your doctor may treat them along with the lung cancer and will take them into account in making treatment choices. If you are having trouble breathing, the doctor may prescribe medication to help open up your breathing tubes. An expectorant may be given to you to make it easier to cough up the mucus in your lungs that can plug up the breathing passages. If shortness of breath becomes a difficult problem, the doctor will probably prescribe oxygen. Influenza and other infections can be difficult for you if you have lung cancer. Your doctor will probably suggest an appropriate flu shot for you in the fall. Other infections can be medicated with antibiotics. Being alert to the possible problems means you can report them to your doctor so that they can be dealt with at an early stage.

What about the patient who continues to smoke even after lung cancer is discovered?

There is no question that cigarette smoking, in the face of lung cancer treatment, makes it more difficult to recover since it cuts back on breathing capacity and increases the risk of pulmonary infections. Studies show that stopping smoking, even after lung cancer is discovered, is beneficial to healing. However, it is helpful to remember that compulsive cigarette smoking is an addictive behavior, not one that results from a lack of willpower. The strongest argument for stopping is the increased feeling of good health that will result once the cravings have started to diminish. It all must ultimately be left up to the patient to make the decision. Interestingly enough, experience shows that 95 percent of those who quit smoking do so on their own without the help of an organized program. If you are the patient and would like to talk with someone about the steps you might take to quit, you can call 1-800-4-CANCER. A trained person will talk with you and help you think through what you may do that can help you to stop smoking. The whole process can be accomplished on the telephone without leaving your home or hospital.

How often do I need to see the doctor after being treated for lung cancer?

The first three years you will need to see the doctor every three to four months and every four to six months thereafter. Chest x-rays will be done at each visit. Blood, urine and CEA (and sputum cytology, if needed) will probably be done every six months during the first year, and yearly thereafter. You should be sure to report any bone pain, appetite loss, cough, suspicious mucus, chest pain, wheezing, hoarseness or swelling of the face and arms to the doctor.

chapter 14

Gastrointestinal and Urinary Cancers

When everything is normal, we take the digestive and urinary systems of our bodies for granted. After all, without thinking about it, our insides have been working without instruction from us for years. Furthermore, most of us consider our gastrointestinal system and bowels an unpleasant topic for conversation. This may explain why it's easy to ignore warning signals and put off seeking help early enough when symptoms occur.

Statistics show that cancers in the colon and rectum are the second most common form of cancer among American men and women in the over-40 age group—so this chapter will focus on colon and rectal cancers, in addition to stomach, liver, pancreatic and esophagus cancers. Urinary tract cancers which include the bladder and kidney are also covered.

- The gastrointestinal system is also called the digestive tract, or it may be referred to as the colorectal system, the intestines or the bowels. We will refer to it as the GI tract or system, since that is what it is commonly called. You go to a GI doctor (a gastroenterologist) to be treated for problems in this part of the body. Cancers of the bladder and kidney, on the other hand, are part of the urinary tract and are the specialty of the urologist.

- The GI tract consists of a large and complex series of twists and turns and is vulnerable to what we eat and to our daily stresses. It can become inflamed and irritable for no known reason, can contract in spasms, develop pouches that become infected or can develop engorged veins that can cause pain and bleeding. And, of course, it is a prime area for cancers to develop and hide. Although cancer is only one of many possible causes for problems, an awareness of the warning signs and appropriate cancer-related checkups can help to catch symptoms at an early stage. When detected early and treated promptly, 75 percent of these digestive tract cancers can be cured.

- The biggest fear of those who are facing the need for surgery in the GI tract is that they will end up with an artificial opening, called a colostomy. This is commonly described as having a "bag." In the majority of cases today, the doctor will usually rejoin the healthy parts of the colon. **It is reassuring to know that about 85 percent of patients will not need to have an artificial opening.** In many cases, the doctor may do a temporary artificial opening to allow healing, which is later reversed with a second procedure to close the opening. Thanks to new techniques and new surgical materials, the number of patients who require permanent colostomies has been greatly reduced.

WHAT YOU NEED TO KNOW ABOUT GASTROINTESTINAL CANCERS

- Anyone with a personal or family history of polyps in the colon, or who has ulcerative colitis or diverticulosis, is at especially high risk for colon cancer and should be examined regularly.

- Early detection and removal of small cancers and polyps reduces the likelihood of major surgery.

- Black males are slightly more likely to have colon cancer than black females or white males or females.

- Doctors estimate they could save many lives each year if persons over 40 would have annual colon and rectal exams.

- Colon and rectal cancer cases are declining in the United States. In 1985, 53 of each 100,000 persons could be expected to have colon-rectal cancer. In 1989, 48 in each 100,000 persons were found to have colon-rectal cancer.

- Thanks to new techniques only 15 percent of colon and rectal cancers will result in the need for a colostomy bag.
- Fewer than 6 percent of all cases of GI cancer occur before the age of 50. The average age at time of diagnosis is over 60.
- Patients have the best chance of survival if the disease is found and treated at an early stage—as it is in about 40 percent of all cases. It is estimated that cure rates of 75 percent or higher could be achieved if these tumors were found and treated before they caused symptoms.
- There appears to be a higher-than-average risk among Americans of Irish, Czech and German ancestry and a low risk among Mormons and Seventh-Day Adventists.
- Large areas in the South and Southwest have significantly lower death rates from colorectal cancer than the average rate for the rest of the country.
- Animal experiments and population studies suggest that the development of colorectal cancer is linked to low intake of dietary fiber and that increased dietary fiber has a protective effect. Other dietary factors, such as high fat and alcohol, appear to be associated with the development of colorectal cancers, especially in women.
- Some studies indicate that aspirin may lower the risk of bowel cancer.
- Among family members of patients with colon cancer, the

SYMPTOMS OF GASTROINTESTINAL CANCER

- Changes in bowel habits, such as constipation or diarrhea.
- Very dark, mahogany-red or bright-red blood in or on the stool. (See the doctor immediately.)
- Abdominal discomfort.
- Gas pains or cramps.
- Constant indigestion or heartburn.
- Persistent narrowing of the stools.
- Urgent, painful need to have a bowel movement.
- Feeling of incomplete emptying following bowel movement.
- Unexplained weight loss, anemia, unusual paleness, fatigue.

risk of developing the disease is three to four times greater than in the general population.

- Those with a history of chronic liver disease (hepatitis) should be aware of an increased risk for gastrointestinal cancer.
- The only kind of cancer classified as liver cancer is one which starts in the liver. These cancers are usually treated differently than cancers in the liver that have spread or metastasized to the liver from another organ.

What kind of doctor should I see if I have symptoms of gastrointestinal cancer?

Gastroenterologists specialize in diseases of the GI tract from mouth to anus, including the small and large intestines, stomach, esophagus, liver, and pancreas.

COLON AND RECTAL CANCERS

WHO IS MOST LIKELY TO GET COLON AND RECTAL CANCERS?

- **Those who have previously had colon or rectal cancers or benign growths (adenomas) removed. For a person with such a history the risk of developing a new cancer of the colon or rectum is roughly three times that of the general population.**
- **Women who have had ovarian, endometrial or breast cancer are more likely to develop colon or rectal cancers.**
- **Those with someone in the immediate family with colon or rectal cancer or adenomas.**
- **Those with a personal history of polyps, ulcerative colitis or hepatitis.**

Where are the colon and rectum situated?

The colon and rectum are different segments of the same organ. The colon, also called the large intestine or bowel, is the final five to seven feet of the intestinal tract. It starts at the right lower part of the abdomen and, defying the laws of gravity, continues upward on the right side of the abdomen, close to the liver under the ribs.

This section is known as the ascending colon. It makes a left turn and crosses to the left side of the abdomen. This two- to two-and-a-half-foot portion is known as the transverse colon. The next portion, called the descending colon, heads down the left side of the abdomen to the pelvis. The final section, which is S-shaped and referred to as the sigmoid colon, along with the final eight or ten

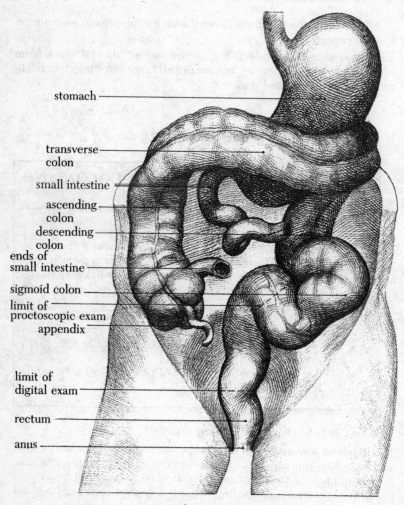

stomach

transverse colon

small intestine

ascending colon

descending colon

ends of small intestine

sigmoid colon

limit of proctoscopic exam

appendix

limit of digital exam

rectum

anus

Colon-rectal area

inches located in the pelvis behind the urinary bladder, are known as the rectum. The final two inches are referred to as the anal region. The colon joins the small intestines to the rectum. The colon and rectum form the lower end of the digestive tract.

Where is the small intestine (bowel) located?

The small intestine, which is also called the small bowel, is part of the digestive tract and consists of three parts. Joining the lower end of the stomach, it is called the duodenum. The jejunum is the portion between the duodenum and the ileum. The ileum joins the large intestine in the lower right side of the abdomen, just above the appendix. The small intestine is longer than the large intestine—about twenty feet in length—but is narrower in width, which is why it is referred to as the "small" intestine. Cancer of the small intestine is rare and treatment is based on the kind of cells found—adenocarcinoma, lymphoma, sarcoma (leiomyosarcoma, angiosarcoma or liposarcoma) and carcinoid tumors.

What kind of tumors develop in the intestinal tract?

There are two kinds of tumors, primarily—benign growths, such as adenomas or polyps, and malignant growths, which are cancer. Most colon and rectal cancers are adenocarcinomas, which are usually found in the lining of the large bowel. Other less common types of cancers of the intestinal tract include sarcomas that begin in the connective tissues, lymphomas that arise in the lymphatic tissues and rarer cancers, such as carcinoid tumors, which are slow-growing.

What tests should I have to assure that cancers in the intestinal tract are discovered early?

There are three tests which are valuable in detecting colon and rectal cancer early in people without symptoms.

1. A digital rectal examination as part of periodic health examination.
2. A fecal occult blood test (stool blood test) annually after age 50.
3. At age 50 and every three to five years thereafter, a sigmoidoscopy.

What kind of warning signs should I watch for?

The most common warning signs are changes in bowel habits, such as constipation or diarrhea, or changes such as persistent narrowing in the size of stools. Some symptoms depend on the location and size of the tumor. Tumors in the right side of the colon sometimes grow large before causing discomfort because the contents of the ascending colon are fluid and can pass through a constricted intestine area. Any discomfort caused by a tumor on the right side is usually dull and vague. A tumor on the left side, where fecal matter is more solid, is likely to cause obstruction symptoms, gas pains, cramps or bleeding. Any symptom that lasts for two weeks or more should be checked by a physician.

What is a polyp?

A polyp is a growth originating from the mucous membranes of the intestine. It grows from the wall into the interior space of the bowel. (Polyps also occur in the bladder, rectum, uterus, nose, etc.) They are very common, occurring in 10 to 15 percent of all adults. Benign polyps, though they may cause intermittent bleeding, the passage of mucus with bowel movements, or, if they are large, obstruct the passage of bowel movements, do not spread to other parts of the body and are most often found during routine intestinal examinations. Cure, through removal, entails little surgical risk. However, some types of polyps that develop in the colon and rectum have the potential to become cancerous as they grow larger. For this reason, it is important to have regular checkups and to be aware of changes in bowel functions so that polyps can be removed when they are in a premalignant stage.

Are there different kinds of polyps?

Yes. The most common colon and rectal polyps, called hyperplastic polyps or hyperplastic mucosal tags, are harmless. Small adenomas, less than one centimeter in size, rarely contain invasive cancer cells. Half of those greater than two centimeters will prove to be cancers. Polyps are described as *pedunculated* when they grow on a stalk that connects the head of the polyp to the bowel wall. Flatter types of polyps that grow directly on the wall of the bowel are known as *sessile* polyps. Polyps differ in their structure, texture and microscopic characteristics, as well as in their potential for cancerous change. About 85 percent of adenomas are tubular, which means that they grow in tubelike patterns. Only about 5 percent of these are likely to develop into cancerous tumors. A very small percentage of adenomas are *villous*, which means that when observed under the microscope they form fingerlike projections. Of these, about 40 percent are likely to develop into cancer. Of the 10 percent of polyps which are classified as a combination of tubular and villous cells (referred to as *tubulovillous*), about 22 percent will develop into cancer. The greater the number of polyps, the greater the risk of cancer, particularly when there are three or more polyps. The doctor will make recommendations about treatment and follow-up treatment based upon the type and number of polyps he finds.

How does the doctor remove a polyp?

It depends on where the polyp is located, what type it is and how large. If it is within eight inches of the rectal opening, it can be removed with a sigmoidoscope through the rectum. It will either be burned off or clipped and removed through the rectum. With today's improved techniques, almost any polyp with a "stalk" can be removed in this manner. Some will still require surgery if they are large or flat. The incision, in such a case, is made at the area of the polyp, the colon is opened, and the polyp is removed. The polyp will be examined under a microscope to see if there are cancer cells. If cancer is found, the segment of the intestine where it grew must be removed.

What are the kinds of intestinal cancers that are considered inherited conditions?

Two types of colorectal cancers are commonly recognized as having a hereditary basis—familial adenomatous polyposis and hereditary nonpolyposis colon cancer. (Very often they are referred to by their abbreviated names, FAP and HNCC.) Familial polyposis is an inherited condition, which means that if members of your family have developed large numbers of polyps in the intestine, you may be at risk for developing this condition. Such polyps grow in the mucous membrane and may become cancerous. People at high risk can protect themselves by having regular checkups starting at an early age and by seeing a doctor immediately if they have any symptoms of bowel problems. They may also be helped by seeing a genetic counselor.

Are there organizations for families with inherited colon cancer?

Intestinal Multiple Polyposis and Colorectal Cancer (IMPACC) is an organization specifically designed to provide support for families with either of the forms of hereditary colon cancer. (See Chapter 26, "Where to Get Help.")

Is there any evidence that colon cancer is carried in the genes?

Research in colon cancer genetics has linked hereditary colon cancer to damage in two genes, with new information being discovered at a rapid rate. Scientists are finding that defects in the DNA repair pathway may set the stage for hereditary nonpolyposis colon cancer. There is more information in Chapter 9, "New Advances and Investigational Trials."

Do hemorrhoids (piles) turn into cancer?

No. However, do not make the mistake of assuming that rectal bleeding is always caused by hemorrhoids, because one of the symptoms of cancer of the colon or rectum is bright-red blood in stools. Rectal bleeding should be checked by a doctor to determine its cause.

TESTS THAT MAY BE USED TO DIAGNOSE COLON AND RECTAL CANCERS

- Health history and physical examination.
- Digital rectal examination.
- Stool blood test (fecal occult blood test).
- Direct visual inspection (proctoscopy, sigmoidoscopy and/or colonoscopy).
- X-ray examination of large bowel, called lower GI series.
- CEA blood test.

How is the digital rectal examination done?

The doctor, wearing thin gloves, puts a greased finger into the rectum and gently feels for lumps. This examination will detect the presence of any abnormalities in the lowest four inches of the rectum. Any stool on the gloved finger will also be checked for blood.

What is the fecal occult blood test?

The fecal occult blood test, also called the guaiac test (pronounced "gwi-yak"), is a simple, inexpensive method of testing stools for traces of blood. Usually stool samples are taken of three consecutive bowel movements so that if there is intermittent bleeding, this can be discovered. To increase the accuracy of the stool analysis, the doctor may ask you to start a meat-free, high-fiber diet (avoiding such vegetables as radishes and red peppers) 48 hours before the collection of the first stool specimen and continuing through the next three days. Vitamin C, iron and aspirin also should be avoided during this time to ensure that the test is accurate. This is a chemical test to find hidden blood in the stool, not a test that directly detects cancer.

What is a sigmoidoscopy?

A sigmoidoscopy is the primary test done to examine the inside of the lower part of the colon. It is sometimes referred to as a "procto" exam. The doctor uses a special instrument, a lighted, flexible, hollow tube called a sigmoidoscope or proctosigmoidoscope which is inserted into the anus. Many doctors use a flexible fiberoptic sigmoidoscope, which allows viewing higher into the colon. At the time of the sigmoidoscopy, a biopsy forceps may be inserted through the inside of the instrument to remove a small piece of tissue for examination. The sigmoidoscopy test is usually done in the doctor's office. To prepare for this examination, the doctor will usually instruct you to have a tapwater enema the night before or the morning of the examination. If bleeding, obstruction or diarrhea is present, the doctor will suggest a less vigorous bowel cleansing. This procedure is best done by a gastroenterologist or a physician who is trained in the procedure. Complications from this examination are rare, but an inexperienced doctor could perforate the bowel, causing serious problems. The procedure may be a bit uncomfortable and you may feel pressure, but in most instances, there is no pain.

What is a colonoscopy?

A colonoscopy is an examination of the colon by means of a flexible, lighted tube, slightly larger in diameter than an enema tube. It permits the doctor to view the entire colon as well as the rectum. Fiberoptic colonoscopy is performed with a longer lighted tube that bends around the curves of the colon so that the doctor can see the entire length of the large bowel, from the anus to the cecum. The instrument allows the doctor to take a biopsy from any part of the colon. The colonoscopy does not replace, but instead complements, the barium enema examination. Before undergoing a colonoscopy, your colon needs to be cleaned. Your doctor will give you instructions on how to do this. The colonoscopy is done under local anesthesia and you will be awake during the procedure. The doctor will insert some air into the colon. Occasionally, the air will cause a feeling of pressure or the same kind of discomfort as gas pain. It is important that the doctor be skilled in the procedure since in the hands of an unskilled physician, perforation and other complications may occur.

Is a lower GI series the same as a barium enema?

The barium enema is done in order to make it possible to take the x-rays of the lower GI or gastrointestinal tract. For this test, a white liquid called barium, that appears white on the x-ray film, is inserted as an enema into the colon. The barium coats the inside of the large intestine and x-rays reveal any polyps, growths or constricted or displaced areas. Air may be pumped into the colon during the test to expand the bowel and make small tumors easier to see. This technique is called an air-contrast or double-contrast barium enema. The barium enema feels much like an ordinary enema, causing a feeling of fullness.

What preparation should be made before these tests?

The doctor will provide you with exact instructions, which usually include a liquid diet and laxatives to help clear the colon of waste so that all areas of the colon can be inspected. (See Chapter 4, "How Cancers Are Diagnosed," for additional information on diagnostic tests).

If tumors are found, must they always be removed?

Yes. Most doctors agree that even benign tumors such as polyps and adenomas should be removed because they may eventually develop into cancer.

QUESTIONS TO ASK YOUR DOCTOR

- Where is the cancer located?
- Is there any sign that it has spread?
- What kind of operation will be performed?
- Will I need blood transfusions during the operation? Should I bank my own blood before going to the hospital?
- How long will I have to be in the hospital?
- How long will the operation take?
- Should I plan on having a nurse with me following the operation?
- Will the operation require that I have a colostomy?
- Will the colostomy be temporary or permanent?
- If permanent, ask: Can you show me exactly where the opening will be? Can I try on the appliance so that I can be sure the opening will be comfortable? What kind of long-term supervision do you give to colostomy patients?
- Will the operation change my eating habits?
- Will there be sexual side effects?
- Will I be scheduled for radiation before or following surgery? (If yes, be sure to read Chapter 7.)
- Will I be scheduled for chemotherapy? (If yes, be sure to read Chapter 8.)
- Who will be performing the surgery? How often do you do this type of operation?
- Is there a patient who has had this operation who could talk with me about it?

- Is there an enterostomal therapy nurse (ET) you recommend?
- Is there a local United Ostomy Association chapter?
- After the operation: What type and stage of cancer do I have?
- Were lymph nodes removed? Am I likely to have lymphedema as a result of the lymph node removal?
- Do you suggest a clinical trial for me?
- How soon will I be able to resume my normal activities?
- When can I start to play golf, or tennis, or resume exercising?

Can cancers of the colon and rectum recur?

Cancer of the colon and rectum can recur at or near the site of the original tumor, and can spread to other parts of the body. Patients treated for large bowel cancer have a 2 to 10 percent chance of developing a new cancer that is not a recurrence of the original tumor in the colon or rectum. Regular follow-up by the doctor is important to detect any recurrences at an early stage.

How serious is surgery for tumors of the colon and rectum?

The surgery varies depending on the location, kind and size of the tumor. Polyps near the rectum can often be removed through the rectum without anesthesia in a surgeon's office, or on an outpatient basis in a hospital, or during an overnight hospital stay. For any benign tumor, the procedure is simple removal of the tumor at its base. If the tumor is cancerous, the tumor as well as a generous portion of the colon above and below must be removed.

What are the stages of colon and rectal cancers?

Once cancer is diagnosed, the doctor needs to know the stage of your disease to plan treatment. Several different methods of staging are used for colon and rectal cancer and you should ask your doctor what stage of cancer you have. If the Dukes staging system is being used, the doctor will indicate that your cancer is a Stage A, B1, B2, C or D. A more recent method of staging is one approved by the American Joint Committee on Cancer and the International Union Against Cancer, which use Stage 0, I, II, III and IV to describe the extent of colon and rectal cancers. Stage 0 indicates early cancer that hasn't spread beyond the limiting membrane of the first layer of colon rectal tissue. Stage IV means that the cancer has spread to other parts of the body—usually the liver or the lungs. (Chapter 4, "How Cancers Are Diagnosed," gives further information on the meaning of staging descriptions.)

What kind of treatment is used for colon and rectal cancers?

Cancers of the colon and rectum differ in their patterns of growth and their response to various treatments. Many factors are involved

STAGES OF COLON AND RECTAL CANCER

STAGE	DESCRIPTION
Stage 0	Very early cancer, found only in innermost lining.
Stage I (Dukes A)	Tumor extends to second or third layers beyond innermost lining and involves inside wall but has not spread to outer wall or outside colon or rectum.
Stage II (Dukes B)	Tumor penetrates to nearby tissue, but has not gone into lymph nodes.
Stage III (Dukes C)	Cancer has spread to nearby lymph nodes but has not spread to other parts of the body.
Stage IV (Dukes D)	Cancer has spread to other parts of the body.
Recurrent	Cancer has recurred after being treated. Recurrence may be in colon or other parts of body—often liver or lungs

in determining treatment, such as the location of the tumor, the stage of the cancer, the type of cancer cells, and your age and general health. The doctor may recommend one or a combination of treatments. The charts include separate information for colon and for rectal cancers.

What is electrofulguration?

Electrofulguration is a kind of surgery that uses an electric current to destroy a tumor.

How are doctors using radiation therapy in treating cancer of the rectum?

Radiation is used in a number of ways in treating rectal cancer. Because rectal cancers sometimes recur at their original site, many doctors are recommending the use of radiation therapy shortly after the surgery as a precaution. Recent research indicates that treatment with radiation before and/or after surgery reduces the risk of the cancer recurring locally. In order to preserve the sphincter muscle, which controls bowel evacuation, one approach is to use high doses of radiation before surgery. Also being evaluated is the use of radiation at the time of surgery, when the tumor is exposed and the surrounding normal tissues can be shielded. This technique is sometimes used in treating tumors that have penetrated the bowel wall and invaded nearby tissue. Another proce-

TREATMENT CHOICES FOR COLON CANCER	
STAGE	**TREATMENT**
Stage 0	Local excision or simple polypectomy or wedge resection.
Stage I	Removal of cancer and section of bowel.
Stage II	Removal of cancer and section of bowel. *Clinical trials:* Chemotherapy, radiation, or biological agents following surgery.
Stage III	Surgery to remove cancer followed by chemotherapy. *Clinical trials:* Chemotherapy, radiation and/or biological therapy after surgery.
Stage IV	Surgery to remove cancer or to make a bypass; **or** surgery to remove parts of other organs such as liver, lungs and ovaries, where cancer may have spread **or** radiation therapy to relieve symptoms **or** chemotherapy. *Clinical trials:* New combinations of chemotherapy or biological therapy.
Recurrent	If recurs in only one part of body, operation to remove cancer. If has spread to several parts of body, chemotherapy or radiation therapy. *Clinical trials:* New chemotherapy drugs or biological therapy.

dure, called endocavitary irradiation, uses a tubular device that is fitted into a special proctoscope. With this technique the radiation can be aimed directly at the tumor. Endocavitary irradiation can be used to cure small, early stage rectal cancers. It is also used for larger tumors when the patient cannot have surgery and for the control of pain and bleeding in large tumors that cannot be removed surgically.

Is chemotherapy being used for patients with colon cancers?

Chemotherapy has been used for some time to treat patients with colon cancers although during early experiments the results were disappointing. Building on the experience of the past, however, new methods are being used which appear to be successful in controlling undetectable cancer cells that remain in the body after surgery. 5-Fluorouracil (5FU) is being used in combination with

TREATMENT CHOICES FOR RECTAL CANCER

STAGE	TREATMENT
Stage 0	Local surgery or simple polypectomy or local excision or electrocoagulation or internal radiation or localized radiation therapy.
Stage I	Surgical bowel resection to remove cancer; **or** internal radiation, electrofulguration or local resection with or without external radiation plus Fluorouracil. *Clinical trials:* Radiation and chemotherapy at time of surgery.
Stage II and III	Surgery to remove cancer followed by radiation therapy and chemotherapy; **or** surgery to remove cancer as well as removal of colon, rectum, prostate or bladder, depending on spread, followed by radiation and chemotherapy; **or** radiation therapy and/or chemotherapy followed by surgery followed by chemotherapy; **or** radiation during surgery.
Stage IV	Bowel resection to remove cancer; **or** if spread to liver, lungs or ovaries, further surgery to remove cancer; **or** radiation therapy; **or** chemotherapy for symptoms. *Clinical trials:* New chemotherapy drugs or biological therapies.
Recurrent	If cancer recurs in one part of body, surgery to remove cancer. Intraarterial chemotherapy or cryosurgery for liver metastases or local recurrence. *Clinical trials:* New chemotherapy drugs or biological therapy.

radiation therapy. Researchers are presently looking at new combinations of chemotherapy drugs as well as new ways of giving adjuvant chemotherapy.

Are blood transfusions recommended during surgery for patients with colon and rectal cancers?

Some studies indicate that packed red blood cells are better than whole blood during surgery for patients with colon and rectal cancers. Many doctors limit the transfusion of blood whenever medically feasible.

What is a stoma?

A stoma is an opening in the skin which allows the end of the small or large intestine to be brought through the abdominal wall and fastened at the skin level. The diameter of the opening may vary from one-half inch to three inches or more.

What is the name of the operation used to create a stoma?

The operation is called an ostomy. Whether permanent or temporary, it takes the name of the area where it is performed. If in the colon, it is called a colostomy and usually means that a portion of the colon and the rectum has been removed. If in the ileum, it is called an ileostomy, and means that the entire colon plus a portion of the small intestine has been removed. A total colectomy means that the entire large intestine and rectum have been removed.

Is a stoma uncomfortable?

A well-cared-for, healthy stoma is comfortable and painless and does not interfere with physical activity. However, much of the success with which a patient is able to handle the stoma is determined by the way in which the surgery is carried out, as well as by the attitude of the patient.

How can I insure a stoma that works well for me?

Many factors contribute to a "good" stoma. First of all, make certain that your surgeon is someone who specializes in this particular type of operation. Some surgeons undertake these operations without the benefit of repeated experience, and though they provide a stoma that is surgically correct, the stoma may not function well from the patient's point of view. Be sure to ask how often the doctor has performed the surgery and what kind of long-term routine supervision will be given. You might ask the doctor if there is a patient who has had the operation who would be willing to talk with you. Be absolutely certain that before the operation, the doctor has marked the site for the stoma so that you know exactly where it will be. It should be located in an area that is free of wrinkles, is slightly convex, away from old scars and creases and can be easily seen by you. Stomas situated in scars, in the navel, or where you wear your belt can be quite unmanageable. Prominent bones, the waistline or rolls of fat can all interfere with the use of ostomy appliances. Of course, the type of ostomy you have determines where the stoma will be to some extent and the nature of the discharge you will have. Your doctor can show you a diagram of the portion of your colon to be removed and where the stoma will be.

What does an enterostomal therapy (ET) nurse do?

The ET nurse is a specialist in ostomy care and rehabilitation. Many times you will be able to speak with an ET nurse before your operation. If not offered, ask the doctor to arrange an appointment with an ET nurse. ET nurses coordinate patient care, teach nursing personnel in hospital and clinics and work closely with the nursing and medical professions to improve the quality of ostomy rehabilitation programs. Your doctor or the United Ostomy Association (see Chapter 26, "Where to Get Help") can refer you to an ET nurse in your area.

How long is the hospital stay for colon or rectal surgery?

The time varies according to the extent of the surgery. Your doctor will be able to tell you what to expect. A simple operation for the removal of polyps is sometimes done on an outpatient basis or may require one or two days of hospitalization. A tumor removed through the abdomen may require four to ten days. As with any surgery, complications can extend this time. In the case of operations which are done in several stages, the patient may have to plan on several hospitalizations, each requiring a varying amount of time in the hospital.

How long does it take to get adjusted to a colostomy appliance?

A great deal depends upon your attitude. There will be mental as well as physical adjustments to be made. After a few months' time, most people become accustomed to the routine and it becomes a normal part of life.

How does the body function without a large portion of the intestines?

Most people find that after the operation they are healthier than they ever were. The problem area has been removed and the intestine that remains is perfectly capable of performing its functions. You have about twenty feet of small intestine and five feet of large intestine. You can live quite normally without a portion of the small intestine and without your entire large intestine. Most digestion actually takes place before food reaches the colon. The colon's function is to absorb the water from the already digested material and to transport waste through its length and store it until it is ready to be expelled from the body. The remaining portions of the colon learn to assume some of the water-absorption role of the intestine that was removed. Even though, to a layman, the removal of a portion of the small intestine or even all of the colon and rectum sounds as though it would be impossible for the body to function, the fact is that after successful surgery, the body adjusts with very little difficulty—and people report that they feel better than they ever did.

What common problems signal that a person with a colostomy should call the doctor?

You should call the doctor when you have:

- Cramps lasting more than two or three hours.
- Severe, unusual odor lasting more than a week.
- Unusual change in stoma size or appearance.
- Obstruction at the stoma or slipping out of place of stoma.
- Excessive bleeding from stoma opening, or moderate amount in pouch in several emptyings. (Eating beets can lead to red discoloration.)
- Injury or cut in stoma.
- Continuous bleeding at junction between stoma and skin.
- Severe watery discharge lasting more than five or six hours.

Where can I get information about living with an ostomy?

A remarkable organization, the United Ostomy Association, exists with the sole purpose of helping people who have had ostomies. So much detailed, informative material has been published that any questions you have are certain to be covered in their publications. The United Ostomy Association offers a variety of booklets compiled from the experiences of many hundreds of patients, nurses and doctors. Local chapters of the United Ostomy Association are located across the country and are listed in the yellow pages under "Associations" or "Social Service Organizations." The American Cancer Society in your area can tell you where the nearest chapter is located and has literature on this subject and often sponsors ostomy meetings (see Chapter 26, "Where to Get Help").

Are there sexual side effects from colon cancer surgery that I should be aware of?

The sexual side effects depend upon the extent of your surgery as well as your treatment. Most people with colon cancer return to normal after recovery from their surgery. Those who have colostomies that are reversed after a period of time may have a longer recovery period, but once the final surgery is done, life can return to normal. If it is necessary to have a total pelvic exenteration, usually for a large, advanced tumor of the colon, both a urostomy and colostomy may be needed. In men, nerves involved with erection will probably be damaged; in women the vagina may be reconstructed so that sexual adjustments must be made. Both men and women, however, find that with patience and understanding, they can make changes in their sexual lives that allow them to find pleasure in less conventional ways. (See Chapter 24, "Living with Cancer," for more information on sexuality problems.)

What kind of periodic checkups should someone with cancer of the colon or rectum have?

It is important for anyone who has been treated for cancer of the colon or rectum to be carefully rechecked on a regular basis by a physician. Follow-up studies may include:

- Complete physical exam every one to two years.
- Stool blood test every year.
- Sigmoidoscopy every six months to three years depending on type of surgery.
- Upper endoscopy every four years.
- CEA tumor marker testing.
- CA 19-9 tumor marker testing.

What is a CEA test?

The CEA test measures the level of carcinoembryonic antigen, which may be found in greater amounts in the blood of patients with colon and rectal cancer. This protein is present in the human embryo but is normally found only in minute amounts in healthy adults. This marker may be useful in showing at an early stage whether cancer has recurred in some patients who had been treated for colorectal cancer previously. This test is not a conclusive test because CEA values are not elevated in all people with the disease. Furthermore, the level of this protein can be abnormally high in the blood of people who do not have cancer, including smokers and those with noncancerous growths or inflammation of the gastrointestinal tract. Because of these facts, the CEA test is used in addition to other tests in making a definitive diagnosis. It does not by itself determine whether or not cancer is present but it may signal the need for further diagnostic tests. The CEA level returns to normal within several weeks after surgery. If the level of CEA begins to rise again, it may mean the cancer has come back. However, other tests must be done, because conditions other than cancer can cause the level to rise.

What is CA 19-9?

This tumor marker, carbohydrate antigen 19-9, is under study for colon and rectal cancer. Alone, the presence of this substance is not a definite signal of recurrence, but when used along with the CEA and other tests, it improves the accuracy in detection of recurrent cancer (see Chapter 9, "New Advances and Investigational Trials" for additional information on tumor markers).

What is the outlook for patients whose colorectal cancers have spread to the liver, lung or ovary?

In certain patients, surgery to remove secondary tumors in the liver may be very beneficial. Surgery is also often successful in treating solitary metastases in the lung or ovary. (See Chapter 25, "When Cancers Recur or Metastasize," for more information.)

STOMACH OR GASTRIC CANCER

The stomach makes up a relatively small part of the intestinal tract. It lies below the diaphragm in the left upper part of the abdomen, crossing over to the right below the liver. It hangs completely free in the abdominal cavity. The stomach is between the esophagus, which connects the stomach to the throat, and the small intestine, which connects the stomach to the colon or large intestine. Unfor-

---

SYMPTOMS OF STOMACH CANCER

- Indigestion.
- A sense of discomfort or vague pain.
- Fullness or bloating or burping.
- Slight nausea, heartburn, indigestion or loss of appetite.

(These are all signs we find easy to ignore. However, if they persist—even intermittently—for a period of two weeks or more you should consult your doctor.)
   Later signs can include:

- Dark stool which may signal blood in the stools.
- Vomiting.
- Rapid weight loss.
- Severe abdominal pain.

(These symptoms may also indicate the presence of an ulcer.)

---

tunately, because there may be no symptoms or the symptoms can be vague, cancer of the stomach can be present for a long period of time and become quite large before it is detected.

How is the diagnosis of stomach cancer made?

A careful history and physical and rectal examination come first. Laboratory tests, such as red and white blood cell counts, and plasma tumor markers will be checked. An upper GI series and gastroscopy with multiple biopsy and brush cytology, in which the stomach lining is gently scraped to give the pathologist material for study, will be done to determine if cancer cells are present.

Do doctors sometimes suspect cancer of the stomach and find a benign tumor?

It is not always easy to distinguish a malignant tumor from a harmless benign tumor even with today's most advanced techniques. It is possible for surgery to uncover an ulcer, a benign tumor or a cancerous tumor.

Do stomach ulcers lead to stomach cancer?

Most doctors feel that the danger of stomach ulcers rests not so much in the possibility that an ulcer may lead to cancer, but rather that it may be cancerous even while being treated as an ulcer.

What is the difference in the usual treatment between a stomach ulcer and a duodenal ulcer?

A duodenal ulcer can be treated conservatively for long periods of time without fear of cancer. A stomach ulcer must be followed closely. A patient is usually put on a strict diet, given appropriate medicine, and subjected to x-ray examination every two to four weeks. If, after a few weeks, there is no change, an exploratory operation is sometimes performed to determine whether cancer is present.

How is cancer of the stomach usually treated?

The usual treatment for cancer of the stomach is prompt surgical removal of the malignant tumor. The operation usually involves the removal of a part or all of the stomach, depending on the location of the malignancy. Sometimes other abdominal organs, such as the esophagus, spleen and pancreas, are removed if they are in the area of the tumor and are believed to be affected. Chemotherapy and radiation are sometimes used in treating cancer of the stomach and biological therapy in combination with chemotherapy and/or radiation is being tested in clinical trials.

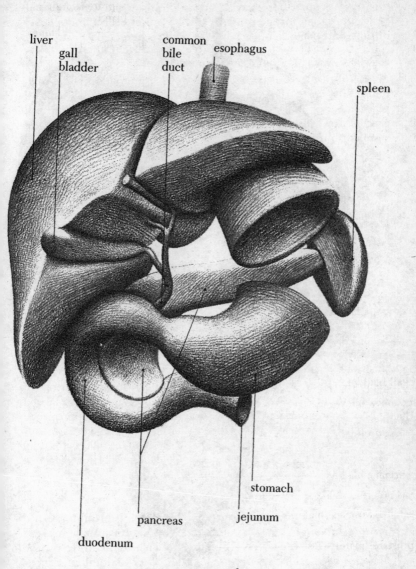

liver

gall
bladder

common
bile
duct

esophagus

spleen

stomach

jejunum

pancreas

duodenum

Front view, major internal organs

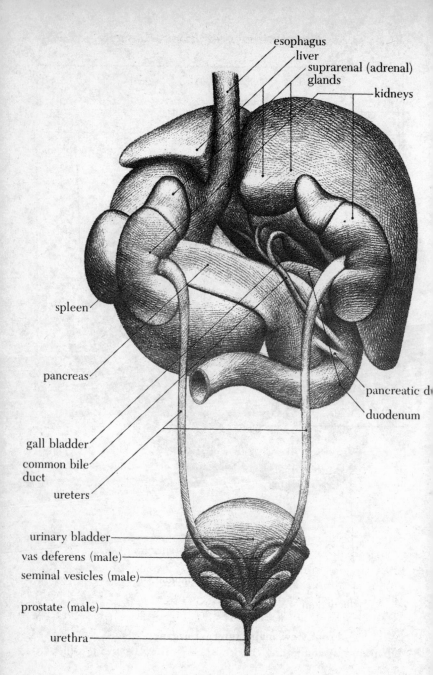

esophagus
liver
suprarenal (adrenal) glands
kidneys
spleen
pancreas
pancreatic d[...]
duodenum
gall bladder
common bile duct
ureters
urinary bladder
vas deferens (male)
seminal vesicles (male)
prostate (male)
urethra

Rear view, major internal organs

STAGES OF STOMACH CANCER (GASTRIC CANCER)	
STAGE	**DESCRIPTION**
Stage 0	Found only in innermost layer of stomach wall.
Stage I	In second and/or third layers of stomach wall but not in lymph nodes or is in second layer of stomach wall and spread to lymph nodes very close to tumor.
Stage II	In second and/or third layer (muscle layer) of stomach wall and spread to lymph nodes away from tumor, or is only in muscle layer but has spread to nearby lymph nodes or is in all four layers of stomach wall but not spread to lymph nodes or nearby organs.
Stage III	In third layer of stomach wall and spread to lymph nodes away from tumor, or in all four layers of stomach wall and spread to lymph nodes or nearby tissues; may or may not have spread to lymph nodes very close to tumor.
Stage IV	Spread to nearby tissues and to distant lymph nodes or spread to other parts of body.
Recurrent	After treatment, cancer recurs in stomach or in other part of body such as liver, bones or lymph nodes.

How can a person live without a stomach?

People who have had all of their stomachs or part of their stomachs removed lead quite normal lives. They usually find it more comfortable to eat smaller, more frequent meals and adjust to this way of life quite easily.

What is the dumping syndrome?

Following the removal of the stomach, some people develop what is referred to as the "dumping syndrome"—nausea, weakness, dizziness, sweating, palpitations—which occurs when the remnant of the stomach empties itself of food too quickly. This can usually be controlled by frequent small feedings and by a high-protein diet with the addition of dry foods and fluids between meals.

What kind of continuing checkups are needed following stomach cancer?

The first and second year, you will probably see your doctor every three months; the third through fifth year, every six months and

TREATMENT CHOICES FOR STOMACH CANCER (GASTRIC CANCER)

Stage	Treatment
Stage 0 or Stage I	Subtotal gastrectomy; **or** total gastrectomy. (Lymph nodes may be removed during surgery.)
Stage II	Subtotal gastrectomy; **or** total gastrectomy. (Lymph nodes may be removed.) *Clinical trials:* Surgery followed by radiation and/or chemotherapy.
Stage III	Total gastrectomy; **or** *Clinical trials:* Surgery followed by radiation and/or chemotherapy; **or** chemotherapy with or without radiation therapy.
Stage IV	Surgery to relieve symptoms, reduce bleeding or remove tumor blocking stomach; **or** chemotherapy to relieve symptoms; **or** *Clinical trials:* New chemotherapy drugs and chemotherapy followed by surgery.
Recurrent	Chemotherapy; **or** *Clinical trials:* New chemotherapy drugs and biological therapy.

yearly thereafter. Stool tests are usually done at each visit. Follow-up CT scans, x-rays, CEA, CBC, panendoscopy, and liver function tests are usually done every six months for the first two years and yearly after that. The GI series is usually done yearly.

ESOPHAGEAL CANCER

What is the esophagus?
The esophagus is the foodpipe. It is a long, hollow muscular tube which goes from the back of the throat down to the stomach, carrying food and liquids.

Are most tumors of the esophagus cancerous?
Most tumors in this area are malignant. More men than women have esophageal cancer, and it occurs most often between the ages of 50 and 70.

What are the symptoms of cancer of the esophagus?
The most common symptom is difficulty in swallowing, sometimes called dysphagia by those in the medical profession. Your food may

seem not to be going down properly, as though it sticks behind the breastbone. There may be sensations of pressure and burning or pain in the upper middle part of the chest, hoarseness, cough, fever or choking. The sensation may seen to get worse and then to get better. Sometimes it comes and goes.

How is cancer of the esophagus treated?

If the cancer is found to be in Stages I or II, surgery is usually the treatment, although chemotherapy and radiation are also sometimes used. Surgery involves the removal of the esophagus in an operation called an esophagectomy. Any remaining part of the esophagus that is healthy may be reconnected to the stomach. A plastic tube or part of the intestine is sometimes used to connect the two parts, so that you can still swallow. Stage III cancers are treated with chemotherapy plus radiation, with surgery being used to relieve symptoms. Stage IV cancers are usually treated with radiation. Sometimes a tube is inserted to keep the esophagus open. Being studied in clinical trials is the use of chemotherapy plus radiation.

How often should you see your doctor after treatment for cancer of the esophagus?

The first year, every three months, the second to fifth year, every four months and after that every six months.

What is Barrett's esophagus?

A syndrome called Barrett's esophagus often occurs in people who suffer persistent heartburn or stomach regurgitations. It can be recognized by the physician by a change in the type of cells lining the esophagus—from the white skinlike tissue that normally coats the area to salmon-colored tissue more closely resembling the inside of the stomach. Although most cases appear to remain benign, scientists say about 90 percent of patients with esophageal cancer begin with Barrett's syndrome. The syndrome is seen mainly in white men—women and black men appear to be less susceptible. It is estimated that a person with Barrett's syndrome has a 10 percent lifetime risk of developing esophageal cancer.

LIVER CANCER

The liver performs many complex functions. It breaks down worn-out red blood cells and converts them into bile, regulates the level of many hormones, stores sugar and regulates the amount which circulates in the blood. It controls the metabolism of cholesterol and stores vitamins A, D, E, and K. Cancer that starts in the liver is uncommon in the United States and Europe, though it is extremely common on a global scale. There is some scientific evidence to show that aflatoxin (a fungal poison which contaminates grain and other foods improperly stored in warm, moist places) and hepatitis B virus may trigger a gene mutation. In addition, a small percentage of those who are diagnosed as having cirrhosis of the liver may eventually develop liver cancer. Many cancers spread or metastasize to the liver, but these are not considered liver cancer and thus are not covered in this chapter.

SYMPTOMS OF PRIMARY LIVER CANCER

- Discomfort in the upper abdomen on the right side, which becomes more acute with deep breathing.
- A hard lump just below the rib cage on the right side.
- Lack of appetite.
- Pain around right shoulder blade.
- Abdominal swelling.
- Feeling full or bloated.
- Episodes of unexplained fever and nausea.
- Jaundice.

Are there different kinds of liver cancer?

There are primary liver cancers which start in the liver and there are cancers that spread from another part of the body or metastasize to the liver. Primary liver cancer is different from cancer that has spread from another part of the body to the liver and is treated differently. (For information about cancers that have metastasized to the liver, see Chapter 25. For information about childhood liver cancer, see Chapter 22.) Most primary liver cancers are adenocarcinomas—either hepatocellular or cholangiocellular. Those which have a fibrolamellar variant have proven to be the most curable.

What kind of doctor treats liver cancer?

Since primary cancer of the liver (which means cancer that starts in the liver as distinguished from cancer that metastasizes to the liver) is a very rare kind of cancer in the United States, it is important for you to seek out a surgical or medical oncologist who treats this type of cancer.

What kind of testing is done to diagnose liver cancer?

A battery of tests will be done to determine the diagnosis. CT scans of the liver will be done. If a lump is detected, the doctor may obtain a small amount of tissue from the liver using a needle biopsy. A laparoscopy also may be done to obtain a tissue biopsy. In addition, an angiography may be needed to determine whether you have a primary liver cancer or whether it is a cancer that has spread from another part of your body. Angiography is also used by the operating surgeon in planning the operation. Blood tests such as AFP and liver function tests are also prescribed.

How is the AFP test used in diagnosing liver cancer?

Alpha-fetoprotein, known as AFP, is a tumor marker which is helpful in diagnosis. Fifty to 70 percent of American patients with hepatocellular cancer have elevated levels of AFP, so this test is significant in making a diagnosis. However, some germ cell cancers and, on rare occasions, pancreatic and stomach cancer patients also have high levels of AFP, so this test is only one indicator, which

STAGES OF AND TREATMENT CHOICES FOR LIVER CANCER

STAGE	TREATMENT
Localized resectable (T1,T2,T3, selected T4; N0; M0)	Surgery to remove cancer from liver; **or** *Clinical trials:* Adjuvant systemic or regional chemotherapy following surgery.
Localized but not resectable (selected T2, T3,T4; N0; M0)	*Clinical trials:* Radiation and chemotherapy followed by radiolabeled antibodies; **or** various types of chemotherapy; **or** some removal of tumor mass followed by chemotherapy and/or hyperthermia, **or** radiation; **or** radiation therapy; **or** liver transplantation in certain patients.
Advanced (Any T, N1 or M1)	*Clinical trials:* Biological therapy; **or** chemotherapy; **or** combination chemotherapy, radiosensitizers, radiation therapy; **or** external radiation and chemotherapy followed by radio-labeled polyclonal antiferritin.
Recurrent	Depends on prior treatment and where located and whether there is cirrhosis of the liver.

is used with other testing, to make a definitive diagnosis (see Chapter 9, "New Advances and Investigational Trials" for more information on tumor markers).

Are chemotherapy drugs being put directly into the liver?

There are devices which allow chemotherapy drugs such as 5-Fluorouracil to be delivered directly into the liver. The device is implanted in the body and includes a catheter which blocks the drug from circulating beyond the liver as well as a filtering device that detoxifies the blood so it can be returned to the patient.

What does the technique called hepatic artery ligation and embolization involve?

In this procedure, being studied, a heavy dose of drugs is injected into the blood vessel leading into the liver. A second tube, or catheter, is inserted into a blood vessel in the groin and guided to the vein leading out of the liver. This catheter has tiny balloons attached to the end of it that block the vessel and prevent the blood from flowing into the rest of the body. The blood flows into the tube through tiny holes and is drawn out of the body, where it is pumped through a carbon filter that removes the drugs before returning the blood to the body. The procedure is done under local anesthesia, takes about two hours and requires the patient to be in the hospital for one or two days.

Are there other new techniques being tried for liver cancer?

Researchers around the world have been experimenting with ways of selectively delivering drugs or radioactive isotopes directly to the liver. Different techniques include the use of polymer beads to deliver antibodies directly to the tumor site.

What kind of checkup schedule should I expect to be on following liver cancer?

You will probably be seeing the doctor for checkups every two to three months for the first two years, then every three to six months for the third through fifth year and yearly thereafter. CT scans and ultrasound tests will probably be done every six months for the first two years, and yearly thereafter. Alpha-fetoprotein, bilirubin and alkaline phosphatase testing will usually be done every two to three months for the first two years, every six months in the third through fifth years and yearly after that.

PANCREATIC CANCER

The pancreas is a key organ in the body and has two important, basic functions. It produces gastric juices that break down your food and it produces hormones that regulate the storage and use of food. Cancer of the pancreas is known as a "silent" disease because it occurs without presenting any real symptoms, usually until it is in a very advanced stage. Recurrence of cancer of the pancreas is the rule rather than the exception. It is important to understand how this translates into the statistics for cure rates. Unless found in an extremely early stage, only 3 percent of patients with pancreatic cancer live for more than five years after diagnosis.

SYMPTOMS OF PANCREATIC CANCER

- Vague discomfort that comes and goes.
- Upper abdominal or lumbar back pain that gradually worsens, often most severe at night.
- Back pain that is aggravated by lying flat and relieved by sitting up or lying in a fetal position.
- Pain that radiates to the back or is limited to the back.
- Pain in the back that is relieved by bending forward or by standing.
- Pain that occurs several hours after meals and is more severe at night.
- Weight loss.
- Change in bowel habits.
- Diarrhea or greasy stools.
- Severe constipation.
- Jaundice.
- Sudden onset of diabetes in a mature person who is not overweight and has no family history of diabetes.

What tests are usually done to diagnose pancreatic cancer?

There are many tests that may be used to diagnose cancer of the pancreas. They include: upper GI barium series, ultrasound, CT scan, MRI, endoscopic retrograde cholangiopancreatography (ERCP), percutaneous transhepatic cholangiography (PTC), angiography, needle biopsy, laparoscopy, and laparotomy.

Are most doctors qualified to diagnose and operate for pancreatic cancer?

Pancreatic cancer is relatively rare. It requires the services of a doctor who has experience in dealing with such cases. Major medical centers, especially those specializing in cancer treatment, have had more experience than most smaller facilities. You should ask your doctor to check if there are clinical trials being done or you can call the Cancer Information Service and ask for information on clinical trials.

Why is cancer of the pancreas difficult to diagnose?

Because the pancreas is hidden behind other organs, it cannot be examined physically, except with surgery. Furthermore, because discomfort at first is vague and comes and goes, early signs may be ignored. The pain may manifest itself as a backache, making it difficult for the doctor to make a diagnosis. Even when the symptoms become more pronounced, physical examination, routine x-rays of the gastrointestinal system and blood tests may fail to indicate the cause of the problem. The upper GI test or barium swallow which outlines the upper digestive tract rarely reveals early pancreatic cancer.

Is ultrasound helpful in detecting pancreatic cancer?

Ultrasound is highly accurate in detecting small tumors at the head of the pancreas but is less accurate in identifying those in the body and tail. It may also help distinguish cancer from pancreatitis but can sometimes suggest the presence of a tumor when there is none. For this reason, ultrasound is usually used in addition to other diagnostic methods.

How are CT scans used in diagnosing pancreatic cancer?

CT scans are more accurate than ultrasound, though they may miss small and early tumors, but are excellent for locating those cancers that have changed the shape of the pancreas and those that have spread beyond its borders.

What does endoscopic retrograde cholangiopancreatography (ERCP) do?

This examination uses a flexible fiberoptic tube which the doctor passes down through the stomach and into the pancreas. A liquid is injected through the tube into the pancreas and x-rays are taken.

It can also be used to obtain a sample of pancreatic cells for examination.

What does percutaneous transhepatic cholangiography (PTC) do?

A fine needle is inserted into the liver and a contrast substance is injected. This substance spreads through the gallbladder and bile ducts to reveal blockages caused by a tumor at the head of the pancreas.

How are laparoscopy and laparotomy used in making a diagnosis?

The doctor can visually examine the pancreas with a laparoscopy through a small incision. He inserts a thin, telescopelike instrument into the abdomen. This procedure, which can be done under local or general anesthesia, poses less risk than a laparotomy but may not confirm the diagnosis. The laparotomy is an operation that enables the doctor to make a conclusive diagnosis, confirming the location and size of the tumor. During the laparotomy, the surgeon may remove the tumor or open blockages caused by the cancer.

Are all tumors and growths in the pancreas cancerous?

It is important to remember that all cysts, tumors, and inflammations of the pancreas do not indicate the presence of cancer. Any growth, whether benign or cancerous, may cause the cells that produce insulin to overproduce, resulting in symptoms that include intense hunger, trembling, fainting, confusion, or convulsions. The operation to remove a cyst is a low-risk one. However, if cancer is found, it may be necessary to operate so as to bypass the obstruction or to remove the entire gland.

What kinds of cancer of the pancreas are there?

There are two major kinds: islet cell cancer of the endocrine pancreas and adenocarcinoma of the exocrine pancreas. Cancers of the endocrine and exocrine pancreas differ in many ways. Cancer of the endocrine pancreas is a highly treatable and often curable collection of tumors. Cancer of the exocrine pancreas, on the other hand, is much more difficult to treat and is not often curable.

What is the most common type of cancer of the pancreas?

The largest percentage of pancreatic cancers are cancers of the exocrine pancreas, and of these, about 90 percent are duct cell cancers that are found in the lining of pancreatic ducts. About three-fourths of exocrine cancers start in the head and neck of the pancreas. Most of the rest begin in the main body of the pancreas

STAGES OF EXOCRINE PANCREATIC CANCER

STAGE	DESCRIPTION
Stage I	Cancer is found only in pancreas or extends to tissues of duodenum, bile duct next to pancreas.
Stage II	Cancer has spread to stomach, spleen, colon or adjacent large blood vessels but not to lymph nodes.
Stage III	Cancer has spread to lymph nodes; may have spread to nearby organs.
Stage IV	Cancer has spread to other organs such as liver or lungs.
Recurrent	Return of cancer after treatment either in pancreas or other part of body.

TYPES OF ENDOCRINE OR ISLET CELL PANCREATIC CANCER

TYPE	DESCRIPTION
Gastrinoma	Increased gastrin, may cause ulcers in stomach.
Insulinoma	Increased insulin, body stores sugar instead of burning it, causing hypoglycemia (often benign).
Miscellaneous— somatostatinoma, pancreatic polypeptide, glucagonoma	Different hormones affected.
Recurrent	Return of cancer after treatment, either in pancreas or other part of body.

and fewer than 10 percent start in the tail. In some patients, cancer is found throughout the pancreas.

What kind of surgery is done to remove cancers of the pancreas?
An operation called the Whipple procedure removes the head of the pancreas, part of the small intestine and some of the tissues around it. Enough of the pancreas is left to continue making digestive juices and insulin. Distal pancreatectomy takes out only the

tail of the pancreas. A total pancreatectomy is a more complex procedure which removes the whole pancreas, part of the small intestine, part of the stomach, the bile duct, the gallbladder, spleen, and most of the lymph nodes in the area. Some doctors believe that a regional pancreatectomy, which is an even more extensive operation, offers a better chance of cure. Early evidence indicates that regional pancreatectomy leads to longer survival than does total pancreatectomy. It seems especially effective for small tumors at the head of the pancreas. The type of operation depends on the stage of the disease, as well as many personal factors such as age and overall condition.

When are bypass operations done for pancreatic cancer?

When the duodenum is blocked, the surgeon may bypass the duodenum and connect the common bile duct with the jejunum, which is below the duodenum.

Is radiation being given during surgery as a treatment for pancreatic cancer?

Intraoperative radiation therapy (IORT), using radiation during surgery, is being studied as a treatment for pancreatic cancer. This permits a greater amount of radiation to be directed at the cancer without significant damage to nearby tissues.

Are biological therapies being used for pancreatic cancer?

Interferon alpha, recombinant IL-2 and combinations of these and other drugs such as 5-FU, cyclophosphamide, leucovorin and granulocyte macrophage-colony-stimulating factor are being tried for patients with pancreatic cancer. Studies also are being conducted to explore the effectiveness of monoclonal antibodies for inoperable pancreatic cancer.

Is tamoxifen being tested for pancreatic cancer?

Some researchers are testing tamoxifen in experimental therapy, giving the drug in addition to the primary treatment.

What are the chances for cure of exocrine cancer of the pancreas?

This type of pancreatic cancer is very difficult to cure because it is usually found after it has spread to nearby organs. The number of cases of exocrine cancer is increasing in the United States and other parts of the world. Though it accounts for about 3 percent of all new cancer cases, it is the fifth leading cause of death from cancer. It is important to understand the seriousness of the condition and the risks.

TREATMENT FOR
EXOCRINE PANCREATIC CANCER

STAGE	TREATMENT
Stage I	Surgery to remove head of pancreas, part of small intestine and some of surrounding tissue (Whipple procedure); **or** total pancreatectomy; **or** surgery to remove tail of pancreas (distal pancreatectomy) if in tail of pancreas; **or** surgery followed by chemotherapy and radiation therapy. *Clinical trials:* Radiation with or without chemotherapy before, during or after surgery.
Stage II	Surgery or other treatments to reduce symptoms; **or** external radiation therapy plus chemotherapy. *Clinical trials:* Radiation therapy plus radiosensitizing drugs; radiation during surgery plus internal radiation therapy; new types of radiation therapy; chemotherapy; surgery followed by external radiation and chemotherapy.
Stage III	Surgery or other treatment to reduce symptoms; **or** external radiation and chemotherapy to reduce symptoms; **or** radiation during surgery, with or without removal of cancer. *Clinical trials:* Surgery plus radiation plus radiosensitizing drugs; radiation during surgery with or without removal of cancer; new types of radiation therapy; chemotherapy.
Stage IV	Surgery or other treatment to reduce symptoms; **or** treatments for pain. *Clinical trials:* Chemotherapy; biological therapy.
Recurrent	Chemotherapy; **or** surgery to reduce symptoms; **or** external radiation to reduce symptoms; **or** treatments for pain. *Clinical trials:* Chemotherapy; biological therapy.

What are the aftereffects when the pancreas is removed?

The recovery period is a long one, and the doctor will prescribe a permanent low-sugar, low-fat diet, often with the addition of vitamin K. Because of the restricted diet, it is difficult to gain weight, which makes recovery slower than usual.

TREATMENT CHOICES FOR ENDOCRINE OR ISLET CELL PANCREATIC CANCER	
TYPE	**TREATMENT**
Gastrinoma	Surgery to remove cancer; **or** surgery to remove stomach (gastrectomy); **or** surgery to cut nerve that stimulates pancreas; **or** chemotherapy; **or** hormone therapy.
Insulinoma	Surgery to remove cancer; **or** chemotherapy; **or** hormone therapy; **or** drugs to relieve symptoms.
Miscellaneous	Surgery to remove cancer; **or** chemotherapy; **or** hormone therapy.
Recurrent	Treatment depends on prior treatment and where it has reappeared.

How often should checkups be scheduled following pancreatic cancer?

Since pancreatic cancer can recur within one to three years, the doctor will usually schedule frequent checkups—every three months for the first and second year, every six months for the third to fifth year and every month thereafter. Ultrasounds and CT scans will usually be done every six months for the first five years, then yearly. Any signs of bile or gastrointestinal obstruction should be reported immediately.

OTHER DIGESTIVE SYSTEM CANCERS

There are other, less often seen, cancers that invade other parts of the digestive system. These include cancers of the gallbladder, bile duct, adrenal gland and anus. All are uncommon, and even rare, cancers and require the services of physicians who are experienced in treating them.

How is cancer of the gallbladder treated?

Surgery is usually done to remove the gallbladder if the cancer has not spread to surrounding tissues, or to relieve symptoms of cancer if it is blocking the ducts. This operation, called a biliary bypass, allows the doctor to do surgery to bypass the blocked ducts. If bile has built up in the area, the doctor may drain the bile through a tube to the outside of your body or he may have the tube go around the blocked area and drain to the small intestine.

High-dose radiation may be used to kill the cancer cells and shrink the tumor. Chemotherapy is also used to relieve symptoms. The use of radiosensitizers is being studied.

How is bile duct cancer treated?

When bile duct cancer is localized to the duct, which connects the gallbladder to the first part of the small intestine, it is surgically removed. If all of the cancer cannot be removed because it has spread, surgery will be done to bypass blockage and radiation will be given. Being studied are the use of radiation therapy with the addition of radiosensitizing drugs and chemotherapy or biological therapy.

Does cancer occur in the adrenal glands?

A rare cancer sometimes occurs on the outer layer of the adrenal glands, which are located above the kidneys. Known as adrenocortical cancer, and sometimes diagnosed through hormone testing, a cancer on this gland may result in hormonal changes such as feminizing changes in men and masculinizing changes in women. Cushing's syndrome, which is usually observed in a rapidly developing fattening of the face and neck, may be caused by either a benign or malignant tumor in the adrenal gland.

What is cancer of the anus?

The anus is the opening at the end of the rectum through which body waste passes. Cancer in the outer part of the anus is more likely to occur in men; cancer in the inner part of the rectum, the anal canal, is more likely to occur in women. There was a time when most of these cancers resulted in the removal of the anus and vulva in women and the anus and scrotum in men, making it necessary for the patient to dispose of waste through a colostomy bag. Some of these cancers can now be treated with an operation that leaves the ring of muscle around the anus so that body wastes can be passed as before. Radiation and chemotherapy are also being used. Internal radiation therapy is used for some patients.

URINARY TRACT CANCERS

The bladder system, or urinary system, includes a number of organs—the bladder, urethra, ureters, and kidneys—and is responsible for eliminating waste products and maintaining stable chemical conditions in the body.

BLADDER CANCER

The bladder, which is a muscular, hollow organ in the lower abdomen, stores urine and increases in size as the urine accumulates. The urine enters the bladder through two tubes called ureters. Urine leaves the bladder through another tube, the urethra. In women, the urethra is a short tube that opens just forward of the vagina. In men, it is longer, passing through the prostate gland and then through the penis. The bladder is the seat of many disorders, including bladder stones, tumors, infections such as cystitis, as well as obstruction and paralysis.

SYMPTOMS OF BLADDER CANCER

- Blood in the urine.
- Pain upon urination.
- Need to urinate often or urgently.

Is blood in the urine always a sign of bladder cancer?

No. Bloody urine may be a first sign, but it can also be a sign of other urinary problems. However, any sign of blood in the urine, even if it happens only once, is a warning to see your doctor immediately. Bloody urine can also be a sign of conditions such as tu-

---

WHO IS MOST LIKELY TO GET BLADDER CANCER?

- People between the ages of 50 and 80.
- Smokers, who are twice as likely as others to have bladder cancer.
- Whites, who have twice as much bladder cancer as those of other races.
- Men, who are twice as susceptible as women.
- Workers in rubber and leather industries and printers, painters, chemical and metal workers, hairdressers, textile workers, machinists and truck drivers.
- Bladder cancer incidence is 40 percent higher in the northern states than in southern states.

mors, infections or bladder stones. Other symptoms of bladder cancer include a change in bladder habits with an increase in the frequency of urination and, rarely, retention of urine or incontinence.

What kind of doctor treats bladder cancer?

Urologists and medical oncologists are the specialists who treat bladder cancers.

What kind of testing is done to diagnose bladder cancer?

The doctor will do a complete physical examination. A bladder tumor can sometimes be felt during a rectal or vaginal exam performed under local anesthesia. Urinary cytology, the examination of urine samples under the microscope, is often done using a saline solution that is inserted and collected through a catheter. Samples of suspicious tissue are obtained with a cystoscope. The patient is anesthetized and the doctor inserts the cystoscope through the urethra, visually observing the inside surface of the bladder, taking small samples of the tissue. An intravenous pyelogram is usually done, in which an opaque dye visible on x-ray film is injected into a vein before x-rays are taken. The x-ray shows an outline of the urinary tract and tumors larger than one centimeter (about half an inch in diameter) can sometimes be seen. Other methods of scanning this area of the body, such as CT scans and ultrasound, are also used to help determine the extent of the cancer. Once bladder cancer is diagnosed, other tests may be performed such as chest x-rays, liver function tests and radioactive liver and bone scans.

What are the major types of bladder cancer?

More than 90 percent of bladder cancers are transitional cell, also known as papillary cancer. A very small percentage are squamous cell carcinomas.

What is papillary cancer of the bladder?

Papillary cancer is the most common type of bladder cancer and the most easily cured. It starts on the bladder wall but grows into the bladder cavity and remains attached to the bladder wall by a mushroomlike stem. This type of tumor may be single or multiple, pea-sized or large enough to occupy the entire bladder. The tumor cells, though they are cancerous, often appear to be almost normal.

Are most bladder tumors found to be cancerous?

Many, if they are confined to the mucosa, are considered to be superficial, which means they are cancerous but not invasive. A high percentage of these will recur in the bladder.

How is bladder cancer treated?

Treatment depends on the stage of bladder cancer, the pathologic grade of the tumor, and the age and health of the patient. It may involve surgery, chemotherapy, immunotherapy, radiation therapy, or a combination of these.

What is photodynamic therapy?

Photodynamic therapy is a new type of treatment being studied in clinical trials for early stages of bladder cancer. A special drug which makes cancer cells more sensitive to light is put into the bladder, and a special light is used to eradicate tumors.

Is laser therapy ever used?

Laser treatment, with the Nd-YAG laser, is sometimes used for superficial tumors. Treatment of these small, superficial tumors of the bladder is usually performed on an outpatient basis, with the patient under local anesthesia. There is a possibility of side effects, including inflammation of the bladder mucosa.

Questions to Ask Your Doctor Before Bladder Surgery

- What sort of operation are you planning?
- Will I be a candidate for continent urinary diversion?
- How often do you perform this kind of surgery?
- Will you use radiation prior to surgery?
- What kind of problems do people you've operated on have after this type of surgery?
- What other options are there for my stage of cancer?
- For men: Do you do nerve-sparing surgery so that I will still be able to have erections after surgery?
- For women: Are you planning to remove part of the vagina? What sort of operation will it be and how will this affect me sexually?

What are the different types of operations used for bladder cancer?

A number of different methods are used depending on where the cancer is located and how far it is advanced. A transurethral resection, segmental cystectomy, cystectomy, radical cystectomy and/or urinary diversion may be performed to remove the cancer.

What is transurethral resection (TUR)?

This is the removal of the bladder growth with a cystoscope inserted into the bladder through the urethra. The doctor then uses electri-

TREATMENT CHOICES FOR BLADDER CANCER

STAGE	TREATMENT
Stage 0: Found only on inner lining of bladder	Transurethral resection with electrofulguration; **or** TUR with electrofulguration followed by chemotherapy or immunotherapy; **or** intravesical chemotherapy; **or** intravesical biological therapy alone; **or** radical cystectomy. *Clinical trials:* Photodynamic therapy.
Stage I or A: Cancer has spread to inner lining of bladder, but not to muscular wall	Transurethral resection with electrofulguration; **or** TUR with electrofulguration followed by intravesical chemotherapy or immunotherapy; **or** intravesical chemotherapy or biological therapy; **or** internal and external beam radiation therapy; **or** segmental cystectomy; **or** radical cystectomy. *Clinical trials:* Chemoprevention or intravesical therapy.
Stage II or B1: Cancer has spread to first lining of muscle layer of bladder	Radical cystectomy with or without node dissection; **or** external beam radiation alone; **or** internal radiation before or after external radiation; **or** internal radiation alone; **or** transurethral resection with electrofulguration; **or** segmental cystectomy. *Clinical trials:* Chemotherapy before cystectomy; chemotherapy plus radiation.
Stage III or B2 or C: Cancer has spread throughout muscular wall and/or to layer of tissue surrounding bladder	Radical cystectomy; **or** radical cystectomy with possible lymph node dissection; **or** external radiation; **or** combination of external and internal beam radiation; segmental cystectomy; **or** internal radiation; **or** external radiation and cisplatin. *Clinical trials:* Chemotherapy before or after cystectomy; **or** chemotherapy and radiation without operation.
Stage IV or D1: Is in nearby tissues and nearby lymph nodes but not in other parts of body	Radical cystectomy with no radiation; **or** external radiation; **or** urinary diversion to reduce symptoms; **or** chemotherapy with or without surgery. *Clinical trials:* Chemotherapy before or after cystectomy; **or** chemotherapy and radiation without operation.

(continued)

TREATMENT CHOICES FOR BLADDER CANCER *(cont.)*	
STAGE	**TREATMENT**
Stage IV or D2: Spread to nearby pelvic organs or to lymph nodes or to other organs	Chemotherapy alone or chemotherapy in addition to surgery; **or** external radiation; **or** urinary diversion *Clinical trials:* Other types of chemotherapy.
Recurrent	Chemotherapy.

cal current to remove superficial bladder tumors and to destroy any cancer cells remaining in the bladder. This treatment is used only on small growths where just the superficial layer of the bladder has been affected. (This treatment is sometimes referred to as "electrofulguration," which means the destruction of living tissue with electrical current.) After this treatment, you will see the doctor regularly every three or four months, because in about one-quarter of all cases, tumors recur in the same vicinity.

What is a segmental resection or partial cystectomy?

This is an operation in which a section of the bladder is removed. A segmental resection is performed only if a tumor is localized in one area of the bladder and is in an area where there is an adequate margin of tissue that can be removed from around the tumor, or with a localized tumor where the area is difficult to reach and cannot adequately be removed with a TUR. Most often, since bladder cancer usually appears on various parts of the bladder at once, more extensive surgery may be necessary.

What is a cystectomy?

A cystectomy is an operation to take out the bladder. A **radical** cystectomy removes the bladder as well as the tissue around it. For males, it means the removal of all of the bladder, its surrounding fatty tissue, the peritoneum over the dome of the bladder, the prostate, the seminal vesicles and pelvic lymph nodes. In women, the entire bladder, the uterus, the ovaries, fallopian tubes, part of the vagina and the portion of the vaginal wall that contains the urethra are usually removed. The surgical incision usually begins at the midline, above the navel, and extends to the level of the pubic bone. The rectum is most often left in place, though it is sometimes necessary, more frequently in men than in women, to remove the rectum if the tumor has grown into that area. Because it can be a complicated operation, it is important to seek out a doctor who is experienced in this type of surgery. Be sure to discuss and understand beforehand exactly how extensive the surgery will be, what other options you might have, and what all the consequences of the surgery are. At the start, when surgery is first being discussed, you may be anxious just to get the surgery over with, and you may not even focus on the sexual side effects because you feel your life is so threatened by the fact that you have cancer. Understanding the consequences of your surgery will help you to plan for your sexual future. Frank discussion with your partner throughout the diagnosis, treatment and recovery process will help to make it possible for you both to learn to deal with the new changes.

What are the sexual side effects of a radical cystectomy?

Since the surgery is very radical, there usually are sexual adjustments to be made. In women, the operation usually removes half of the vagina and the urethra. Usually the surgeon uses the remaining back wall of the vagina to rebuilt the vaginal tube. When reconstructed, this means that the vagina is narrower than normal. Another method used is the separation of the back wall of the vagina from the rectum behind it, creating a vaginal tube that may be normal in width but more shallow than normal. Men should ask their doctors if nerve-sparing surgery is possible. As explained in Chapter 12, "Prostate and Other Male Cancers," the surgery may be done so that nerves surrounding the prostate can be spared so normal erection is still possible. Both men and women should discuss the pros and cons of each type of surgery with the physician or other health professional. Besides changes in the functioning of sexual organs, both men and women who have radical cystectomy may require an ostomy—an outside-the-body pouch for collection of urine. Again, it is important to discuss with your health care team what will be involved in your case, since many new methods are being used.

How can a person live without a bladder?

Many people live without a bladder. And many new techniques are being used to remove urine when the bladder has been eliminated. One new method uses a part of the small intestine to make a new urine storage pouch that is connected to the remaining part of the urethra. Urine then passes out of the body through the urethra, making it unnecessary to have an opening outside the body. When this solution is not possible, the surgeon may use part of the small intestine to make a tube through which urine can pass out of the body through an opening (stoma). This procedure is called a urostomy. Another method is to use part of the small intestine to make a storage pouch inside the body where the urine collects. This makes it possible to use a tube or catheter to drain the urine through a stoma, eliminating the need for a collection bag on the outside of the body.

Where can I get information about living with bladder surgery?

Please be sure to write or call the United Ostomy Association (see Chapter 26, "Where to Get Help"). You can also look in the white pages of your telephone directory or call your American Cancer Society office to find the nearest chapter. There are over 700 United Ostomy Association chapters in the United States and Canada. They offer a tremendous amount of very specific information about urostomy surgery and dealing with life after a urostomy. There is an ostomy visitor service which provides preoperative and postoperative visits at home or in the hospital. In addition, enterostomal therapy (ET) nurses specialize in ostomy care and rehabilitation. Ask your doctor to arrange an appointment for you with an ET nurse.

Is it usual for a patient to be depressed after this kind of operation?

It is not unusual to feel depressed. It is important for everyone to understand that this is a temporary but normal feeling. An inability to cope with the new way the body functions may reinforce the thought that you may never be able to cope with anything again. The depression is usually short-lived and subsides once you learn the new patterns of life. Again, we cannot stress strongly enough the wisdom of contacting the United Ostomy Association. Their material is very specific, covering care of the stoma, helpful ideas and practical tips, complications, types of appliances, social and sexual questions, as well as coping with skin problems, odor and injury.

What other kinds of treatments are used besides surgery?

Chemotherapy may be prescribed either before surgery to try to improve results or to preserve the bladder. Internal or external radiation, biological therapy (such as interferon) and photodynamic therapy all may be used depending upon the stage of your cancer, your age and your overall condition. There are a number of treatment options for each stage of bladder cancer. You would be wise to study them and discuss the pros and cons of each with a well-qualified doctor.

What are bladder washings?

Bladder washings, or intravesical chemotherapy, are used to attempt to kill any cancer cells before or after surgery. These include anticancer drugs such as Thiotepa, mitomycin-c, Bleomycin (Blenoxane), doxorubicin (Adriamycin), and Bacillus Calmette-Guerin (BCG). All are introduced into the bladder by catheter and held by the patient for two hours. There are usually four to eight weekly treatments.

Does bladder cancer metastasize to other parts of the body?

Many bladder cancers are slow-growing and do not spread to other parts of the body. Metastases, when they do occur, usually are found in the pelvic nodes and usually remain localized initially. Early detection and removal is the surest cure, since cancers which are not removed can spread to the lung, bones and liver.

How often should I see my doctor after treatment for bladder cancer?

It is important to see your doctor regularly—every three months for the first year, every six months for the second year and every year thereafter.

Do bladder tumors tend to recur?

Bladder tumors have a tendency to recur either in the same location or in some other part of the bladder. Most of these growths are noninvasive. Most recurrences can be treated successfully if they are found in an early stage.

KIDNEY CANCER (RENAL CELL CANCER)

Kidneys come in pairs—one on each side of the back portion of the abdomen. They are located on each side of your body, toward the back, just above the waist on either side of the spine. An adrenal gland is located on the top of each kidney. The kidney is encased in a membrane called a capsule. Inside each kidney are tiny tubules that filter and clean the blood, take out waste products and make urine. Although the kidneys are best known for producing urine, besides filtering waste products from the blood and returning to the circulating blood those substances that are necessary for normal chemical balance, they also make an important hormone that helps regulate the formation of new red cells in the bone marrow. Overall, the role of the kidney is to monitor the body's internal environment—keeping fluids and chemicals in balance. The central part of each kidney is hollow and receives the bódy fluids. The urine leaves the kidney and passes down the ureter—a long tube—which connects with the bladder.

SYMPTOMS OF KIDNEY CANCER

- Blood in the urine.
- Persistent ache or pain in the area over the kidneys, either in the back or along the side of the body.
- A feeling of a lump or mass in the kidney region.
- Weight loss.

What kind of doctor should be used for kidney cancer?

It is important to choose a board-certified urologic surgeon to treat kidney cancer and a hospital or medical center which is experienced in dealing with kidney cancer.

What tests are done to diagnose kidney cancer?

The doctor will order a blood test, a urine test and a variety of imaging tests such as intravenous pyelogram (IVP), CT scan and ultrasound imaging. Additional tests may include a selective renal arteriography or inferior venacavagram. Kidney cancer is difficult to diagnose and requires careful and thorough testing and because of this has been labeled the "internist's tumor."

Do abnormal liver function tests before an operation mean the cancer has spread to the liver?

Abnormal liver function tests before surgery may be due to a paraneoplastic syndrome that is reversible with the removal of the tumor.

Are all kidney tumors cancerous?

No. Many are benign. The benign growths often are filled with fluid and can be classified as cysts. They vary in size. However, whether the tumor is cancer cannot always be determined without surgery.

What are the different types of kidney cancers?

There are several kinds of kidney tumors. Over eight out of ten are renal adenocarcinomas or renal cell cancers. These tumors start in the lining of the tubules of the kidney. The remaining 20 percent of kidney cancers begin in cells in other parts of the kidney. Transitional cell cancers, oncocytomas, papillary adenocarcinomas, fibrosarcomas or other sarcomas and Wilms' tumors are other rarer kinds of kidney cancers. (For more information on Wilms' tumor, which is a childhood kidney tumor, please see Chapter 22, "Childhood Cancers.")

Do kidney cancers ever disappear spontaneously?

Kidney cancer is one of the few tumors in which the unexplained disappearance of tumors is well documented. This occurs very rarely and tumors sometimes reappear. In most cases surgery is the most successful treatment for kidney cancers.

What is a kidney removal called?

In medical terminology, the removal of the kidney is known as a nephrectomy. Thousands of such operations are performed each year for cancer as well as for other reasons. There are few complications unless the tumor has spread beyond the kidney. A radical nephrectomy means that the kidney as well as the adrenal gland above the kidney, the surrounding fatty tissue and the lymph nodes adjacent to the kidney are removed. A partial nephrectomy means that only the part of the kidney around the cancer is removed. This type of operation is usually performed when the other kidney has poor function or has previously been removed. A simple nephrectomy means that only the kidney is removed, leaving the surrounding area intact.

Can one live normally if a kidney is removed?

Fortunately, people can live perfectly normal lives with only one good kidney.

What is arterial embolization?

This is a procedure which is designed to block the flow of blood to the tumor in the kidney. The doctor injects small pieces of a special gelatin sponge or alcohol into the artery that provides the blood supply to the tumor. It is a method usually used only in patients who cannot have surgery or to relieve symptoms.

Is it important for me to donate blood before my operation?

Since it may be necessary to give you a blood transfusion during the operation, your surgeon may want three or four units of blood on hand for the operation. Because you may not be able to delay the operation, and there may not be time for you to donate your

TREATMENT CHOICES FOR KIDNEY CANCER

STAGE	TREATMENT
Stage I: Cancer is found only in the kidney	Radical nephrectomy; **or** simple nephrectomy; **or** partial nephrectomy; **or** if surgery is inadvisable: external radiation; **or** arterial embolization.
Stage II: Cancer has spread to fat around kidney but not beyond capsule that contains kidney	Radical nephrectomy; **or** external radiation before or after operation; **or** partial nephrectomy; **or** if surgery is inadvisable: external radiation; **or** arterial embolization.
Stage III: Cancer has spread to renal vein or to inferior vena cava (vein that carries blood from lower part of body to heart)	Radical nephrectomy with possible removal of lymph nodes and/or renal vein or vena cava; **or** arterial embolization followed by radical nephrectomy; **or** external radiation to relieve symptoms; **or** simple or radical nephrectomy to relieve symptoms. *Clinical trials:* External radiation before and after surgery with radical nephrectomy; adjuvant alpha interferon.
Stage IV: Cancer has spread to nearby organs such as bowel or pancreas or to distant parts such as lungs, bone or skin	Interleukin-2; **or** alpha interferon; **or** external radiation to relieve symptoms; **or** simple nephrectomy to relieve symptoms; **or** if spread to area around kidney, radical nephrectomy; **or** if spread further, nephrectomy plus limited surgery where it has spread.
Recurrent: either in original area or other parts of body	Interleukin-2; **or** alpha interferon; **or** external radiation; **or** vinblastine.

own blood (the process takes several weeks), you may want to ask family members or friends to donate blood on your behalf. You should discuss this with your doctor.

Is there an organization which acts on behalf of kidney cancer patients?

The National Kidney Cancer Association provides information to patients and physicians, sponsors research on kidney cancer and acts as an advocate on behalf of patients. (See Chapter 26, ''Where to Get Help.'') You can also get information on kidney cancer from the Cancer Information Service and from the American Cancer Society.

How long will it take before I can return to work?

Many patients return to work about three weeks after surgery. It is wise to "baby" yourself a bit. It usually takes about three full months for your muscles to heal completely. After about two months, you should be ready to build up your level of exercise to help restore your muscle tone.

Are there any new treatments that are being used for kidney cancer?

A new injectable drug (proleukin or IL-2) is the first drug approved by the FDA to be used to treat kidney cancer that has spread beyond the kidney. Though the drug is not effective on every patient, for those it helps, the results are significant. The drug works by stimulating the immune system, but can have very serious side effects. Patients are hospitalized during treatment. Numerous clinical trials using this drug are being done and offer another treatment possibility for kidney patients who have cancer which has spread beyond the kidney.

What kind of continuing checkup schedule should I follow?

After diagnosis and a nephrectomy, you should receive regular medical follow-up and supervision for the rest of your life. The doctor will usually schedule you for checkups every three months for the first year; every four months for the second to fifth year and yearly thereafter. Recurrences have been found most often within the first three years after surgery at the original site or in the lung, bone, liver and sometimes in the brain. Usually, when discovered early before further spread, surgery will be done to remove the new cancer. If you experience problems with weight loss, loss of appetite, weakness, headache, changes in your mental status, fevers or high temperatures, abdominal pain or skeletal pain, cough, shortness of breath, enlarged lymph glands or blood in your urine, you should be sure to let your doctor know. Even though, most times, the symptoms may not have anything to do with your past history, it is wise to have them checked out immediately for your own peace of mind.

Do tumors sometimes occur in the ureter?

Tumors can occur in the ureter, but they are quite uncommon. This type of tumor is similar to bladder cancer and usually necessitates the removal of the kidney on the same side as the affected ureter.

chapter 15

Skin Cancer

Most skin cancers are very visible so they are easier to identify early than many other kinds of cancer. Many people have a number of small, colored spots on their bodies—moles, freckles, birthmarks, or liver spots. Some are present at birth. Others develop at different times throughout life. Almost all of these spots are normal and remain that way. But when there are changes in existing moles and other skin spots or when new spots appear, action should be taken.

Cancer of the skin is the most common kind of cancer—and, because it is easy to see, it can be diagnosed and treated at an early stage. Over 700,000 skin cancers are reported annually. Most of these are categorized as basal cell or squamous cell cancers or nonmelanoma cancers. However, about 32,000 of the skin cancers are cutaneous melanomas—serious skin cancers that arise in moles or in the tanning cells of the skin and which, in later stages, can spread or metastasize to other parts of the body.

What You Need to Know About Skin Cancer

- Skin cancer has a better prognosis than most other types of cancer. It is curable in over 95 percent of cases.

SKIN CANCER RISK FACTORS

RISK FACTOR	DESCRIPTION
Ultraviolet radiation	Exposure to ultraviolet radiation from the sun and other sources.
Skin color	People with light skin and blue eyes who sunburn easily are more susceptible than those with naturally dark skin.
Sun exposure	People who were severely sunburned as children. People who have intense sun exposure once in a while as opposed to outdoor workers who are constantly exposed
Occupational	Exposure to coal tar, pitch, creosote, arsenic compounds or radium.
Moles	A very large number of very large moles present from birth.
Genetics	*For melanoma:* Two or more first-degree relatives—parents, children, brothers, sisters—who have had melanoma.
Age	Risk increases with age. Peak age for discovery is in the 40s. Those diagnosed younger than 50 have a better prognosis.

- There are three major types of skin cancer. The two most common types, **basal cell** and **squamous cell,** rarely spread. **Melanoma,** the third type, is a serious condition. It has a greater tendency to metastasize to other parts of the body.
- All skin cancers do not look the same. Some are small, smooth, shiny, pale or waxy lumps. Others are rough, red or brown scaly patches. Still others look like flat or raised moles.
- Most true moles tend to be symmetrical. Suspicious moles usually are uneven—with one half not matching the other.
- Most true moles have a clear-cut border. Suspicious moles have a notched, scalloped or indistinct border.
- True moles may be dark or light—but they are usually uniform in color. Suspicious moles have uneven or variegated color. Shades of black, brown and tan, white, gray, red or blue may be seen.
- Most moles are smaller than the size of a pencil eraser. Suspicious moles tend to be larger and may change in size.
- The cure rate for skin cancer could be 100 percent if all

skin cancers were brought to a doctor's attention before they spread.

- If caught early and surgically removed, melanoma has a cure rate of more than 99 percent.
- Even if caught later, when the melanoma is invading nearby tissue, the cure rate is more than 90 percent.
- Scientists are researching proteins that elicit natural immunity against melanoma. A gene, MART-1, has been identified that could potentially be used to produce a melanoma vaccine.
- Melanoma can occur on any skin surface.
- Melanoma occurs most commonly on the lower extremities in women and on the back in men.
- Melanoma is rare in black people and others with dark skin. When it does develop in dark-skinned people, it tends to occur under the fingernails or toenails or on the palms or soles.
- Any sore, blister, patch, pimple, mole or other skin blemish that does not heal within two or three weeks should be examined by a doctor.

SKIN CANCER PREVENTION HINTS

Sensible precautions can help protect you from skin cancers and help you find skin cancers early, before they have a chance of doing permanent damage. Since we know that the sun is a contributing factor in over 90 percent of skin cancers, it is wise to take precautions against the damaging rays of the sun on a year-round basis.

- Do a monthly skin exam. Become familiar with your skin and the pattern of moles, freckles and beauty marks.
- If you detect any changes in your skin, see your doctor right away.
- Find a doctor with experience in dealing with skin cancer, one who understands the importance of family history and who is willing to remove any changing skin lesions early.
- Spend as little time in the sun as you can. Ultraviolet rays of the sun are the most frequent cause of cancer. Deliberate, repeated suntanning increases the incidence of skin cancer. Sun exposure has a cumulative effect. Infants should always be kept out of the sun, and young children should be taught sun protection early.
- Use a 15 SPF-rated sunscreen, especially between 10 A.M. and 3 P.M. Reapply the sunscreen after swimming or sweating.

Remember that UV rays can pass through clouds or be reflected by snow or water. Wear tightly woven protective clothing such as sun hats, long sleeves, pants and gloves, which help reduce the penetration of ultraviolet rays.

- Do not use indoor sunlamps or tanning parlors.

KNOW THE SIGNS OF SKIN CANCER

- A skin growth that increases in size and appears pearly, translucent, tan, brown, black or multicolored.
- A mole, birthmark or beauty mark that changes color, increases in size or thickness, changes in texture, is irregular in outline.
- A spot or growth that continues to itch, hurt, crust, scab, erode or bleed.
- An open sore or wound on the skin that does not heal or persists for more than four weeks, or heals and then reopens.

If you have any of these symptoms, see your doctor immediately.

Are sunlamps and suntanning booths safe?

All tanning devices produce ultraviolet radiation that, like ultraviolet rays from the sun, can cause eye injuries, skin burns and may help to promote cancer. The long-term effects of ultraviolet tanning devices are unknown.

Are skin lightener creams dangerous?

Skin bleaches are linked to skin problems like abnormal darkening. Animal studies suggest a possible cancer risk. The ingredient hydroquinine suppresses production of melanin, which produces skin pigmentation.

Do some medications increase the effects of sunlight and ultraviolet radiation?

There are some substances that are photosensitizing—-that is, you can get a serious sunburn with relatively little exposure when these substances are in your system. Among them are birth-control pills, diuretics (used for high blood pressure), oral hypoglycemics (antidiabetic drugs), phenothiazines (tranquilizers such as Thorazine), sulfa drugs (used for bacterial infections), and antibiotics ending with the suffix -cycline. Saccharin, halogenated slicylanilides, oil of bergamot and essenses of lemon and lime also have been implicated. Persons taking many of the chemotherapy drugs or who have had radiation must also be aware of the effects sunlight has on these substances.

How do skin cancers grow?

Skin cell growth begins deep below the surface of the skin, in the epidermis, where basal cells divide to produce new cells. New cells push mature cells upward to the skin's surface, where they die and flake off. In this way, the skin constantly repairs itself, as new cells grow and multiply in a controlled, orderly manner to replace dying cells. The outermost layer of the skin is made up mostly of flat, scalelike cells called squamous cells. The deepest part of the epidermis also contains melanocytes, the cells that produce the pigment called melanin. Sometimes any of these cells may begin to grow in an uncontrolled manner, leading to an overgrowth of tissue, or a tumor. The tumors may be either benign or malignant.

What are the different kinds of skin cancer?

There are a number of different kinds of skin cancer which behave in different ways. The most common type is basal cell cancer. Squamous cell cancers are the next most common. These two types of skin cancer are referred to as non-melanoma skin cancers. Melanoma (sometimes called cutaneous melanoma or malignant melanoma) is not as common as basal cell and squamous cell cancers, but it is much more serious.

What is hyperkeratosis?

This is a precancerous condition that appears as a scaly patch or small scab of skin in a sharply limited, usually small area. Hyperkeratoses are usually caused by exposure to direct stong sunlight and hot drying wind. They are nearly always found on the face, neck and hands.

What is keratoacanthoma?

This is an unusual skin lesion which appears in a sun-exposed area and may grow rapidly to substantial size over a short period of time. It is usually a smooth, red nodule, sometimes with a central umbilical spot, which is often difficult to distinguish from other skin cancers. Keratoacanthomas do not metastasize, but careful diagnosis is important because they are similar in appearance to squamous cell carcinoma, which, in some cases, can metastasize. A biopsy is needed to determine the cell type.

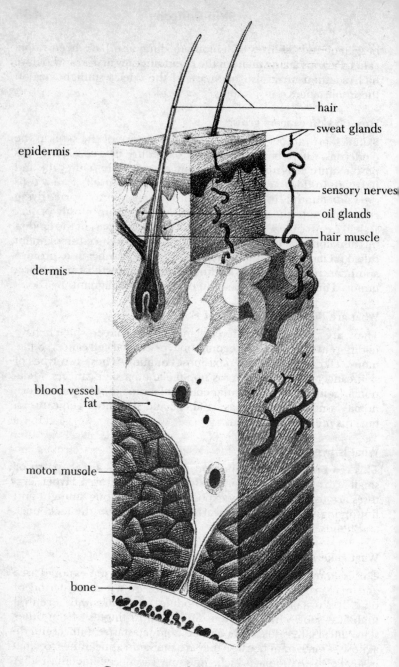

hair

sweat glands

epidermis

sensory nerves

oil glands

hair muscle

dermis

blood vessel

fat

motor muscle

bone

Cross-section of skin (enlarged)

What is sweat-gland cancer?

This is a very rare kind of cancer that may metastasize to the lymph nodes or to distant sites. It can originate from any gland but usually occurs near the anus, eyelids, ears, armpits and scrotum.

What is xeroderma?

Xeroderma is an inherited condition. It is thought to be a precancerous disease. The skin is irregularly pigmented and scaly and later becomes thin, ulcerated, and scarred. It is strongly sensitized to sunlight, and cancer occurs on the areas which have been exposed to it, even briefly.

What is a limpoma?

A limpoma is a soft, fatty, noncancerous tumor that lies directly beneath the skin. It can be as small as a pea or as large as a grapefruit. Limpomas feel soft and move freely under the skin. If they are in a visible spot, or if they show signs of growth, they should be removed.

Do warts ever become cancerous?

Warts do not turn into cancer.

Do hemangiomas become cancerous?

Hemangiomas, blood vessel tumors of the skin, are usually not malignant. They may appear at any time from birth to old age on any part of the body. They range from the size of a pinhead to the size of a nickel. Sometimes they bleed if they are in an area that becomes irritated, such as on a man's face. Most are harmless and do not grow. Doctors usually do not remove them unless they are unsightly.

What is a ganglion?

A ganglion is not a cancer. It is a thin-walled cyst which appears in the tendons or joints, filled with a colorless, jellylike substance. Ganglions are usually seen on the inside wrists of children and young adults.

What is a sebaceous cyst?

Sebaceous cysts, also known as wens, occur when sebaceous glands become clogged and develop into cysts. These rarely turn into cancer. When they increase in size over a period of weeks or months, they should be checked by a dermatologist, who will usually remove them.

What is a fibroma?

Skin fibromas very rarely become cancerous. They are small, hard lumps about the size of a cherry pit. They are not usually removed. Another type, pediculated fibromas, little tags that dangle on stalks from the skin, are common on necks and armpits and are fully treated by electrocautery.

Do tattoos cause skin cancer?

Tattoos usually do not cause cancer. However, if there is any sign of itching or bubbling around the edges, the tattoo should be checked by a physician.

What other skin conditions are there that are not cancerous?

There are a number of other skin conditions that may look suspicious, but which are harmless. Seborrheic keratoses (raised, warty-looking, appear to be stuck onto the skin's surface, easy to scrape off with a fingernail), skin tags (papillomas—little outpatchings of skin), syringomas (benign tumors caused by an enlarged sweat gland—different from the rare kind of sweat gland cancer that is known to metastasize), histiocytomas (solitary, well-rounded firm nodules), snile lentigo (liver spots), and sebaceous hyperplasia (shiny, yellow, waxy-oily tumors) are skin conditions that are almost always benign and rarely turn into cancer.

How can I tell whether or not a growth is cancerous?

You cannot. You should bring any skin change to the attention of your doctor. Only a trained physician can determine the nature of an abnormal skin growth—whether it is benign, precancerous, or malignant. If you have any questions or doubts, seek out the opinion of a qualified dermatologist who has had experience dealing with skin cancers.

QUESTIONS TO ASK YOUR DOCTOR ABOUT SKIN CANCER

- What kind of skin cancer do I have?
- What kind of treatment will you prescribe for me?
- What are the pros and cons of this treatment?
- What other alternatives are there to this treatment?
- Will I have a scar? How large will it be?
- Will I need a skin graft?
- Who will do it?
- What are the side effects of this treatment?
- How often will I need to return for checkups?

NON-MELANOMA SKIN CANCERS

How does basal cell cancer behave?

Basal cell cancer is the most common and the least lethal form of skin cancer. It accounts for 90 percent of all skin cancers in the southern states and 47 percent in the northern states. It usually occurs on areas of the skin that have been in the sun—the face, head, neck, arms, hands and back. Often it will appear as a small, raised bump that has a smooth, pearly appearance. Another type looks like a scar, and it is firm to the touch. Basal cell cancer is very slow growing, may spread to the tissue around the cancer, but seldom spreads to other parts of the body. If not treated properly, however, it can invade and destroy nearby bone and cartilage. **Following treatment for basal cell cancer, you should have a clinical examination every six months for five years. It has been found that 36 percent of those with basal cell cancers will develop a second basal cell cancer within five years. Thereafter, yearly examinations should be done.**

What is squamous cell cancer?

Squamous cell skin cancer is the second most common type of skin cancer, after basal cell cancer. It rarely spreads, but it does so more often than basal cell cancer. Most of the epidermis is composed of squamous cells, which are flat. Squamous cell cancers are faster growing than basal cell. Overall, only about 2 percent of squamous cell cancers spread to other parts of the body. However, about 20 percent of squamous cell cancers that develop on the lips or in burn scars or x-ray scars are known to metastasize. Squamous cell cancer is two to three times more common in men than in women. Studies indicate that the risk of developing this type of skin cancer is related to the cumulative amount of sun exposure and the degree of skin pigmentation. **Since squamous cell cancers have a potential to metastasize, if you have squamous cell cancer, you should be reexamined every three months for the first several years and then followed indefinitely at six-month intervals.**

What are precancers?

Precancers are abnormal skin conditions that tend to become cancerous at a later date. The most common are senile or actinic keratosis, actinic cheilitis and hyperkeratosis. Actinic cheilitis is a related condition that usually appears on the lower lips. These are skin conditions that appear as rough, red or brown, scaly patches. These often develop in older persons whose skin has been exposed for many years to the ultraviolet rays of the sun, although some types occur on unexposed parts of the body such as the chest, back or arms. These different types of keratoses are not considered to be cancer, but can change into basal cell or squamous cell skin cancer. Since keratoses can become malignant, these precancerous conditions should be checked regularly. Premalignant conditions may be treated with topical agents, cryosurgery, electrosurgery, dermabrasion, shave excision or carbon dioxide laser.

What is leukoplakia?

Leukoplakia is a condition resembling keratosis, which occurs as a white thickening on the lip, tongue or mouth. It frequently occurs in heavy pipe smokers and tobacco chewers.

What is Bowen's disease?

Bowen's disease is a rare form of squamous cell skin cancer, sometimes referred to as precancerous dermatitis. It often occurs in several primary sites. The growth is reddish-pink and raised, with scaling. It usually occurs on the unexposed areas of the skin. Sometimes it is associated with internal malignancies.

TREATMENT CHOICES FOR NON-MELANOMA CANCER

TYPE	TREATMENT
Basal cell	Micrographic surgery, simple excision with margin evaluation, electrosurgery, cryosurgery, radiation therapy, laser therapy, topical chemotherapy. *Clinical trials:* Photodynamic therapy, chemoprevention, biological therapy.
Squamous cell	Micrographic surgery, simple excision, electrosurgery, cryosurgery, radiation therapy, topical 5-FU, carbon dioxide laser, alpha interferon.
Actinic keratosis	Topical agents, cryosurgery, electrosurgery, dermabrasion, shave excision or carbon dioxide laser.

What type of doctor should I see if I have suspicious skin spots?

Although your family doctor usually will check your skin during regular physical exams, especially if you ask to have this done, it is wise to see a dermatologist if you have suspicious skin spots. If you have malignant melanoma, it is important that you see a surgeon who specializes in cancer treatment or an oncologist who is familiar with melanoma treatment. If you need reconstructive work done as a result of skin cancer, a plastic surgeon, dermatologist, otolaryngologist, or maxillofacial surgeon would be the doctor of choice.

Can a doctor tell the difference between the different kinds of skin cancers by looking at them?

A skilled dermatologist or a doctor experienced in detecting skin cancer usually can tell the difference by looking at the spot in question. However, skin cancer specialists say that what sometimes looks like a benign growth can prove to be cancerous when biopsied. The only way to really know is to have the biopsy.

What kind of treatment is used in treating skin cancers?

There are a number of ways to treat skin cancer, including surgery, micrographic surgery, electrosurgery, cryosurgery, radiation therapy, carbon dioxide laser, topical fluorouracil, systemic retinoids, alpha interferon and photodynamic therapy.

When is surgery used for non-melanoma skin cancers?

Surgery is used to remove many non-melanoma skin cancers. Usually, surgery is performed under local anesthesia and the cancer is taken out completely at the time of biopsy with no further therapy required. In some cases, cancers are larger than they appear on the skin's surface and more tissue must be removed than might seem necessary. Many surgeons use margins of three to five millimeters for small, well-defined tumors and margins of at least one centimeter for large or more aggressive types of tumors.

When is cryosurgery used for skin cancers?

Cryosurgery, which uses extreme cold to freeze off the lesions, is sometimes considered for actinic keratoses, small basal cell and squamous cell tumors. Liquid nitrogen is applied with a special spray device or a cotton-tipped applicator. The treatments can be done without anesthesia and can be performed efficiently during a routine office visit. There may be some swelling of the area following treatment and it may take about four weeks before the area treated with cryosurgery heals. Cryosurgery can result in permanent pigment loss—the area may appear pink or white when healed. Cryosurgery should not be used for sclerosing basal cell cancers or for tumors of the scalp, nose, lip, eyelid margins or lower legs, cancers fixed to the underlying bone or cartilage, at the margins of the fingers, the elbow, or for cancers previously treated with surgery.

Is electrosurgery used for skin cancer?

This method, which the doctors call electrodesiccation and curettage, dehydrates the tumor with high-frequency electrical current and removes the tumor. You will usually have an anesthetic injected to numb the area and the cancer is scooped out with a sharp instrument with a spoon-shaped end called a curette. It is the most common method of removing basal cell cancers. In treating squamous cell tumors, the doctors use this method for very small cancers. Though it is a quick method for destroying the cancer, this method is not totally satisfactory since the adequacy of treatment cannot be assessed immediately because the doctor cannot visually detect the depth of microscopic tumor invasion. Usually it is necessary to repeat the procedure two to three times, or more, if the tumor is large. Since distortion can occur on healing with electrosurgery, it is not recommended for use around the eyes and mouth. The treatment may leave a white scar.

Is simple surgery with biopsy examination of the margins of the skin cancer a safe method?

This is a traditional surgical treatment sometimes used for basal cell and squamous cell cancers. However, this method allows only a small fraction of the total tumor margin to be examined pathologically, and studies show that recurrence is more likely with this method.

What is Mohs' micrographic surgery?

Mohs' technique is a precise method of surgically removing a cancer one thin layer at a time, until only healthy tissue remains. This method, though it is complicated, expensive and requires a specially trained physician, ensures that the entire cancer is removed while taking as little healthy tissue as possible. It has the highest cure rate for both primary and recurrent non-melanoma skin cancers because the cancer is microscopically delineated until it is completely removed. It is used for recurrent basal cell and squamous cell cancers as well as for initial basal and squamous cell cancers when they occur at sites which have a high treatment failure rate. It is also used for those tumors with poorly defined borders, diameters larger than two centimeters, or cancers in such difficult areas as the eyelid, nose, finger and genitalia. You will sometimes hear this treatment referred to as chemosurgery because when it was first used, the growth was treated with a chemical such as zinc chloride paste before surgery.

When is radiation therapy used for skin cancers?

Radiation therapy is sometimes used to treat skin cancer that occurs in areas such as eyelids, nose or ears, that are hard to treat with surgery. Radiation may also be used for people who cannot tolerate surgery. It is sometimes used for cancers that have grown deep into tissue, are too large to be removed completely by other means, or have recurred. Several treatments may be needed. Changes in skin color and texture may occur and may become more noticeable many years after treatment. Experience has shown that following treatment with radiation, tumors of the nose and the ears have the highest recurrence rates within five years.

Is topical fluorouracil (5-FU) used in skin cancer treatment?

This simple treatment, in which 5-FU cream or solution is applied for four to six weeks, is effectively used for actinic keratoses. Superficial basal cell carcinomas and squamous cell cancers in situ sometimes are treated with topical 5-FU as well. However, careful and prolonged follow-up is essential, since deeply embedded portions of the cancer may escape treatment and result in future recurrences. Swelling is common, especially the first week after treatment is begun, often becoming marked and progressing to oozing, crusting or ulceration. Itching and burning often occur, and healing usually takes three to six weeks once treatment is stopped. You usually do not have a scar as a result of this treatment.

Are retinoids being used for skin cancer treatment?

There are some current studies being done to determine whether retinoids are successful for skin cancer treatment. Some clinical trials using a combination of alpha-interferon and retinoids appear to be effective in treating squamous cell cancers. However, the short-term side effects and long-term effects of these agents presently exclude them as the treatment of choice for most patients.

Is carbon dioxide laser used to treat skin cancers?

Carbon dioxide laser is sometimes used for superficial types of basal cell cancers, as well as for selected squamous cell in situ cancers, especially if bleeding is present. The laser light beam, which produces a powerful, narrow beam of light at one wavelength, can be used to vaporize the abnormal growth. It is sometimes used in conjuction with curettage.

MELANOMA

What is melanoma?

Melanoma (referred to medically as cutaneous melanoma or malignant melanoma) is the most serious type of skin cancer. It occurs most frequently in white women and men over the age of 40 who have a lot of moles on their body, who have light complexions, red or blond hair, and skin that freckles and burns easily. Women most often get melanoma on the arms and legs. In men, it is most often seen on the trunk, head or neck. **Half of all melanomas begin in a previously benign mole. Early signs of change in the mole, such as a darkening or a change in color, an increase in size, or an itching sensation should be immediately checked by a doctor. Bleeding and ulceration of the mole are later signs of possible problems.** Melanoma is best treated when it is found early, as it can spread quickly to other parts of the body through the lymph system or through the blood.

How do melanomas start?

Melanomas develop when a melanocyte, which is a cell that produces melanin, begins to behave abnormally. Melanin is the pigment which gives our skin its natural color. Healthy cells normally grow, divide, and replace themselves in an orderly fashion. Sometimes melanocytes grow in a cluster. These benign clusters of melanocytes are called moles. (Doctors sometimes refer to them as nevi; one mole is called a nevus.) Moles are very common. They may be present at birth or may appear later on—usually before age 40. They generally grow or change only slightly over time. When they are taken off, they normally do not return. Melanomas occur when the melanocytes become maligant. Often the first sign is a change in the size, shape or color of an existing mole. Or it may appear as a new, abnormal lump in normal skin or as a new, ugly-looking mole. If a melanoma is not removed early, cancer cells may grow downward from the skin surface, invading healthy tissue. When a melanoma becomes thick and deep, the disease often spreads to other parts of the body and is difficult to control.

What are atypical moles?

Some people have certain abnormal-looking moles (sometimes called dysplastic nevi) that may be more likely than normal moles to develop into melanoma. Most people with atypical moles have just a few of these abnormal moles; others have many. Atypical moles often look very much like melanoma.

Should all moles be removed?

Moles are very common. Since melanoma is relatively rare—about 1 to 2 percent of all human cancers—the odds that any one mole will become malignant melanoma are less than one in several million. Moles on the palms of the hands, the soles of the feet, or the genitalia are more apt to turn into malignant melanoma than are moles elsewhere. In addition, if you have a mole in a location that is likely to be irritated, such as where a brassiere strap rubs, or where it might be nicked in shaving, it is wise to have it removed. Usually it will be examined to make certain it is not cancerous.

Do moles get darker during pregnancy?

Moles on a woman's body may become darker than usual during pregnancy. This is normal and not a sign of melanoma, but it is wise to have them checked by the gynocologist.

Is melanoma inherited?

About 10 percent of all people who have melanoma have family members who also have had melanoma. There appears to be a predisposition to melanoma in some families. Genetic studies are learning more about the location of abnormalities in the DNA that make some people predisposed to melanoma cancers.

Are there different kinds of melanoma?

There are four fairly distinct forms of primary melanoma. They are:

1. **Superficial spreading melanoma,** which starts from a preexisting or new mole.
2. **Nodular melanoma,** which also starts from a preexisting or new mole.
3. **Lentigo maligna melanoma,** also known as Hutchinson's melanotic freckle, which tends to occur on the face or in areas of the body exposed to the sun.
4. **Acral lentiginous melanoma,** which appears as a dark mark on the palms, soles, or around nails.

In addition, there are some miscellaneous unusual types: mucosal lentiginous melanoma, which appears on the mouth and genitals; desmoplastic melanoma, which causes fibrous adhesions; and verrucous melanoma, which is rough and warty.

What do physicians look for when determining whether a mole is a melanoma?

Physicians refer to the **ABCD** of melanoma: **A**symmetry, **B**orders that are irregular, **C**olor variability and **D**iameter (greater than six millimeters).

How should the biopsy for melanoma be done?

A properly performed biopsy is critical in diagnosing melanoma. Ideally, the biopsy should be performed in such a way that the complete melanoma is removed and examined for cancer.

Is it easy to diagnose melanoma?

Diagnosis of melanoma requires the services of physicians and pathologists who are experienced in this type of cancer diagnosis. If there is any doubt at all about the diagnosis, the biopsy should be reviewed by several pathologists before any decisions about treatment are made.

What tests are done once melanoma is diagnosed?

Your doctor will prescribe a series of tests to determine if cancer cells have spread to other parts of the body to stage the disease. Staging considers how deeply the cancer has penetrated the skin and subcutaneous tissue, how widely it has grown and whether it has metastasized. Staging procedures may include a thorough physical examination, chest x-rays, blood tests, and liver function tests.

How is staging determined for malignant melanoma?

Staging is determined either by the vertical thickness in millimeters (called Breslow's classification) or by the anatomic level of the tumor (known as Clark's classification). Stages are further classified by other classifications that indicate the thickness of the tumor and the level of invasion. Since staging is of primary importance in determining the treatment to be used, these classifications are very specific. Accurate staging of the original melanoma requires careful inspection of the entire specimen by an experienced pathologist. (For further information on staging and classifications, please refer to Chapter 4, "How Cancers Are Diagnosed.")

What treatments are used for malignant melanoma?

The treatment for malignant melanoma depends upon the location, extent and stage of the disease. The depth to which the skin has been invaded determines the extent of the treatment. Some melanomas that have spread to nearby lymph nodes may be curable with wide surgery of the tumor and removal of the involved nearby lymph nodes. Melanoma that has spread to other areas, such as the liver, lungs, bone, brain and internal organs, is more difficult to cure, although surgical removal of the metastasized cancer is sometimes successful. When a large amount of skin is removed, grafting may be necessary. Skin may be taken from another part of the body and grafted to the area where the cancer was removed.

Malignant melanoma is the single most common tumor reported to spontaneously regress, although this occurs in less than 1 percent of cases.

How extensive should surgery be for small melanomas?

According to the National Cancer Institute, removal of only the cancerous tissue and a small (one centimeter) margin is needed to treat early melanoma—without more extensive surgery. Furthermore, in many cases of small melanomas, there is no need for removal of nearby lymph nodes, nor for expensive scanning diagnostics, such as CT scans.

Is chemotherapy used for melanoma?

Chemotherapy using isolated arterial perfusion may be used, especially if the cancer occurs on an arm or leg. In this method, in order to allow the drug to reach the tumor directly, chemotherapy drugs are put into the bloodstream of the arm or leg where the melanoma is found. Chemotherapy may also be prescribed after surgery to kill any undetectable cancer cells that might still remain in the body. Chemotherapy appears to have better results in melanoma occurring in childhood.

How does arterial perfusion work?

Arterial perfusion, sometimes called isolated limb perfusion, is a method of administering high doses of chemotherapy only to the affected limb. As a result, many of the side effects that are common with systemic chemotherapy are avoided. Blood circulation to and from the arm or leg is temporarily stopped with a tourniquet. Blood is withdrawn from the patient and pumped through a machine that adds oxygen and anticancer drugs. The blood is then pumped back into the major artery supplying the limb being treated. Often the blood is heated to enhance the effects of the drugs. The most common drug used in this method of treatment is melphalan. Another technique, known as intraarterial regional infusion, is sometimes used when the cancer is limited to an arm or a leg. Again, normal blood circulation to and from the limb is stopped. Anticancer drugs are infused directly into the main artery of the limb. Most commonly used drugs are dacarbazine (DTIC) and cisplatin.

Are some of the newer biological treatments being used for melanoma?

A number of different types of biological therapies are being tested in clinical trials for melanoma in Stages II, III, IV and for recurrent melanoma.

Is radiation used for melanoma?

Radiation is sometimes used to treat local recurrences of melanoma that cannot be removed surgically. In cases in which the disease has spread to the lung, gastrointestinal tract, bone, or brain, radiation may provide relief from symptoms.

TREATMENT CHOICES FOR MALIGNANT MELANOMA

STAGE	TREATMENT
Stage I pT1, N0, M0 or pT2, N0, M0	Conservative surgery after biopsy; **or** wide surgical excision, skin grafting to cover wound and lymph nodes around tumor may be removed.
Stage II pT3, N0, M0	Wide surgical excision; **or** wide surgical excision of tumor and removal of nearby lymph nodes. *Clinical trials:* Wide excision followed by adjuvant chemotherapy or biological therapy; **or** wide surgical excision followed by chemotherapy given directly into the arm or leg (isolated arterial perfusion).
Stage III pT4, N0, M0, **or** any pT, N1, or N2, M0	Wide surgical excision. Skin grafting if needed. Nearby lymph nodes may be removed. *Clinical trials:* Wide surgical excision, chemotherapy given directly into arm or leg (isolated arterial perfusion); **or** wide surgical excision, followed by adjuvant chemotherapy or biological therapy or immunotherapy.
Stage IV any pT, any N, M1	Surgery to remove lymph nodes that are cancerous or tumors that have spread to other areas of the body; **or** radiation therapy to relieve symptoms; **or** systemic chemotherapy. *Clinical trials:* Newer types of systemic chemotherapy or biological therapy; **or** biological agents injected directly into tumors that have spread.
Recurrent	Dependent on many factors, including prior treatment and site of recurrence. No accepted standard treatment. *Clinical trials:* Systemic chemotherapy and/or biological therapy such as alpha interferon, IL2, high-dose cisplatin, other chemotherapy combinations, combined hyperthermia and radiation.

Are skin grafts common following surgical removal of malignant melanoma?

Skin grafts may be necessary following the removal of skin cancers, depending upon the location and extent of the surgery. A portion of healthy skin is taken from one area of the body and moved to another area. In skin cancer, such grafts cover the areas that have been left bare by the surgical removal of portions of the skin. The replacement skin is usually taken from the back or thigh or other part of the body and stitched to the wound.

Is it painful to have a skin graft?

There is usually only a little pain and a burning sensation in the area from which the skin was removed and no pain at the site where it is applied.

Will the grafted skin look like normal skin?

The match of normal and grafted skin depends upon where the graft comes from. The doctor will try to match it as closely as possible—in color and texture. In a few months, the graft develops sensation. It is wise to protect the skin from the sun as the new skin can become sunburned, but will probably not darken as much as surrounding skin. The new skin will grow hair only if it came from a location where hair was originally growing.

What kind of doctor should I use for a skin graft?

This will depend upon the location of the graft, the size and the type being done. Facial procedures are done by dermatologists, otolaryngologists, maxillofacial surgeons and plastic surgeons.

How often should someone who has had melanoma have a checkup?

Since anyone who has had melanoma is at increased risk for developing new melanomas as well as for a recurrence of the original melanoma, they should be checked regularly. The chance of recurrence is greater for those whose melanoma was thick or had spread to nearby tissue than for someone with a very thin melanoma. In general, recurrences of melanoma may occur within 18 to 24 months after treatment. You should see your doctor every three months for the first year, every four months until the fifth year, and every 6 months thereafter. Depending on your stage of disease, you may have yearly chest x-rays or CT scans of the chest and liver. It is especially important for those who have had melanoma to thoroughly examine their own skin on a monthly basis.

UNUSUAL SKIN CANCERS

What is ocular melanoma?

Ocular melanoma, like melanoma of the skin, originates in melanocytes, the pigmented cells that give the eye its color. Ocular melanoma may grow in any of the uveal structures of the eye (the iris, ciliary body or choroid). Melanoma that develops in the iris may produce a pigmented spot, changing to translucent or pink, which you often discover yourself. Other signs include distortion of the pupil, presence of new blood vessels, curling of the iris near the pupil, and cataract formation. If tumors reach a large size, you may have symptoms such as loss or deterioration of vision and floating spots. Cataracts, secondary glaucoma, and inflammation also may occur.

Should I go to a specialized center for treatment for ocular melanoma?

Since side effects accompany each form of treatment, it is important to have an open and complete discussion with well-qualified doctors, including an ophthalmologist and oncologist, to develop the treatment plan best suited to the patient. Before making any decisions about treatment, anyone with this unusual type of cancer should seek out second opinions and consider the possibility of having treatment at one of the leading cancer centers.

How is ocular melanoma treated?

Only a dozen years ago, melanoma of the eye meant taking out the eye and a diminished chance for long-term survival. Today, treated in few specialized radiotherapy centers, using proton beams, melanoma patients may be able to keep not only their eyes, but also their vision to such an extent that they can drive a car. Ocular melanomas usually are managed with radiation or with surgery to remove either the tumor (resection) or the entire eye (enucleation). In cases of choroid and ciliary body melanomas, there are more treatment options available, including localized radiation using a method where radioactive pellets are enclosed in a plastic disk covered on one side with a gold plate. The radiation released by the plaque is directed to the tumor, while the gold plate protects the surrounding tissues and the brain from receiving radiation.

Are there any ocular melanomas that do not need treatment?

Small ocular melanomas that are not growing and do not interfere with vision may not be treated, but they do require close observation.

What is Merkel cell carcinoma?

This is an unusual type of skin cancer that often spreads to the lymph nodes in the area of the tumor. High-power electron microscopes make it possible to identify this cell type, which is most commonly found on the scalp, neck, face and fingertips. It occurs most often in older patients, generally between the ages of 50 and 90. Unlike some skin cancers that appear as a sore that does not heal, Merkel cell cancers begin as painless lumps on the surface of the skin. Treatment includes removal of the tumor and a wide margin of healthy tissue. Radiation therapy or removal of lymph nodes is sometimes recommended.

NOTE: Information on Kaposi's sarcoma can be found in Chapter 19, "Bone and Soft Tissue Sarcomas."

chapter 16

Adult Leukemia

Many people think that leukemia is a children's disease. In fact, many more adults have leukemia than children. Of the more than 29,000 new cases of leukemia that occur each year, fewer than 10 percent affect children. The rest occur in adults, many of them over the age of 60.

Leukemias in adults are of both the acute and chronic types, approximately evenly divided between the two types. Leukemia strikes both sexes and all ages. Although the causes of leukemia are not fully understood, certain factors are known to increase the risk of developing the disease. They include genetic factors such as Down's syndrome as well as exposure to high or repeated doses of radiation, genetic changes, exposure to some chemicals and infections from certain viruses. Over the last thirty years, there has been a dramatic improvement in survival of patients with acute lymphocytic leukemia. In the early 1960s, the five-year survival rate was 4 percent, in the early 1970s it was up to 28 percent, and in the mid-1980s it was 51 percent. (Please see Chapter 22, "Childhood Cancers," for information on childhood leukemias.)

WHAT YOU NEED TO KNOW ABOUT LEUKEMIA

- Leukemia is a cancer of the organs that make blood—the lymph system and the bone marrow. The number of cells produced, the rate at which they are produced and their ability to function are altered.

- There are four major types of leukemia, each with its own individual characteristics and treatments.
- Improvements in treatments over the last decade have made it possible for physicians to treat the disease aggressively—and in some cases to cure it.
- More than half of all leukemias occur in people over 60 years of age.
- Acute leukemia means it is a rapidly progressing type. Chronic leukemia usually progresses more slowly, but can be unpredictable. Many times there are no symptoms for many years. Other times it may progress more rapidly.

WHO IS MOST LIKELY TO GET LEUKEMIA?

- White people more often than blacks.
- People of Jewish ancestry more often than other whites.
- Males more often than females.
- Those exposed to high or repeated doses of ionizing radiation.
- Patients who received at least two grays (a measure of radiation) as treatment for ankylosing spondylitis, a spinal condition.
- Some patients with Hodgkin's disease who received radiation and chemotherapy.
- Those with some genetic abnormalities, such as Down's and Bloom's syndromes, Fanconi's anemia, neurofibromatosis, and Philadelphia chromosome.
- Those who have had long-term exposure to certain chemicals and drugs, such as benzene, chloramphenicol and phenylbutazone, and chemotherapy drugs such as alkylating agents.
- If one identical twin develops acute leukemia before 6 years of age, there is a 20 percent chance the other twin will develop it within a few months. Fraternal twins and siblings of those with leukemia are at greater risk than the normal population.
- Though not confirmed by studies, there is suggestive evidence that those living near high-voltage transmission lines (especially children) may be at risk.

What kind of doctor is best for treating someone who has leukemia?

Leukemia can be a very difficult disease to treat, so it is essential that a qualified hematologist or oncologist who is experienced in dealing with leukemia is involved in making your treatment plans. Another important factor to be considered is the hospital. Facilities with extensive supportive care capabilities that have access to blood products and a multidisciplinary team of physicians, nurses and pharmacists assure that the patient receives the best treatment possible.

SYMPTOMS OF ACUTE LEUKEMIAS (ALL AND AML)

- Fever and flulike symptoms.
- Changes in energy level, appetite and temperament.
- Joint and bone pain.
- Joint tenderness or swelling.
- Paleness, dizziness, weakness.
- Tendency to bruise or bleed easily.
- Unexplained bleeding.
- Recurrent infections in skin, gums, lung, urinary tract.
- Tiny red or brown spots on skin.
- If central nervous system is affected: headache, blurred vision, confusion, unexplained fever.

Because symptoms may be vague it is often difficult to make an early diagnosis of acute leukemia. Sometimes symptoms may be present for less than three months, sometimes for only a few days.

What is leukemia?

Leukemia is cancer of the blood-forming cells. It occurs when immature or mature cells multiply in an uncontrolled manner in the bone marrow.

How do the blood-forming cells work?

The three major types of cells in the blood are red blood cells (erythrocytes), white blood cells (leukocytes) and platelets (thrombocytes). All of these cells are produced in the bone marrow. Most blood cells mature in the bone marrow, but some also mature in the thymus, spleen, lymph nodes, and tonsils. After maturing, the adult cells slowly seep into the blood vessels and become part of the blood.

What is the function of red blood cells?

Red blood cells act as a transportation system. They carry oxygen from the lungs to the other cells of the body and bring back waste products or carbon dioxide. If there are too few red blood cells, it is difficult for cells to get enough oxygen. This causes what we call anemia and results in weakness, lack of energy, dizziness, headache and irritability. Red blood cell counts are part of the blood counts monitored in blood tests.

What do white blood cells do?

White blood cells are the main components of the immune system. Their primary role is to fight infection. There is normally only about one white blood cell for every five hundred red blood cells. If a bacterial infection is present, the number may increase dramatically. They are produced by stem cells in the bone marrow, though some mature outside the marrow in the lymph nodes, spleen, tonsils, and thymus. If the white blood cell count is abnormally low, a person's chance of developing an infection increases.

Are there different kinds of white blood cells?

There are several major types, each with a specific function. Granulocytes, one type of white blood cells, fight infections. It takes nine to ten days for immature cells formed in the bone marrow to become mature granulocytes. Because granulocytes circulate for only six to ten hours, any interruption in their production quickly places you at risk for developing an infection. There are three different kinds of granulocytes: neutrophils, basophils and eosinophils. Mononuclear cells destroy invading antigens, particularly viruses. There are two different kinds of mononuclear cells: lymphocytes and monocytes (macrophages). In doing blood counts, laboratory tests measure the levels of these different types of white blood cells. You may hear some of these cell types referred to by other names:

- Neutrophils are also called polymorphonucleacytes, PMN, or polys. Immature neutrophils are sometimes called bands or stabs.
- Eosinophils may be referred to as "eos."
- Lymphocytes as lymphs.
- Monocytes as monos.

What do platelets do?

Platelets are essential in clotting of blood. Checking the platelet count is part of the testing done for those who are suspected of having or who have leukemia. An abnormally low platelet count (called thrombocytopenia) may result in excessive bleeding from wounds or in mucous membranes, skin, or other tissues.

What are blasts?

Blasts, or leukemic cells, are immature white blood cells. In normal marrow, less than 5 percent of these abnormal cells are present.

What are petechiae?

Petechiae (pronounced "pe-te-ke-eye") is the medical jargon for small red and/or brown spots on the skin, which are actually tiny hemorrhages. They can look like a rash. They are caused by a low blood count and decreased clotting function and are often seen in conjunction with leukemia.

TESTS THAT MAY BE USED TO DIAGNOSE ADULT LEUKEMIA

- Physical examination.
- Laboratory tests that include blood counts, chemistries and urine tests.
- Diagnostic x-rays.
- Bone marrow biopsy and aspiration.
- Spinal tap.

What is a peripheral blood smear?

This is a blood test in which a drop of blood is smeared on a glass slide, fixed, stained and examined under a high-power microscope. The size and shape of a large number of red blood cells, the numbers of the different types of white blood cells and the number of platelets are examined and recorded.

Why is there so much emphasis on blood tests?

When you have leukemia, blood tests become a part of your life. Since leukemia means that there is an abnormality in the production of blood, the blood counts tell the doctor about the state of your health. Blood checks help to determine how you are progressing.

What is the total white blood cell count?

The white blood cell count or leukocyte count measures the total number of circulating leukoctyes.

What is the differential white blood cell count?

The differential white blood cell count gives the percentage of each type of white cell that makes up the total white blood count. Alone, this count has limited value—it must always be interpreted in relation to the total leukocyte count. If the percentage of one type of cell is increased, it can be inferred that cells of that type are relatively more numerous than normal. This is not always the case, because it is not known if this reflects an absolute decrease in cells of another type or an actual absolute increase in the number of cells that are relatively increased.

BLOOD COUNTS

NOTE: Values may vary according to age and individual laboratory standards.

CELL TYPE	NORMAL VALUES
Differential white blood cell count (leukocyte count)	
Neutrophils	50–60%
Eosinophils	1–4%
Basophils	0.5–1%
Lymphocytes	20–40%
Monocytes	2–6%
Platelets	150,000–350,000 per cubic millimeter
Hematocrit (% of cells in volume of blood)	
Males	40–54%
Females	37–47%
Hemoglobin **NOTE: If blood-drawing tourniquet is left on too long, may produce abnormally high values**	
Males	14–18 grams per deciliter
Females	12–16 grams per deciliter

What is the hematocrit count?

The hematocrit count gives the percentage of red cells in a volume of whole blood. The test separates the plasma and blood cells.

How is a bone marrow biopsy done?

A bone marrow biopsy takes a small sample of bone marrow through a needle inserted into a bone—either the hip, or less frequently, the breastbone. (In a bone marrow aspiration, a fluid specimen is drawn out.) In a needle biopsy, a core of solid cells is removed. (In infants or small children, bone marrow samples are sometimes taken from the shinbone just below the knee.) A local anesthetic is injected to numb the tissue over the biopsy site. The biopsy needle is inserted into the bone. The core of the needle is removed and the needle is advanced and rotated in both directions, forcing a tiny core of bone into the needle. Each test takes about ten to twenty minutes. You will feel a dull to sharp pain that will last as long as the needle is being advanced and removed. The local anesthetic does not affect the deeper bone pain, but the pain lasts only a minute or less. There may be soreness at the biopsy site for several days. Test results are usually available in several days.

What are spicules?

When doing a bone marrow test, the doctor wants to be certain to retrieve bone marrow. Spicules are bits of bone marrow with fat in them, which give a representative sample of marrow cells. Without enough spicules, it is impossible to make an accurate diagnosis of the bone marrow cells.

QUESTIONS TO ASK YOUR DOCTOR BEFORE AGREEING TO START LEUKEMIA TREATMENT

- What kind of leukemia do I have?
- Is it a chronic or acute type of leukemia?
- Which cells are affected?
- Is this a very unusual type of leukemia?
- Can you explain the blood counts and tell me what is normal for me?
- Has the diagnosis been checked by a hematopathologist?
- Do you suggest that this diagnosis be confirmed by getting a second opinion at one of the large centers which specializes in this type of cancer?
- Would it be wise for me to get my treatment at one of the major cancer centers?

- How many cases like mine do you treat each year?
- What kind of treatment are you planning for me?
- Is bone marrow transplantation a choice for me after initial treatment?

How is leukemia classified and what is the difference between acute and chronic leukemia?

Broadly, acute and chronic leukemia is classified as lymphocytic or myeloid, according to the type of cell that is multiplying abnormally. Acute means that it is progressing rapidly with a large number of highly immature cells. Chronic means that it is progressing slowly with greater numbers of more mature cells.

Why is supportive care during treatment so essential for leukemia patients?

Patients with leukemia have very low platelet and white blood cell counts and are at great risk of life-threatening infection and bleeding. The purpose of supportive care is to prevent or reduce the effects of anemia, bleeding and infection.

ACUTE LEUKEMIAS

What are the two types of acute leukemias?

In adults, the most common type of acute leukemia is acute **myeloid** leukemia or **AML**, which accounts for more than half of all adult leukemias. The other type of acute leukemia is acute **lymphocytic** leukemia or **ALL**. This is the adult version of the most common childhood leukemia. It is more difficult to control in adults than in children. It accounts for only a small percentage of adult leukemias. Some leukemias, classified as biphenotypic, have both lymphoid and myeloid features. Some show no differentiation of either cell type and are classified as undifferentiated. It is sometimes difficult to distinguish between the two types of acute leukemias, so it is essential that proper laboratory studies be done and confirmed so that the correct diagnosis is made.

How is the diagnosis made for the acute types of leukemia?

Often blood tests will show a low hemoglobin count, a low level of normal white blood cells or platelets or the presence of leukemic

TYPES OF LEUKEMIA

Type	Description
Acute lymphocytic leukemia (ALL)	Begins in immature B or T lymphocytes. Accounts for only 6% of adult leukemias. (75% of childhood leukemias are ALL. Treatments for children are different than for adults. See Chapter 22.)
Acute myeloid leukemia (AML); also called **acute nonlymphocytic leukemia** (ANLL); there are also a number of subtypes of AML	Begins in immature myeloid cells. Accounts for 54% of adult leukemias and 20% of childhood leukemias. (See Chapter 22 for more information on childhood AML.)
Chronic lymphocytic leukemia (CLL)	Begins in the B lymphocytes, rarely in T lymphocytes. 25% of adult leukemias are this type and less than 1% of childhood cancers fall into this category.
Chronic myeloid leukemia (CML); also called **chronic granulocytic leukemia**	Begins in immature myeloid cells that would normally develop into granulocytes. Accounts for 15% of adult leukemia.
Polycythemia vera (not a true leukemia)	Too many red blood cells made in bone marrow.
Agnogenic myeloid metaplasia	Improper maturing of red blood cells and white blood cells called granulocytes.
Essential thrombocythemia (not a true leukemia)	Number of platelets in blood much higher than normal, but other blood cells are normal. Extra platelets make it hard for blood to flow normally.
Hairy cell (HCL); also called **leukemic reticuloendotheliosis**	Involves blood and bone marrow, affects mostly middle-aged and older men.
Preleukemia or **smoldering leukemia** (myelodysplastic syndrome); may progress to acute nonlymphocytic leukemia (ANLL)	Bone marrow does not function normally and not enough normal blood cells are made. Occurs most often in older people, but sometimes seen in younger persons.

blasts. As many as 10 percent of patients, however, have normal blood counts at the time of diagnosis. In such cases, the diagnosis can be confirmed with a bone marrow biopsy. Many laboratory tests are conducted using the bone marrow sample. The cell's origin is identified so that the leukemia can be properly classified. Tests using stains and dyes help identify types of cells, certain cell surface markers and other cell characteristics.

ACUTE LYMPHOCYTIC LEUKEMIA

How are acute lymphocytic leukemias classified?

Acute lymphocytic leukemias are classified by an L designation:

- L1: Lymphoblasts tend to be small, with little cytoplasm, regularly shaped nuclei, more mature cells.
- L2: Lymphoblasts are more mature, varying in size and nuclear shape.
- L3: Large lymphocytes, abundant cytoplasm, similarly shaped nuclei.

What kind of treatment is used for ALL?

Although great strides have been made in the treatment of childhood ALL, which is now considered one of the most curable forms of cancer, the advances in treatment of adult ALL have been more difficult. Treatment for adult ALL uses chemotherapy. This treatment is divided into three phases: remission induction, central nervous system prophylaxis and postremission treatment.

What is remission induction?

Remission induction is the attempt to destroy all detectable leukemic cells and to reduce the number of blasts in the bone marrow to 5 percent. It is an intensive stage of treatment in the hospital and usually lasts four to seven weeks. The patient must be very carefully monitored to prevent or reduce the effects of anemia, bleeding, and infection. Patients may need periodic transfusions with red blood cells to control anemia. Transfusions of platelets reduce the rate of hemorrhage, allowing treatment with anticancer drugs to continue even when the platelet count has been very low. Sometimes patients become resistant to platelets obtained from persons with a different platelet type. When this occurs the body recognizes the transfused platelets as foreign and rapidly destroys them, which then causes bleeding. Methods of comparing human leukocyte antigens (HLA) on the surface of white blood cells now make it possible for closer matches of donated white blood cells, reducing the chances of rejection. Even patients who previously had developed resistance to nonmatched platelets can be helped when platelets are HLA-matched. Corticosteroids are sometimes given prior to transfusion to improve the body's ability to use red blood cells and platelets. As you can see from the possible complications of this treatment, carefully supervised supportive care is an important component during this stage of treatment.

What is central nervous system prophylaxis?

A small percentage of adults with ALL have evidence of leukemia in the central nervous system at the time of diagnosis and about 40 percent may develop central nervous system disease as time goes on. Researchers have found that treatment can often prevent this complication. Chemotherapy with or without radiation of the brain are the possible treatments.

What is postremission treatment?

After remission has been achieved, further treatment is essential to make sure that there is not a relapse. Maintenance programs for adults are similar to those for children, using a variety of drug combinations and schedules. Usually this treatment is given for one and one-half to three years. It is started either immediately after remission or may be delayed for nine months. Bone marrow transplantation as a treatment has been investigated, but it has not, at this time, been shown to have an advantage over chemotherapy alone. However, patients at high risk of relapse may be considered for either allogeneic or autologous bone marrow transplant clinical trials either during the first remission or a subsequent one. (More information on bone marrow transplants can be found in Chapter 9, "New Advances and Investigational Trials.")

What treatments are used when an ALL patient has a relapse?

Treatment for relapsed ALL depends on many factors, including the length of the previous remission and the site of the relapse. Clinical trials are under way testing the use of high-dose combination chemotherapy, with or without radiation, followed by bone marrow transplant; use of new anticancer drugs and drug combinations; and biological therapy with monoclonal antibodies.

ACUTE MYELOID LEUKEMIA (AML OR ANLL)

What is acute myeloid leukemia?

Acute myeloid leukemia (AML), which is also known as acute non-lymphocytic leukemia (ANLL), is leukemia in which abnormal, immature white blood cells are produced in the bone marrow. Normally, the bone marrow makes cells called blasts that mature into several different types of blood cells that have specific jobs to do in the body. In AML, the blasts do not mature but continue to reproduce and become too numerous. AML is the most common form of adult leukemia and affects people aged 40 and over. There are a number of subtypes of AML which are treated in a similar manner as AML. If left untreated, death can occur within a few months due to infection or uncontrolled bleeding.

How is the diagnosis made?

Blood tests, blood and human leukocyte antigen (HLA) typing and tests to determine the blood's ability to clot are all needed to make an accurate diagnosis. In some instances, an analysis of spinal fluid may be necessary. Treatment of AML is different from treatment for ALL. Therefore, laboratory diagnostic tests must be carefully done to distinguish between the two before any treatment is begun.

How are the different leukemic cells of AML classified?

The different subtypes are classified by an M designation:

- M0: Undifferentiated leukemia.
- M1: Acute myeloblastic leukemia with immature cells.
- M2: Acute myeloblastic leukemia with some mature cells.
- M3: Acute promyelocytic leukemia. ·
- M4: Acute myelomonocytic leukemia.
- M5: Acute monocytic leukemia.
- M6: Erythroleukemia (immature red and white blood cells).
- M7: Acute megakaryocytic leukemia (immature platelets).

How is acute myeloid leukemia staged?

Staging systems are not used for acute myeloid leukemia. Treatment depends upon whether the leukemia is untreated, in remission or relapsed.

What kind of treatments are used for AML?

Chemotherapy combinations bring about complete remission in approximately 65 percent of patients. During this period, known as remission induction, the two major potential complications are infection and bleeding. Frequent transfusions may be needed and broad-spectrum antimicrobial therapy—treatment to kill microorganisms, such as bacteria or fungi, or to suppress their growth—is used to treat these problems. Additional treatment following the achievement of remission induction is necessary. No one treatment is considered standard. It is unclear whether longer term therapy at lower doses, called maintenance therapy, or shorter term intensive therapy, known as consolidation therapy, is preferable. Both have been demonstrated to prolong remission.

What therapy is used if there is a relapse after the original treatments?

Clinical trials are testing the use of new agents. Allogeneic bone marrow transplants are being used and autologous bone marrow transplants are being evaluated.

What does refractory disease mean?

Refractory disease means the leukemia has not responded to treatment and therefore has not gone into remission.

Do most acute myeloid leukemias go into remission?

Advances in the treatment of AML have resulted in substantially improved remission rates. With the aggressive treatments now prescribed, about 60 to 70 percent of adults with AML can expect a complete remission. The results are even better for those under age 60.

Does AML affect the central nervous system?

Central nervous system relapse occurs in only a small percentage of patients, although certain types of AML and patients with high white blood cell counts are at greatest risk. An analysis of a sample of spinal fluid may be taken for evaluation in these cases. Spread to the central nervous system is treated with chemotherapy.

What are myelodysplastic syndromes (MDL)?

This is a group of blood disorders which have an increased risk of becoming AML. About half of patients diagnosed with AML initially were diagnosed as having one of these myelodysplastic syndromes—also known as preleukemia anemia or smoldering anemia. In the final analysis, these syndromes may be different stages of the same disease, since often one type of MDS will change to another type before finally becoming AML. Even when the final evolution to AML does not occur, there may be life-threatening anemia, a drop in platelet levels, infections and ulceration of the mucous membranes. While most often seen in older people, these syndromes can occur in younger people as well. They may develop following treatment with drugs or radiation therapy for other diseases (called secondary myelodysplastic syndromes), or may develop without any known cause (called de novo myelodysplastic syndromes). The mainstay of treatment is transfusions of blood cells or platelets for relief of anemia or bleeding. Vitamins and other drugs may also be used. Clinical trials of chemotherapy or biological therapy are underway. Allogeneic bone marrow transplants are being used for patients under 40 with de novo myelodysplastic syndromes.

CHRONIC LEUKEMIAS

What are chronic leukemias?

In chronic leukemia, too many mature white blood cells are produced and build up in the body. They develop slowly, often with no symptoms at first, and may remain undetected for a long time. There are two types of chronic leukemias, classified by the type of cell in which they begin. Chronic lymphocytic leukemia, known as CLL, is twice as common in men as in women. The average age of diagnosis is 60. CLL is rare before age 30 and it almost never occurs in children. Chronic myelocytic leukemia, CML, is slightly more common in men than in women. The average age of diagnosis is 45. CML accounts for only about 5 percent of children's leukemias.

SYMPTOMS OF CHRONIC LEUKEMIA—CLL, CML AND HCL

- General feeling of ill health.
- Fatigue.
- Lack of energy.
- Fever.
- Loss of appetite.
- Night sweats.
- Enlarged lymph nodes in neck or groin.
- Enlarged spleen.
- Anemia

CML: Pain in the left upper quadrant, vague feeling of abdominal fullness

---

CHRONIC LYMPHOCYTIC LEUKEMIA (CLL)

What is chronic lymphocytic leukemia (CLL)?

Chronic lymphocytic leukemia is a cancer in which lymphocytes multiply very slowly but in a poorly regulated manner, live much longer than normal and are unable to perform their proper function. About one-quarter of all CLL patients have no symptoms and the disease often is diagnosed as a result of a routine blood test. Some patients may have enlarged lymph nodes in the neck or groin or show signs of anemia. The average age at diagnosis is 60. The course of the disease varies a great deal from person to person. Some people remain without symptoms for many years. In other people, CLL may progress more rapidly.

How is CLL diagnosed?

Blood tests are used, as well as bone marrow biopsy and more sophisticated chromosomal tests. CLL is suspected when blood tests reveal an increase in the number of lymphocytes in the blood to more than 15,000 per cubic millimeter as well as the presence of certain identifying characteristics on the lymphocytes' outside surface. CLL may be confused with other related diseases, especially non-Hodgkin's lymphoma.

What kind of treatment is used for CLL?

Treatment for CLL can range from periodic observation for patients who have no symptoms to treatment of complications such as infections or to a variety of investigation treatments. Because CLL often progresses slowly and cannot currently be cured with standard chemotherapy, it is generally treated in a conservative manner. Corticosteroids are used for many patients, sometimes in combination with chemotherapy. In later stages, if the spleen is very enlarged and is destroying large numbers of normal blood cells, the spleen may be removed. Removal of the spleen does not interfere with normal living. Its functions are taken over by other components of the body.

What is leukapheresis?

Luekapheresis is a procedure that transfuses white blood cells from healthy donors into patients whose low white blood cell count puts them at risk for infections.

CHRONIC MYELOGENOUS LEUKEMIA (CML)

What is chronic myelogenous leukemia (CML)?

Chronic myelogenous leukemia is one of the four major types of leukemia, and accounts for about 20 percent of leukemia cases. It affects the cells that are developing into white blood cells, called granulocytes. It is associated with a unique chromosomal abnormal-

STAGES OF AND TREATMENT CHOICES FOR CHRONIC LYMPHOCYTIC LEUKEMIA (CLL)

STAGE	TREATMENT
Stage 0: More than 15,000 lymphocytes per cubic millimeter (absolute lymphocytosis). No other symptoms.	No treatment needed in most cases. Doctor will follow you closely to initiate treatment if needed. Chemotherapy may be used.
Stage I: Absolute lymphocytosis and enlarged lymph nodes. No other symptoms.	If no other symptoms, may not need treatment. Close follow-up; **or** external radiation to swollen lymph nodes; **or** chemotherapy.
Stage II: Absolute lymphocytosis, enlarged lymph nodes, as well as enlarged liver *or* spleen.	If few or no symptoms, may not need treatment. Close follow-up; **or** chemotherapy; **or** *Clinical trials:* Biological therapy; **or** external radiation to spleen.
Stage III: Absolute lymphocytosis and anemia. Symptoms due to enlarged lymph nodes, liver or spleen.	Alkylating agents plus corticosteroids; **or** removal of spleen; fludarabine; **or** combination chemotherapy; **or** Whole body radiation; **or** external radiation to spleen. *Clinical trials:* Biological response modifiers.
Stage IV: Absolute lymphocytosis and fewer than 100,000 platelets per cubic millimeter with or without enlarged lymph nodes, liver or spleen or anemia.	Same as Stage III.
Not responsive to treatment.	Treatment will depend on numerous factors. May consider clinical trial of new chemotherapy drugs.

ity called the Philadelphia chromosome. It is one of the types that eventually progresses to a more acute form. CML is very difficult to treat since present treatments do not cure the disease or prevent blastic crisis.

What is the Philadelphia chromosome?

The Philadelphia chromosome is an abnormal chromosome that is found in more than 90 percent of people who have chronic myelogenous leukemia (CML). This chromosome was the first to be identified for a specific cancer. The cause of the chromosomal defect and its influence in the course of the disease is not known. But it has been seen in all phases of the disease and is rarely affected by treatment. It may sometimes be seen in the acute leukemias and other diseases, but much less commonly. (Incidentally, this abnormality is an acquired genetic defect present only in the blood cells and cannot be transmitted to offspring.)

How is CML diagnosed?

CML is usually diagnosed with the help of a complete blood count and bone marrow biopsy.

What are the symptoms of CML?

About 90 percent of patients complain of fullness in the upper abdomen. This is caused by a swollen spleen, which may fill most of the abdomen.

What are the phases of CML?

CML has three distinct phases: chronic, accelerated and blast. In the chronic phase, the most common at diagnosis, there are few blast cells in the blood and bone marrow, and there may be no symptoms of leukemia. This phase can last from several months to several years. In the accelerated phase, more blast cells and fewer normal cells are found in the bone marrow and blood. In the blast phase, 30 percent of the cells in the blood or bone marrow are blast cells and these collections of cells may form tumors in the bones or lymph nodes. Transition from phase to phase may occur gradually over a year or more, or it may occur abruptly. The blast phase or blast crisis, as it is sometimes called, usually occurs three to five years after diagnosis and is very similar to aggressive acute leukemia but is more difficult to treat.

What treatment is used for CML?

Those who have blood counts that are nearly normal may receive no treatment. They will be checked often so that treatment may be given if the disease begins to progress. Surgery to remove the spleen is sometimes done to relieve physical discomfort or other problems resulting from a severely enlarged spleen. Many people in the chronic phase of CML respond well to treatment and live normal lives. Patients with newly diagnosed CML are urged to consider participating in clinical trials exploring the new therapeutic approaches using bone marrow transplants, biological response modifiers, and combination chemotherapy.

STAGES OF AND TREATMENT CHOICES FOR CHRONIC MYELOGENOUS LEUKEMIA (CML)

STAGE	TREATMENT
Chronic: Few blast cells, no symptoms	None if blood counts are near normal or stable. Careful follow-up by doctor; **or** chemotherapy to lower white cell count; **or** surgery to remove spleen; **or** bone marrow transplant; **or** *Clinical trials:* Biological therapy with or without chemotherapy or after bone marrow transplant.
Accelerated: More blast cells	Chemotherapy to lower white cell count; **or** transfusions of blood or blood products to relieve symptoms; **or** drugs used in chronic phase; **or** *Clinical trials:* Bone marrow transplant or autologous marrow transplant.
Blast: More than 30% of cells are blast cells; tumors in bone or lymph nodes	Chemotherapy (new drugs being studied); **or** radiation, if tumors in bone; **or** *Clinical trials:* Bone marrow transplant.

What are myeloproliferative disorders?

This is a group of diseases in which too many of certain types of blood cells are made in the bone marrow. They include: polycythemia vera, agnogenic myeloid metaplasia and essential thrombocythemia as well as chronic myelogenous leukemia (CML).

What is polycythemia vera?

This disorder is characterized by the uncontrolled production of red blood cells. The spleen may swell because the extra blood cells collect there. Itchiness all over the body is one of the symptoms of polycythemia vera. In order to lower the amount of blood in the body, a needle may be placed in a vein and blood is removed. This is called phlebotomy. Chemotherapy or radiation is also sometimes used to lower the number of red blood cells. New chemotherapy drugs are being studied for use in treating polycythemia vera. With treatment, many patients live with this condition for years. There is a possibility that polycythemia vera can progress to a more acute form of leukemia, so close follow-up is necessary.

What is agnogenic myeloid metaplasia?

In this disorder, red blood cells and certain white blood cells called granulocytes do not mature properly. The spleen may swell and there may be too few mature red blood cells to carry oxygen, causing anemia, which may require red blood cell transfusions. Usually, if there are no symptoms, the doctor will follow your case closely so you can be treated if symptoms develop. Treatments include: external radiation to the spleen or chemotherapy to reduce swelling of the spleen or hormone therapy to increase the number of red blood cells or surgery to remove the spleen. Clinical trials of biological therapy are being done.

What is essential thrombocythemia?

In essential thrombocythemia, the number of platelets in the blood is much higher than normal, although the other blood cells are normal. The extra platelets make it hard for blood to flow normally. Treatment for this condition includes plateletpheresis, in which a special machine is used to filter platelets from the blood. Chemotherapy may be used to lower the number of platelets in the blood. New drugs and biological therapy are being studied in clinical trials.

What is hairy cell leukemia?

Hairy cell leukemia is a form of chronic leukemia that involves an unusual type of B lymphocyte that has hairlike projections. It is five times more common in males than in females. The average age at diagnosis is 54. It usually begins slowly, with undramatic symptoms which may include weakness caused by anemia, development of infections and pain or discomfort due to enlargement of the spleen. Hairy cell leukemia is easily controlled and may be cured in most patients. About one-tenth of patients require no treatment. Your doctor's decision whether or not treatment is necessary is based on blood counts, spleen enlargement, indications that the disease is progressive, or other complications. Surgical removal of the spleen may be recommended as the initial treatment. About half of the patients who have their spleens removed need no additional treatment. Interferon therapy may be used, but many patients relapse when it is stopped. New drugs are being tested, as is bone marrow transplantation for younger patients who are in good health but have not responded to other treatments.

chapter 17

Lymphomas and Multiple Myeloma

> The term *lymphoma* is a general term for cancers that develop in the lymph system, a part of the body's immune defense system. Lymphomas are among the most difficult cancers to understand and to categorize. Some remain dormant, with few symptoms for many years, while others are extremely aggressive types.

Lymphomas are divided into two major types: Hodgkin's disease and non-Hodgkin's lymphoma. Although the two types have some similarities, they differ widely in cell origin, how they spread and how they are treated. The most common type of lymphoma is called Hodgkin's disease. All other lymphomas are grouped together and are called non-Hodgkin's lymphomas. In diagnosing lymphoma, the doctor will need to know the number and location of affected lymph nodes, the type of lymphoma, and whether the disease has spread to the bone marrow or organs outside the lymphatic system.

> Multiple myeloma begins in the plasma cells and other white blood cells that are part of the immune system. It weakens and damages bones, destroying the normal bone tissue. Most often seen in older adults, it is a slow-growing, treatable kind of cancer.

Multiple myeloma is a type of cancer in which the body produces more white blood cells (plasma cells) than normal. These unneeded plasma cells all look exactly alike and are all abnormal. Called myeloma cells, they collect in the bones, forming tumors and causing other problems. Multiple myeloma is a highly treatable kind of cancer.

LYMPHOMAS

WHAT YOU NEED TO KNOW ABOUT HODGKIN'S DISEASE AND NON-HODGKIN'S LYMPHOMA

- Lymphoma is a general term for cancers that develop in the lymph system. They account for about 3 percent of all cases of cancer in this country.
- The cure rate for early stage Hodgkin's disease is nearly 90 percent in some treatment centers.
- Many special tests are needed to diagnose and stage lymphoma.
- Because treatment decisions for lymphomas are very complex, it is especially important that treatments be carried out at institutions that have skilled pathologists, modern radiation equipment and a team of physicians who are expert in treating the disease.
- Treatments usually include radiation and chemotherapy. Bone marrow or peripheral stem cell transplants are sometimes used in treating lymphomas (please see Chapter 9, "New Advances and Investigational Trials").

What is the lymph system?

The lymph system is made up of a network of thin tubes that branch, like blood vessels, into the tissues throughout the body. The tubes carry lymph, a colorless, watery fluid that contains infection-fighting white blood cells, called lymphocytes, to all parts of the body. Situated along this network of vessels are groups of small glands, called lymph nodes. Other parts of the lymphatic system include the spleen, thymus, and bone marrow.

What is the role of the spleen?

The spleen, located on your left side near the stomach, is an organ that produces lymphocytes, filters the blood, stores blood cells and destroys those that are aging. It is the only organ capable of mount-

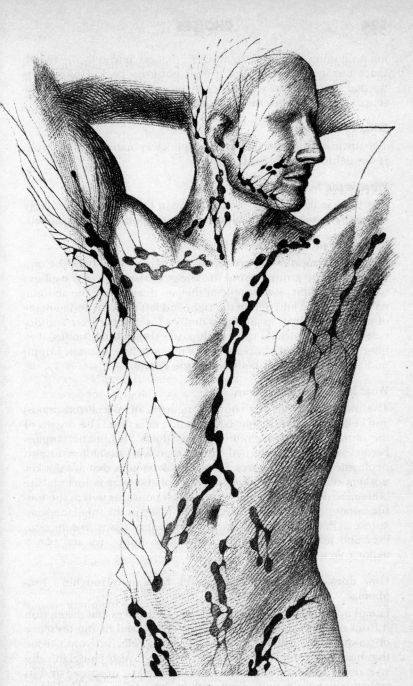

Lymph system

ing an immune response to antigens that are borne by the blood. Once the spleen is removed it does not grow back. However, its normal functions are taken over by other body tissues and its absence does not interfere with normal living.

What is the thymus?

The thymus is an organ in which lymphocytes mature and multiply. It lies behind your breastbone.

What is the bone marrow?

The bone marrow is soft, spongy tissue in the center of your large bones that produces white blood cells, red blood cells and platelets.

Where are the lymph nodes found?

Clusters of lymph nodes are found throughout your body: behind the ears, in the groin, behind the knees, in the front of the elbow, under the armpit, at the angle of the jaw, deep inside the abdominal cavity, at the junction of the right and left bronchi and in many other areas. They trap and help destroy foreign particles and disease-causing agents. As the lymph passes through the nodes, they filter out foreign substances and pick up more lymphocytes. Lymph nodes are part of your body's immune system.

What is the immune system?

The immune system is a complex network of specialized organs and cells that defends your body against infection. The organs of the immune system are often referred to as "lymphatic" organs because they are concerned with the growth, development and deployment of lymphocytes, the white blood cells that are the key workers of your immune system. Lymphatic organs include the bone marrow, thymus, spleen and lymph nodes, as well as the tonsils, appendix and clumps of lymphatic tissue in the small intestine known as Peyer's patches. Some nonlymphatic organs, like the skin, liver and lungs, also contain circulating lymphocytes and play a major role in immunity.

How does Hodgkin's disease differ from non-Hodgkin's lymphoma?

Hodgkin's disease has unique microscopic features that distinguish it from other lymphomas. Often, it is recognized by the presence of unique cells, called the Reed-Sternberg cells, in lymph tissue that has been removed by surgery for biopsy. Also Hodgkin's disease tends to follow a more predictable pattern of spread and its spread is generally more limited than that of the non-Hodgkin's lymphomas. By contrast, the non-Hodgkin's lymphomas are more likely to begin in sites like the liver and bones than in the lymph nodes.

What are the symptoms of lymphoma?

The most common symptom is a painless swelling in the neck, underarm or groin, caused by enlarged lymph glands. The affected lymph node is usually painless, firm, rubbery in consistency, and freely movable.

If I have an enlarged lymph gland should I see a doctor immediately?

Lymph glands may be enlarged as a result of infections or other illnesses such as mononucleosis or rheumatoid arthritis—but if you have a lymph gland in the neck, armpit or groin that remains enlarged for three weeks or longer, you should check with your doctor. If you have had a recent infection or another problem that could cause an enlarged lymph gland, the doctor may decide to delay doing the biopsy for a few days or a few weeks, while watching to see if it clears up. When lymph node swelling lasts more than six weeks and does not respond to antibiotics, it is suggestive of lymphoma. The only sure way to determine whether or not you have lymphoma is for the doctor to examine lymph tissue that has been surgically removed by biopsy.

Why is staging so important?

Because the symptoms, rate and pattern of spread and the treatment of lymphomas vary greatly, it is important that the disease be accurately diagnosed by an experienced pathologist (or hematopathologist) who can recognize subtle cellular distinctions among the various lymphatic cancers. The nature and extent of your first treatment influences and can severely limit future treatments. Therefore, it is important for the doctor to stage your condition correctly before beginning treatment. The staging procedure may take from one to three weeks.

QUESTIONS TO ASK YOUR DOCTOR IF YOU HAVE HODGKIN'S DISEASE OR NON-HODGKIN'S LYMPHOMA

- Is the disease confined to one area or more than one area?
- What are my treatment choices?
- Can you explain the cell type and how my disease has been staged?

- Would a clinical trial be appropriate for me?
- Will I become sterile as a result of the treatment? Is there anything I can do to avoid sterility?
- If I am pregnant, must my pregnancy be terminated? Will I be able to have children?
- Will I be able to continue to work? Will I be able to continue to exercise?
- Will I have long-term side effects as a result of the treatment?

Can sterility occur in a male as the result of treatment for lymphomas?

Yes, and this issue should be discussed with your doctor at the outset, because some of the treatments are known to cause sterility. There may be changes in sperm due to drugs and radiation therapy and sperm banking may be needed.

Can treatment for lymphoma affect a woman's menstrual cycles and her fertility?

Radiation therapy in the abdomen or pelvic area can result in loss of ovarian function. Women may wish to have an oophoropexy (an operation to move the ovaries behind the uterus) before beginning radiation therapy. This helps preserve ovarian function by shielding the ovaries from exposure to radiation during treatment.

Can lymphoma occur during pregnancy?

It is very rare, but both Hodgkin's and non-Hodgkin's lymphoma can occur during pregnancy. If the lymphoma is in the neck or underarm area only, it can usually be treated with radiation therapy, with the fetus shielded. If the disease is more extensive and the pregnancy is in its first four and a half months, a therapeutic abortion is usually suggested. During the last half of pregnancy, treatment will depend on the stage of the pregnancy and the aggressiveness of the disease. Sometimes treatment is delayed.

Can I have a baby after I've been treated for lymphoma?

Lymphoma itself does not need to have an adverse effect on fertility, the course of pregnancy, labor or the baby. The treatment and its side effects, however, must be taken into consideration in making a judgment. If you have lymphoma, you should consult with your doctor about family planning, an important issue, because it is difficult to predict when treatment may be needed. The doctor usually will advise that you wait for a period of time after remission before you become pregnant. Women have become pregnant and delivered normal children after they have had intensive treatment for lymphoma.

Are there other long-term side effects as a result of the treatment?
It depends upon the treatment being given. Some patients find they have relatively minor long-term complications. For others, the side effects may be severe. Organs such as the lungs, heart or kidneys may be affected. You may be at higher risk for leukemia in the future. You need to discuss the risks and management of these risks with your health care team.

HODGKIN'S DISEASE

The most common type of lymphoma is called Hodgkin's disease. Before 1970, most people with Hodgkin's disease often died within two years of diagnosis. Today, Hodgkin's disease is usually curable, particularly if it is discovered early. More than 75 percent of all newly diagnosed patients with Hodgkin's disease are curable with modern radiation therapy, chemotherapy or a combination of the two treatments. Both adults and children are diagnosed with Hodgkin's disease. (Treatment of Hodgkin's disease in children is discussed in Chapter 22, "Childhood Cancers.")

What is Hodgkin's disease?
Hodgkin's disease is a type of lymphoma. In Hodgkin's disease, cells in the lymphatic system grow abnormally and the disease can spread to other organs. As the disease progresses, the body is less able to fight infection. Hodgkin's disease is rare. It accounts for less than 1 percent of all cases of cancer in this country.

WHO GETS HODGKIN'S DISEASE?

- Younger people, with the peak age between 15 and 34.
- People over the age of 54.
- More common in males than in females.
- Family history of Hodgkin's disease increases risk for other brothers and sisters.

What causes Hodgkin's disease?
The causes of Hodgkin's disease are not fully understood. There are many theories that have been explored, such as viruses, environ-

ment and genetics. However, what causes the disease or what is required to prevent it are not known. Hodgkin's disease usually starts in one lymph gland and spreads in an orderly pattern to nearby chains of lymph nodes.

What kinds of doctor and hospital are best for treating Hodgkin's disease?

It is important to be in the hands of a team that has experience in treating this disease. A multidisciplinary team of cancer specialists, including radiation oncologists, surgeons, pathologists, and medical oncologists, should be consulted so that a proper treatment plan can be made. The high cure rates for this cancer are due to excellent results achieved with modern radiation therapy and effective combination chemotherapy. Be sure you are treated at a major institution that has modern linear accelerators and treatment planning simulators.

SYMPTOMS OF HODGKIN'S DISEASE

- **Painless swelling in the neck, armpit or groin.**
- **Fevers, night sweats, fatigue and weight loss.**
- **Itching and reddened patches on the skin.**

Are fever, weight loss and night sweats often symptoms of Hodgkin's disease?

Fever, weight loss and night sweats are symptoms often seen in Hodgkin's disease. A pattern of high fever alternating with normal or subnormal body temperature may also be seen.

Is itching a common symptom for those with Hodgkin's disease?

Sometimes itchy skin—or pruritus, as it is sometimes referred to by the medical profession—marks the early stages of Hodgkin's disease. You can have it in one place or all over the body. It usually disappears with treatment of the disease and some relief may be possible with antihistamines. You may get it again at a later time. If that occurs, you should report it to your doctor.

How is Hodgkin's disease diagnosed and staged?

Hodgkin's disease has special characteristics that distinguish it from the other lymphomas. It needs to be carefully staged because the extent of disease strongly influences the choice of treatment. Many

TESTS THAT MAY BE USED TO DIAGNOSE HODGKIN'S DISEASE

- Complete history with special attention to unexplained fever, night sweats or weight loss of more than 10 percent in prior six months.
- Physical examination with particular attention to lymph nodes, liver, spleen and bone tenderness.
- Chest x-ray.
- CT scan.
- Ultrasound.
- Blood and urine tests.
- Bone marrow tests.
- Lymphogram.
- Gallium scan may be done.

Depending on condition, these may also be needed:

- Liver, spleen and bone scans.
- Splenectomy.
- Liver biopsy.
- Kidney tests.
- Staging laparotomy (in selected patients only).

different kinds of tests are involved. If Hodgkin's disease is suspected, the doctor will ask about your medical history and will do a thorough physical exam. In addition, blood tests, tests of the liver and urine, x-rays and scans of the chest or abdomen, and a lymphogram may be ordered. A gallium scan may also be used. The doctor will perform a biopsy, removing tissue from an enlarged lymph node. It is important that the disease be accurately diagnosed by an experienced pathologist who can recognize subtle cellular distinctions among the various lymphatic cancers. The pathologist will look at the tissue under the microscope for abnormal cells, called Reed-Sternberg cells, that are usually found with Hodgkin's disease.

What are Reed-Sternberg cells?

These are abnormal cells that help confirm a diagnosis of Hodgkin's disease, but in general they are difficult to detect. They are named for the two scientists who first identified them. Finding the

Reed-Sternberg cells alone is not enough to diagnose Hodgkin's disease, because they have been found in other diseases.

Why is the diaphragm important in diagnosis?

The diaphragm, a thin muscle below your lungs and heart that separates the chest cavity from the abdominal cavity, is important for determining treatment. You will hear the doctor talking about your disease being above or below the diaphragm or on one side or both sides of it. If you have it on one side of the diaphragm, either below or above it, it will be treated differently than if it is found on both sides.

What are the cellular classifications of Hodgkin's disease?

There are four classifications: lymphocyte predominance, nodular sclerosis, mixed cellularity and lymphocyte depletion. Nodular sclerosis and mixed cellularity are the most common.

What is a lymphogram?

A lymphogram or a lymphangiogram is an x-ray of the abdomen, pelvis or chest. It shows the size of the lymph nodes and detects abdominal lymph node involvement which may not be seen through other tests. In some institutions CT scans are used instead of or in addition to the lymphogram.

How is a lymphogram done?

The test is done under local anesthesia. Small incisions are made at the tops of the feet. An oil-based dye is injected into the lymph system at the top of the feet. The lymph system carries the dye up the legs and into the abdominal lymph nodes. When the x-rays are taken, the dye outlines the lymphatic system. It shows the size of the various lymph nodes, their shape and even their internal structure. This allows the doctor to identify abnormal nodes. The patterns of lymph flow that show up on the x-rays are also important, because lymph does not pass easily through the nodes that are filled with cancerous cells, so abnormal patterns of lymph flow develop. From this test, the doctor is able to identify involved nodes and to choose several lymph nodes to remove and examine. Because the dye remains in the lymph vessels for a long period of time after a lymphogram, x-rays can be taken during and after treatment to monitor the effects of treatment on the cancer.

How long does it take to do a lymphogram?

The lymphogram takes several hours the first day, with follow-up x-ray films on the second day. Further testing is usually done and the dye remains in the lymph nodes for months to more than a year.

Is there anything special I can do during or after the test?

Be sure to tell the doctor or nurse if you feel any shortness of breath after the dye has been injected. Wear loose shoes to avoid irritating the area where the incisions are made. Do not put your feet in water until the stitches have been taken out. Clean the area of the stitches every day with alcohol. Report any signs of redness or swelling to the nurse or doctor. You can have some possible side effects. They include: a bluish color in your feet and your urine, allergic reaction to the dye, infection where the incision was made, fever within 24 hours of the injection and pulmonary oil embolism.

How will the biopsy be done?

Usually, the biopsy is done under local anesthesia in a doctor's office or in a one-day surgery center. After the operation, depending on its location, you will need to wear loose-fitting clothing over the surgical site. You will also need to wait until the stitches are removed before bathing the area.

What is a laparotomy?

A laparotomy is an operation to explore the entire abdomen. It allows the doctor to determine the extent of disease and if it has spread to the abdomen.

Is a laparotomy routinely used to diagnose lymphoma?

No. Several years ago, laparotomy was a routine procedure for diagnosing Hodgkin's disease. Today, it is done only if the information gained will actually change the treatment being given. It is usually restricted to patients in whom radiation alone will be used for treatment.

What are the stages of Hodgkin's disease?

After the initial tests have been completed, the extent of disease is staged by a widely used system called the Ann Arbor Staging Classification of Hodgkin's disease. It divides Hodgkin's disease into stages:

Stage I: Cancer is found in only one lymph node area or in only one area or organ outside of the lymph nodes.

Stage II: Cancer is found in two or more lymph node areas on the same side of the diaphragm or cancer is found in only one area or organ outside of the lymph nodes and in the lymph nodes around it. Other lymph node areas on the same side of the diaphragm may also be found to be cancerous.

Stage III: Cancer is found in lymph node areas on both sides of the diaphragm. The cancer may also have spread to an area or organ near the lymph node areas and/or to the spleen.

Stage IV: Cancer has spread to more than one spot to an organ or organs outside the lymph system. Cancer may or may not be found in the lymph nodes near these organs, or cancer has spread to only one organ outside the lymph system, but lymph nodes far away from that organ are involved.

Relapsed: Cancer has come back after it has been treated. It may come back in the area where it first started or in another part of the body.

What does an A, B or E added to the stage mean?

An "A" designates there are no general symptoms. A "B" designates that the patient has any of the following symptoms: unexplained loss of more than 10 percent of body weight in the six months before diagnosis, unexplained fever, or drenching night sweats. Thus, your stage could be designated as IA or IB, depending upon the absence or presence of symptoms. An "E" denotes that the disease has extended into nearby tissues.

How and where does Hodgkin's disease spread?

Hodgkin's disease begins in a lymph node, often in the neck, and spreads in a predictable pattern from the original site to lymph nodes in other areas. It usually spreads first to nearby lymph nodes and then to the nearby organ. In advanced Hodgkin's disease, the lungs, spleen, liver and bone marrow may also be affected.

How is Hodgkin's disease treated?

The treatment depends upon the person's medical history, age, type and stage of disease. The usual treatment for most patients with early Hodgkin's disease is high-energy radiation. Combination chemotherapy also is effective in the treatment of early stage Hodgkin's disease, as well as for advanced Hodgkin's disease and for patients who have relapsed after radiation therapy. Drugs and radiation are sometimes given together, mainly in treating patients with tumors in the chest or abdomen. Bone marrow or peripheral stem cell transplants are being studied in clinical trials for certain patients. (Please see Chapter 9, "New Advances and Investigational Trials," for information on these transplants).

How successful are the treatments for Hodgkin's disease?

The success of the treatment for Hodgkin's disease has improved dramatically over the past thirty years. Before 1970, few patients

STAGES OF HODGKIN'S DISEASE

STAGE	DESCRIPTION
Stage I	Cancer is found in only one lymph node area (I) or in only one area or organ outside of the lymph nodes (IE).
Stage II	Cancer is found in two or more lymph node regions on the same side of the diaphragm (II); **or** cancer is found in only one area or organ outside of the lymph nodes and in the lymph nodes around it. Other lymph node areas on the same side of the diaphragm may also have cancer (IIE).
Stage III	Cancer is found in the lymph node regions on both sides of the diaphragm (III). The cancer may also have spread to an area or organ near the lymph node areas (IIIE), or to the spleen (IIIS) or both (IIIE + S). Stage III-1 indicates the cancer is limited to the upper abdomen. Stage III-2 indicates involvement of pelvic and/or para-aortic nodes. Zero to four nodules on the spleen are classified as minimal disease in the spleen. Five or more nodules constitute extensive disease in the spleen.
Stage IV	Cancer has spread in more than one spot to an organ or organs outside the lymph system. Cancer cells may or may not be found in the lymph nodes near these organs; **or** cancer has spread to only one organ outside the lymph system, but lymph nodes far away from that organ are involved.
Relapsed	Cancer has come back after it has been treated. It may come back in the area where it first started or in another part of the body.

with advanced Hodgkin's disease recovered from their illness. Most died within two years. Today the outlook is much brighter. More than half of all patients with advanced Hodgkin's disease are disease-free after follow-up of more than ten years. For early stage Hodgkin's patients, the news is even better. The cure rate has risen to nearly 90 percent in major cancer centers. This success has been due mainly to modern radiation treatment techniques that allow large doses of radiation to be given, while shielding normal tissues to prevent unnecessary damage. In addition, combination chemotherapy has cured many patients with more involved disease.

How is radiation treatment planned?

A technique, called a treatment planning simulator, is used to plan your radiation treatment. The simulator takes detailed x-rays of you

TREATMENT CHOICES FOR HODGKIN'S DISEASE

STAGE	TREATMENT
Stage IA	*If your cancer is above the diaphragm and does not involve a large part of your chest, your treatment may be one of the following:* Radiation to upper part of the body (mantle field) and to the lymph nodes in the upper abdomen; **or** radiation to mantle field only (in selected patients); **or** radiation to mantle field, the lymph nodes in the upper abdomen and the spleen; **or** chemotherapy with or without radiation. *If your cancer is above the diaphragm but involves a large part of your chest, your treatment may be one of the following:* Radiation to the upper body (mantle field) plus chemotherapy; **or** radiation therapy to mantle field and to the lymph nodes in the upper abdomen; **or** *Clinical trials:* New methods of treatment. *If your cancer is below the diaphragm, your treatment may be one of the following:* Radiation to the lymph nodes in the upper abdomen and pelvis. The spleen or the groin may also be treated if needed; **or** total nodal radiation; **or** chemotherapy with or without radiation to areas that contain cancer.
Stage IB	*If your cancer is above the diaphragm and does not involve a large part of your chest, your treatment may be one of the following:* Radiation to the upper body (mantle field) and to the lymph nodes in the upper abdomen or total nodal radiation; **or** radiation to mantle field plus chemotherapy; **or** *Clinical trials:* Chemotherapy alone. *If your cancer is above the diaphragm but involves a large part of your chest, your treatment may be one of the following:* Radiation to mantle field plus chemotherapy; **or** chemotherapy plus radiation to the area where the cancer is found; **or** radiation to mantle field, the lymph nodes in the upper abdomen and the spleen. *If your cancer is below the diaphragm, your treatment may be one of the following:* Total nodal radiation or radiation to lymph nodes in the upper abdomen and pelvis; **or** chemotherapy plus radiation therapy to the upper abdomen and pelvis, to the areas that contain cancer or to the spleen.
Stage IIA	*If your cancer is above the diaphragm and does not involve a large part of your chest, your treatment may be one of the following:* Radiation to the upper body (mantle field) and to the lymph nodes in the upper abdomen; **or** radiation to mantle field only (in certain patients); chemotherapy with or without radiation; **or** *Clinical trials:* New methods of treatment. *If your cancer is above the diaphragm, but involves a large part of your chest, your treatment may be one of the following:* Radiation to upper body (mantle field) plus chemotherapy; **or** radiation to mantle field and to the lymph nodes in the upper abdomen. *If your cancer is below the diaphragm, your treatment may be one of the following:* Radiation to the lymph nodes in the upper abdomen and pelvis. The spleen or the groin may also be treated if needed;

Stage IIB	*If your cancer is above the diaphragm and does not involve a large part of your chest, your treatment may be one of the following:* Radiation to the upper body (mantle field) and to the lymph nodes in the upper abdomen or total nodal radiation **or** chemotherapy alone or followed by radiation to mantle field. *If your cancer is above the diaphragm but involves a large part of your chest, your treatment may be one of the following:* Chemotherapy plus radiation to upper body (mantle field); **or** chemotherapy plus radiation to the area where the cancer is found. *If your cancer is below the diaphragm, your treatment will probably be:* Chemotherapy with or without radiation.
Stage IIIA	*If your cancer does not involve a large part of your chest, your treatment may be one of the following:* Total nodal radiation. Radiation may also be given to the liver; **or** chemotherapy plus radiation; **or** chemotherapy. *Clinical trials:* Chemotherapy. *If your cancer involves a large part of your chest, your treatment will probably be:* Chemotherapy plus radiation. *Clinical trials:* Chemotherapy.
Stage IIIB	Chemotherapy; **or** chemotherapy and radiation to areas where the cancer is found or to more extended areas. *Clinical trials:* Chemotherapy.
Stage IV	Chemotherapy; **or** chemotherapy with total nodal radiation or with radiation to places with large amounts of cancer. *Clinical trials:* Bone marrow or peripheral stem cell transplantation and/or chemotherapy.
Relapsed disease	Treatment depends on where disease has returned and treatment received before. If previous treatment was radiation therapy without chemotherapy, treatment may be chemotherapy. If treatment was chemotherapy without radiation therapy and cancer comes back only in lymph nodes, treatment may be radiation therapy to the lymph nodes with or without more chemotherapy. If disease comes back in more than one area, treatment may be more chemotherapy **or** chemotherapy with or without bone marrow or peripheral cell transplantation. *Clinical trials:* High doses of chemotherapy with or without bone marrow or peripheral cell transplantation.

in the position you will be in when you get your treatment so that the radiation fields can be designed to conform to your body. Individually shaped protective blocks are made to shield your normal tissues. The planning simulator is essential in treating Hodgkin's disease.

What is the mantle field?

This is a term used by the radiation oncologists to describe the part of the upper area of the body to be treated by radiation. It is almost the shape of an arrow, with the point starting at the neck and the base extending to the diaphragm. It encompasses the lymph nodes in the upper part of the body. The heart and lungs are protected during treatment by lead shields, to reduce the risk of complications to these organs.

What is the inverted Y?

This term is used to describe the part of the lower area of the body to be treated by radiation. Shaped like an upside-down Y, it extends from the diaphragm to the lower border of the pelvis and includes the lymph nodes in the lower part of the body.

What kind of chemotherapy treatments are used to treat Hodgkin's disease?

The first effective chemotherapy treatment for advanced Hodgkin's disease, known as the MOPP program, was developed by researchers at the National Cancer Institute and is considered to be one standard treatment. MOPP consists of four anticancer drugs in combination: mechlorethamine (nitrogen mustard), vincristine (Oncovin), procarbazine and prednisone. A second drug combination, ABVD (doxorubicin, bleomycin, vinblastine and DTIC), is also considered to be a standard treatment. Sometimes, MOPP and ABVD are given as alternating treatments. In addition, there are other combinations that have proved to be effective and are now also considered standard options when chemotherapy is needed.

How long will it take after all these treatments for my energy level to return?

It depends on your age, stage of disease and intensity of the treatment. It takes longer for older patients and patients with advanced disease who received combined treatments. The return to normal energy levels may take up to a year or more.

Will there be sexual side effects?

Impotence and inadequate sperm counts have been reported in men even before treatment begins. Radiation to the pelvic area and some of the chemotherapy drugs can cause sexual problems for both men and women, including infertility, low sexual desire, erection problems, weaker orgasm, vaginal dryness and painful intercourse and reduced vaginal size. There is more information on side effects in Chapter 7, ''Radiation Treatment,'' and Chapter 8, ''Chemotherapy.'' Sexuality is discussed in Chapter 24, ''Living with Cancer.''

Is there any long-term danger to this intensive radiotherapy and chemotherapy?

In spite of the effectiveness of the treatments, some have been shown to have long-term effects. Several studies have shown an association between certain therapies and the development of leukemia many years later. The risk of leukemia is about 5 percent at ten years according to most studies. It seems to be highest in patients over 40 who have been treated with both intensive radiotherapy and intensive chemotherapy. Recent research at the National Cancer Institute indicates that the risk of leukemia seems to decline after ten years. In the past, women treated for Hodgkin's disease with radiation before the age of 30 were at a markedly increased risk for breast cancer, with the risk increasing dramatically more than twenty-five years after therapy. It is hoped that new treatment methods will decrease many of these risks.

Do people who have AIDS get Hodgkin's disease?

Some people with AIDS (Acquired Immunodeficiency Syndrome) also have Hodgkin's disease. This may be explained by the fact that many AIDS patients are young or because AIDS patients have a weakened immune system. AIDS patients usually have a Stage III or IV Hodgkin's disease when they are diagnosed. The disease may be found in the skin or bone marrow, which is not usual in other patients.

Is the treatment different for persons with AIDS?

The treatment is similar, but it depends on the health of the patient. Most patients with AIDS do not tolerate the chemotherapy drugs as well as other patients. They get more infections during treatment. While their remission rates are similar to other patients, because of their other complications, they live a shorter time than is usually expected for persons with the same stage of disease.

What treatment is available for a patient who relapses after the first set of treatments?

It depends on the first treatment and also on the stage of the disease. If the treatment was radiation, chemotherapy may be administered. If chemotherapy had been given, another combination of drugs might be tried. A bone marrow transplant or peripheral stem cell support might be considered. (There is more information on bone marrow transplants and peripheral stem cell support in Chapter 9, "New Advances and Investigational Trials.")

How often should I see a doctor for checkups after being treated for Hodgkin's disease?

Careful follow-up will be needed and may vary for different types and stages of Hodgkin's disease. Generally, you will have regular visits with your doctor every month or two for the first year, then every three to six months for the next four years and every year after that. Chest x-rays and blood tests will probably be done at every visit. At the end of the first year, your doctor may order CT scans of the chest and abdomen. The critical time is the first five years. If you are disease-free after five years, you are usually considered to be cured.

Are there any symptoms I should report to the doctor?

Yes. You should report fever, itching, night sweats, lumps or breathing problems.

NON-HODGKIN'S LYMPHOMA

Lymphomas, other than Hodgkin's disease, are grouped together and are called non-Hodgkin's lymphomas. There are about ten different types of non-Hodgkin's lymphomas. Some types spread more quickly than others and are more difficult to treat. Major advances have been made in treating the non-Hodgkin's lymphomas.

What is non-Hodgkin's lymphoma?

Non-Hodgkin's lymphoma is a cancer that develops in the lymph system—but can spread to organs other than lymph nodes, such as the liver or the bones. There are at least ten types of non-Hodgkin's lymphomas. Often they are grouped by how fast they grow—low grade (slow growing), intermediate grade and high grade (rapidly growing).

Who is most likely to have non-Hodgkin's lymphoma?

More males than females get non-Hodgkin's lymphoma. It can strike people as young as age 40, although those between the ages of 60 and 69 are at highest risk. Those with deficiencies in their immune system, whether inherited (Wiskott-Aldrich syndrome and Bloom's syndrome), a result of autoimmune disease (rheumatoid arthritis, systemic lupus erythematosus) or acquired (organ transplant patients, AIDS patients) are at increased risk for developing the disease. For reasons not understood, the incidence of lymphoma is increasing yearly, especially in people with autoimmune deficiencies, such as AIDS.

What causes non-Hodgkin's lymphoma?

The cause of non-Hodgkin's lymphoma remains unknown. It is thought that certain viruses, deficiencies in the immune system and chromosome abnormalities play a part. Burkitt's lymphoma, which is found in Africa, is associated with the Epstein-Barr virus, but the precise role of this virus in unknown. Some people who have had long-standing Sjögren's syndrome develop diffuse aggressive lymphomas or immunoblastic lymphomas. It is believed that there may be an association between the two diseases.

SYMPTOMS OF NON-HODGKIN'S LYMPHOMAS

- Painless swelling in the neck, armpit or groin.
- Fevers, night sweats, fatigue and weight loss.
- Itching and reddened patches on the skin.
- Nausea and vomiting or abdominal pain.

What kind of doctor is best for treating non-Hodgkin's disease?

The treatment planning for non-Hodgkin's disease is complex. It should be carried out by a well-trained multidisciplinary team of cancer specialists, including radiation oncologists, surgeons, pathologists, and medical oncologists. Since the treatment is influenced by the cell type, it is important that the biopsy results be carefully reviewed by a pathologist who is experienced in diagnosing lymphoma. Be sure that the institution where you are being treated has modern linear accelerators and treatment planning simulators, as well as medical oncologists who are experts in chemotherapy treatment.

How is non-Hodgkin's disease diagnosed and staged?

Non-Hodgkin's disease needs to be carefully staged because the extent of disease strongly influences the choice of treatment. Many

---

TESTS THAT MAY BE USED TO DIAGNOSE NON-HODGKIN'S LYMPHOMA

- Complete history with special attention to unexplained fever, night sweats or weight loss of more than 10 percent in prior six months.
- Physical examination with particular attention to lymph nodes, liver, spleen and bone tenderness.
- Chest x-rays.
- Abdominal CT scan.
- Ultrasound tests.
- Blood and urine tests.
- Liver and kidney function tests.
- Bone marrow tests.
- Liver, spleen and bone scans.
- Gallium scan (in selected patients).
- Lymphogram (in patients with abdominal CT scans that are negative).

---

different kinds of tests are involved. If non-Hodgkin's disease is suspected, the doctor will ask about your medical history and will do a thorough physical exam. The doctor will perform a biopsy of an enlarged lymph node, removing tissue that will be examined under the microscope. In addition, blood tests, tests of the liver and urine, x-ray of the chest, CT scan of the abdomen and biopsy of the bone marrow, liver and other accessible sites will be done. A gallium scan may also be used.

How will the lymph node biopsy be done?
Usually, the lymph node biopsy is done under local anesthesia in a doctor's office or in a one-day surgery center.

What is a lymphogram?
A lymphogram, or a lymphangiogram as it is sometimes called, is a test done to look for evidence of lymphoma in the abdominal lymph nodes, which usually cannot be felt.

When is a lymphogram used in non-Hodgkin's lymphoma?
It is a rarely used procedure in some patients to verify early stage disease in the lower abdomen. It is not used in patients whose disease is more advanced. (You will find details on how a lympho-

gram is done in the section on Hodgkin's disease earlier in this chapter.)

Is a laparotomy used to stage non-Hodgkin's disease?

No. A laparotomy, an operation to explore the entire abdomen to determine the extent of disease, is not routinely used in non-Hodgkin's lymphoma because the majority of non-Hodgkin's lymphoma patients have disease below the diaphragm and do not require it for staging the disease. Laparotomy, if used, is reserved for the few patients with early stage disease in whom evidence of the disease in the abdomen would change the treatment from radiation therapy to chemotherapy.

How are the different types of non-Hodgkin's lymphoma classified?

Around the world there are six different systems to classify the more than ten different types of non-Hodgkin's lymphomas. Some of the systems place major emphasis on the structure of the cell that becomes cancerous; others on the arrangement of the cells when examined under the microscope. In 1981, an international panel of expert pathologists developed a new classification system, called the International Working Formulation, to help standardize terms and apply new knowledge gained from the science of immunology. In the Working Formulation, lymphomas are classified depending upon the type of cell found in the cancer and on the arrangement of the cells. The types fall into three basic groups: low grade, intermediate grade and high grade.

What types are low-grade lymphomas?

The low-grade lymphomas are small lymphocytic, follicular small-cleaved cell and follicular mixed cell.

What types are intermediate-grade lymphomas?

The intermediate-grade lymphomas are follicular large cell, diffuse small-cleaved cell, diffuse mixed cell, and diffuse large cell.

What types are classified as high-grade lymphomas?

The high-grade lymphomas are immunoblastic large cell, lymphoblastic convoluted or nonconvoluted cell, small-cleaved cell (Burkitt's or non-Burkitt's) and HTLV-I.

Who is at highest risk for intermediate and high-grade lymphoma?

Intermediate and high-grade lymphomas are often seen in patients with Acquired Immunodeficiency Syndrome who require special treatment.

What is the Rappaport system?

Although many doctors are using the Working Formulation, you may hear references to the Rappaport system. In this system, a non-Hodgkin's lymphoma is described as either nodular or diffuse, based on the growth pattern of the cancer cells as seen through the microscope. The disease is further classified by cell type. If the cancer cells are small and resemble lymphocytes, it is called lymphocytic lymphoma. If the cancer cells are large and resemble macrophages or histiocytes, it is called histiocytic lymphoma. If the cells have both features, it is called mixed lymphoma. The Rappaport system also describes lymphoma cells as either poorly differentiated or well differentiated. Poorly differentiated cancer cells have poorly defined borders and are irregular in structure and size. Cancer cells that are more normal when looked at under the microscope are referred to as well differentiated.

What is meant by an indolent lymphoma?

Indolent lymphomas spread slowly and often take years to develop into aggressive disease. Most nodular lymphomas are called indolent or favorable histiocytic lymphomas.

What are aggressive lymphomas?

Most of the diffuse types, which tend to progress rapidly, are called aggressive or unfavorable histology lymphomas. Without treatment, these rapidly growing lymphomas can progress very quickly and become fatal. However, these lymphomas can respond favorably to chemotherapy treatment.

What is primary CNS lymphoma?

CNS is shorthand for central nervous system. Primary CNS lymphomas are tumors of the lymph system that begin in the brain. You also can have a lymphoma that begins in another part of the body and spreads to the brain. The primary CNS lymphomas that are not AIDS related are usually B-cell lymphomas that begin in the central nervous system. They occur at random in the general population and in patients with deficiencies in their immune systems.

Are there any other types of lymphomas?

There are certain types of non-Hodgkin's lymphomas that have unique features that distinguish them from the others. They include Burkitt's lymphoma (a childhood B-cell lymphoma generally found in tropical Africa), lymphoblastic lymphoma (a childhood lymphoma most often of T-cell origin) and cutaneous T-cell lymphoma (originally called mycosis fungoides). Cutaneous T-cell lymphoma is discussed later in this chapter.

TYPES OF NON-HODGKIN'S LYMPHOMA AND HOW THEY ARE REFERRED TO UNDER TWO SYSTEMS

WORKING FORMULATION	RAPPAPORT SYSTEM
Low grade Small lymphocytic (SL) Follicular, small-cleaved cell (FCS) Follicular, mixed cell, cleaved and large cell (FM)	Diffuse lymphocytic, well differentiated (DLWD) Nodular lymphocytic, poorly differentiated (NLPD) Nodular mixed, lymphocytic and histiocytic (NM)
Intermediate grade Follicular, large cell (FL) Diffuse, small-cleaved cell (DSC) Diffuse, mixed cell, small and large cell (DM) Diffuse, large cell, cleaved or noncleaved cell (DL)	Nodular histiocytic Diffuse lymphocytic, poorly differentiated (DLDP) Diffuse mixed, lymphocytic and histiocytic (DM) Diffuse histiocytic (DH)
High grade Immunoblastic, large cell (IBL) Lymphoblastic, convoluted or nonconvoluted cell (LL) Small non-cleaved cell, Burkitt's or non-Burkitt's (SNC) HTLV-I	Diffuse histiocytic (SH) Diffuse lymphoblastic (DL) Diffuse undifferentiated, Burkitt's or non-Burkitt's

What are the stages of non-Hodgkin's disease?

After the initial tests have been completed, the extent of disease is staged by a widely used system called the Ann Arbor Staging Classification, It divides non-Hodgkin's disease into stages:

Stage I: Cancer is found in only one lymph node area or in only one area or organ outside of the lymph nodes.

Stage II: Cancer is found in two or more lymph node areas on the same side of the diaphragm or cancer is found in only one area or organ outside of the lymph nodes and in the lymph nodes around it. Other lymph node areas on the same side of the diaphragm may also have cancer.

Stage III: Cancer is found in lymph node areas on both sides of the diaphragm. The cancer may also have spread to an area or organ near the lymph node areas and/or to the spleen.

Stage IV: Cancer has spread to more than one spot to an organ or organs outside of the lymph system. Cancer may or may not be found in the lymph nodes near these organs or cancer has spread to only one organ outside of the lymph system, but lymph nodes far away from that organ are involved.

Relapsed: Cancer has come back after it has been treated. It may come back in the area where it first started or in another part of the body.

What does an A, B or E added to the stage mean?

An "A" means there are no general symptoms. A "B" designates that the patient has any of the following symptoms: unexplained loss of more than 10 percent of body weight in the six months before diagnosis, unexplained fever, or drenching night sweats. Thus, your stage could be designated as IA or IB, depending upon the absence or presence of these symptoms. An "E" denotes that the disease has extended into nearby tissues.

Are there any other factors used for staging non-Hodgkin's lymphoma?

Several other factors are taken in account by the doctor when staging non-Hodgkin's lymphoma. These include the grade of disease, its cell type, bulk of disease and sites of involvement.

How and where does non-Hodgkin's lymphoma spread?

Non-Hodgkin's disease is likely to begin in organs other than lymph nodes, like the liver and the bones. In many cases, by the time non-Hodgkin's lymphoma is diagnosed, cancer cells often have already spread throughout the body, including abdominal lymph nodes, liver, bone marrow and the gastrointestinal tract.

How is non-Hodgkin's disease treated?

The treatment depends upon the person's medical history and age, the type, grade and stage of disease and whether or not it has been found above or below the diaphragm. The treatment can include radiation of the lymph nodes, combination chemotherapy or drugs and radiation given together. Bone marrow and peripheral stem cell transplants are being studied in clinical trials for certain patients (please see Chapter 9, "New Advances and Investigational Trials," for information on these treatments).

How is primary CNS lymphoma treated?

Primary CNS lymphoma is treated either with radiation or radiation and chemotherapy. Clinical trials with different kinds of chemotherapy treatment are also under study.

STAGES OF NON-HODGKIN'S DISEASE	
STAGE	**DESCRIPTION**
Stage I	Cancer is found in only one lymph node area (I); **or** cancer is found in only one area or organ outside of the lymph nodes (IE).
Stage II	Cancer is found in two or more lymph node regions on the same side of the diaphragm (II); **or** cancer is found in only one area or organ outside of the lymph nodes and in the lymph nodes around it. Other lymph node areas on the same side of the diaphragm may also have cancer (IIE).
Stage III	Cancer is found in the lymph node regions on both sides of the diaphragm (III). The cancer may also have spread to an area or organ near the lymph node areas (IIIE), or to the spleen (IIIS) or both (IIIS + E).
Stage IV	Cancer has spread in more than one spot to an organ or organs outside of the lymph system. Cancer cells may or may not be found in the lymph nodes near these organs; **or** cancer has spread to only one organ outside of the lymph system, but lymph nodes far away from that organ are involved.
Relapsed	Cancer has come back after it has been treated. It may come back in the area where it first started or in another part of the body.
Primary CNS lymphoma	Tumors of the lymph system that begin in the brain.

What kinds of lymphoma are most common in persons infected with HIV?

Persons who test positively for HIV are four times more likely to develop non-Hodgkin's lymphoma than is the general public. Most of these persons will have high-grade B-cell lymphoma (small non-cleaved Burkitt's and non-Burkitt's or immunoblastic), intermediate-grade B-cell lymphoma (large cell) or central nervous system lymphoma. In over 50 percent of patients, the lymphoma will be found after AIDS has been diagnosed. The lymphomas are found in all of the major risk groups.

Is the treatment for patients with AIDS-related lymphoma different?

Both the treatment and the response to the treatment are different. Because the persons with AIDS-related lymphoma are usually diag-

TREATMENT CHOICES FOR LOW-GRADE NON-HODGKIN'S DISEASE

STAGE	TREATMENT
Low-grade Stage I	*If your cancer is above the diaphragm and does not involve a large part of your chest, your treatment may be one of the following:* Radiation to the area where cancer cells are found, **or** radiation to upper part of the body (mantle field) or to only the neck, upper chest and the lymph nodes under the arms; **or** *Clinical trials:* New methods of treatment. *If your cancer is below the diaphragm, your treatment may be one of the following:* Radiation to the area where the cancer cells are found; **or** radiation to the lymph nodes in the abdomen and pelvis; **or** *Clinical trials:* New methods of treatment.
Low-grade Stage II	*If your cancer is above the diaphragm, your treatment may be one of the following:* Radiation to the area where the cancer cells are found; **or** radiation to the upper body (mantle field) or only to the neck, upper chest and the lymph nodes under the arms. *If your cancer is below the diaphragm, your treatment may be one of the following:* Radiation to the area where the cancer cells are found **or** radiation to the lymph nodes in the upper abdomen and pelvis; **or** *Clinical trials:* New methods of treatment.
Low-grade Stage III	If you do not have symptoms, you may not need treatment. Your doctor will watch you closely so that you can be treated if symptoms develop; **or** combination chemotherapy; **or** single-agent chemotherapy; **or** radiation. *Clinical trials:* Observation plus radiation; **or** chemotherapy and radiation followed by bone marrow transplant or new agents.
Low-grade Stage IV	If you do not have symptoms, you may not need treatment. Your doctor will watch you closely so that you can be treated if symptoms develop; **or** combination chemotherapy; **or** single-agent chemotherapy; **or** *Clinical trials:* Bone marrow or peripheral stem cell transplantation.
Low-grade relapsed	*If it is still a low-grade lymphoma, your treatment may be one of the following:* Radiation and/or combination chemotherapy.

TREATMENT CHOICES FOR INTERMEDIATE-GRADE NON-HODGKIN'S DISEASE

STAGE	TREATMENT
Intermediate-grade Stage I	*If you did not have surgery to determine the stage of your cancer (thus were clinically staged), your treatment may be one of the following:* Chemotherapy plus radiation therapy; **or** chemotherapy alone. *If you had surgery (including laparotomy) to determine the stage of your cancer (thus were pathologically staged), your treatment may be one of the following:* Radiation therapy to mantle field (if your cancer is above the diaphragm); **or** radiation to the abdomen and pelvis (if your cancer is below the diaphragm); **or** radiation plus chemotherapy; **or** chemotherapy alone; **or** *Clinical trials:* New methods of treatment.
Intermediate-grade Stage II	Combination chemotherapy; **or** combination chemotherapy and radiation to places where large amounts of cancer are found; **or** radiation alone (in selected patients); **or** if cancer is found in the digestive tract, surgery plus chemotherapy; **or** *Clinical trials:* New methods of treatment.
Intermediate-grade Stage III	Combination chemotherapy; **or** combination chemotherapy and radiation to places where large amounts of cancer are found; **or** *Clinical trials:* Chemotherapy followed by bone marrow transplant.
Intermediate-grade Stage IV	Combination chemotherapy; **or** combination chemotherapy plus radiation to places where large amounts of cancer are found; **or** combination chemotherapy plus intrathecal chemotherapy (injected into the spinal fluid); **or** *Clinical trials:* Chemotherapy followed by bone marrow transplant.
Intermediate-grade relapsed	Combination chemotherapy and/or total body radiation and bone marrow transplant; **or** *Clinical trials:* Bone marrow transplant with or without colony-stimulating factors.

TREATMENT CHOICES FOR HIGH-GRADE NON-HODGKIN'S DISEASE

STAGE	TREATMENT
High-grade Stage I	*If you have lymphoblastic lymphoma:* Intensive combination chemotherapy, sometimes with radiation. *Immunoblastic lymphoma:* Combination chemotherapy alone or with radiation. *Diffuse undifferentiated lymphoma or Burkitt's lymphoma:* Multidrug therapy. *Clinical trials:* Bone marrow transplants.
High-grade Stage II	*If you have lymphoblastic lymphoma, your treatment may be one of the following:* Combination chemotherapy plus intrathecal chemotherapy (injected into the spinal fluid); **or** combination chemotherapy plus intrathecal chemotherapy and radiation to the brain. Radiation therapy is also given to places in the body with large amounts of cancer. *If you have immunoblastic lymphoma,* you will probably be treated as if you had Stage II intermediate-grade lymphoma (see previous page). *If you have small noncleaved cell lymphoma, including Burkitt's lymphoma, your treatment may be one of the following:* Combination chemotherapy; **or** *Clinical trials:* New methods of treatment, including bone marrow transplant.
High-grade Stage III	*If you have lymphoblastic lymphoma, your treatment may be one of the following:* Combination chemotherapy plus intrathecal chemotherapy (injected into spinal fluid); **or** combination chemotherapy plus intrathecal chemotherapy and radiation to the brain. Radiation is also given to places in the body with large amounts of cancer. *If you have immunoblastic lymphoma,* you will probably be treated as if you had Stage III intermediate-grade lymphoma (see previous page). *If you have small noncleaved cell lymphoma, including Burkitt's lymphoma, your treatment may be one of the following:* Combination chemotherapy; **or** *Clinical trials:* New methods of treatment, including bone marrow transplant.
High-grade Stage IV	*If you have lymphoblastic lymphoma, your treatment may be one of the following:* Combination chemotherapy plus intrathecal chemotherapy (injected into the spinal fluid); **or** combination chemotherapy plus intrathecal chemotherapy and radiation to the brain. Intrathecal chemotherapy and radiation is also given to places in the body with large amounts of cancer. *If you have immunoblastic lymphoma,* you will probably be treated as if you had Stage IV intermediate-grade lymphoma (see previous page). *(continued)*

TREATMENT CHOICES FOR HIGH-GRADE NON-HODGKIN'S DISEASE (cont.)

STAGE	TREATMENT
High-grade Stage IV (continued)	*If you have small noncleaved cell lymphoma, including Burkitt's lymphoma, your treatment may be one of the following:* Combination chemotherapy; or *Clinical trials:* New methods of treatment, including bone marrow or peripheral stem cell transplant.
High-grade relapsed	*Clinical trials:* New methods of treatment, including continuous infusion chemotherapy and bone marrow or peripheral stem cell transplant.

nosed with advanced disease that has spread outside of the lymph nodes, the treatment is more aggressive, the disease is more extensive and is less responsive to chemotherapy. In addition, because of deficiencies in their immune system and in their blood cells, they are at increased risk for infections, which makes it difficult for these patients to endure aggressive treatments.

What factors need to be considered when selecting treatment for AIDS-related lymphoma?

Several factors need to be considered, such as how severe the deficiency of the immune system is, what kind of infectious illnesses the person has had, whether the bone marrow and other organs are involved, and how healthy the patient is at the present time.

What other areas are usually involved in AIDS-related lymphoma?

The most common sites are the GI (gastrointestinal) tract, central nervous system, bone marrow and liver. Some patients have involvement of the rectum, heart or the sac around it, lungs, bile ducts, mouth or soft tissues.

How often should I see a doctor for checkups after being treated for non-Hodgkin's lymphoma?

Careful follow-up will be needed and may vary for different types and stages of non-Hodgkin's disease. Generally, you will be checked every three months for the first year, every four months for the second to the fifth years, then yearly thereafter. You will probably have chest x-rays and blood tests at every visit. Every year, you may have ultrasound or CT scans of the abdomen and pelvis.

What symptoms should I be looking for to report to the doctor?

You should report loss of appetite or loss of weight, fever, pain, lumps, difficulty in breathing, intestinal symptoms, problems with your balance or a change in personality.

CUTANEOUS T-CELL LYMPHOMA

What is cutaneous T-cell lymphoma?

Cutaneous T-cell lymphoma is a rare chronic type of malignancy (also known as mycosis fungoides) which appears on the skin and can be present for many years. In its early stages it usually affects the skin and may stay confined to one area for long periods of time, sometimes for years. The disease is slowly progressive, and patients may live for many years with localized disease. Eventually the lymph nodes and internal organs may become involved. When large numbers of the tumor cells are found in the blood, the condition is called the Sezary syndrome. Cutaneous T-cell lymphoma is frequently difficult to diagnose in its initial stages and several biopsies may be required before it is accurately diagnosed.

Is cutaneous T-cell lymphoma a fungus?

The disease was named mycosis fungoides several centuries ago when it was thought to be caused by a fungus. It has long been recognized that it is a disease primarily affecting the reticuloendothelial system—cells scattered throughout the body which destroy other cells, bacteria, and fragments of foreign materials, and form antibodies.

What kind of doctor should be treating cutaneous T-cell lymphoma?

It is a rare disease and needs to be treated in a major medical center, involving the joint decisions of dermatologist, medical oncologist and radiation oncologist.

What are the symptoms of cutaneous T-cell lymphoma?

Reddish plaquelike tumors of scaly, thickened skin may develop. They may resemble eczema or psoriasis and may be found on the back, arms, stomach, face, scalp or other parts of the body. They may itch or spread and ulcerate. In the next stage, called the infiltration stage, lymph nodes may be enlarged and the skin becomes infiltrated with an overgrowth of reticuloendothelial cells of several kinds which allows a microscopic diagnosis to be made. In the third stage the tumors on the skin may become painful, itchy, uncomfortable and may become infected. In the fourth stage, the lymph nodes, liver, or lung may be involved.

How is cutaneous T-cell lymphoma staged?

Staging depends on how the cancer has spread. In Stage I, the cancer only affects parts of the skin. There are red, dry, scaly patches, but no tumors. The lymph nodes are not enlarged. In Stage II, the skin has scaly patches but no tumors; lymph nodes are larger than normal but do not contain cancer cells, or there are tumors on the skin but the lymph nodes do not contain cancer cells. In Stage III, nearly all the skin is red, dry and scaly. The lymph nodes are either normal or are larger than normal, but do not

STAGE	TREATMENT
TREATMENT CHOICES FOR CUTANEOUS T-CELL LYMPHOMA (Mycosis Fungoides)	
Stage I	Total skin electron beam (TSEB) radiation; **or** topical chemotherapy; **or** phototherapy (PUVA); **or** local electron beam or x-ray therapy. *Clinical trials:* TSEB radiation plus topical or systemic chemotherapy; **or** TSEB radiation plus x-ray therapy to lymph nodes or total body irradiation; **or** PUVA plus biological therapy, chemotherapy or total body irradiation.
Stage II	Topical chemotherapy; **or** phototherapy (PUVA); **or** total skin electron beam radiation (TSEB); **or** local electron beam or x-ray therapy. *Clinical trials:* TSEB radiation plus topical or systemic chemotherapy; **or** TSEB radiation plus x-ray therapy to lymph nodes or total body radiation **or** phototherapy plus interferon, chemotherapy, or total body radiation **or** interferon.
Stage III	Topical chemotherapy; **or** phototherapy (PUVA) **or** TSEB radiation therapy; **or** local electron beam or x-ray therapy; **or** systemic chemotherapy; **or** *Clinical trials:* Biological therapy; **or** phototherapy.
Stage IV	Systemic chemotherapy; **or** topical chemotherapy; **or** total skin electron beam radiation; **or** phototherapy (PUVA); **or** local electron beam or x-ray therapy. *Clinical trials:* Biological therapy, new chemotherapy combinations; **or** photochemotherapy.
Relapsed	Depends upon many factors, including previous treatment; may be: TSEB radiation therapy; **or** local electron beam or x-ray therapy; **or** topical chemotherapy; **or** systemic chemotherapy. *Clinical trials:* Interferon, new chemotherapy, biological therapy or phototherapy plus chemotherapy or new chemotherapy combinations.

contain cancer cells. In Stage IV, cancer cells are found in the lymph nodes or the cancer has spread to other organs, such as the liver or lung. Sometimes after being treated, there can be a relapse which requires further treatment.

MULTIPLE MYELOMA
(PLASMA CELL NEOPLASMA)

Is multiple myeloma the same as bone cancer?

No, it is not. Although multiple myeloma (the most common of a group of plasma cell neoplasma) affects the bone marrow, it begins in the cells of the immune system. Bone cancer, on the other hand, begins in the cells that form the hard, outer part of the bone. Multiple myeloma is treated differently than bone cancer.

What is plasmacytoma?

If the myeloma cells are collected in only one bone and form a single tumor, it is called plasmacytoma. Some people with plasmacytoma may develop multiple myeloma eventually. Extramedullary plasmacytoma patients have isolated plasma cell tumors of soft tissues, usually in the tonsils or tissues around the nose.

What is macroglobulinemia?

This is a type of plasma cell neoplasm in which lymphocytes that make an M-protein buildup in the blood. (It is sometimes called Waldenstrom's.) Lymph nodes and liver and spleen may be swollen.

Who usually gets multiple myeloma?

Multiple myeloma is most often seen in adults between the ages of 50 and 70. More men then women have multiple myeloma and it is more common among blacks than whites.

What are the symptoms of multiple myeloma?

The main symptom is bone pain, often in the back or ribs. Broken bones may also occur. Weakness, a tired feeling, weight loss, nausea, vomiting, constipation, problems with urination, repeated infections and weakness or numbness in the legs are all possible symptoms.

What kind of doctor treats multiple myeloma?

Treatments for multiple myeloma are complex. You need to be under the care of an oncologist or a hematologist who has experience in treating this disease.

How does the doctor diagnose multiple myeloma?

X-rays may show the patches of bone that have been destroyed, along with the number and size of tumors in the bones. Blood and urine tests are used to detect whether they contain high levels of antibody proteins (M proteins) which suggest the presence of this disease. A bone marrow aspiration or a bone marrow biopsy is often done to check for myeloma cells. In the bone marrow aspiration, the doctor inserts a needle into the hipbone or breast bone to withdraw a sample of fluid and cells from the bone marrow. To do a bone marrow biopsy, the doctor uses a larger needle to remove a sample of solid tissue from the marrow (more detailed descriptions of these tests are in Chapter 4, "How Cancers Are Diagnosed"). In some cases, you will have magnetic resonance imaging (MRI) to give close-up views of the bones.

Are most myeloma patients anemic?

Since cancer cells may prevent the growth of new red blood cells and disease-fighting white blood cells, people with multiple myeloma may be anemic and susceptible to infections, such as pneumonia. They may also have too much calcium in their blood (hypercalcemia), causing loss of appetite, nausea, thirst, fatigue, muscle weakness, restlessness and confusion. In addition, multiple myeloma patients may have serious problems with their kidneys because they are not filtering and cleaning the blood properly.

STAGES OF MULTIPLE MYELOMA

STAGE	DESCRIPTION
Stage I	Relatively few cancer cells have spread throughout body. Number of red blood cells and amount of calcium in blood are normal. No tumors (plasmacytomas) found in bone. Amount of M protein in blood or urine is very low. There may be no symptoms of disease.
Stage II	A moderate number of cancer cells have spread throughout the body.
Stage III	A relatively large number of cancer cells have spread throughout the body. One or more of the following may also be present: a decrease in the number of red blood cells, causing anemia; the amount of calcium in the blood is very high; more than three bone tumors are found; high levels of M protein are found in the blood or urine.

TREATMENT CHOICES FOR MULTIPLE MYELOMA AND PLASMA CELL NEOPLASMS

STAGE	TREATMENT
Stage I	*If you have no symptoms:* Careful monitoring to see if disease progresses. *If you have symptoms:* Chemotherapy, with localized radiation therapy, if needed to treat bone tumors; **or** *Clinical trials:* New methods of treatment, including biological response modifiers (including interferon) plus chemotherapy.
Stage II	Combination chemotherapy, with radiation therapy, if needed to treat bone tumors; **or** *Clinical trials:* Biological response modifiers, multidrug treatment, bone marrow transplantation.
Stage III	Combination chemotherapy, with radiation therapy, if needed to treat bone tumors; **or** *Clinical trials:* Multidrug treatment, biological response modifiers, bone marrow transplantation.
Isolated plasmacytoma of bone	External radiation therapy to tumor. If other symptoms appear, chemotherapy may be needed.
Extramedullary plasmacytoma (usually in tonsils or sinuses)	External radiation therapy to tumor; **or** surgery to remove tumor, usually followed by external radiation therapy or surgical removal plus radiation. If other symptoms appear, chemotherapy may be needed.
Macroglobulinemia (Waldenstrom's)	*If you have no symptoms:* Careful monitoring to see if symptoms develop. *If you have symptoms:* Chemotherapy treatment; **or** for temporary symptoms, plasmapheresis to filter cells from blood. *Clinical trials:* New chemotherapy drugs and combinations of drugs.
Monoclonal gammopathy of undetermined significance	Close monitoring to see if symptoms of plasma cell neoplasm or lymphoma develop.
Refractory plasma cell neoplasm	Chemotherapy; **or** *Clinical trials:* New drugs and combinations of drugs.

How is multiple myeloma treated?

If you have more than one tumor, the treatment will depend on your medical history, age, type and stage of disease. If you have multiple myeloma but do not have symptoms of the disease, you will probably not get any treatment. Rather, the doctor will watch you to see if there are any changes. Chemotherapy is the usual treatment for multiple myeloma. Among the drugs being used are L-PAM, melphalan, and cyclophosphamide, alone or in combination with prednisone. Sometimes radiation therapy will also be used, especially to treat local symptoms in the bone. Biological therapy (interferon and interleukin-2), bone marrow transplantation, peripheral stem cell support, and treatment with colony-stimulating factors are being studied in clinical trials for certain patients.

How is plasmacytoma of the bone treated?

If you have a single tumor of the plasma cells that found in the bone, with no M protein found in the blood or urine, you will probably be treated with radiation therapy.

Is exercise important to the myeloma patient?

It is important to try to prevent bone fractures. Exercise can reduce the loss of calcium from the bones. Talk to your doctor and nurses about what kind of exercise you can do. A cane or a walker can help provide a wider base of support for you. Drinking plenty of fluids is also important, since it helps the kidneys to get rid of excess calcium in the blood and prevents problems that occur when calcium collects in the kidneys.

What can be done to relieve the bone pain?

If you have bone pain, make sure you discuss it with your health team so that they can find ways to relieve it. You can take pain medicine. Some people have found that relaxation and imagery can help reduce their pain. Radiation therapy may be used to control severe bone pain and to stabilize areas that are likely to fracture. There is more information on controlling pain in Chapter 24, "Living with Cancer."

Can I do anything to prevent infections?

There are some things that you can do. Be sure not to get any inoculations of vaccines made with live materials. Make sure you drink plenty of liquids and eat a diet high in calories and proteins. Tell your doctor if you have signs of infection, such as a fever, sore throat, rash, tired feeling, or difficult or painful discharge of urine. Get enough sleep. Nap if you feel tired.

chapter 18

Gynecological Cancers

The female reproductive system still remains a mystery to many women, even though we are reminded of its existence by monthly menstrual periods. Although most women know that a lump in the breast is not to be ignored, many of us remain uninformed about the danger of ignoring symptoms of problems in the reproductive tract. Since so many of the cancer problems that occur in this part of a woman's body are silent, regular checkups are a wise insurance policy. Though many women consider the pelvic examination a nuisance at best and an embarrassing experience at worst, the examination takes on a whole different aspect when you stop to appreciate the incredible biological design of this part of the body. The better we understand how it all works, the better able we are to listen to our bodies and detect problems at a point when something can be done.

In whatever part of the reproductive system your cancer is located, it is helpful to know as much as you can about it so you can ask the right questions and make the right decisions about your treatment.

What You Need to Know About Cancers of the Female Reproductive Organs

- Many operations for these kinds of cancers affect your ability to have children. They also may affect your ability to have sexual relations.
- Since each part of the female reproductive system is unique, treatment varies depending upon the location of the tumor.
- Make sure you understand exactly what is going to be done to you, what organs will be affected and what side effects to expect before you have any treatments.
- A Pap test can accurately detect cancer of the cervix. It is not a test for detecting cancer of the endometrium, fallopian tubes, or ovaries.

Where do female reproductive system cancers occur?

The areas involved include:

- Cervix.
- Endometrium (also called the uterus or womb).
- Ovaries and fallopian tubes.
- Vagina.
- Vulva.

What is the doctor looking for when doing a pelvic exam?

The pelvic exam lets the doctor see the vagina and cervix. The doctor can also feel the uterus, vagina, ovaries, and fallopian tubes and can take a Pap smear. The doctor uses a speculum to widen the opening of the vagina to make it easier to see the upper part of the vagina and cervix. Once this portion of the examination is complete, the doctor usually examines the rectum. By inserting one finger into the rectum and one finger into the vagina, the physician is actually examining both areas at the same time, providing another opportunity to feel the uterus and ovaries. The doctor is looking for irritations, infections, and warts, as well as any abnormalities in shape and size.

How often should a woman have a pelvic examination?

Between the ages of 18 and 40, a pelvic examination, along with a Pap test, should be done every one to three years. Over 40, it should be done each year.

WHO IS AT RISK?

Site	Age	Risk and Possible Preventive Factors
Cervix	30–60	Sexual intercourse before age 18; multiple sex partners; younger women whose mothers took DES; genital herpes virus; papillomaviruses; genital warts; smoking; possibly oral contraceptives. *Possible preventive factors:* Estrogen replacement; vitamin A (retinoids), vitamin B.
Endometrium (uterus or womb)	55–70	Heavy women with large body frames; high-calorie, high-fat diets; infertility due to ovulation failure; family history; few or no children; early menstruation; late menopause; estrogen replacement therapy without progestational modification (used in 1960s and 1970s). *Possible preventive factors:* Birth control pills, especially pills containing both estrogen and progestin.
Ovaries	40–70	History of breast cancer; no pregnancies; family history of several members with ovarian cancer—mother, sister, daughter. *Possible preventive factors:* Multiple pregnancies; oral contraceptives; early menopause; diet rich in vitamin A and fiber.
Vagina	60–80 (12–30 if mother took DES)	Genital viruses; chronic irritation; women who have had hysterectomies. Mother who took DES during pregnancy.
Vulva	Fifty percent with preinvasive are 20–40; older women (60 and over) at risk for invasive	Chronic vulvar disease; previous malignancy of lower genital tract; history of breast cancer; herpes papilloma virus; herpes simplex 2; exposure to coal tar derivatives.

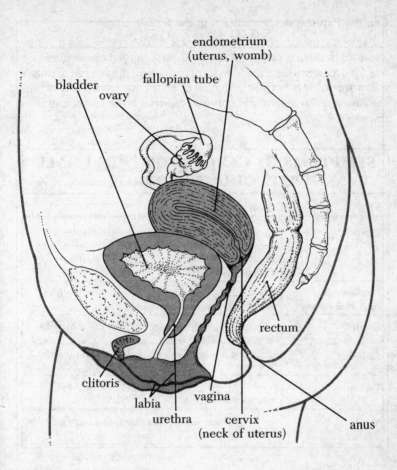

Female reproductive organs
(Illustration by Dolores Bego)

Can the Pap test detect cancers in the female tract?

A Pap test can accurately detect cancer of the cervix, but it is not a test for detecting cancer of the endometrium, fallopian tubes, or ovaries. In cases where these types of cancer are discovered through a Pap smear, it is because the cancer cells have passed down into the cavity of the uterus and continued through the cervix and into the vaginal discharge.

SYMPTOMS OF CANCERS OF THE FEMALE REPRODUCTIVE TRACT

Site	Symptom
Cervix	Abnormal bleeding, may start and stop between regular periods, or may occur after intercourse, douching or pelvic exam. Increased vaginal discharge. Often **no** symptoms.
Endometrium (uterus or womb)	Abnormal bleeding after menopause. May begin as watery, blood-streaked discharge.
Ovaries	Swelling, bloating, discomfort in lower abdomen; loss of appetite, feeling of fullness, even after light meal; gas, indigestion, nausea, weight loss. Often no **early** symptoms.
Vagina	Vaginal bleeding, vaginal discharge, pelvic pain. Often **no** symptoms.
Vulva	Intense itching; lesions sometimes seen, may be white, red or darkly pigmented.

What kinds of sexual side effects can result from treatment of cancers of the female reproductive organs?

Side effects vary, depending upon the location of the cancer and the type of treatment. Some treatments have little or no effect on sexuality. Some women find that after a hysterectomy, for example, they are more relaxed and enjoy sex because they are no longer worried about becoming pregnant. Other women report vaginal problems that may be associated with surgery, radiation or chemotherapy. Sexual problems are covered under the specific treatments in Chapters 6 through 8 and in Chapter 24, "Living with Cancer."

What can be done if the vagina becomes narrowed after treatment for gynecological cancer?

Treatments for cancers in the gynecological area sometimes result in a condition called vaginal stenosis which causes the narrowing of the muscles and tissues that form the walls of the vagina. Vaginal stenosis can result from the formation of scar tissue, making it difficult for you to have essential pelvic exams or sexual intercourse. Information on using a dilator to prevent vaginal stenosis can be found in Chapter 7, "Radiation Treatment."

CANCER OF THE CERVIX

WHAT YOU NEED TO KNOW ABOUT CERVICAL CANCER

- The number of deaths from cancer of the cervix has **decreased more than 70 percent** during the last forty years, mainly due to the Pap test and regular checkups.
- In its early stages, cancer of the cervix is a highly curable disease—almost 100 percent curable, in fact.
- The accuracy of your Pap test depends on the quality of the laboratory interpreting the slide your doctor sends. You can ask for a reading from another lab or for a second pathology report before action is taken.
- To help insure a more accurate reading it is wise to arrange your appointment between days 15 and 20 of your menstrual cycle. The day your period starts counts as day 1.
- Do not douche for at least three days before your Pap test. If you do, there won't be enough loose cells in your vaginal fluid for an accurate test.
- Don't use birth control foam or jelly for five days before the test.

Where is the cervix located?

The cervix connects the uterus (or womb, where a baby develops) with the vagina (birth canal).

Is the cervix part of the uterus?

The cervix is the lower part or neck of the uterus. It protrudes into the vagina and is the segment of the uterus which can be seen by the doctor during a pelvic examination. Cancer of the cervix, or neck of the uterus, and cancer of the endometrium, or body of the uterus, present two very different sorts of problems. It is important for you to know exactly where your particular cancer is. We

UNDERSTANDING THE MEANING OF GYNECOLOGICAL OPERATIONS

OPERATION	PROCEDURE	WHAT YOU SHOULD KNOW
Laparoscopy	Small incision in lower abdominal wall to obtain a biopsy.	Sometimes used in diagnosis in ovarian, fallopian tube and uterine cancers or to remove organs in abdomen or pelvis. General anesthesia used.
Conization	Removal of localized preinvasive lesion.	More extensive than simple biopsy. Performed under general anesthesia. May be done instead of hysterectomy. Pregnancy may still be possible.
Subtotal or **supracervical hysterectomy**	Uterus is removed, but cervix remains.	Will be unable to have children. Normal sexual relations.
Vaginal hysterectomy	Uterus removed through vagina.	Not advisable if uterus is enlarged or not fully movable. More difficult to perform than hysterectomy.
Total hysterectomy	Removal of cervix and uterus.	No longer fertile. Will not menstruate. Normal sexual relations.
Radical hysterectomy; also called **Wertheim's operation**	Removal of uterus, fallopian tubes, and ovaries as well as much of tissue surrounding uterus, regional lymph nodes and part of vagina.	Because of extent of operation, may have postoperative complications which involve vital body systems, bladder, bowel dysfunctions. If premenopausal, causes abrupt menopause and menopausal symptoms. No longer fertile. Sexual relations still possible.

(continued)

UNDERSTANDING THE MEANING OF GYNECOLOGICAL OPERATIONS *(cont.)*

OPERATION	PROCEDURE	WHAT YOU SHOULD KNOW
Myomectomy	Fibroid tumors removed from wall of uterus but uterus left intact.	Recommended for younger women with fibroid tumors who wish to retain ability to become pregnant.
Oophorectomy or **ovariectomy**	Removal of one or both ovaries.	Abrupt menopause if both ovaries removed. If only one removed, may continue to menstruate and can become pregnant. Normal sexual relations.
Salpingectomy or **bilateral salpingo oophorectomy**	Removal of fallopian tubes and ovaries.	Menstruation ceases. No longer fertile. Normal sexual relations.
Simple vulvectomy	Removal of skin of major and minor lips of vulva and clitoris.	Sexual relations still possible.
Radical vulvectomy	Removal of vaginal lips, clitoris, skin surrounding vulva and lymph glands.	Preoperative radiation often prescribed prior to operation. Sexual relations still possible.
Vaginectomy	Removal of vagina.	Vagina may be smaller or shorter after surgery. Plastic surgery may be necessary.
Pelvic exenteration	Radical hysterectomy plus removal of rectum and bladder.	For very advanced cancer of cervix. Leaves patient with both bowel and urinary openings on abdomen. Very extreme operation.

Subtotal, supracervical, or partial
Removes uterus

Total or complete
Removes uterus and cervix

Total plus unilateral salpingo-oopherectomy
Removes uterus, cervix, one fallopian tube, and one ovary

Radical
Removes uterus, cervix, fallopian tubes, ovaries, part of vagina, and regional lymph nodes

Types of hysterectomies
(Illustrations by Dolores Bego)

will be referring to the cervix and the endometrium (instead of uterus) in this chapter since those are more accurate descriptions.

What is the papilloma virus?

This is a general term—its full name is human papilloma virus. It is often referred to by its initials, HPV. HPV includes 70 similar viruses that tend to cause warts, including the fairly common warts that grow on hands and feet. About 25 of the wart strains are found in the genital tract. Two of the wart strains, numbers 16 and 18, are high-risk strains and are found in most cancers of the cervix. Many people who harbor the genital wart virus do not develop warts or the precancerous condition known as dysplasia. The highest levels of HPV infection are found among teenage girls and young women. It is estimated that a third of college-age women are infected with the virus. The virus appears to enter the cervix through tiny injuries sustained during sexual intercourse. Frequent sex with an infected partner increases the odds of the virus causing problems. In girls under 18, the cervix is much less mature and is more vulnerable to wart virus infection. Studies consistently find many fewer infections in older women.

Is HPV the cause of cervical cancer?

Researchers estimate that at least 90 percent of all cervical tumors contain the wart virus. These papillomas have been invading animal cells since the beginning of time. They infect almost every animal on earth, although a virus that infects one animal may not infect another. The viruses come in about 70 different strains—each of which specializes in infecting one type of skin cell. One will cause warts only between the fingers, others invade other parts of the body. About 25 strains infect the genital area and can be sexually transmitted. Oral sex can transmit them to similar tissues in the vocal cords.

What is done if there are visible genital warts?

Usually the doctor will recommend removal. Repeated treatments may be needed to remove all of the warts. Recurrences are possible. Sexual partners also should be checked for warts and treated. If further tests reveal mildly abnormal cells, close follow-up may be recommended. Often the tissue will return to normal on its own. At present, there is no treatment for the virus itself.

Do dysplasia or hyperplasia always lead to cancer in the female organs?

These precancerous conditions do not necessarily lead to cancer. Often they revert to normal without any treatment. However, since there is, as yet, no way of telling which will turn cancerous and which will revert to normal, it is important to be examined by a physician at regular intervals so that any changes can be detected at an early stage.

Is human papilloma virus (HPV) DNA typing done if there are abnormal cells in the cervix?

HPV DNA typing may be helpful in determining who is at high risk and may need more aggressive evaluation and follow-up. However, this procedure is presently available generally only at medical centers.

At what age do women usually get cervical cancer?

The age varies, with the peak for cancer in situ being between 30 and 40 and for invasive cancer between 40 and 60. However, cervical cancer may occur at any age. About 25 percent is seen in women under the age of 35.

What kind of cancer are most cancers of the cervix?

Most cancers of the cervix are squamous cell cancers. Some are adenocarcinomas or squamous cell tumors with some adenocarcinoma cells. Both are treated in the same manner, although those with adenocarcinoma cells appear to be more aggressive.

What are the symptoms that alert me to cervical cancer?

There are usually no visible symptoms or signs in the early stages of cervical cancer. As the cancer grows, there may be unusual bleeding or discharge. You may have longer menstrual periods, a heavier flow, bleeding between periods or after intercourse, or bleeding after menopause. The bleeding is usually bright red and unpredictable as to when it appears, its amount, or its duration. Although these symptoms may not be cancer they should be checked by the doctor. Cancer of the cervix is usually detected through a Pap smear. It is almost 100 percent curable in its earliest stages. Thanks to the Pap smear, more than two-thirds of cervical cancers are now detected in the early, in situ stage.

How is the Pap test done?

The Pap smear is a simple, painless test that can be done in a doctor's office, a clinic, or a hospital. Its purpose is to detect abnormal cells in and around the cervix. While a woman lies on an examining table, a speculum is inserted into her vagina to widen the opening. Living cells are collected in and around the cervix, usually with a small cervical brush. The specimen is put on a glass slide and sent to a medical laboratory for evaluation. The test is usually done by a gynecologist or other specially trained health care professionals, such as physician assistants, nurse midwives and nurse practitioners. The interpretation of the slide by the laboratory is an important factor in the diagnosis. The percentage of misinterpretations has been shown to be quite high, so it is important to have the test verified before any treatment is undertaken.

When should the first Pap test be done?

The recommendation of the American Cancer Society is that all women who have had sexual intercourse should begin a regular screening program for cervical cancer.

Is it necessary to have a Pap test every year?

Women who are, or who have been, sexually active, or have reached age 18, should have an annual Pap test and pelvic examination. After a woman has had three or more consecutive satisfactory normal annual examinations, the Pap test may be performed less frequently at the discretion of the physician.

Should older women continue to have Pap tests?

Yes. There is no upper age limit for Pap tests. Older women should continue to have regular physical exams, including a pelvic exam and Pap test. Some doctors recommend that women should continue to have Pap tests until menopause and every three to five years beyond 65.

Is it necessary to have a Pap test after a woman has had a hysterectomy?

A woman who has had a hysterectomy should continue to have Pap tests. Her doctor may do the test less frequently, depending on the type of hysterectomy she has had.

When you get the result of the Pap test, what is the meaning of the classifications used by the laboratory?

A number of classifications are used and may vary from one laboratory to another. Normally, your physician will discuss the findings with you. Rarely would you be given a numerical classification without an explanation. However, the chart on the next page explains the meaning of some of the most widely used classifications.

Where are tests and procedures used to evaluate the extent of abnormal cell change detected by a Pap smear done?

Many are done in the physician's office. Colposcopy usually is done in the doctor's office. Cervical biopsy and endocervical curettage,

WHAT A PAP SMEAR RESULT MEANS

Class	What It Means	What Your Doctor May Do
Class I	Negative or normal, no cell changes apparent.	Routine follow-up
Class II	Atypical. Slightly abnormal. May be due to mild infection.	Examine for lower genital infection; repeat Pap smear in 3–4 months. If condition persists, colposcopic examination. If abnormal, cervical biopsy.
Class III	Suspicious dysplasia. There are three stages—see below.	Must be diagnosed with cervical biopsy (Class III, IV and V).
Class III-CIN-1	Mild dysplasia. Abnormal cells in lower third of cervical surface.	Cryocautery—freezing of abnormal cells.
Class III-CIN-2	Moderate dysplasia. Abnormal cells in lower two-thirds of cervical surface.	Cryocautery or laser therapy. Pap smear should be repeated.
Class III-CIN-3	Severe dysplasia. Entire thickness of cervical surface cells involved.	Conization or other treatment.
Class IV & V	Positive. Smear contains cells that are suspicious of cancer.	Biopsy needed to determine if in situ or invasive.

which is the scraping of tissue to remove cells for microscopic examination, are done either in the doctor's office or the hospital. Conization or cone biopsy, which is the surgical removal of a cone-shaped piece of cervical tissue for examination under a microscope, is done in the hospital. This biopsy may also serve as a treatment to remove suspicious cancer cells.

Why must a biopsy be done if the Pap smear already indicates there are cancerous cells?

The Pap smear is only a screening tool. Although it is very accurate as a screening device, a biopsy must be done to give a definite diagnosis of cancer so that treatment can be properly staged.

Can cancer of the cervix progress from dysplasia to invasive cancer?

If untreated, 30 to 70 percent of in situ cancer will develop into invasive cancer over a period of ten to twelve years. In about 10 percent of patients the in situ cancer, if it goes untreated, will become invasive in the period of under one year.

QUESTIONS TO ASK YOUR DOCTOR BEFORE BEING TREATED FOR CERVICAL CANCER

- Has my Pap test been rechecked to make absolutely certain that I do have a cancerous condition?
- What kind of cancer is it and where is it located?
- Has there been any spread?
- What kind of treatment are you planning?
- Is this treatment necessary or is it elective?
- Is there an alternative way of treating this condition?
- Will this treatment mean I can't have a baby?
- Will this treatment affect my sexual functioning?
- Will it affect my urinary function or control?
- If radiation therapy is being used, what complications will these treatments cause in my case?

What is a colposcopy?

If the Pap smear indicates that there are suspicious cells, the doctor will usually examine your vagina and cervix with a colposcope. The colposcope is basically a microscope on a stand. It gives a lighted, magnified view showing greater detail than can be seen with the naked eye. The procedure is known as a colposcopy. At the same time, the doctor may remove tissue for a biopsy.

Is the colposcopy painful?

If tissue is removed for a biopsy, you may have some minor discomfort. The procedure takes ten or fifteen minutes and is usually done in a doctor's office. You may have a brown vaginal discharge for a few days.

What is the Schiller test?

The Schiller test is a diagnostic test for cells in the vagina and cervix. It is done by swabbing the area with a brown liquid which makes abnormal areas stand out as white or yellow spots.

What is the loop electrosurgical excision procedure (LEEP)?

This is a relatively new surgical procedure for treating abnormal, precancerous tissue in the cervix (cervical intraepithelial neoplasia), using an electrified wire loop through which high-frequency current passes. This technique is also referred to as LOOP diathermy, or LLETZ, large loop excision of the transformation zone. Your cervix is numbed, the loop is inserted into the vagina and the precancerous cells are removed, producing a button-size sample of tissue. Your wound is packed with a medicinal paste that hastens healing and the tissue is sent to a pathologist for further analysis. After two or three months, your cervix is completely healed. This technique is less costly, can be done in a doctor's office, has a shorter recovery time and, when done by a well-trained physician, fewer complications.

How is cryosurgery done?

Cryosurgery or cryocautery uses liquid nitrogen or carbon dioxide to destroy tissue by freezing. The substance is placed in a hollow metal probe that is inserted into the tumor or applied to its surface. The one drawback to cryosurgery is that the surgeon cannot control the precise width and depth of the area being frozen. It is important that the mucus-secreting glands that are involved in pregnancy not be destroyed. The treatment is painless. There may be a watery discharge for two to four weeks after treatment.

Is laser surgery used in treating CIN?

Yes. The laser is mounted on the colposcope and the laser beam is directed at the affected area. The laser allows for great accuracy in removal of the diseased tissue, sparing disease-free tissue. There may be some discomfort but there is little vaginal discharge and healing occurs in about two weeks. There may be thermal damage to tissue, which may make future detection of invasive cancer difficult.

What is conization?

Conization, also called cone biopsy, is the surgical removal (referred to also as cold-knife conization or surgical conization) of a cone-shaped piece of tissue from the cervix. It is sometimes used to diagnose cervical cancer or to treat early cervical cancer. It is usually performed in a hospital or a surgical center, since it requires general anesthesia. It may result in infertility. With newer methods available for detection, conization is less often used. In some places, LEEP (loop electrosurgical excision procedure) is replacing the use of cryosurgery, laser therapy and cold-knife conization to remove precancerous cells.

When is conization or laser used for early stage cervical cancer?

If your cervical canal is involved and you wish to preserve the uterus and avoid radiation therapy and/or more extensive surgery, laser or cold-knife conization may be used. If you are past childbearing age, you may be treated by total abdominal or vaginal hysterectomy.

What are the treatments for Stage I-A cervical cancer?

There are three treatments : total hysterectomy, intracavitary radiation (see Chapter 7, "Radiation Treatment"), or conization. Radiation may be used when surgery is not advisable. If there is no vascular or lymphatic spread, conization may be appropriate.

What are the treatments for Stage I-B cervical cancer?

Radiation therapy or a radical hysterectomy are the usual treatments, the choice depending upon the size of the tumor and the age and preferences of the patient. Radiation therapy is usually the choice if the cancer has expanded the cervix greater than 3.0 centimeters. For those with three or more lymph nodes that are affected, postoperative total pelvic radiation is suggested.

Is treatment different for those with Stage II-A cervical cancer?

Either radiation therapy or radical hysterectomy with pelvic lymphandectomy may be used. The size of the tumor is the most important factor. For tumors 6.0 centimeters or larger, radiation appears to be comparable to radiation plus hysterectomy. Sometimes surgery following radiation is used if the tumors in the cervix are not responding to radiation. If the lymph nodes are found to be positive, radiation may be scheduled for that area following surgery.

What are the standard treatments for Stage II-B and Stage III cervical cancer?

The usual treatment is external beam radiation with the addition of radiation implants (brachytherapy) and chemotherapy. A number of clinical trials are testing radiation plus chemotherapy as well as surgery to determine the stage of the disease as well as the removal of lymph nodes thought to be cancerous, followed by external radiation therapy.

How is Stage IV-A cervical cancer usually treated?

Radiation or surgery is the usual treatment. Some clinical trials are using radiation therapy and chemotherapy, or chemotherapy followed by radiation.

What treatments are used for Stage IV-B cervical cancers?

Usually radiation therapy is used to relieve the symptoms of cervical cancer. A number of chemotherapy drugs are also used instead of radiation.

What is the SCC antigen test used for?

The squamous cell carcinogen (SCC) antigen test is a tumor marker test which reflects the success or failure of treatment of cervical cancer. It is used to determine whether the treatment has been successful in treating the cancer.

Are there sexual side effects to treatment for cervical cancer?

There can be sexual side effects, depending upon the extent of the disease and the type of treatment. Some treatments, such as radiation, can shorten the vagina, and some cancers of the cervix may extend into the vagina. For information on sexual side effects, see information under cancer of the vagina as well as in Chapter 7, "Radiation Treatment."

What treatment is used if cervical cancer recurs?

If the cancer recurs in the pelvis, surgery may be done to remove the area where the cancer has spread, as well as to remove the cervix, uterus and vagina (called an exenteration). Or further radiation therapy and chemotherapy may be used. If the cancer has recurred outside the pelvis, combination chemotherapy may be used and there are clinical trials available which are testing new drugs or combinations of drugs.

What are the consequences of a total pelvic exenteration?

This surgery, which includes the removal of the lower colon, rectum, or bladder as well as the cervix, uterus and vagina, is the most radical kind of pelvic surgery. Two ostomies are usually created, one for urine and one for bowel functions. In addition, the vagina is usually reconstructed. The clitoris and outer genitals are usually not removed, so that many women find they can still have sexual desire, pleasure and orgasm.

What kind of checkups should be scheduled following treatment for cancer of the cervix?

The first year, you will probably see the doctor every three months and your Pap smear will be repeated at six, nine and twelve months. Chest x-rays and CT scans will be done at the end of the first year. The second to fifth year, checkups will probably be scheduled each six months and after that yearly checkups should suffice. Tell you doctor if you have vaginal discharge or bleeding, bone pain, weight or appetite loss, bowel or bladder problems or swelling of the legs. Lifelong follow-up on a regular basis is important.

TREATMENT CHOICES FOR CERVICAL CANCER

STAGE	WHAT IT MEANS	TREATMENT
Stage 0	Cancer in situ, very early stage found only in first layer of cells of lining of cervix.	Cryosurgery; or laser surgery; or diathermy; or conization; or total abdominal or vaginal hysterectomy (for women who cannot have, or no longer want, children). Properly treated, cure rate can be 100 percent.
Stage I-A	Cancer is found throughout cervix with small amount of cancer found deeper in tissues of cervix	Hysterectomy plus removal of ovaries (ovaries not usually removed in younger women); or internal radiation therapy; or conization.
Stage I-B	Larger amount of cancer in tissues of cervix.	Internal and external radiation combined; or radical hysterectomy to remove uterus, cervix, ovaries, part of vagina, and lymph nodes in pelvic area; or same as above with addition of radiation therapy.
Stage II-A	Cancer has spread beyond cervix to upper two-thirds of vagina but has not extended to pelvic wall.	Combined internal and external radiation; or radical hysterectomy with lymph node dissection; or radiation followed by surgery. *Clinical trials:* Radical hysterectomy, lymph node dissection followed by radiation.
Stage II-B	Cancer has spread to tissue around cervix.	Combined internal and external radiation plus antimetabolic anticancer drug (hydroxyurea). *Clinical trials:* Sequential or concurrent radiation and chemotherapy; neoadjuvant chemotherapy; altered radiation fractionation; brachytherapy. *(continued)*

TREATMENT CHOICES FOR CERVICAL CANCER (*cont.*)

STAGE	WHAT IT MEANS	TREATMENT
Stage III	Spread extends to pelvic wall or involves lower third of vagina and/or ureters.	Combined internal and external radiation plus antimetabolic anticancer drug (hydroxyurea). Radiation plus chemotherapy concurrently or in sequence. *Clinical trials:* Neoadjuvant chemotherapy; altered radiation fractionation; brachytherapy.
Stage IV-A	Cancer spread to organs close to cervix such as bladder or rectum.	Combined internal and external radiation. *Clinical trials:* Radiation and chemotherapy concurrently or in sequence; neoadjuvant chemotherapy; altered radiation fractionation; brachytherapy.
Stage IV-B	Cancer spread to faraway organs such as lungs.	Radiation therapy to relieve symptoms such as pain; **or** systemic chemotherapy.
Recurrent	Depends upon where recurrence occurs.	*In pelvis:* Surgery to remove lower colon, rectum, or bladder—depending on where cancer spread—along with cervix, uterus and vagina plus radiation therapy and chemotherapy or chemotherapy.

CANCER OF THE ENDOMETRIUM (LINING OF UTERUS OR WOMB)

What is the endometrium?

The endometrium is the lining of the uterus or womb. The body or corpus of the uterus is a muscular, hollow, pear-shaped organ which is lined with epithelial cells. Cancer in this area is referred to as uterus or uterine cancer or endometrial cancer. The endometrium is made up of several layers of glands, blood vessels and tissue. When a woman is menstruating, the endometrial tissue grows and thickens in preparation for receiving a fertilized egg. Menstruation occurs when this tissue is not used and passes out through the vagina. Endometrial cancer develops in the epithelial layer. It is in this lining area where the most common type of female genital cancer occurs.

WHO GETS ENDOMETRIAL CANCER?

Endometrial cancer most often affects women after menopause. Seventy-five percent of all cases occur after the age of 50 and only 4 percent before the age of 40. Women who may be at risk for endometrial cancer include:

- Heavy women with large body frames.
- Women who are 50 pounds overweight (nine times more likely to develop problems than women of average weight).
- Women who have a history of diabetes and hypertension.
- Women who have had infertility problems due to failure of ovulation.
- Women who had unusual bleeding during menopause indicating overstimulation of the endometrium by irregular estrogen secretion.
- Women who had late menopause (after age 52).
- Women who had prolonged estrogen replacement treatment. NOTE: Use of "combination" oral contraceptives (estrogen plus progesterone or progestins) appears to *lower* risk of endometrial cancer.
- Women in families where other members have had this type of cancer.
- White women (at higher risk than black women).

What is endometriosis?

Endometriosis is a condition in which the kind of tissue that normally lines the uterus is found in abnormal places, such as on the outside of the uterus, the surface of the ovaries, in tissues between the vagina and rectum, in tissue in the lower abdomen. It is not a cancerous condition, but it does cause painful menstrual periods, abnormal bleeding and general discomfort. Treatment may be with medication or surgery.

Do fibroid tumors become cancerous?

Fibroid tumors (sometimes called leiomyomas) are noncancerous tumors in the uterus, usually found in women over 35 years of age. Often fibroids do not cause symptoms and do not need to be treated, although they should be checked often. When a woman stops having menstrual periods, fibroids may become smaller, and sometimes disappear. Symptoms of fibroids depend on the size and location of the tumors and may include irregular bleeding, vaginal discharge, and frequent urination. When fibroids press against nearby organs and cause pain, surgery may be needed. It is estimated that about 20 percent of women over 30 have fibroid tumors. Only about three cases in every thousand fibroid tumors become cancerous.

What is endometrial hyperplasia?

Endometrial hyperplasia is an abnormal increase in the number of endometrial cells and of stromal cells—cells that support endometrial tissue. Many scientists regard it as a precancerous condition. Severe hyperplasia is often called in situ cancer of the endometrium. Symptoms may include heavy bleeding during menstruation, erratic bleeding between periods or abnormal or heavy bleeding during menopause. Though every case of hyperplasia does not develop into cancer, uterine cancer goes through a hyperplastic stage before becoming cancerous. Therefore, hyperplasia is a warning that cancer may develop. Endometrial hyperplasia may be mild, moderate or severe. Endometrial hyperplasia can occur in menopausal and postmenopausal women as well as in young women who have irregular menstrual cycles.

What is the treatment for endometrial hyperplasia?

Treatment depends upon age and how advanced the hyperplasia is at the time it is diagnosed. For younger women who wish to remain fertile, endometrial hyperplasia may be treated with dilation and curettage (D&C). For women with severe hyperplasia and those for whom fertility is no longer a concern, hysterectomy may be recommended. If surgery is not possible because of other medical problems, progesterone may be prescribed.

What are the symptoms of endometrial cancer?

Abnormal bleeding after menopause is the most common symptom. The bleeding may begin as a watery, blood-streaked discharge. Later, the discharge may contain more blood. If there is reappearance of bleeding around the time of menopause, it is important to be checked as soon as possible by the doctor. Cancer of the endometrium usually occurs in women of this age group, so any abnormal bleeding should be diagnosed.

What causes endometrial cancer?

The causes of endometrial cancer are not well understood, but there are a number of factors that seem to increase the risk of developing it. One factor that appears to be related is hormone production. It is known that fatty tissue converts certain hormones into estrone, a form of estrogen. Scientists believe that an elevated estrogen level may be the reason why heavy women are twice as likely to develop endometrial cancer as are women of normal weight. Many studies suggest that the development of endometrial hyperplasia, which often precedes endometrial cancer, is related to hormones. Women who develop two kinds of tumors of the ovary—theca cell, which is benign, and granulos cell, which is malignant—are at a higher-than-average risk for endometrial cancer.

Who is at risk for endometrial cancer?

Women who have taken estrogen replacement therapy have a two to eight times greater risk of developing endometrial cancer than those who have not taken estrogen. The risk increases after two to four years on estrogen and seems to be greatest when large doses are taken. Today, few women receive treatment with estrogen alone. In addition, studies now indicate that premenopausal women who have taken oral contraceptives containing estrogen and progesterone seem to be at *less* risk for endometrial cancer than a similar-aged group of women who have never taken them. Diabetes and high blood pressure have also been listed as risk factors, but these relationships may not be as clear-cut as they appear, since scientists feel that it may be the effect of obesity on the estrogen level, rather than diabetes or high blood pressure, that increases the risk of endometrial cancer.

What are the major types of cancer that develop in the endometrium?

There are two major types. The most common type, which we will focus on in this chapter, is endometrial cancer which develops in the endometrium. These cancers are classified by the type of cells found. Three-quarters are adenocarcinomas. Other cell types include adenosquamous carcinoma, which accounts for 18 percent; papillary serous carcinoma, which is seen in 6 percent of cases; and clear cell carcinoma, which is responsible for 1 percent. The second type of endometrial cancer is uterine sarcoma, which develops in the uterine connective tissue.

How is endometrial cancer diagnosed?

The diagnosis usually begins with a review of symptoms and medical history. The physician will perform a pelvic exam, checking the uterus, vagina, ovaries, fallopian tubes, bladder and rectum. Routine laboratory tests, including blood tests and urinalysis, also are done. A Pap test may also be done, although it is not a specific test for uterine cancer because it detects only those cancer cells from the endometrium that have passed through the cervix into the vaginal discharge. The only way to get a definitive diagnosis is by taking a sample of the cells from the uterine wall. This is usually done with aspiration curettage or with a D&C (dilation and curettage).

How is aspiration curettage done?

This procedure is usually done in the doctor's office with an endometrial aspirator which consists of a disposable tube connected to a syringe. The tube is inserted through the cervix into the uterus and a piece of tissue is taken from the uterine lining. The tissue samples are studied to see if there are abnormal cell changes. If analysis of the tissue shows an overgrowth of lining cells (hyperplasia), a D&C may be advised to prevent future problems.

What is a D&C (dilation and curettage)?

This is a minor surgical procedure in which the uterus is scraped with an instrument, known as a curette, to obtain a sample of tissue. (The procedure is also sometimes used to remove the cancerous cells in cases of hyperplasia.) It is usually done on an outpatient basis, either in the doctor's office or in the hospital. Local or general anesthesia is used.

What is the next step if a biopsy confirms endometrial cancer?

Additional tests are needed to determine the extent of the disease. Several x-ray exams, such as intravenous pyelography (IVP), CT scans, ultrasound, MRI and bone scanning may be done before surgery.

QUESTIONS TO ASK YOUR DOCTOR ABOUT ENDOMETRIAL CANCER TREATMENT

- How extensive do you think the surgery will be?
- What grade and stage is it?
- Will you show me exactly what the operation entails and what will be removed?

- Where will the scar be? Will the scar be vertical or horizontal?
- Will this operation change my bowel functions, urinary control, or sexual life in any way?
- Is there an alternative way of treating this condition?
- Has it spread? Is it in the lymph nodes?
- Have the progesterone and estrogen receptor levels been checked?
- What are the risks and what side effects should I expect?
- How long will it be before I can return to normal activities?

What kind of surgery is done for endometrial cancer?

A hysterectomy, the surgical removal of the uterus, is the most common treatment for endometrial cancer. Usually, if the cancer has not spread beyond the endometrium, the uterus as well as the fallopian tubes and ovaries will be removed. Radiation therapy, internal and external radiation, and hormone therapy are also used for later stages of endometrial cancer.

Is it important to have progesterone and estrogen receptors checked?

It has been found that progesterone receptor levels are an important part of the evaluation process for treatment of those with Stage I and Stage II endometrial cancer. Progesterone levels greater than 100 were found to be a good sign that the cancer probably would be contained.

Does it make a difference whether the cancer cells are well or poorly differentiated?

Besides being staged, endometrial cancers are also grouped according to their degree of differentiation. Grade 1 means the cells are well differentiated. They resemble normal cells. Grade 2 means they are moderately well differentiated. Grades 3 and 4 (sometimes called stage 0 carcinoma of the endometrium) refer to poorly differentiated cells. Poorly differentiated cells are abnormally shaped and bear little resemblance to normal cells. These cells often spread more rapidly than those that are well differentiated. For example, treatment for Stage I cancer depends on the location of the tumor and whether the cells are well or poorly differentiated. When only part of the myometrium is affected and cells are reasonably well differentiated, and when the tumor is not invasive, hysterectomy and removal of the ovaries and fallopian tubes are recommended. In addition, a few lymph nodes in the adjacent areas are removed

TREATMENT CHOICES FOR ENDOMETRIAL CANCER

Stage	What It Means	Treatment
Stage 0	In situ, very early, inside uterus only, on surface.	D&C followed by hormone therapy; **or** hysterectomy if fertility is not a factor.
Stage I	Found only in main part of uterus, not in cervix.	Total hysterectomy, plus removal of ovaries, fallopian tubes and lymph nodes sampling; If nodes are positive, same as above with addition of postoperative radiation therapy to pelvis. *Clinical trials:* Radiation alone for selected patients.
Stage II	Cancer cells have spread to cervix.	Total hysterectomy, plus removal of ovaries, fallopian tubes and lymph nodes sampling followed by radiation or preoperative internal and external radiation followed by total hysterectomy plus removal of ovaries, fallopian tubes and lymph node sampling or radical hysterectomy and pelvic lymphandectomy.
Stage III	Spread outside uterus but not to pelvis.	Radical hysterectomy, plus ovaries, fallopian tubes, ovaries and part of vagina; lymph node dissection followed by radiation; **or** internal and external beam radiation; **or** hormone therapy.
Stage IV	Spread beyond pelvis to other body parts or into lining of bladder or rectum.	Internal and external radiation; **or** hormone therapy. *Clinical trials:* Chemotherapy.
Recurrent	Cancer returns after being treated.	Radiation to relieve pain, nausea and abnormal bowel functions; **or** hormone therapy. *Clinical trials:* Chemotherapy.

to determine whether cancer has spread. If no cancerous cells are found in the nodes, no further treatment is necessary. However, in all other cases and cell types, a more drastic node dissection is done and radiation therapy may follow the surgery.

What kind of follow-up exams will be needed after being treated for endometrial cancer?

The doctor will probably schedule follow-up visits every three months for the first year, every six months for the second to fifth year and yearly thereafter. Examination will probably include pelvic exam, stool, blood, urine tests, and a Pap test. Tumor markers, like CA-125, which can detect a protein shed by cancerous tissue, will usually be done at each visit. Chest x-rays are done yearly. Tell your doctor if you have any vaginal bleeding, pelvic pain, change in the size of your stomach, or swelling of the legs. The most crucial follow-up time is the first three years, but lifetime follow-up is important.

What is sarcoma of the uterus?

Sarcoma of the uterus is a very rare kind of cancer in which cancer cells grow in the muscles or connective tissues of the uterus. These include carcinosarcoma, leiomyosarcoma, endometrial stromal sarcoma, and mullerian adenosarcoma. Uterine sarcomas sometimes develop in women who had very high doses of radiation administered for benign uterine bleeding five to twenty-five years ago. A radical hysterectomy, with surgical removal of the uterus, fallopian tubes and the ovaries, and some of the lymph nodes in the pelvis and abdomen, may be necessary. Sometimes this is followed by radiation therapy. Clinical trials of surgery followed by chemotherapy or hormone therapy are also being done.

OVARIAN CANCER

Where are the ovaries located?

The ovaries are located in the pelvis, one on each side of the uterus. Each of these female reproductive organs is the size and shape of an almond. During each monthly menstrual cycle, one ovary releases an egg. The ovaries are the body's main source of female hormones—estrogen and progesterone—which regulate the menstrual cycle and pregnancy. These hormones control the development of female body characteristics, such as the breasts, body shape, and body hair.

What are the symptoms of ovarian cancer?

Often there are no symptoms of early ovarian cancer, which makes it difficult to detect ovarian cancer at an early stage when there is the greatest chance of cure. An ovarian tumor can grow for some time before pressure or pain can be felt. Symptoms, when they do occur, can include:

- Abdominal swelling or bloating.
- Discomfort in the lower part of abdomen.
- Feeling full after a light meal.
- Nausea or vomiting.
- Lack of appetite.
- Gas or indigestion.
- Unexplained weight loss.
- Diarrhea, constipation or frequent urination.
- Shortness of breath.
- Bleeding that is not part of regular menstruation pattern.

Who is most likely to develop ovarian cancer?

Most cases of ovarian cancer are found in women over the age of 50. But the disease is also sometimes found in younger women. Ovarian cancer is relatively rare, affecting about one in seventy women. Risk rises with age, with most cases occurring after menopause. Risk doubles for older women who have never had children or who have previously had breast or endometrial cancer. The highest risk appears to be in women with two or more first-degree relatives—mother, daughter, or sister—with the same problem. Eighty-five to 90 percent of cancers that have not spread beyond the ovary are curable. The real problem is that they are difficult to detect at an early stage, since often there are no symptoms in the early stages, and even when they appear, they may be ignored because they are so vague. Often when cancer of the ovary is found, it has spread to other organs.

What kind of tests are used to detect ovarian cancer?

The first step is usually a pelvic exam with a Pap smear being done at the same time. The Pap smear, however, is a test for cancer of the cervix and should not be depended upon to find or to accurately diagnose ovarian cancer. An ultrasound may be done of the ovaries to help differentiate between healthy tissues, fluid-filled cysts and tumors. CT scans may be ordered as well as a lower GI series and an IVP. A blood test to measure a substance that is produced by ovarian cancer cells, called CA-125, may be ordered. If these tests raise the suspicion that cancer may be the problem, the only sure way is to examine a sample of the ovarian tissue under the microscope, called a biopsy. This requires surgery.

What is the CA-125 blood test?

This cancer antigen blood test has proved useful for monitoring the success of ovarian cancer treatment, indicating whether a tumor has shrunk or if it has recurred. It works less well at detection and misses about half of all early tumors. In addition, endometriosis and fibroids, both of which are benign uterine tumors, can also elevate CA-125 levels.

What kind of surgery will be required for the biopsy?

The entire ovary must be removed because, if the problem is cancer, cutting through the outer layer of the ovary may cause spread. If the pathology report shows that the ovary is cancerous, further surgery is usually necessary. The second ovary, the uterus and the fallopian tubes are usually removed. In addition, the surgeon will also take samples of nearby lymph nodes and check the diaphragm and fluid from the abdomen to determine whether or not the cancer has spread.

What kind of cancers develop in the ovaries?

Epithelial ovarian cancer occurs in the lining of the ovary, and accounts for 90 percent of all ovarian cancers. Of these epithelial ovarian cancers, about 15 percent are called tumors of low malignant potential, and are treated differently from the more common and more invasive ovarian cancers of the epithelium. Other ovarian cancers include germ cell cancer and stromal tumor (sex cord tumor), which are quite rare. Germ cell tumors affect the egg-making cells in the ovary and most often affect young women. Stromal tumors affect the sex cord and include granulosa cell tumors and Sertoli-Lydig tumors.

QUESTIONS TO ASK YOUR DOCTOR BEFORE BEING TREATED FOR OVARIAN CANCER

- What kind of operation will I have?
- Exactly what parts of my reproductive tract will you be taking out?
- How long will I have to be in the hospital? Recuperating at home? When will I be able to get back to my normal routine?

- Will I have pain after the operation? For how long? How will it be treated?
- Will I still be able to have sex after the operation?
- Will I need chemotherapy or radiation treatment after the operation? When will it start? For how long? Will I be able to continue my normal activities?
- Will you be planning to do second-look surgery?

How is ovarian cancer treated?

Surgery is the most common treatment. The type of surgery depends upon the extent of the cancer. A *total abdominal hysterectomy and bilateral salpingo-oophorectomy* means that the ovaries, fallopian tubes and uterus are removed. If the area that stretches from the stomach to the nearby organs in the abdomen is affected, this operation is called an *omentectomy*. If only one ovary is removed along with the fallopian tube on the same side of the body, the operation is called a *unilateral salpingo-oophorectomy*. *Tumor debulking* means taking out as much of the cancer as possible. *Laparotomy* refers to any surgical procedure in which the abdominal cavity is opened either to examine it (*exploratory surgery*) or to perform surgery. Radiation is also used in treating ovarian cancer. It may be *external radiation*, from a machine, or it may be put directly into the sac that lines the abdomen in a liquid that is radioactive, called *intraperitoneal radiation*. Chemotherapy is also used. It may be taken by pill, put into the bloodstream intravenously or given directly to the affected area.

Will I still have menstrual periods after the operation?

It depends on whether both ovaries are taken out, your age and your general condition. If both ovaries are removed, you will begin to have symptoms of menopause soon after the operation, no matter what age you are. Since the use of hormone replacement therapy, which is usually given to women for symptoms such as hot flashes and vaginal dryness, has not been studied in women who have had ovarian cancer, you need to discuss the risks and benefits of using hormones with your doctor.

What happens to me sexually when the ovaries are removed?

Because the ovaries are not the only production site for estrogens—the adrenal glands also produce androgens which govern sexual desire—there should be no change in your desire. A decrease in vaginal lubrication may make it necessary for you to use extra lubrication during intercourse.

TREATMENT CHOICES FOR EPITHELIAL OVARIAN CANCERS

STAGE	WHAT IT MEANS	TREATMENT
Stage IA	Cancer in one ovary; capsule intact.	Total abdominal hysterectomy, bilateral salpingo-oophorectomy with omentectomy with lymph node sampling; **or** total abdominal hysterectomy as above followed by intraperitoneal radiation; **or** total abdominal hysterectomy as above followed by chemotherapy; **or** total abdominal hysterectomy as above followed by external radiation to abdomen and pelvis. *For selected IA patients who hope to remain fertile:* Ovary and fallopian tube on affected side removed, (unilateral salpingo-oophorectomy), lymph nodes in pelvis and abdomen biopsied. *Clinical trials:* Internal radiation or chemotherapy.
Stage IB	Growth limited to both ovaries; capsules intact.	
Stage IC	Tumor on surface of one or both ovaries or capsule ruptured or fluid contains malignant cells.	
Stage IIA	Cancer in one or both ovaries and/or spread to uterus, and/or fallopian tubes.	Total abdominal hysterectomy and bilateral salpingo-oophorectomy with tumor debulking. Lymph node sampling. Following operation either: systemic chemotherapy; **or** external beam radiation to abdomen and pelvis; **or** intraperitoneal radiation if only small amount of cancer. For residual disease (over 2 cm.) combination chemotherapy. *Clinical trials:* Internal radiation, high-dose chemotherapy with autologous bone marrow transplant.
Stage IIB	Cancer extends to other part of pelvis.	
Stage IIC	Tumor either IIA or IIB but on surface of one or both ovaries or capsule ruptured or fluid contains malignant cells.	

(continued)

TREATMENT CHOICES FOR EPITHELIAL OVARIAN CANCERS *(cont.)*

STAGE	WHAT IT MEANS	TREATMENT
Stage IIIA	Cancer in one or both ovaries, spread to lymph nodes or other parts of abdomen or surface of liver or intestines.	Total abdominal hysterectomy as above followed by: systemic chemotherapy; **or** external beam radiation to abdomen and pelvis (If residual disease is less than 0.5 cm.). *Clinical trials:* New chemotherapy drugs; **or** intraperitoneal chemotherapy; **or** Taxol.
Stage IIIB	Cancer in one or both ovaries with spread to peritoneal surfaces, none exceeding 2 centimeters diameter, nodes negative.	
Stage IIIC	Cancer in one or both ovaries with larger than 2 centimeter spread and/or positive nodes.	
Stage IV	Cancer in one or both ovaries and spread outside abdomen or inside liver.	Tumor debulking followed by systemic chemotherapy. *Clinical trials:* Taxol; **or** new chemotherapy drugs or combinations of drugs.
Recurrent	Cancer recurs after treatment, either in remaining ovary or elsewhere.	Systemic chemotherapy; **or** Taxol; **or** surgery to improve quality of life; **or** chemotherapy drug combination; **or** Tamoxifen. *Clinical trials:* Intraperitoneal chemotherapy; **or** high-dose chemotherapy drugs with autologous bone marrow or new anticancer drugs and biologicals.

What is second-look surgery?

Following radiation or chemotherapy, an operation called a second-look laparotomy is sometimes done. During the second-look operation, the doctor will take samples of lymph nodes and other tissues in the abdomen to see if the treatment has been successful. This operation should be performed only for patients on clinical trials or for those in whom the surgery will change the treatment. This operation is usually performed through a vertical incision in the abdomen.

Is taxol being used for ovarian cancers?

Taxol, an anticancer drug originally derived from the bark of Pacific yew trees and now being made synthetically, is being studied for its use in the treatment of ovarian cancers. In early trials it has demonstrated a 30 percent response in patients who had been treated previously with other regimens. (See Chapter 8, "Chemotherapy.")

What kind of follow-up is recommended for women who have had ovarian cancer?

Your doctor will probably ask you to come back every three months for the first year, and every six months thereafter. You will have blood, urine and Pap tests every six months, tests for tumor marker CA-125 every six months and chest x-rays or CT scans every year. You should tell the doctor if you notice changes in the size of your stomach, pain in your pelvic area, bleeding in the vagina, swelling of the legs, or signs of masculinization.

What is an ovarian low malignant potential tumor?

It is an ovarian epithelial cancer but its potential to become malignant is much lower than for the usual epithelial cancer. About 15 percent of all epithelial cancers fall into this category. Because these tumors are not as malignant as the other epithelial cancers, they are treated differently. In Stages I and II, a unilateral salpingo-oophorectomy is considered adequate treatment by some physicians. In cases where there is only one ovary or where the second ovary is cystic, partial oophorectomy may be considered if fertility is to be preserved. If childbearing is not a consideration, a total abdominal hysterectomy and bilateral salpingo-oophorectomy is usually recommended. Once a woman has completed having children, most, but not all, physicians favor removal of the remaining ovarian tissue as it may be at risk of recurrence. For patients with a more advanced stage of low malignant potential tumor, chemotherapy and/or radiation is sometimes used.

TREATMENT CHOICES FOR OVARIAN GERM CELL CANCERS

STAGE	WHAT IT MEANS	TREATMENT
Stage I	Cancer in one or both ovaries.	**Dysgerminoma:** Surgery to remove affected ovary and fallopian tube on same side (unilateral salpingo-oophorectomy) followed by radiation therapy or by chemotherapy if you wish to remain fertile. If tumor has ruptured, radiation therapy is preferred. **Other cell types:** Surgery as above followed by chemotherapy; **or** surgery as above with no further treatment.
Stage II	Cancer in one or both ovaries and/or spread to uterus, and/or fallopian tubes and/or other part of pelvis.	**Dysgerminoma:** Surgery to remove uterus and both ovaries and fallopian tubes (total abdominal hysterectomy and bilateral salpingo-oophorectomy) followed by radiation therapy; **or** if cancer is only in ovary and fallopian tube on same side and you wish to remain fertile, unilateral salpingo-oophorectomy followed by chemotherapy. **Other cell types:** Total abdominal hysterectomy and bilateral salpingo-oophorectomy. If cancer cannot be totally removed, tumor debulking will be done followed by chemotherapy; **or** if cancer is only in ovary and fallopian tube on one side and you want to remain fertile, unilateral salpingo-oophorectomy can be done followed by chemotherapy; **or** total abdominal hysterectomy and bilateral salpingo-oophorectomy plus tumor debulking followed by chemotherapy. If cancer remains following chemotherapy, further surgery to remove as much of tumor as possible.

Stage III	Cancer in one or both ovaries, spread to lymph nodes or to other parts of abdomen or to surface of liver or intestines.	**Dysgerminoma:** Total abdominal hysterectomy and bilateral salpingo-oophorectomy and tumor debulking. If remaining cancer is very small, external radiation following surgery; **or** same as above, but if remaining cancer is large, systemic chemotherapy following surgery; **or** if you wish to remain fertile, surgery to remove only ovary and fallopian tube involved, followed by chemotherapy. **Other cell types:** Total abdominal hysterectomy and bilateral salpingo-oophorectomy and tumor debulking, followed by chemotherapy. If cancer remains following chemotherapy, further surgery to remove tumor followed by further chemotherapy if there is still active cancer; **or** systemic chemotherapy followed by total abdominal hysterectomy, bilateral salpingo-oophorectomy and tumor debulking. Possible further chemotherapy; **or** if cancer found only in ovary and fallopian tube on same side and you want to remain fertile, unilateral salpingo-oophorectomy followed by chemotherapy.
Stage IV	Cancer in one or both ovaries and spread outside abdomen or inside liver.	**Dysgerminoma:** Total abdominal hysterectomy and bilateral salpingo-oophorectomy plus tumor debulking. Chemotherapy following surgery. If cancer remains, additional chemotherapy with different drugs; **or** if cancer found only in ovary and fallopian tube on same side and you want to remain fertile, unilateral salpingo-oophorectomy followed by chemotherapy. **Other cell types:** Total abdominal hysterectomy and bilateral salpingo-oophorectomy plus tumor debulking. Chemotherapy following surgery. If cancer remains, further surgery plus additional chemotherapy with different drug; **or** systemic chemotherapy followed by total abdominal hysterectomy and bilateral salpingo-oophorectomy and tumor debulking. Possible further chemotherapy; **or** if only in one ovary and fallopian tube on same side and you want to remain fertile, unilateral salpingo-oophorectomy followed by chemotherapy.
Recurrent	Cancer recurs after treatment, either in remaining ovary or elsewhere.	**Dysgerminoma:** Systemic chemotherapy with or without radiation. **Other cell types:** Systemic chemotherapy.

What is the difference between ovarian epithelial cancers and ovarian germ cell cancers?

Germ cell cancers, of which there are a number of different types, appear to be more aggressive than epithelial cancers, and therefore different treatments are prescribed. The most common type of germ cell cancer is the dysgerminoma. These rare tumors are seen most often in young women or adolescent girls and usually affect only one ovary. They are generally curable if found and treated early. The use of chemotherapy after initial surgery is very successful in treating germ cell cancers of the ovary. Dysgerminomas, when they are confined to the ovary, are less than ten centimeters in size and have an intact, smooth capsule unattached to other organs, have a high cure rate when treated with conservative surgery. One or more successful pregnancies following unilateral salpingo-oophorectomy have been reported by women who were treated.

Is chemotherapy successful in treating ovarian germ cell cancers?

Almost all patients who have ovarian germ cell cancers can benefit from postoperative chemotherapy. The use of platinum-based combination chemotherapy has improved the treatment of many types of ovarian germ cell cancers such as endodermal sinus tumors, immature teratomas, embryonal carcinomas, choriocarcinomas and mixed tumors containing one or more of these elements.

Do primary cancers grow in the fallopian tubes?

Cancer that starts in the fallopian tubes is the rarest cancer of the female genital tract and is often difficult to distinguish from ovarian cancer. Symptoms can include excessive bleeding, vaginal discharge or pains in the abdomen or pelvis. Diagnosis is usually only possible with exploratory surgery. Usually treatment is hysterectomy with removal of the ovaries and fallopian tubes with lymph node dissection. Radiation is usually given following surgery. Chemotherapy is sometimes used.

CANCER OF THE VAGINA

What is cancer of the vagina?

Cancer of the vagina is an uncommon, highly treatable, often curable cancer which grows in the passageway between the cervix and the vulva. This part of the body is often referred to as the birth canal. Squamous cell vaginal cancer is most often found in women over the age of 50. An even rarer type of vaginal cancer is clear cell adenocarcinoma, found most often in young women between the ages of 17 and 21. This type of cancer is associated with DES (diethylstilbestrol). It is believed that daughters of women who took DES to prevent miscarriage between 1945 and 1971 are at a risk of developing clear cell adenocarcinoma. (Treatment for adeno-carcinoma may differ from treatment for squamous cell vaginal cancer and treatment should be handled by someone experienced in this field.

TREATMENT CHOICES FOR VAGINAL CANCER (SQUAMOUS CELL)

STAGE	TREATMENT
Stage 0 or in situ, found inside vagina only, early	Removal of vagina with or without skin grafting; **or** partial or total removal with skin grafting; **or** intravaginal chemotherapy with 5% fluorouracil cream; **or** laser surgery; **or** intracavitary radiation.
Stage I, not spread outside vagina.	*If less than 0.5 cm thick:* Intracavitary radiation; **or** surgery with skin grafting. *If greater than 0.5 cm thick:* Radical vaginectomy with lymph node dissection; **or** internal radiation; **or** external radiation.
Stage II, spread outside vagina, but not to bones of pelvis	Radiation, both internal and external; **or** surgery plus radiation.
Stage III, spread to bones of pelvis, other organs and lymph nodes	Combination internal radiation and external radiation; **or** surgery may be combined with above.
Stage IV-A, spread to bladder or rectum	Combination internal and external radiation; **or** surgery may be combined with above; **or** clinical trials.
Stage IV-B, spread to other parts of body, such as lungs	Radiation; **or** clinical trials.
Recurrent, comes back in vagina or another place	Difficult to treat. Clinical trials should be considered.

What kind of follow-up is needed for vaginal cancers?
Lifelong follow-up is important for women with vaginal cancers. For the first year, follow-up will probably be every three months.

Pap smears and tumor markers should be checked at this time with chest x-rays, urine and stool testing every three months for the first six months and then at six-month intervals until the fifth year. Thereafter, yearly checkups should be scheduled. Tell the doctor if you have vaginal discharge or bleeding, bone pain, weight or appetite loss, bowel or bladder problems or swelling of the legs. Routine examinations are an important factor in detecting problems early and raising the cure rates for vaginal cancer.

Must special care be taken after having a radiation implant in the vagina?

The procedure for radiation implants is explained in Chapter 7, "Radiation Treatment." However, there are a few additional points which you will need to know about if you are having vaginal radiation implant treatments. For two to three weeks following the implant, you should not use tampons, should not have intercourse and should not douche or take tub baths. After the this period, it is necessary, in the interest of proper healing, for you either to use a dilator or to have intercourse in order to prevent the vaginal cavity from closing and/or forming adhesions. Since the implant often causes vaginal dryness, use of a water-soluble lubricant may make intercourse more comfortable. It is advised that you have intercourse two or three times a week or use a dilator to help the tissues begin to stretch. Some degree of discomfort and perhaps a little bleeding may be noticed. The use of the vaginal dilator is described later in this chapter in the section entitled "Sexual and Urinary Problems Following Gynecological Treatments."

Is it normal for intercourse to hurt following vaginal surgery?

Intercourse may cause you some pain following this surgery. The cause may be a combination of physical and psychological factors. You should first check with your doctor or nurse whether there are physical reasons why you feel pain. The use of medicine, including antispasmodics and analgesics, may be advised to help you relax before intercourse and prevent a tightening of your pelvic muscles, which can make intercourse uncomfortable. Touching and exploring the vaginal area with your fingers may help you gain confidence. Short-term behavioral sexual therapy, with instruction in relaxation and desensitization techniques, or consultation with a sex therapist, may be helpful.

Is reconstruction done following vaginal cancer surgery?

If possible, plans for reconstruction should be made before original surgery, although reconstruction may be possible at a later date even if not preplanned. Just as women who have undergone mastectomies may have breast reconstruction, women who have vaginal surgery (or colpectomies) may have plastic surgery to reconstruct the vagina. Women who have had this reconstruction say it is possible to regain former sensations and feelings. Partners report pleasurable, successful sexual relations following this surgery. Reconstruction is often done in stages, and may involve several separate surgeries done several weeks or months apart. Consultation with a reputable plastic surgeon who will do the reconstruction, as well as with the surgeon who performs the surgery, is necessary.

CANCER OF THE VULVA

What is cancer of the vulva?

The vulva is the outer part of the vagina and looks much like a pair of lips. It is made up of several structures including the clitoris, labia, and the hymen. Cancer in this area is rare, most often occurs in women over 50, although it can sometimes occur in women under the age of 40. Most of these cancers are found to be of the squamous cell type. Women who have constant itching and changes in the color and texture of the vulva are at high risk for getting cancer of the vulva. Surgery is the most common treatment for vulvar cancer. Vulvar cancer is highly curable when diagnosed in an early stage, before nodes become involved.

QUESTIONS TO ASK YOUR DOCTOR BEFORE BEING TREATED FOR VULVAR CANCER

- How extensive will the surgery be?
- What exactly will be removed?
- Will the clitoris be removed?
- Where will the scars be located?
- Will this procedure change my normal urination, voiding and sexual patterns?
- How long will I be in the hospital?
- How long will recovery take?
- How long will the surgery take?
- How long before stitches are removed?
- Following surgery, what kinds of complications should I report to the doctor and what doctor will I report to?

TREATMENT CHOICES FOR VULVAR CANCER

STAGE	WHAT IT MEANS	TREATMENT
Stage 0 or in situ; very early stage	Found only in vulva on surface of skin.	Surgery with wide localized excision; **and/or** laser surgery. (NOTE: if a simple vulvectomy, the removal of the entire vulva, is suggested, you should know that more limited surgical procedures, such as skinning or partial vulvectomy, produce equivalent results and are less drastic. Topical fluorouracil is **not** a reliable first choice of treatment.)
Stage I	Found only in vulva and/or in perineum (between opening of rectum and vagina); two centimeters (one inch) or less in size.	Wide localized surgery; **or** radical local surgery with removal of all lymph nodes in groin on same side; **or** radical vulvectomy and lymph node removal in groin and upper part of thigh on both sides; **or** if unable to tolerate surgery, radiation therapy.
Stage II	Found in vulva and in perineum (between opening of rectum and vagina); larger than two centimeters (one inch) in size.	Modified radical vulvectomy, removal of lymph nodes in groin and upper part of thigh on both sides; **or** if unable to tolerate surgery, radiation alone.
Stage III	Found in vulva and/or perineum (space between rectum and vagina) and has spread to lower part of urethra and/or vagina and/or anus and/or has spread to nearby lymph nodes.	Modified radical or radical vulvectomy, removal of lymph nodes in groin and upper thigh on both sides of body. Radiation given to pelvis if cancer found in lymph nodes; **or** radiation followed by radical vulvectomy and removal of lymph nodes on both sides of body; **or** radiation with or without chemotherapy (selected patients). *(continued)*

TREATMENT CHOICES FOR
VULVAR CANCER *(cont.)*

STAGE	WHAT IT MEANS	TREATMENT
Stage IV	Spread beyond urethra, vagina and anus into lining of bladder and bowel or spread to lymph nodes in pelvis or other parts of body.	Radical vulvectomy and removal of lower colon, rectum or bladder, depending on location of cancer, along with removal of uterus, cervix and vagina (pelvic exenteration); **or** radical vulvectomy followed by radiation; **or** radiation therapy followed by radical vulvectomy; **or** radiation therapy (selected patients) with or without chemotherapy.
Recurrent	Cancer returns after treatment.	Surgery to remove new cancer; **or** radical vulvectomy plus pelvic exenteration; **or** radiation plus chemotherapy; **or** clinical trials.

- Should I expect swelling in my legs, groin, and feet due to the lymph node dissection?
- How long will it be before swelling from lymph node dissection ceases?
- Will my sexual responses be changed by the surgery?
- How long before I can resume sexual intercourse?
- How long before I can use tampons?
- Is it wise for me to use a vaginal douche?
- How long before I can resume normal activities?

What are the surgical procedures used for cancer of the vulva?

The technical terms for the various operations include: wide local excision, which removes the cancer and some of the skin around it; skinning vulvectomy, which removes only the skin of the vulva; partial vulvectomy, which takes out less than the entire vulva; simple vulvectomy, which takes out the entire vulva, but no lymph nodes; and radical vulvectomy, which removes the entire vulva and the lymph nodes around it. If the cancer has spread outside the vulva and the other female organs, the doctor may have to perform a pelvic exenteration—the surgical removal of the lower colon, rectum, or bladder as well as the cervix, uterus and vagina. Following surgery, reconstruction with plastic surgery and skin grafts may be done to create an artificial vulva or vagina.

What are the possible complications of a radical vulvectomy?

Following the operation, because of the removal of a large number of lymph nodes, fluid collects under the skin and may be a problem until other lymph channels have become established. For this reason, deep breathing, coughing and leg exercises are started immediately after surgery. Frequent irrigations with sterile saline solution, heat lamp treatments and sitz baths are also used to promote healing.

Is sexual intercourse possible after vulvectomy?

Intercourse is still possible though you may have to change position or technique. Removal of the vulva may cause the remaining vaginal tissues to tighten, making intercourse and physical examination more difficult. Intercourse and/or stretching of the vagina right after the operation is important to make sure that the tissues will remain supple and elastic.

Is laser beam therapy used for cancer of the vulva?

Laser beam therapy may be used either alone or with wide local excision for Stage 0 vulvar cancer.

Is radiation treatment used for cancer of the vulva?

Radiation treatment is sometimes done, followed by surgery, or in some cases the surgery is followed by radiation.

SEXUAL AND URINARY PROBLEMS FOLLOWING GYNECOLOGICAL TREATMENTS

What sexual changes can I expect after treatment for gynecological cancer?

First and foremost, you should have a frank discussion with your doctor before the surgery, if possible, so that you know what to expect and so that you can mentally start dealing with the issues. When you first have sexual intercourse after having had treatment, you will probably worry about pain and think that your sexual life will never be the same as it was before. Don't be surprised if your first attempt is disappointing. You will probably have to make adjustments. Talk with your doctor or nurse about sex and discuss what the doctor tells you with your partner. Good communication is essential at this time. Tell your partner if you hurt and what feels good or painful. Remember that no matter what kind of cancer treatment you have had, the ability to feel pleasure from being touched almost always remains. Even if some aspects of sexuality have changed, pleasure is still possible.

What are the most common symptoms that interfere with sexual functioning following gynecological treatment?

Lack of desire and pain are two of the most commonly heard problems. Lack of desire immediately after treatment may be caused by worry, depression, and pain. Pain during intercourse can be caused by changes in the body as the result of treatment. Pain can occur after surgery, radiation or other treatment that affects the hormonal balance. The pain can set off a series of further problems. Sometimes just one incidence of painful intercourse can cause the muscles around the opening of the vagina to tense up and make intercourse impossible and unpleasant.

How can I learn to relax my vaginal muscles?

There are a set of exercises called Kegel exercises, which can help teach you to relax and thus lessen pain during intercourse.

- The muscles around the entrance to the vagina are the same ones that stop the flow of urine. When you urinate, try stopping the flow of urine for a few seconds. Be aware of the muscles you use to make this happen. Relax your muscles and let the urine flow again.
- Practice using those muscles when you are not urinating. First, tighten the muscles in the genital area. To check whether you are tightening the right muscles, try slipping one finger about two inches into your vagina. When you tense your vaginal muscles, you will feel a slight twitch of the vaginal walls around your finger.
- Once you know the muscles that need relaxing you can do the exercise anywhere—while reading, sitting in the car or watching television. Just tighten your vaginal muscle, count to three and relax. Do this ten times in a row, several times a day.
- During intercourse, make sure you are well lubricated. Use the same technique to tense and relax your vaginal muscles. The action will help you focus on your excitement and will add to your partner's pleasure.
- If you begin to feel tightness or pain, stay still for a moment while you gently squeeze your vaginal muscles around your partner's penis. Notice the looseness when you relax your muscles.
- If you still have pain, you may need the help of your gynecolo-

gist or a sex therapist. Some doctors recommend using a series of vaginal dilators in different sizes to stretch the vagina.

How is a vaginal dilator used?

A vaginal dilator can be helpful in stretching the vagina. Dilators are cylinder- or tube-shaped and usually made of plastic. They come in various sizes. Your doctor will prescribe the correct size for you. Usually you will start with one about the size of a finger, then the size is increased until the vagina has stretched enough to allow a man's penis to enter without pain. To use the dilator, lubricate it well with a water-based gel. Lie down in bed or put your foot up on the toilet and gently and slowly insert the dilator into the vagina. If you feel tight, tense and relax your muscles, then put the dilator farther into the vagina. You may need to squeeze and relax a few times before the dilator is fully inserted. Sometimes it is helpful to bear down as if having a bowel movement. When the dilator is in as far as possible, leave it in your vagina for about ten minutes. NOTE: When the vagina has been rebuilt with skin grafts, a special dilator may be prescribed to be worn 24 hours a day for a period of time.

What is the effect of premature menopause on sexual intercourse?

Premature menopause, as caused by the removal of the ovaries, triggers severe and abrupt changes in the body. Besides causing hot flashes, the loss of estrogen causes the vagina to become tight and dry. Understanding the consequences of this type of treatment and compensating for it with the use of extra lubrication can help to make intercourse more comfortable. There are many water-based gel vaginal lubricants available. You may find that a vaginal moisturizer can help relieve dryness. There are many on the market, such as Astroglide, K-Y Jelly, Lubrin or Condom Mate, Ortho Personal Lubricant, Replens, Surgilube and Today Personal Lubricant. Replens, which is used three times weekly, keeps the vagina moist at all times, helps normalize the PH balance and helps prevent yeast infections.

How does a radical vulvectomy affect sexual functioning?

When the whole vulva, including the inner and outer lips and the clitoris, and sometimes lymph nodes in the area are surgically removed, there may be a problem with reaching orgasm. The outer genitals, especially the clitoris, are the centers of sexual sensitivity. Additionally, there may be a feeling of numbness in the genital area, which may return over the period of a few months. When scarring is severe, the surgeon may do reconstructive surgery with skin grafts to correct the problem of a narrowed vaginal entrance.

How is a vagina reconstructed?

Several methods are used. Skin grafts are the most common method. Following such a reconstruction, a special vaginal mold is designed to be worn internally. At first it is worn 24 hours a day. Gradually, it is worn for part of the day. In about three months, regular sexual intercourse or the use of a plastic tube (dilator) to stretch out the vagina for a short time daily is enough to keep the vagina open. Without dilation, the vagina will shrink and close. If the entire vagina needs to be rebuilt, flaps of muscle and skin from both inner thighs are used. The surgeon forms the flaps from each side into a closed tube which is lined by the skin surface and then is sewn into the area where the vagina was removed. When the new vagina heals, it is similar in size and shape to the one which was surgically removed. Learning to live with a redesigned vagina means that couples need to make adjustments in their sexual patterns. Different intercourse positions may need to be tried to bring pleasure since the muscles ringing the vaginal entrance no longer can be contracted at will and nerve sensations are connected to the original nerve supplies at the inner thigh. Some women who have had the surgery say that changes in sensations due to the surgery can be sexually interesting and stimulating.

What is the result of lymph node removal in the genital area?

When lymph nodes in the groin are removed, swelling can occur in the genital area and in the legs. The problems, referred to as lymphedema, can be similar to those described in Chapter 11, "Breast Cancer," except that they occur in another part of the body. For more information about this side effect, get in touch with the Lymphedema Network. See Chapter 26, "Where to Get Help," for address and telephone.

PREGNANCY AND GYNECOLOGICAL CANCERS

What happens if you get cancer in the reproductive area when you are pregnant?

Pregnancy complicated by a diagnosis of cancer in the reproductive organs is very rare indeed, but when it happens, it creates an incredible range of multiple problems, both physical and emotional. In general, most cancers do not, in and of themselves, impact on the outcome of the pregnancy, although the pregnancy is certainly complicated by the diagnosis of cancer. Unless continued pregnancy will compromise treatment and thus prognosis, therapeutic abortion has not been shown to be of benefit in altering the progression of the cancer. The risks of abortion and fetal malformation from radiation and chemotherapy are highest during the first trimester and vary with treatments used. During the second and third trimesters, the evidence of increased risk appears to be minimal. Most doctors feel that if cure is a reasonable goal, treatment should not be compromised by modification or delay. However, if treatment for cure or significant relief is not possible, the goal must then shift to these altered priorities. (There is information concerning breast cancer and pregnancy in Chapter 11, "Breast Cancer.") The discovery of cancer during pregnancy is a highly traumatic event that needs to be carefully evaluated before any decisions are made.

What happens when cancer of the cervix is found during pregnancy?

Most of the cancers of the cervix found during pregnancy are Stage 0 or in situ cancers. Invasive cancer of the cervix is seen in only 2 to 5 percent of all cases. Symptoms are similar to those found in nonpregnant women. Very often, with Stage 0 or in situ cancers, pregnancy is allowed to continue and treatment delayed until after delivery, unless the disease appears to be spreading. If invasion is found during the first two trimesters, surgery or radiation therapy without therapeutic abortion is usually the treatment. During the third trimester, the baby, when viable, may be delivered by cesarean section, with appropriate treatment undertaken after the delivery. There is an unresolved controversy over the safety of vaginal delivery versus cesarean delivery. Some doctors recommend cesarean delivery because they feel that vaginal delivery may disseminate the cancer or cause hemorrhage or infection. One study reported recurrence in an episiotomy after vaginal delivery. Other doctors suggest that vaginal delivery actually may be beneficial and should be planned if possible. Careful follow-up is essential.

What is done when ovarian masses appear during pregnancy?

Though ovarian masses are common during pregnancy, only about 2 to 5 percent become malignant. There are several approaches to treatment. Some doctors feel that a mass that is larger than five centimeters that continues into the second trimester should be explored. Others feel that a mass over six centimeters should be evaluated immediately. Yet others feel that a single, encapsulated, movable mass under ten centimeters can wait until the second trimester for evaluation. However, if the mass is found to be cancerous, treatment should continue just as it would in someone who is not pregnant. Early stage disease may be managed by removal of the affected ovary and biopsy of the other ovary. The pregnancy may be allowed to continue. If the patient is near delivery, a cesarean section, followed by the appropriate therapy, is usually the choice. For other stages and scenarios, standard treatment should be followed. As in the treatment of all cancers, the wishes of the patient will be considered. It is not uncommon for a pregnant woman with advanced disease to delay treatment until the fetus is viable. In every case, treatment should be started at the earliest possible time.

What are gestational trophoblastic tumors?

A group of rare cancers known as gestational trophoblastic tumors grow in the uterus in the tissues that are formed after a woman conceives. Hydatidiform moles and choriocarcinoma are the two most common of these cancers. Hydatidiform mole, sometimes called molar pregnancy, occurs when the sperm and egg cells join but do not succeed in forming a fetus. The tissue that grows in the uterus resembles grapelike cysts and does not spread outside the uterus. Choriocarcinoma may develop from a hydatidiform mole or from tissue that remains in the uterus following an abortion or delivery of a baby. It can spread outside the uterus to other parts of the body. A third, very rare type of gestational trophoblastic tumor, which starts where the placenta was attached in the uterus, is known as placental-site trophoblastic tumor. Before chemotherapy, many of these cancers were considered fatal. Choriocarcinoma was the first malignancy which proved to be curable by chemotherapy after it had metastasized. Today, the cure rate is 97 to 100 percent for those which have not metastasized, and 75 percent for those listed as metastatic with poor prognosis. The major factors are early diagnosis, proper treatment and careful follow-up.

What is the HCG ?

The HCG measures serum beta human chorionic gonadotropin, which is produced normally during pregnancy. In patients with gestational trophoblastic tumors, HCG is abnormally elevated in the blood and urine. The doctor measures the HCG titer level, which serves as a sensitive marker to indicate the presence or absence of activity of the cancer before, during, and after treatment.

TREATMENT CHOICES FOR GESTATIONAL TROPHOBLASTIC TUMOR (MOLES AND CHORIOCARCINOMA)

TYPE	WHAT IT MEANS	TREATMENT
Hydatidiform mole	Confined to inside of uterus, does not spread outside uterus. If found in muscle of uterus, called invasive mole (chorioadenoma destruens).	D&C, suction evacuation, preservation of childbearing ability; **or** hysterectomy, ovaries not removed. Close monitoring. Chemotherapy if levels of BHCG rise, tissue diagnosis shows choriocarcinoma or postevacuation hemorrhage not caused by retained tissues occurs.
Placental-site trophoblastic	Found where placenta was attached and in muscle of uterus, very rare.	Hysterectomy. (These tumors are relatively resistant to chemotherapy.)
Nonmetastatic choriocarcinoma (chorioadenoma destruens) (these are the most common types, considered 100 percent curable)	Found inside uterus from tissue remaining following hydatidiform mole or following abortion or delivery. Has not spread outside uterus.	Single-agent chemotherapy; **or** hysterectomy if fertility is no longer desired.
Good-prognosis metastatic (gestational trophoblastic choriocarcinoma)	As above, but spread to other parts of the body but last pregnancy less than 4 months prior, beta HCG level is low, has not spread to liver or brain, has never had chemotherapy.	Single-agent chemotherapy; **or** hysterectomy followed by chemotherapy; **or** chemotherapy followed by hysterectomy if cancer remains following chemotherapy.

(continued)

TREATMENT CHOICES FOR GESTATIONAL TROPHOBLASTIC TUMOR (MOLES AND CHORIOCARCINOMA) *(cont.)*

TYPE	WHAT IT MEANS	TREATMENT
Poor prognosis metastatic, choriocarcinoma*	As above, with spread to other parts of the body and if any of the following: pregnancy more than 4 months ago, beta HCG level high, cancer spread to liver or brain, have had chemotherapy which did not eradicate cancer or tumor began after normal pregnancy.	Multiple-agent chemotherapy. Radiation to places where cancer has spread, such as to brain. Radiation to liver not recommended, can lead to myelosuppression that may make administration of chemotherapy more difficult.
Recurrent	Cancer returns after treatment, either in uterus or other part of body.	Chemotherapy.

* Any patient with a poor prognosis metastatic gestational trophoblastic tumor needs therapy quickly. There are hospitals with trophoblastic centers where there are physicians with experience in treating this type of cancer.

What kind of follow-up is suggested for gestational trophoblastic tumors?

Careful follow-up is essential—a pelvic examination every other week and a chest x-ray every four to six weeks. Beta HCG testing should be done weekly until it has fallen to normal levels, then every two weeks for three months, then every six months for three years.

DES-RELATED CANCERS

What is DES and what is its connection to cancer of the cervix and vagina?

DES is a synthetic form of estrogen, also known as diethylstilbestrol. It was prescribed from the early 1940s until 1971 to help women with certain complications of pregnancies. It has been found that when given during the first five months of pregnancy, DES interfered with the development of the reproductive system in a fetus.

A link has been found between DES exposure before birth and an increased risk of developing abnormal cells in the tissue of the cervix and vagina. These abnormal cells resemble cancer cells in appearance. However, they do not invade nearby healthy tissue the way cancer cells do. They usually occur between the ages of 25 and 35 in women whose mothers took DES. DES-exposed daughters may also have structural changes in the vagina, uterus, or cervix. Most of these changes do not cause medical problems but some women may have irregular menstruation and an increased risk of miscarriage and premature delivery. There is some evidence that DES-exposed sons may have testicular abnormalities, such as undescended testicles or abnormally small testicles, although the risk of testicular cancer or infertility has not shown an increase.

Where can DES-exposed people get additional information?

DES Action is a consumer group organized by individuals who were exposed to DES. DES Cancer Network provides information about DES-related cancer. See Chapter 26, " Where to Get Help," for addresses and telephone numbers.

chapter 19

Bone and Soft Tissue Sarcomas

Bone and soft tissue sarcomas are cancers of the structural and connective tissues of the body. They include bone (osteosarcoma), cartilage (chondrosarcoma), fibrous connective tissue (fibrosarcoma), fat (liposarcoma), muscle (myosarcoma), and blood vessels (angiosarcoma). While most of these can appear at any age, osteosarcoma is most common in young people between 10 and 25 and chondrosarcoma is more common between 30 and 60. Bone cancers are extremely rare—only about 2,000 new cases are diagnosed each year. Soft tissue cancers are also quite unusual, with a total of about 6,000 new cases each year. Molecular genetics are being studied in musculo-skeletal tumors, and perhaps in the future, genetic therapy will help to alleviate some bone cancers.

For those who are dealing with a diagnosis of sarcoma, it is reassuring to know that increased knowledge about bone and soft tissue sarcomas and a multidisciplinary approach to treatment have improved the results of bone and soft tissue tumor treatment in recent years. (Osteosarcoma, Ewing's sarcoma, and rhabdomyosarcoma are discussed in Chapter 22, "Childhood Cancers." Multiple myeloma is covered in Chapter 17, "Lymphomas and, Multiple Myeloma.")

WHAT YOU NEED TO KNOW ABOUT BONE AND SOFT TISSUE CANCERS

- Sarcomas are cancers that begin in the structural and connective tissues. They are divided into two groups: those that begin in the bone and those that begin in the muscles, fat and other connective or supportive tissues of the body (soft tissue sarcomas).

- Cancers that begin in the bone are quite rare. (Cancers that spread to the bone are more common. This chapter deals only with cancers that **start in the bone,** not those that have spread to the bone.)

- Because these cancers are rare, it is important to be seen at a major medical or research center where there are specialists with expertise in diagnosing and treating these cancers.

- Most tumors in the bone are found to be benign. A very small percentage are cancerous.

- Cancer can occur in any of the 206 bones in the body—but it occurs most often in the arms and legs.

- Children and young people are more likely than adults to have primary bone cancers.

- Surgery is the most common treatment for most bone cancers (except for Ewing's sarcoma).

- Until recently, amputation was considered the best treatment for bone cancers in the arm or leg. Today, limb-sparing surgery is possible in many cases with the use of preoperative or postoperative chemotherapy. Even high-grade soft tissue sarcomas in the arms and legs can often be treated while preserving the limb.

- **Inappropriately performed biopsy must be avoided** since it can ruin chances of having limb-sparing surgery.

- Soft tissue sarcomas can grow anywhere in the body. The largest percentage develop at or above the knee or in the trunk. Fifteen percent develop in arms and hands, 10 percent in the head and neck and about 10 percent in the back wall of the abdominal cavity. Some of these are so well hidden by overlying normal tissue that they may become quite large before being noticed.

- When bone cancers spread, they do so through the bloodstream, since bones do not have a lymph system.

SYMPTOMS

BONE CANCER

- Pain.
- Swelling or mass.
- Stiffness or tenderness in the affected area.
- Loss of bladder or bowel function (if cancer is in pelvic bones or base of spine).
- Bone fractures.

SOFT TISSUE SARCOMAS

- Enlarging, nontender swelling or mass.
- Pressure against nearby nerves and muscles.

Are sarcomas difficult to diagnose?

Because they are seen infrequently, sarcomas may be misdiagnosed, confused with benign disease or overlooked. CT scans, MRI and ultrasounds will show changes in bone or cartilage. They also can show abnormal changes in softer tissues. A bone scan can detect sarcomas of the bone. Arteriograms or angiograms depict blood vessels, showing whether they are pushed aside or whether the tumor has an abnormal blood supply. Chemical changes in the blood are often found in sarcomas of bone. Chest x-rays are important in evaluating sarcomas because these cancers have a tendency to spread to the lungs. The biopsy is the final diagnostic procedure. It is usually done as an open biopsy rather than as a needle biopsy to get an adequate piece of tumor so that treatment can be properly staged. **If the sarcoma affects a bone in the arm or leg, the biopsy should be done by the surgeon who will be doing the limb-sparing surgery. An inappropriately done biopsy can make it impossible to achieve limb-sparing surgery.**

Is there a blood test that can detect cancer of the bone?

A blood test to determine the level of alkaline phosphatase, an enzyme produced by cells that form new bone tissue, is often used in detecting bone tumors. However, this enzyme is also found in large amounts in the blood for other reasons, for instance when children or adolescents are growing, when a bone is mending or when a disease causes the production of an abnormal amount of bone tissue. Therefore, this blood test can be used only as an indicator, not as a definitive diagnostic test.

What kind of doctor should be treating bone or soft tissue sarcomas?

Since these two types of cancers are extremely rare, specialists experienced in treating these types of cancer are most likely to be found at large cancer treatment and research centers. Since the selection of treatment is determined by the information gleaned from a biopsy, careful review of the biopsy tissue by a pathologist experienced in these types of cancers is important. Complete staging and planning treatment by a multidisciplinary team of cancer specialists—pathologists, surgeons, radiation oncologists and medical oncologists—who can review all of the information gathered in the diagnostic and staging procedures, will assure that the very latest and best treatment is given.

Why is the biopsy so important in staging bone and soft tissue sarcomas?

Treatment will be based on the type of cells found in the biopsy tissue. Having the advice of an orthopedic surgical oncologist **before** biopsy is important since the biopsy may have an impact on how subsequent surgery is performed.

What causes bone and soft tissue sarcomas?

Relatively little is known regarding the cause of these cancers. It does appear that prior cancer therapy in the form of high-dose radiation and some chemotherapy drugs (the alkylating agents) may be linked to the development of primary bone cancer. Osteosarcoma, the most common type of bone cancer that occurs frequently in adolescents during peak years of bone growth, may be triggered by overactivity of bone cells. A small number of families in which siblings have developed osteosarcoma are being studied to see if there is a genetic defect. Children with hereditary retinoblastoma also are at high risk for developing osteosarcoma. Doctors stress that sarcomas are definitely not related to common injuries, although athletic injuries in children often bring about discovery of a sarcoma. The single exception appears to be the more-than-coincidental occurrence of sarcomas in the scars of serious burns. In experimental animals, both chemicals and viruses cause sarcomas.

What kind of follow-up is recommended for sarcomas?

Because these tumors are unusual, follow-up must be customized. However, during the first two years, repeat visits to the physician will probably be scheduled for every three months. The third year, every four months, the fourth and fifth year, every six months, and thereafter every year.

BONE CANCERS

What is bone cancer?

Bone cancer occurs when the cells in the bone begin to grow in a disorderly or uncontrolled way. Tumors in bones may be benign or cancerous. Benign tumors are more common than cancerous ones. Both grow in the same way, compressing adjacent healthy bone tissue, sometimes absorbing the healthy tissue and replacing it with abnormal tissue. A benign tumor is limited to the bone in which it develops. Bone cancers destroy the outer layer of the bone and can invade surrounding soft tissues and other bones. Sometimes cells from bone cancers, like all other types of cancer, break away from the primary tumor and spread.

How are bone cancers staged?

Information collected from the physical examination, laboratory tests, x-rays and, finally, from the biopsy, reveal the location and size of the tumor and whether it has spread. For some bone cancers, the pathologist's determination of the grade of the cancer cells is done to help predict the aggressiveness of a tumor based on the appearance of the cells. Bone cancers have two grades. Low-grade tumors are likely to spread outward from the original tumor but are not likely to metastasize. High-grade tumors grow rapidly, spread to surrounding tissues and metastasize to other parts of the body. Stage I disease includes low-grade tumors without metastases; Stage II, high-grade tumors without metastases; Stage III, any grade tumors with metastases. In general, the type of bone cancer is not as important in selecting treatment as its location, size and extent of spread.

What is osteosarcoma?

Osteosarcoma, the most common type of bone cancer, originates in the newly forming tissue of the bone and develops in the long bones of the arms and legs. It contains immature bone cells that destroy and replace normal tissue, weakening the bone.

MAJOR TYPES OF BONE CANCER

TYPE	DESCRIPTION
Osteosarcoma or **osteogenic sarcoma** (also discussed in Chapter 22, "Childhood Cancers")	Most common type, contains immature bone cells which destroy and replace normal tissue, weakening bone. Usually occurs in large bones of upper arm and leg; 10–25 age group.
Chondrosarcoma	Made up of abnormal cartilage. Usually occurs in pelvis, upper leg, shoulder; 30–60 age group.
Ewing's sarcoma (see Chapter 22)	Begins in immature nerve tissue, usually in bone marrow. Occurs in leg, hip, arm; 10–20 age group.
Malignant giant cell tumor	Begins in connecting tissue of bone marrow. Weakens knee or vertebra, causes bone fractures. Occurs in 40–55 age group.
Fibrosarcoma of bone	Begins in connective tissue within bone marrow cavity. Seen in leg, arm, hip. Occurs in 30–40 age group.
Chordoma	Cellular remnants of fetal spinal cord. Occurs in upper or lower end of spinal column or skull; 55–65 age group.
Parosteal sarcoma	Involves mid shaft of bone. Can often be cured by removing affected section of bone. Slow growing.
Adamantinoma and a group of types previously known as **reticulum cell sarcomas of the bone** now referred to as **malignant fibrous histiocytoma, small round cell sarcomas,** and **diffuse large cell lymphona of bone**	Rare.

Has treatment and outlook for those with osteosarcoma changed in the last twenty years?

Twenty years ago, only about 20 percent of patients with osteosarcoma lived five years or more after diagnosis. The only effective treatment was amputation and there was no known way to control metastasis. With the advent of adjuvant chemotherapy for this disease, five-year survival rates for osteogenic bone cancer patients who have no signs of metastasis at diagnosis are now up to 60 to 80 percent. Preoperative chemotherapy followed by surgery and postoperative chemotherapy are also being used. For tumors that cannot be removed, clinical studies are being conducted on the use of intensive chemotherapy and high-dose localized radiation. Osteosarcoma is discussed in more detail in Chapter 22, "Childhood Cancers."

What is chondrosarcoma?

Chondrosarcomas are sarcomas that grow in the cartilage. They can often cause swollen joints or restrict motion. They are found in the pelvic bone, long bones, scapula and ribs and less frequently in the bones of the hand, foot, nose and base of the skull. They can remain rather slow-growing, but when they become aggressive can metastasize to the lungs and heart.

What is fibrosarcoma?

This is a very rare form of bone cancer which may occur at any age but is rare in children. It is felt that Paget's disease is a predisposing factor in the development of fibrosarcoma. Fibrosarcomas may also develop in persons who have had radiation or at the site of a past bone fracture.

What is the usual primary treatment for most bone cancers?

Except for Ewing's sarcoma, the primary treatment is surgery. The most important consideration in planning surgery is to be certain that the primary tumor and all surrounding tissue where it may have begun to spread are removed. Whenever possible, a margin of healthy tissue also is removed to further reduce the chance that tumor cells remain. For the cancers that occur in the arm and leg, amputation was once considered the best treatment. However, preoperative and postoperative chemotherapy now make it possible to perform limb-sparing surgery in many cases. Some bone cancers are also treated with radiation therapy. (Treatment for Ewing's sarcoma is discussed in Chapter 22, "Childhood Cancers.")

What is a skip metastasis?

A skip metastasis is a tumor nodule located in the same bone as the main tumor but not in continuity with the tumor. It is usually located in the joint adjacent to the main tumor and is most often a high-grade sarcoma.

How are metastases to the lung treated in bone cancer?

If bone cancer does metastasize, more than 50 percent of the time it will occur in the lung. Surgery may be possible, depending on the size and number of metastatic tumors in the lung. Usually this surgery is preceded or followed by chemotherapy. Ifosfamide is also being used for recurrent osteoscarcoma.

What steps are necessary in limb-sparing operations?

A limb-sparing operation requires three steps. First, the tumor must be removed, along with a margin of healthy tissue. The removed segment is replaced with a bone graft or a metal prosthetic bone. The final step is the replacement of the removed margin tissue, usually muscle, with healthy tissue taken from another part of the body.

What circumstances might require amputation of a leg or arm?

Although every effort is made to avoid amputation and to preserve as much normal function as possible, there are some cases where it becomes necessary to amputate. For example, if it is impossible to remove an adequate amount of healthy tissue to assure that the tumor is totally removed, or if the neurovascular bundle is involved by the tumor, amputation may be necessary. Amputation also is recommended if a nonfunctional limb would result from the operation. Sometimes in children younger than 10 years of age, amputation is recommended because of skeletal development problems, although new expandable prostheses and rotationplasty are possible options that should be explored.

How is reconstruction accomplished when amputation occurs?

The doctor will explain the different kinds of reconstruction that are possible, and decisions must be made depending on the patient's functional needs. Fusion (called arthrodesis) may result in a stiff joint, but permits activities such as running and jumping. Arthroplasty with metallic or bone allograft is another choice. The implant, however, is an artificial joint that will not tolerate activities such as jogging, racquet sports or heavy lifting. The third choice is intercallary allograft reconstruction. Transplants of bone, tendon, ligaments and connective tissue are used. (Transplants are donated from accident victims and frozen.) Often a cast or brace must be worn for six to twelve months until the allograft is healed to the host bone.

Is it wise before having surgery to meet with someone who has had the same operation?

It may be helpful and encouraging to talk with someone who has been through such a surgery. Your doctor or the social workers at the hospital may be able to put you in touch with someone. The American Cancer Society also may be helpful. Rehabilitation requires patience, cooperation, coordination, and tremendous physical energy.

ADULT SOFT TISSUE SARCOMA

What is adult soft tissue sarcoma?

Soft tissue sarcomas are cancers that are found in the soft tissues of the body—the muscles, connective tissues or tendons, the vessels that carry blood or lymph, joints, and fat. Because these tissues are found in all parts of the body, the treatment can vary depending upon the location of the tumor. Since many soft tissue sarcomas are found in areas close to the bones of extremities, the hard decision of whether or not to amputate an arm or a leg must sometimes be made. However, even high-grade sarcomas of the arm and leg can often be effectively treated while preserving the limb, with pre- or postoperative radiation playing an important role.

What happens if a tumor is removed and then it is discovered to be a sarcoma?

It is not uncommon for this to happen. In this situation, surgery will need to be performed again to take a wider margin around the tumor. This is done to take out any microscopic tumor cells remaining, to lessen the likelihood of a local recurrence and the possibility of spread.

TYPES OF SOFT TISSUE SARCOMA

Type	Description
Fibrosarcoma	Often located deep in thigh or arms or trunk; may be large when found; 45–50s age group.
Synovial cell sarcomas; also called **synoviomas**; this type has tendency to spread to lymph nodes	Most commonly in leg, between thigh and knee, also hands and feet; 20–30 age group.
Rhabdomyosarcoma; has tendency to spread to lymph nodes	Usually found in thigh, shoulder, upper arm; may be large when found; 40–50 age group.
Liposarcoma	Often found in fatty tissue of thigh, also arms, legs or trunk; middle-aged men.
Leiomyosarcoma	Develop in smooth muscles of uterus, back part of abdominal cavity; very rare.
Hemangiosarcoma	Originates in blood vessels, found in arms, legs, trunk.
Lymphangiosarcoma	Develops in lymph vessels, usually in the arms.
Neurofibrosarcoma	Develops in peripheral nerves; arms, legs, trunk.
Chondrosarcoma	Usually seen in legs. Develops in cartilage and bone-forming tissue.

How are sarcomas staged?

Although the size of a soft tissue sarcoma is important, the kind of cell that makes up the tumor is a key factor in determining the stage. The more different the cancer cells look from normal cells, the higher the stage. Well-differentiated cancer cells (which means they resemble their normal counterparts) are considered low-grade. Since high-grade tumors are more likely to spread than low-grade ones, it is important for the physician to know this before making recommendations for treatment.

What tests may be used to determine treatment?

X-rays and scans of the affected area must be done so that the exact location and dimensions of the tumor can be determined. Possible tests, in addition to laboratory studies and a thorough physical examination, may include:

- X-ray called a xerogram or soft tissue radiograph.
- CT scans to give three-dimensional map of tumor and surrounding tissues.
- Tomogram.
- Arteriogram.
- MRI.
- Ultrasound.
- Biopsy (should be done in conjunction with surgical oncologist for best possibility of sparing limb).

<table>
<tr><td colspan="2" align="center">**TREATMENT FOR
ADULT SOFT TISSUE SARCOMA**</td></tr>
<tr><td>**STAGE**</td><td>**TREATMENT**</td></tr>
<tr>
<td>Stage I: Cells look quite normal (well differentiated); tumor less than 5 cm in size or if larger, has not spread to lymph nodes or other parts of body; not likely to metastasize but may recur locally if inadequately treated</td>
<td>*If in arm or leg:* Surgery to remove cancer; **or** radiation therapy followed by surgery; **or** surgery followed by radiation; **or** radiation before and after surgery. If inoperable, high-dose radiation.
If in head, neck, abdomen or trunk: Surgery with or without radiation; **or** radiation before and after surgery.</td>
</tr>
<tr>
<td>Stage II: Cells less normal looking (moderately well differentiated); tumor may be any size, but has not spread to lymph nodes or other parts of body. **CAUTION:** tumor may be surrounded by pseudocapsule containing tumor cells and surgery must remove adequate margins</td>
<td>*If in arm or leg:* Surgery to remove cancer with pre- or post-operative radiation; **or** surgery followed by radiation; **or** radiation alone; **or** radiation before and after surgery; **or** *Clinical trials:* New forms of radiation; **or** regional chemotherapy followed by limb-sparing surgery; **or** surgery with or without radiations therapy and adjuvant chemotherapy; **or** chemotherapy.
If in head, neck, abdomen or trunk: Surgery with or without radiation after surgery **or** radiation before and after surgery; **or** *Clinical trials:* Radiation during surgery; **or** surgery and adjuvant chemotherapy **or** chemotherapy.　*(continued)*</td>
</tr>
</table>

TREATMENT FOR
ADULT SOFT TISSUE SARCOMA *(cont.)*

STAGE	TREATMENT
Stage III: Cells are poorly differentiated or undifferentiated; tumor may be any size, but has not spread to other parts of body (See **CAUTION** on previous page)	*If in arm or leg:* Surgery; **or** surgery followed by radiation; **or** radiation alone; **or** radiation before and after surgery; **or** *Clinical trials:* New forms of radiation; **or** systemic or regional chemotherapy followed by surgery; **or** surgery with or without radiation followed by adjuvant chemotherapy. *If in head, neck, abdomen or trunk:* Surgery with or without radiation after surgery **or** Radiation before and after surgery; **or** *Clinical trials:* Radiation during surgery; **or** surgery followed by adjuvant chemotherapy.
Stage IV A: Cancer has spread to lymph nodes in area but not to other parts of body	Surgery to remove cancer and lymph nodes (lymph node dissection); **or** surgery as above followed by radiation; **or** radiation before and after surgery to remove cancer and lymph nodes (lymph node dissection).
Stage IV B: Cancer has spread to other parts of body such as lungs	Surgery to remove cancer with or without radiation after surgery; **or** radiation before and after surgery; **or** radiation alone; **or** chemotherapy to relieve pain and discomfort; **or** *Clinical trials:* New chemotherapy drugs; **or** biological therapy; **or** adjuvant chemotherapy.
Recurrent: Cancer has come back after being treated, either in tissues where it began or another part of body	Depends on previous treatment. Surgery to remove cancer; **or** surgery followed by radiation therapy; **or** preoperative radiation and surgery; **or** *Clinical trials:* chemotherapy.

KAPOSI'S SARCOMA

What is Kaposi's sarcoma?

Kaposi's sarcoma is a cancer that is found in the tissues under the skin or mucous membranes. It causes red-brown or purple patches on the skin, often on the legs, without other symptoms. It spreads to other organs in the body, such as the lung, liver, or intestinal tract. Until the early 1980s, Kaposi's sarcoma was considered a very rare disease that was found mainly in older men, patients who had organ transplants, or African men. In people who do not have AIDS, the disease develops slowly.

How does Kaposi's sarcoma differ in AIDS patients?

In the 1980s, doctors began to see many cases of Kaposi's sarcoma in people with AIDS. In these cases, Kaposi's sarcoma may be found in the mouth, nose, lymph nodes, gastrointestinal tract, lung, liver and spleen. Kaposi's sarcoma usually spreads more quickly in patients with AIDS. It may produce significant deterioration in the organ affected. About 30 percent of AIDS patients develop Kaposi's sarcoma. It is also sometimes seen in homosexual men who have no evidence of HIV infection.

How is Kaposi's sarcoma staged?

There is no true staging for Kaposi's sarcoma at this time. Patients are grouped according to one of three types of Kaposi's sarcoma—classic, immunosuppressive treatment related, epidemic (AIDS related) or recurrent. Treatment depends upon the type.

What is classic Kaposi's sarcoma?

This is considered a rare disease, usually found in older men (50 to 70) of Jewish, Italian, or Mediterranean heritage. The disease is usually limited to one or two patches, usually localized in one or both legs, often at the ankle or sole. It progresses slowly, sometimes over ten to fifteen years. The lower legs may swell and the blood may not be able to flow properly. After some time, it may spread to other organs and there is a possibility that another type of cancer may develop later on in life. Usually, the doctor will check the skin and lymph nodes of the patient at regular intervals.

What is immunosuppressive related Kaposi's sarcoma?

This type may occur in people who are taking immunosuppressants. It may occur in patients who have had kidney or liver transplants. In some cases, when patients were able to reduce or change the dosage of immunosuppressive drugs, the disease was controlled. In some cases, the Kaposi's sarcoma regressed.

TREATMENT CHOICES FOR KAPOSI'S SARCOMA

TYPE	TREATMENT
Classic: Progresses slowly, sometimes over 10–15 years	For solitary or limited lesions, radiation therapy; **or** local surgery. For widespread skin disease, radiation or chemotherapy. For lymph and gastrointestinal involvement, chemotherapy plus local radiation therapy for individual lesions.
Immunosuppressive: May occur in people taking drugs to suppress immune system for liver or kidney transplant	May be controlled if able to cease taking immunosuppressive drugs. If not or if does not work, radiation therapy if confined to skin; **or** *Clinical trials:* Chemotherapy.
Epidemic: Found in patients with AIDS; this type spreads more quickly than other kinds of Kaposi's sarcoma and often is found in many parts of body	Surgery, using local removal, electrodesiccation and curettage or cryotherapy; **or** intralesional chemotherapy; **or** systemic chemotherapy; **or** *Clinical trials:* New chemotherapy drugs, antiretroviral therapies; **or** biological therapy.
Recurrent: Kaposi's sarcoma which has come back after being treated, either in same area or another part of body	Depends on type, past treatment response and general health. May wish to take part in clinical trial.

chapter 20

Brain and Spinal Cord Cancers

The specter of brain cancer is one of the most terrifying of nightmares. We all instinctively fear any tampering with the the brain because of its role as the center for controlling thought, emotion and feeling. Yet the incidence of brain cancer remains very low for the population as a whole, accounting for about 1.5 percent of all cancers. With the aid of advanced imaging methods like magnetic resonance imaging (MRI), PET and CT scans, doctors are now able to diagnose and treat brain cancers that in the past often were classified as strokes, senility or other neurological disorders.

New techniques in identifying a brain tumor before the operation allow neurosurgeons to approach surgery with greater information, thereby making it possible to establish a firm diagnosis, relieve symptoms and in the case of some tumors, accomplish cures. Fortunately most central nervous system tumors in adults develop in accessible parts of the brain—the frontal, parietal, occipital and temporal lobes. Extensive surgery can be done on these important centers with good results. In many instances, where surgery is not curative, other treatments, including radiation therapy and chemotherapy, are being used. New developments in immunotherapy and gene therapy are being tested and promise to deliver even more effective treatment of brain tumors.

There is no doubt that cancers of the brain and central nervous system represent a complex problem for the patient, family and the medical team. The biggest fear people have is that they will lose their minds or become "vegetables" as the result of an operation. The outlook for recovery today is not as bleak as might be believed. Progress is being made in many areas. The length of survival as well as the quality of life is improving for most people who have brain cancers. Unlike a generation ago, medical specialists now have a spectacular array of powerful scanning machines to see inside the brain, new computerized diagnostic tools and new methods of tumor removal, which help minimize damage to normal tissues. As with other types of cancer, many factors determine the outcome of brain cancer, including the type and grade of tumor, the location of the tumor and how it affects the tissues that surround it.

WHAT YOU NEED TO KNOW ABOUT BRAIN TUMORS

- There is a major difference between cancers *of* the brain and cancers *in* the brain. Tumors *of* the brain originate there. Tumors *in* the brain come from other organs through the invasive process known as metastasis. (For information on tumors that metastasize, see Chapter 25, "When Cancers Recur or Metastasize.")
- Brain tissue does not regenerate but the brain is a remarkably adaptable organ. One part of the brain can take over the functions of a disabled or missing part. Extensive surgery can be done on many accessible parts of the brain without causing severe neurological damage.
- Nearly half of all primary brain tumors can be cured by appropriate therapy, usually neurosurgery.
- Scientific advances, coupled with technological advances, are leading to better and better cure rates.

Who is most likely to get brain cancer?

Those most likely to have brain tumors include young children and young adults to age 20 and people over age 40, with peak ages between 50 and 60. New studies show dramatic increases in brain cancers in older persons. Among people over the age of 75, the incidence of brain tumors more than doubled from 1968 to 1985. For people over 80, the rate of increase soared by as much as 23

SYMPTOMS OF BRAIN CANCER

- Headache, usually after waking and lessening as the day goes on.
- Seizures.
- Vomiting, usually after waking, with or without nausea.
- Weakness or loss of feeling in the arms or legs.
- Lethargy or mental sluggishness.
- Uncoordinated, clumsy movements (ataxic gait).
- One-sided muscle weakness (hemiparesis).
- Difficulty in swallowing (dysphagia) or with speech (dysarthria).
- Ringing or buzzing in the ear (tinnitus).
- Dizziness (vertigo).
- Drowsiness.
- Loss of sense of smell (anosmia).
- Abnormal eye movements or changes in vision.
- Changes in personality or memory.

percent a year. For the 2,000 new cases of childhood brain tumors, there is especially good news, thanks to improved diagnostic and surgical techniques. (See Chapter 22, "Childhood Cancers.")

Are there different types of brain cancer?

Brain cancers are divided into two types—those which start in the brain, and those which metastasize to the brain from cancer in some other part of the body. There are estimated to be about 17,000 cases of primary brain cancers and cancers of the central nervous system and as many as 80,000 to 100,000 cases of cancer that has metastasized to the brain. This chapter will deal with brain tumors which start in the brain, referred to as *primary brain tumors*, although much of the information will also be of interest to those with metastatic brain tumors. (Also see Chapter 25, "When Cancers Recur or Metastasize.")

What causes brain cancer?

The cause of primary brain cancer is unknown. In most cases it appears that patients with a brain tumor have no clearly defined reason why they should be at risk. However, some studies have linked the risk for brain cancer to exposure to high doses of ionizing radiation—such as x-rays and gamma rays, which can cause chromosomal changes. Occupational exposure to organic solvents and some pesticides, and employment in electrical and electronic-related jobs, as well as oil refining, rubber manufacturing and drug manufacturing, have been studied. Other studies have shown that chemists and embalmers have a higher incidence of brain tumors. Genetic factors, including the familial Li-Fraumeni syndrome and neurofibromatosis, have also been implicated. Studies in laboratory animals have found that certain chemicals and DNA viruses can cause brain tumors.

Do cellular phones cause brain cancer?

At this point, there are no definitive studies which link brain cancer and the potential risk from nonionizing electromagnectic radiation released by cellular telephones. However, studies are under way to research this question. The phones in question are hand-held cellular phones, the kind that have a built-in antenna that is positioned close to the user's head during normal telephone conversations. You should be aware that the safety of so-called "cordless phones," which have a base unit connected to the telephone wiring in a house and which operate at far lower power levels and frequencies, has not been questioned.

What kind of doctor should be treating someone with brain cancer?

Initially, most people see their family doctors. This is where a diagnosis of brain tumor usually begins. A basic neurological examination usually follows the taking of a complete history of the symptoms. If the results of this examination lead your physician to suspect a brain tumor, you will probably be referred to a specialist in the brain tumor field, commonly a neurosurgeon. Diagnosis and treatment are best handled in a major cancer center, many of which have brain tumor centers with multidisciplinary teams with diverse expertise, the very latest equipment and doctors who are trained in the use of the new techniques. Experts in such specialties as neurology, neurosurgery, oncology, pathology, diagnostic radiology, imaging, and radiation therapy pool their cooperative efforts to provide the best coordinated services.

What are the parts of the brain and what does each part do?

The brain is a soft grayish-white spongy mass of nerve and supportive tissue that is enclosed inside the inpenetrable bony helmet known as the skull. The bony casing that protects the brain from all outside matter is the reason why even the tiniest growth can cause serious trouble inside the skull. In the simplest of terms (hardly adequate to cover a complex subject), the brain has three major parts: the cerebrum, the cerebellum and the brain stem. The

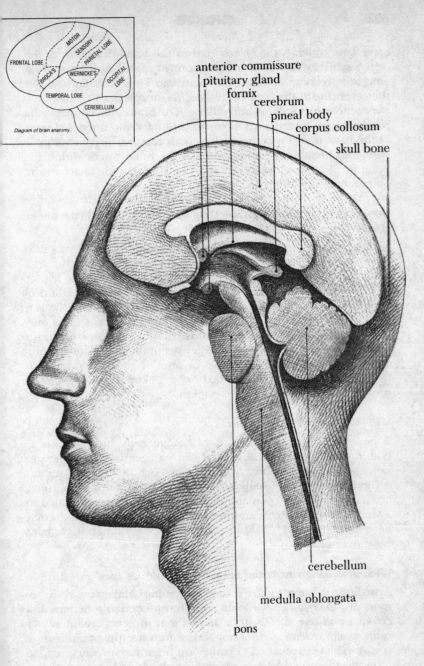

Diagram of brain anatomy.

FRONTAL LOBE
BROCA'S
MOTOR
SENSORY
PARIETAL LOBE
WERNICKE'S
OCCIPITAL LOBE
TEMPORAL LOBE
CEREBELLUM

anterior commissure
pituitary gland
fornix
cerebrum
pineal body
corpus collosum
skull bone

cerebellum

medulla oblongata

pons

Brain

cerebrum, which is the largest part of the brain, fills most of the upper skull. Its functions include control of the muscles, speech, emotions, reading, thinking and learning. The cerebellum, under the cerebrum at the back of the brain, controls balance and complex actions like walking and talking. The brain stem connects the brain with the spinal cord. It controls hunger and thirst and most of the basic body functions such as body temperature, blood pressure, and breathing. The location of the brain tumor within the brain is, of course, the most important determining factor in the outcome of any surgery or treatment.

Do some symptoms relate directly to the part of the brain the tumor is in?

Sometimes the symptoms are produced by the tumor pushing into a particular area of the brain. Tumors that are located in the area controlling motion can produce weakness in the arm, the leg, or both. A tumor located in the cerebellum, for instance, might produce loss of coordination, balance, or the ability to walk. However, since symptoms are usually difficult to pinpoint, may appear only occasionally, and are similiar to those of other diseases, diagnosis may be delayed. For example, the key symptom in olfactory meningioma is loss of smell. Since loss of smell is considered a minor problem by many people, it could be overlooked and not diagnosed until other symptoms become evident.

What is a benign brain tumor?

A benign brain tumor consists of benign cells and has distinct boundaries. Usually these tumors can be removed, and they are not likely to recur. Surgery alone may cure this type of tumor. Although it may not invade nearby tissue, it can press on sensitive areas of the brain. When an otherwise benign tumor is located in a vital area of the brain and interferes with vital functions, it may be treated as though it were malignant, even though it contains no cancer cells.

What is a malignant brain tumor?

A malignant brain tumor is life-threatening. Malignant brain tumors are likely to grow rapidly, interfere with vital functions and crowd or invade the tissue around them. If a malignant tumor remains compact and does not spread into healthy brain tissue it is said to be encapsulated. A malignant brain tumor may spread to other locations in the brain or spinal cord, but seldom metastasizes outside the brain and spinal cord.

What are metastatic brain tumors?

Metastatic brain tumors are different from primary brain tumors because they are cancerous tumors that start somewhere else in the body and spread to the brain. Because cancers can spread through the blood, it is not surprising that the brain is a frequent site of spread. The brain receives 20 percent of the blood flow of the heart, and the arteries within the brain have an "end-artery" pattern that can trap cancer cells, which then multiply and form a new cancer. Metastatic tumors are treated in a similar fashion to the primary cancer from which they spread. (See Chapter 25, "When Cancers Recur or Metastasize," for more information.)

Why are brain tumors sometimes hard to diagnose?

Brain tumors may be difficult to diagnose because the bones of the skull hide brain tumors. The doctor cannot feel or see them during a routine examination. Scans are done to view the tumor, but only a sample biopsy of the tumor examined microscopically can provide an exact diagnosis.

Why are brain tumors so dangerous?

Often, the damage done by brain tumors is due to their size. The skull cannot expand to make room for even a small mass growing within it. As a result, the tumor presses on and displaces normal brain tissue. This pressure may damage or destroy delicate brain tissue. Many of the symptoms of a brain tumor are caused by this pressure. Sometimes, a tumor may cause blockage of fluid that flows around and through the brain. This blockage can also create increased pressure. Some brain tumors also cause swelling due to accumulation of fluid. The tumor may also grow into other areas of the brain and the mass effects of size, pressure and swelling combine to make them destructive to the most sensitive areas of the brain.

Why are some brain tumors inoperable?

Brain tumors sometimes occur in a part of the brain that is inaccessible to the neurosurgeon. The brain stem, thalamus, motor area, and deep areas of gray matter are often considered to be inoperable areas. Biopsy alone for diagnosis may be performed if the tumor cannot be removed. Occasionally, biopsy may not be possible or advisable, even with the most advanced techniques. Treatment is then based on the assumed type of tumor.

What are the most common primary brain tumors?

About half of all primary brain tumors in adults are gliomas. These tumors begin in the glial tissue, which is the supportive tissue of the brain. They are divided into several types—astrocytomas, brain stem gliomas, epedymomas, and oligoendrogliomas. Glial cells, the supporting cells of the brain, are numerous and fulfill many structural and metabolic functions, including protecting and maximizing the efficiency of the neurons, and assuring their nourishment and stability. These cells are responsible for a variety of tumors which are capable of behaving in a benign or malignant fashion.

What are the characteristics of astrocytomas?

Astrocytomas may grow anywhere in the brain or spinal cord. They are recognized by the fact that they arise from small, star-shaped cells called astrocytes. In adults, they are most often found in the cerebrum. In children, they occur in the brain stem, the cerebrum and the cerebellum. Noninfiltrating astrocytoma is a relatively slow-growing tumor that usually does not grow into the tissues around it. Well-differentiated mild and moderately anaplastic astrocytoma is slow growing, but the tumor may start to grow into other tissues around it. A Grade III astrocytoma is sometimes called anaplastic astrocytoma and grows more rapidly. A Grade IV astrocytoma is usually called glioblastoma multiforme. It grows very rapidly.

What are brain stem gliomas?

These cancers occur in the lowest, stemlike part of the brain. The brain stem controls many vital functions. Tumors in this area generally cannot be removed. Most brain stem gliomas are high-grade astrocytomas.

What are ependymomas?

Ependymomas usually develop in the lining of the ventricles, though they also occur in the spinal cord. Although these tumors can develop at any age, they are most common in childhood and adolescence.

What are oligodendrogliomas?

These tumors arise in the cells that produce myelin, the fatty covering that protects nerves. They grow slowly and usually do not spread to surrounding brain tissue. They occur most often in people of middle age, but have been seen in people of all ages.

What are medulloblastomas?

These tumors are usually found in the lower part of the brain. They arise from developing nerve cells that normally do not remain in the body after birth. Medulloblastomas are sometimes called primitive neuroectodermal tumors. Although they are sometimes found in adults, they are found more often in children and are more common in boys than in girls.

What are meningiomas?

Meningiomas are common tumors, accounting for about 20 percent of adult primary brain tumors. They are usually benign and the majority are surgically curable. They grow in the meninges and because they grow very slowly, the brain may be able to adjust to their presence. They grow in such a way that they usually indent the brain and cause symptoms by pressure or by producing a reaction in adjacent brain tissue in the form of irritation or edema. When they begin to cause symptoms, they are often quite large. They occur most often in women between 30 and 50 years of age.

What is acoustic neuroma?

These benign tumors begin in Schwann cells, which produce the myelin that protects the acoustic nerve. The most common of these tumors is acoustic neuroma, sometimes called vestibular schwannoma, which causes hearing loss as the earliest symptom. Schwannomas may also develop on other nerves—the trigeminal, facial or vagal.

What are craniopharyngiomas?

Craniopharyngiomas start in the area of the pituitary gland near the hypothalamus. They are usually benign, but are sometimes considered malignant because they can press on or damage the hypothalamus and affect vital functions. They occur most often in children and adolescents.

What are germ cell tumors?

These tumors arise from primitive, developing sex cells known as germ cells. The most frequent type of germ cell tumor in the brain is the germinoma. Embryonal carcinoma, choriocarcinoma, and teratomas also fall into this category.

What are pineal region tumors?

These tumors occur in or around the pineal gland, a tiny organ near the center of the brain. The tumor may be slow growing (pineocytoma) or fast growing (pineoblastoma). The pineal region is a very difficult one to operate on and these tumors often cannot be removed. Sometimes they are called pineal parenchymal tumors.

How are brain tumors diagnosed?

The diagnosis of brain tumors has been made more accurate and more precise by the enormous advances that have occurred in neu-

TESTS THAT MAY BE USED TO DIAGNOSE BRAIN CANCER

Depending on results of physical and neurologic examinations, testing may include:

- MRI.
- CT scan.
- PET scan (where available).
- X-ray of skull, using radioactive dye.
- Angiogram or arteriogram.
- Myelogram.
- EEG (electroencephalogram, used for seizure disorders).
- Tumor and cerebral fluid markers.
- Vision and hearing tests.

roimaging. At one time, lumbar puncture with examination of the fluid, x-ray visualizations of the fluid structure, and brain wave readings (EEG) were the only tools available for diagnosis. Today, much more sophisticated diagnosis is available thanks to magnetic resonance imaging (MRI). Tremendous advances in MRI diagnosis have even overtaken many of the advantages of angiography. Reactions to tumors, such as the swelling (edema) that forms as a result, can be assessed. The nature and extent of the blood flow of the tumor can be measured. CT scanning of the head is useful in the diagnosis of certain brain tumors and in instances where MRI is not available or feasible. Angiography is used, particularly in vascular tumors, where, in some cases, the procedure may be used to block blood vessels prior to surgery. As you can imagine, diagnosis of brain tumor requires the skills of highly qualified specialists. The doctor may order MRI and CT scans, PET scans and/or radionuclide scans. A lumbar puncture or spinal tap and electroencephalogram may be needed. All of these diagnostic techniques help to establish a tentative diagnosis.

How is the final diagnosis made?

The final diagnosis of brain cancer can be made only with a sample of the tumor tissue. The neurosurgeon submits samples of the tumor tissue to a neuropathologist who can then establish an exact diagnosis.

How is a diagnosis established if an open biopsy is not possible?

For those areas that cannot be reached easily through an open biopsy, a surgeon can, through a small hole made in the skull, use stereotactic instrumentation to obtain a biopsy.

How are brain tumors graded?

Some brain tumors are graded from low grade (Grade I) to high grade (Grade IV). The grade refers to the way the cells look under the microscope. Cells from higher grade tumors are more abnormal looking and generally grow faster than cells from lower grade tumors. Higher grade tumors are more malignant than lower grade tumors.

What kind of treatments are used for brain cancers?

Surgery, radiation, chemotherapy and immunotherapy are all being used to treat brain cancers. Nearly half of all primary brain tumors can be cured with appropriate treatment.

QUESTIONS TO ASK YOUR DOCTOR BEFORE STARTING TREATMENT FOR CANCER OF THE BRAIN OR SPINAL CORD

- Where is the tumor located?
- What kind of tumor is it?
- What is the plan for surgery?
- What kind of diagnostic tests will I still need? How painful or dangerous are they?
- Will you have to drill a hole in my skull?
- What are the expected benefits of treatment?
- Will there be side effects?
- What can be done about side effects?
- What are the risks?
- How long will I be in the hospital?
- Will I need special nursing care?
- How soon after the operation will we know how successful it was?
- Will there be any treatments following surgery? What kind and for how long?
- Where can I go for another opinion?
- Who is the most skilled doctor in dealing with this type of cancer?
- Where is the nearest hospital with a brain tumor center?
- Are there any clinical trials being done for my kind of cancer?
- Will I need to change my normal activities? For how long?

ADULT BRAIN TUMORS

COMMON TYPES OF BRAIN TUMORS	FEATURES	SYMPTOMS	POSSIBLE TREATMENT
Acoustic neurinoma (neurilemoma, schwannoma neurinoma)	Benign tumor of acoustic or eighth cranial nerve. Very slow growing. Occurs in adults in middle years.	Loss of hearing in one ear, buzzing or ringing in ear, if seventh nerve affected, facial paralysis and loss of facial sensation. Difficulty swallowing, impaired eye movement, unsteadiness.	Total surgical removal is often possible. Radiation may be used.
Adenoma (see Pituitary adenoma.)			
Astrocytoma—tumors that arise from astrocyte cells, part of supportive tissue of brain. If mixed with oligodendroglioma and/or ependymoma, they are referred to as mixed gliomas. **(See page 635.)**	Different classification systems used. In I–IV system, Grade I is benign, Grade IV (glioblastoma multiforme) is most malignant; other systems separate them into distinct types—cerebral gliomas, noninfiltrating, well-differentiated anaplastic, anaplastic and glioblastoma multiforme.	Depend on nervous system location in which they occur.	Location often determines treatment. See below and oligodendroglioma and ependymoma.

(includes juvenile pilocytic astrocytomas, subependymal astrocytomas)	metastasis is rare. Slow growing, but may invade large area.	location in which they occur.	curable with surgery alone or surgery followed by radiation to residual tumor; some form cysts or are enclosed in a cyst. Metastasis is rare. *Clinical trials:* Reoperation and radiation therapy, chemotherapy, new drugs and biologicals.
Astrocytoma: well-differentiated, moderate anaplastic (includes gemistocytic, anaplastic and malignant astrocytoma)	Grow more rapidly than low-grade and tend to invade nearby healthy tissue. Recur more frequently than lower grade because spread to surrounding tissues makes it difficult to remove completely.	Depend on nervous system location in which they occur.	Treatment based on extent of spread of tumor. Surgery plus radiation or surgery only if patient is under 35 years old. *Clinical trials:* Radiation with or without chemotherapy for residual tumor, deferred radiation or varying radiation doses.
Astrocytoma: anaplastic (includes glioblastoma multiforme and gliosarcoma)	Rapid growth, difficult to remove and cure. Middle-aged adults. Mixed cell types make it difficult to treat.	Symptoms vary depending on location. Cells often stray throughout brain.	Treatment based on extent of spread. Surgery and radiation; or surgery, radiation and chemotherapy. *Clinical trials:* Hyperfractionated irradiation, accelerated fraction radiation, stereotactic radiosurgery, radiosensitizers, hyperthermia, interstitial brachytherapy, intraoperative radiotherapy, new drugs or biologicals.

(continued)

ADULT BRAIN TUMORS *(cont.)*

COMMON TYPES OF BRAIN TUMORS	FEATURES	SYMPTOMS	POSSIBLE TREATMENT
Brain stem glioma	May be an astrocytoma, anaplastic astrocytoma, glioblastoma multiforme, or mixed tumor. More common in children than adults.	Vomiting, headache, uncoordinated walk, muscle weakness of one side of face, swallowing or speech difficulty, hearing loss.	May be inoperable. Cure difficult. Radiation. Being studied for recurrence: biological modifiers and new drugs.
Chordoma	Usually benign but frequently invades adjacent bone. Most often found in people aged 21–40. Base of skull or end of spine.	Headache, double vision, neck pain, facial numbness.	Complete removal often possible. Charged particle radiation rather than conventional radiation often used.
Central Nervous System (CNS) germ cell tumors—germinoma, embryonal carcinoma, choriocarcinoma and teratoma	These arise from the sex cells.	Headache, nausea, vomiting, lethargy, double vision.	Depends on cell type, location, biological markers and surgical resectability.

Cysts—dermoid and epidermoid—usually benign	Dermoid usually appear in lower spine except in young children, where brain incidence is greater. Epidermoid cysts most common in adults.	Depends upon location.	Surgical removal.
Craniopharyngioma	Benign, congenital tumor, occurs in children and adolescents. Some grow rapidly. Often curable.	Obesity, delayed development, decreased vision, swollen optic nerve.	Surgery; **or** surgery plus radiation if not completely removed. (For children under 3, radiation delayed if possible.)
Ependymoma (well differentiated and myxopapillary ependymoma)	Occur in lining of ventricles and central canal of spinal cord. Benign type most common. Myxopapillary is found in spine. Occasionally metastasizes to other locations in central nervous system.	Headache, nausea, vomiting dizziness, impaired muscular coordination, swollen optic nerve.	Surgery alone if totally resectable; **or** surgery followed by radiation if residual tumor. *Clinical trials:* At recurrence, reoperation and radiation, if not previously used. Chemotherapy, new drugs and biologicals. *(continued)*

ADULT BRAIN TUMORS (cont.)

Common Types of Brain Tumors	Features	Symptoms	Possible Treatment
Ependymoma, malignant (anaplastic and ependymyoblastoma)	Anaplastic ependymomas grow more quickly than do the well-differentiated tumors. Ependymyoblastomas are rare cancers that usually occur in children and grow quickly.	Occasionally metastasizes to other locations in central nervous system.	Surgery plus radiation; **or** *Clinical trials:* Adjuvant chemotherapy before, during and after radiation. *Recurrence:* Chemotherapy. Clinical trials of new drugs and biological response modifiers.
Glioblastoma multiforme (refer to Astrocytoma)			
Medulloblastoma	Grows rapidly. Children and young adults. Invasive, frequently metastasizes, may even spread outside brain and spinal cord.	Impaired muscular coordination, walking, speech. Though located in the cerebellum, tumor may metastasize via spinal fluid.	Surgical removal of bulk of tumor plus craniospinal radiation. Tumor very responsive to radiation. *Clinical trials:* Addition of chemotherapy.

Meningioma, benign	Slow-growing, benign tumor with borders. Commonly occurs in middle-aged adults in cerebral hemispheres, midline and spine.	Symptoms caused are due to compression rather than invasion.	Usually curable if tumor is accessible and resectable, surgery. Surgery and radiation if not entirely removable.
Meningioma, malignant (hemangiopericytoma, papillary meningioma, meningeal sarcoma)	These types are difficult since complete removal is less common and proliferative capacity is greater.	Loss of vision, seizure, headache, swollen optic nerve, loss of smell, hearing loss.	Surgery plus radiation; or *Clinical trials*: Interstitial brachytherapy, radiosensitizers, hyperthermia, intraoperative radiotherapy with external beam radiation, and new drugs and biological response modifiers following radiation.
Mixed glioma (astrocytoma/ependymoma; **or** mixed astrocytoma/oligodendroglioma; **or** mixed astrocytoma/ependymoma/oligodendroglioma)	Similar to anaplastic astrocytomas.	Seizures are common.	Surgery plus radiation; **or** surgery plus radiation plus chemotherapy. *Clinical trials*: Interstitial brachytherapy, radiosensitizers, hyperthermia, intraoperative radiation in conjunction with external beam radiation to improve local control of tumor and/or new drugs and biological response modifiers following radiation. *(continued)*

ADULT BRAIN TUMORS *(cont.)*

Common Types of Brain Tumors	Features	Symptoms	Possible Treatment
Oligodendroglioma, well differentiated	Occur in supportive tissue of brain.	Seizures are common.	Surgical removal and radiation. Often surgery only if patient is under 45; **or** *Clinical trials:* Radiation with or without chemotherapy if not completely removed.
Oligodendroglioma, anaplastic	Middle-aged adults. Astrocytoma cells may be present. Often grows for many years before diagnosed.	Seizures are common.	Surgery plus radiation; **or** surgery plus radiation and chemotherapy. *Clinical trials:* Interstitial brachytherapy, radiosensitizers, hyperthermia, intraoperative radiotherapy combined with external beam radiation to improve local control of tumor; **or** new drugs and biological response modifiers. May recur.
Optic nerve glioma	Usually occurs in children under 10. Slow growing.	Loss of vision, rapid movement of eyeballs, crossed eyes, developmental delay, abnormal thinness.	If no symptoms, observation; if growing, radiation **or** surgery. *Clinical trials:* Chemotherapy to delay radiation.

Pineal parenchymal tumors (pineocytoma—slow growing; pineoblastoma—more rapid growing; and pineal astrocytoma, which varies depending on degree of cell differentiation)	Vary in prognosis depending on degree of anaplasia. Higher grades more difficult to cure.	Headache, nausea, vomiting, lethargy, double vision.	Surgery plus radiotherapy for pineocytoma and lower grades of astrocytoma; **or** surgery plus radiation plus chemotherapy for pineoblastoma and higher grades of astrocytoma; **or** *Clinical trials:* Radiosensitizers, hyperthermia, intraoperative radiation in conjuction with external beam; **or** new drugs and biological response modifiers after radiation.
Pituitary adenoma	Benign, slow growing, most common in young or middle-aged adults. Classified as secreting and non-secreting and by type of hormone secreted. Can affect brain and optic nerves.	Depends upon type of hormone secreted. Impotence, stoppage of menstruation, excessive activity of thyroid, enlargement of hands and feet or excessive size. If optic chiasm affected by pressure—visual loss and headache.	*Secreting type:* Complete surgical removal, with or without radiation. Responds well to treatment. *Nonsecreting type:* Radiation may follow partial surgical removal.
Spinal tumors	Primary cancers of the spinal cord are usually intradural and extramedullary.	Muscle weakness, pain if spinal cord is infiltrated.	Surgery usually used for intradural, extramedullary tumors. Treatment for other spinal cord tumors depends on whether tumor is primary or metastatic, exact location and type.

What kind of surgery is used in treating brain cancers?

Surgery is one of the oldest techniques for treating brain cancers. Fortunately, researchers are continuing to develop new techniques which make it possible for the physician to perform the delicate job of tumor removal more accurately, with fewer surgical risks and better long-term results. Neurosurgical tools, such as ultrasound equipment which uses sound waves to bounce off tumor tissue and give accurate boundaries, are being used in many medical centers. Ultrasonic aspirators are now used to break up and suction out tumor particles, assisting the surgeon in tumor removal.

What is the aim of brain surgery?

The purpose of the surgery is to remove the entire tumor if possible, or as much tumor as possible. Even partial removal of the tumor provides relief of symptoms, and the smaller amount of tumor left after surgery makes it possible to treat it more easily with other forms of treatment. Surgery is also performed to establish an exact diagnosis, to determine the full extent of the tumor and to provide access for other treatments, such as radiation implants or radiation.

Is laser surgery being used to remove brain tumors?

Laser surgery is used by some neurosurgeons to vaporize tumor tissue. During the surgical procedure, the neurosurgeon removes as much tumor as possible without causing undue neurologic damage. After this debulking, the laser may be used to remove remaining tumor cells. Lasers are sometimes used to remove an entire tumor by breaking up the tumor into pieces and vaporizing the pieces.

How is stereotactic surgery used in treating brain tumors?

Stereotactic surgery uses computer-assisted techniques to allow the surgeon to remove tumors in some parts of the brain which are difficult to reach manually. CT scanning and MRI, in conjunction with special computer techniques, may allow a tumor to be seen in three dimensions. Attached to special computer-assisted stereotactic instruments, this equipment may allow the physician to surgically remove a deep or difficult-to-reach tumor.

What is evoked-potential testing?

Evoked-potential testing uses small electrodes to measure the electrical activity of nerves. The test can be used to determine areas controlled by an individual nerve. This testing may serve as a guide during the surgical removal of tumors growing around important nerves.

How is intraoperative brain mapping used in treating brain tumors?

This technique involves mapping out areas of the brain that control vital functions such as areas of the brain involved in speech and language. Performed during a surgical procedure, this technique allows the removal of more tumor while minimizing damage to critical brain tissue.

What is a craniotomy?

The most common treatment for both benign and malignant brain tumors is complete surgical removal. A craniotomy is the operation for exposing the brain so the surgeon can remove the diseased tissue. A craniotomy is usually performed under general anesthesia, although sometimes local anesthesia is used. Despite improved technological methods for detecting brain cancer, opening the skull is still the only way to obtain tumor tissue for pathology tests or to remove the tumor.

What preparations are necessary before the operation?

The head is shaved in the area of the operation, and the scalp is cleaned with soap and water. An antiseptic will be used and all but the portion to be operated on will be covered with sterile drapes.

How will the operation be done?

Usually, the doctor makes an incision in the shape of a semicircle on the affected part of the scalp. The skin will be flapped down and holes drilled in the skull. The doctor will then connect the holes by sawing with a wire, air, or electric saw so that a block of bone (called a bone flap) can be removed from the skull. In effect, a window will have been made into the skull through which to work. Directly underneath are the membranes which cover the brain. These will be cut so that the physician can see the brain.

Is the bone replaced after the operation?

After the operation, the doctor will return the bone flap to its location in the skull and stitch the skin back in place. Sometimes a metal or fabric mesh is used to close the opening. In some cases, replacing the bone is not necessary. Muscles in the back of the head, for example, are very strong and can protect the brain.

Can the exact location of the tumor usually be determined before the operation?

With the advanced technology now available, the exact location can be pinpointed.

Can the doctor tell before the operation whether a brain tumor is malignant or benign?

The doctor may suspect what type of tumor is involved but the final diagnosis depends upon a careful study of biopsy samples taken from various parts of the tumor.

Do brain operations take a long time to perform?

The delicate surgery required to perform a brain operation requires the skills of highly trained surgeons. The location and complexity of the tumor, the procedure being used and the surgeon's dexterity all have a bearing on the length of time involved. Some operations are complete within an hour or two. Others may take three, four or more hours.

Can biopsies be performed in most parts of the brain, even when surgery is not possible?

Computer-guided stereotactic methods now allow needle biopsies to be obtained safely in virtually any part of the brain.

Will I have intravenous feedings following brain surgery?

Sometimes feedings are through a tube in the stomach or vein. Often you can be fed by mouth.

Should I plan to have special nurses after brain surgery?

It depends upon the hospital where you have your surgery. Most large hospital centers use intensive care centers where patients are monitored constantly by nurses with clinical expertise in caring for patients who have had this kind of surgery. Otherwise, it is advisable to have special nurses for several days.

What are the aftereffects of brain surgery?

Many people who have brain surgery are back to normal very soon after surgery. Usually the doctor will be able to give you some indication before the operation as to how long your recovery time will be, if you will have any defects after the operation—such as poor vision, hearing loss, difficulty in speaking, or problems with use of arms or legs. The operation itself usually does not cause the problems; the problems are usually caused by the location of the growth in the brain.

Are a number of samples of the brain tissues taken during the operation?

A number of samples, sometimes as many as a dozen or more, are taken from around the edges of tumors. These are sent from the operating suite to the surgical pathology laboratory, where, within fifteen minutes, the operating surgeon knows whether there are malignant cells. The remainder of the tumor tissues are processed for more extensive analysis.

How effective is radiation therapy for brain tumors?

Radiation therapy has been proven effective for most malignant brain tumors, including metastatic cancers. The effect of radiation on the immature brain has led to the need to limit this treatment for young children. In adults, reactions may occur during or shortly after radiation therapy, or within a few weeks to two or three months after radiation. Late-delayed reactions may develop even years after treatment and sometimes may be indistinguishable from tumor recurrence on CT and MRI scans. Newer forms of focused radiation are being developed. (For more information on radiation, see Chapter 7.)

How is interstitial radiation being used for brain cancer?

This type of radiation, which involves the computer-directed placement of radioactive pellets directly into tumor tissue, is sometimes referred to as brachytherapy, tumor seeding or radioactive pellets. This is a local form of therapy that uses such sources as Iodine-125, Iridium-192 or Californium-252 (neutron). Sometimes interstitial radiation is used as a boost following conventional radiation or in place of it. Several different courses of implantation are being investigated—radioactive pellets removed in three to five days, pellets removed in a few months and permanent implantation. This method is being used to treat recurrent tumors in adults, but it is also being investigated as an initial treatment.

How are radiosensitizers used for brain cancer?

It is thought that cells exposed to oxygen are more responsive to radiation therapy. Radiosensitizers are usually given through an artery, followed by a course of conventional radiation. A number of different agents are under investigation.

How is stereotactic radiation used to treat brain cancer?

This method delivers a high, single dose of radiation to a small, precisely defined area. It lessens the exposure of normal brain tissue to radiation. This treatment is most appropriate for small, benign brain tumors and vascular abnormalities.

What is hyperfractionation?

Hyperfractionation is a method of giving smaller daily doses of radiation more frequently—often twice a day—without a change in the overall treatment length.

What is photodynamic therapy?

Photodynamic therapy uses a drug that concentrates in tumor cells. During a surgical procedure, laser light activates the drug. When activated, the drug kills the tumor cells. Studies are being done to find drugs that will be absorbed evenly through the tumor, excreted rapidly from the body and which absorb light well.

Is hyperthermia being used in brain cancer treatment?

Heat therapy (hyperthermia) is being investigated as a treatment. Several devices are used, including radiofrequency, microwaves, ultrasound and electromagnetic equipment. This treatment is under investigation as an individual treatment as well as for use in combination with interstitial radiation.

Is chemotherapy used in treating brain cancers?

A group of anticancer drugs known as alkylating agents can cross the blood-brain barrier. Included are carmustine (BCNU) and lomustine (CCNU). (For more information about chemotherapy drugs, see Chapter 8.)

What is the role of steroids in treating brain tumors?

Steroids can control the swelling due to accumulation of fluids often associated with brain tumors. Dexamethasone, prednisolone and prednisone are some types of steroids used. They may be prescribed temporarily following surgery or during radiation because these treatments often cause swelling.

Are anticonvulsants given to all brain cancer patients?

At one time all patients with brain tumors were given anticonvulsants as a preventive measure. Today anticonvulsants are used primarily in patients who have had a seizure, and only in special circumstances as a preventive treatment.

Is gene therapy being used for brain tumors?

Many new approaches are being tested. One new treatment involves the injection of a gene that produces an enzyme called thymidine kinase. The presence of the enzyme makes the infected tumor cells susceptible to the potent antiherpes drug ganciclovir. The treatment is presently in clinical trials on a small number of patients.

What kind of medical follow-up will I have for my brain cancer?

You will usually have follow-up visits, including a complete checkup, at three-month intervals for the first year, six-month intervals for the second to fifth year and yearly thereafter. During the first year, the doctor will check carefully for any physical changes, asking you questions about headaches, seizures, speech or mental changes, motor deficits and balance problems. Every six months you will have a complete physical, a chest x-ray, CBC, CT scan or MRI of the brain. If indicated, an EEG or skull x-ray will be done.

SPINAL CORD TUMORS

Does cancer occur in the spinal cord?

Sometimes tumors of the brain extend down into the spinal cord. Other tumors start in the spinal cord. More often, cancers in the spinal cord have metastasized from another part of the body. (See Chapter 25, "When Cancers Recur or Metastasize.")

Are most spinal cord tumors cancerous?

Tumors which grow within the spinal cord (referred to as primary spinal cord tumors) are more often cancerous than those which start outside the cord itself.

What are the symptoms of spinal cord tumors?

Spinal cord tumors may stop the flow of communication between the body and the brain in either one or both directions, similar to spinal cord injuries which occur as a result of accidents. Symptoms vary depending upon the location of the tumor. Some symptoms can mimic other diseases such as multiple sclerosis or cervical disk disease.

How are spinal cord tumors diagnosed?

Spinal cord tumors usually are diagnosed through the use of magnetic resonance imaging (MRI), spinal puncture and myelogram. The spinal puncture will usually show an obstruction to the free flow of spinal fluid. Chemical analysis of the fluid often provides additional useful information. The myelogram is performed with the injection of radioactive substance into the spinal fluid so that x-rays can pinpoint the location of the tumor.

How are primary spinal cord tumors treated?

Spinal cord tumors are difficult to remove surgically without destroying a section of the spinal cord. Proton-beam radiation, which is available in only a few major centers, may destroy spinal cord tumors without damaging surrounding tissue.

What is the treatment for primary spinal cord tumors that start in the membrane around the cord or in the spinal nerve?

Many of these tumors are not cancerous. They cause pressure on the cord and the nerves. They can usually be removed by surgery.

How are spinal cord tumors that have metastasized from somewhere else treated?

Radiation treatment is sometimes used for metastasized spinal cord tumors.

PITUITARY GLAND

What is pituitary adenoma?

Pituitary adenoma is a growth in the pituitary gland, a small organ, about the size of a pea, in the center of the brain just above the back of the nose. It is sometimes referred to as the master gland because it influences body growth, metabolism and other functions. Depending upon where the tumor is growing, different hormones are affected. ACTH-producing tumors can result in a fat buildup in the face, back and chest with the arms and legs becoming very thin—sometimes referred to as Cushing's disease. High blood pressure, weakness in muscles and bones and high blood sugar are other symptoms. Prolactin-producing tumors of the pituitary gland cause the breasts to produce milk and menstrual periods to stop when a woman is not pregnant and cause impotence in men.

chapter 21

Head and Neck Cancers

There have been significant advances in the treatment of head and neck cancers with combinations of radiation and surgery, the use of laser surgery and a variety of new reconstructive procedures that make it possible for better results to be achieved. In dealing with head and neck cancers which may be disfiguring, it is important to look for a doctor who is committed to providing <u>the best possible treatment that causes the least functional disability.</u> Don't hesitate to explore all your options before committing to treatment.

Cancer can affect any part of the head and neck area—from the *oral cavity,* which includes the lips, hard and soft palate, tongue, gums and tonsils, to the *nasal area,* which includes the nose, nasal cavity and sinuses, as well as the *upper respiratory,* which includes the larynx, trachea and muscles in the neck and upper back. In addition, the *ear* and the thyroid areas also are susceptible to cancerous growths. Although these cancers account for very small percentages of the total number of cancers each year, because they affect such vulnerable and visible parts of the body, we are all very aware of them.

What is head and neck cancer?

Cancer of the head and neck is a catchall phrase for an assortment of cancers which occur in the parts of our bodies that are responsible for speech, chewing, swallowing, seeing and hearing. Some of the most common areas affected are:

- Larynx (glottic, supraglottic, pharynx).
- Mouth and oral cavity (tongue, gums, floor of mouth, lip, cheek, oropharynx, soft palate, tonsil, walls of pharynx and back of tongue).
- Nose (nasopharynx, nasal cavity, paranasal sinus).
- Salivary gland (parotid gland).
- Thyroid.

Are most of these cancers difficult to treat?

Depending on the type of cancer and where it is located, you may be facing a simple operation or one that is quite complex. It is important to know, before you begin any kind of treatment, exactly what you are dealing with.

What kind of doctor should I go to for treatment for head and neck cancers?

Careful examination and diagnosis are essential before any treatment is agreed upon for cancers of the head and neck. A multidisciplinary team approach is important since this is such a specialized area. Your treatment team may include a head and neck surgeon (also called an otolaryngologist), radiation oncologist, medical oncologist, oral surgeon, dentist, speech therapist and psychological counselor. Most of the major cancer centers around the country specialize in treating these cancers (see Chapter 26, "Where to Get Help," for more information).

QUESTIONS TO ASK YOUR DOCTOR ABOUT TREATMENT

- What are my treatment choices?
- What are the risks and side effects I can expect?
- Will surgery be necessary?
- What other alternatives are there?
- Where will the incision be and what will the scar look like?
- Will a modified or radical neck dissection be done?
- How will the surgery affect the way I eat, talk and swallow?
- Can radiation or radium implants be used instead of surgery? Is laser surgery an option?

- Will radiation or chemotherapy be used in addition to surgery?
- What kind of reconstructive surgery can be done?
- How many operations will that entail?
- What are the effects?
- How long will it all take?
- Will it cure me?
- How expensive will it be?
- Who will be doing the surgery?
- Who else will be on my treatment team?
- Can I talk with them before I have my operation?
- How many patients with head and neck cancer are you treating?
- Can you put me in touch with a support group?
- Do you know anyone who has had this treatment who I can talk with about it?
- What kind of follow-up will I have after treatment?

What are the most common types of cancers that occur in the head and neck area of the body?

The most common sites of head and neck cancer are those that occur in the mouth (oral cavity), pharynx (throat), larynx (voice box), thyroid and sinuses.

What is a radical neck dissection?

Between 150 and 350 lymph nodes can be found in the head and neck above the collarbone, which is nearly one-third of the total number of lymph nodes in the body. A radical neck dissection is performed along with the removal of the cancer, to remove the lymph nodes in the neck when cancers in the head and neck are found to have spread to the area. The operation is a major one and may require up to five or six hours to perform, when it is done along with the removal of the primary cancer. The surgery is done on one or on both sides of your neck depending on where the cancer has spread. You should know that in a radical neck dissection, the nerves and muscles which serve your neck and upper back and are responsible for arm motion are involved. For some time after surgery, you may find it difficult to raise your arms and to keep your shoulders from falling forward. Special exercises will be prescribed by the doctor or hospital therapist to help you regain your strength in these muscles.

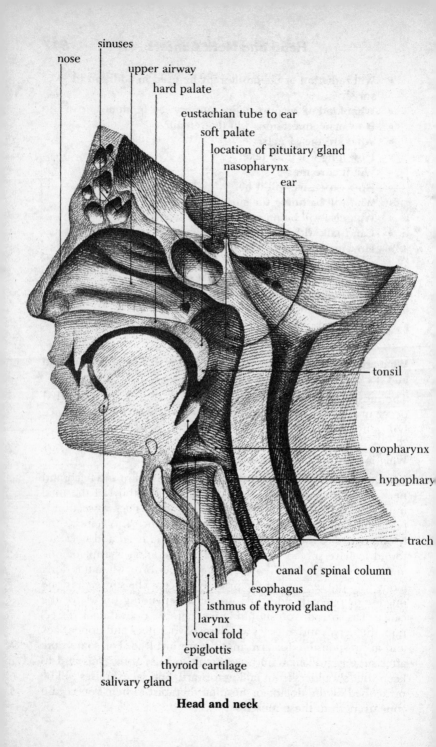

nose

sinuses

upper airway

hard palate

eustachian tube to ear

soft palate

location of pituitary gland

nasopharynx

ear

tonsil

oropharynx

hypophary

trach

canal of spinal column

esophagus

isthmus of thyroid gland

larynx

vocal fold

epiglottis

thyroid cartilage

salivary gland

Head and neck

What kinds of facial changes might a patient with head and neck cancer have?

Because of the delicate areas where surgery is needed for head and neck cancers, changes in various facial structures, including mouth, lips, cheek, neck, ears, nose and eyes, may be necessary.

POSSIBLE SIDE EFFECTS	
LOCATION OF CANCER	POTENTIAL PROBLEMS
Larynx	Speech
Tongue, palate, lips	Indistinct speech, drooling, eating
Jaw, salivary glands, muscles	Chewing, drooling
Tongue, palate, pharynx, salivary glands	Swallowing, speech
Larynx	Airway opening care
Larynx, trachea	Breathing, feeding tube
General	Appearance, nutrition

What is done to help correct these changes?

Reconstructive surgery is often done to minimize the effects of the drastic surgery needed. Another option may be maxillofacial prosthetics, which are sculpted silicone, urethane and acrylic artificial parts, used to restore facial features changed by cancer surgery. You may need a maxillofacial prosthesis to speak or eat or swallow. Or it may be necessary because you have lost an eye, your nose, or a portion of your face, jaw, or teeth and gums.

What is reconstructive surgery?

Reconstructive surgery is the reconstruction of features from the patient's own tissue. The reconstructive surgeon is familiar with the use of skin, cartilage, and bone grafts and plays a key role in planning, initiating, and coordinating the process of rehabilitation.

What kind of doctors create maxillofacial prosthetics?

A maxillofacial prosthodontist is a physician who is a specialist in evaluating and restoring facial and oral features following surgery. The skills required by these doctors lie in being able to restructure the face from both a cosmetic and functional point of view.

Are there hospitals which specialize in doing reconstructive work in the head and neck area?

Some centers specialize in the delicate reconstructive work necessary in treating unusual cancers in the head and neck area. Some of the centers with special expertise include: Memorial Sloan-Kettering Cancer Center in New York, Roswell Park Cancer Institute in Buffalo, Indiana University in Indianapolis, the University of Chicago, the University of California at Los Angeles, the University of Michigan, the University of Texas M.D. Anderson Cancer Center, and the Mayo Comprehensive Cancer Center in Rochester, Minnesota.

How expensive is it to have a prosthetic device made?

Prices vary, of course. An external facial prosthetic device, such as a jaw, for example, ranges between $1,800 and $2,500. Plastic and reconstructive surgery can cost three to four times as much and require multiple operations. There are, of course, pros and cons for either choice. There are still problems with matching color tone of the prostheses to skin color and the self-adhesives used in prosthetic devices may not be totally satisfactory. But advances are constantly being made and there are talented and devoted doctors who are dedicated to this field and to their patients.

Are there organizations that can help me with information and resources?

Let's Face It is an international information and support organization for people with facial difference and their families. It provides mutual support, educational services and an annual resource listing for individuals who are facially disfigured. The National Oral Health Information Clearinghouse, a service of the National Insitute of Dental Research, is a resource for patients, health professionals and the public seeking information on the health of people with oral health problems. For addresses and telephone numbers, see Chapter 26, "Where to Get Help."

What kind of studies are being done with vitamins and their effect on head and neck cancers?

Many scientists are conducting studies on the use of vitamins for prevention as well as following treatment for some types of head and neck cancers. Beta-carotene and vitamin E are the two substances most commonly being tested. Vitamin E and beta-carotene are antioxidants, which means they neutralize the unpaired electron in the inlet oxygens known as free radicals, which can damage DNA and are believed to help cause cancer. Vitamin E works by

TYPES OF OPERATIONS USED FOR HEAD AND NECK CANCERS

TYPE	DESCRIPTION
Cordectomy	Vocal cord is removed.
Supraglottic laryngectomy	Supraglottis, located above the true vocal cords, is taken out.
Hemilaryngectomy; also called partial laryngectomy	Part of larynx is removed.
Total laryngectomy	Entire larynx removed. Permanent hole in front of neck, called a tracheostomy, for breathing.
Laryngopharyngectomy or partial laryngopharyngectomy (partial may leave some voice use)	Larynx and all or part of hypopharynx removed. Since hypopharynx is involved with breathing, eating and talking, all may be affected. Plastic surgery may be needed.
Radical or modified neck dissection	Lymph nodes removed on one or both sides of neck; back and arm movement may be affected.
Lobectomy (hemithyroidectomy)	One lobe of thyroid, sometimes isthmus and tissue connecting lobes also removed.
Near-total thyroidectomy	Removal of parts of both lobes and isthmus of thyroid tissue; or removal of whole lobe and part of another.
Total thyroidectomy	Removal of all thyroid tissue.

protecting the fatty acids in cell membranes against free radical peroxidation—and appears to have some effect on the epithelial tissues that line the mouth, esophagus and intestines. The studies being done use these substances in greater doses than the levels usually taken in accordance with U.S. Recommended Daily Allowances.

What kind of follow-up checkups are needed for those who have had cancer of the head and neck?

Monthly checkups are usually recommended for the first year, every two months the second year and every three months the third year. After that, you should continue to see the doctor every six months.

Usually, the doctor will do a careful physical checkup of the head and neck area and cervical nodes. A chest x-ray and barium swallow will be ordered on a yearly basis and, if needed, a CT scan may be done as well.

LARYNX

What is the larynx?

The larynx is the voice box. It is the upper part of the windpipe above the trachea. The esophagus is just behind the trachea and the larynx. The openings of the esophagus and the larynx are very close together in the throat. The larynx forms the Adam's apple in the neck. Air coming in passes through the larynx to the lungs. In front of the larynx are the vocal cords. Muscles move the vocal cords, which are made to vibrate by air exhaled from the lungs.

Who is most likely to get cancer of the larynx?

Men are almost nine times more likely to develop cancer of the larynx than women, although the incidence in females is now rising, possibly due to increased smoking among women. Cancer of the larynx occurs most often in people over the age of 55. It is more common among black Americans than among whites. One known cause of cancer of the larynx is cigarette smoking. The risk is even higher for smokers who drink alcohol to excess as well as for asbestos workers or those who have been exposed to nickel or mustard gas.

What are symptoms of cancer of the larynx?

The symptoms of cancer of the larynx depend on the size and location of the tumor. Since most tumors begin on the vocal cords, they almost always cause hoarseness or other changes in the voice. Tumors in the area above the vocal cords may cause a lump in the throat, difficult or painful swallowing, a cough that persists, a sore throat, or an earache. Tumors that begin in the area below the vocal cords, which are rare, can cause shortness of breath or harsh, noisy breathing. Larger tumors may cause swollen neck glands, pain, weight loss, bad breath, and frequent choking on food. Hoarseness that lasts for more than three weeks should be checked by a doctor.

Are all growths on the larynx cancerous?

No. Most tumors of the larynx are benign. Noncancerous growths may be caused by allergy, irritation, infection or overuse of the voice. They can be removed and the voice restored to normal.

Sometimes, especially if the growths are wartlike, they may recur and will be operated on again. Cancer of the larynx can be removed by surgery when found early, and the voice may be saved.

Where does cancer of the larynx occur?

Cancer of the larynx cannot be considered one disease but rather three different, distinct types, depending upon where the cancer is. The three main parts of the larynx are: the glottis (true vocal cords), the supraglottis (area above the vocal cords) and the subglottis (the area below the vocal cords). Cancers in each region involve different symptoms, treatments and rehabilitation methods.

What is the meaning of the different stages of cancer of the larynx?

If your cancer is Stage I, this means that the cancer is confined to the area where it started and that the vocal cords can move normally. In Stage II, the cancer is only in the larynx and has not spread to lymph nodes in the area or to other parts of the body. Stage III means that the cancer has not spread outside the larynx, but the vocal cords cannot move normally, or that the cancer has spread to the tissues next to the larynx. Also included in Stage III are those larynx cancers where the cancer has spread to one lymph node on the same side of the neck as the cancer. The lymph node measures no more than three centimeters, or just a little over 1 inch. In Stage IV, the cancer has spread to tissues around the larynx, such as the pharynx or the tissues in the neck. The lymph nodes in the area may or may not contain cancer. Also considered Stage IV is cancer which has spread to more than one lymph node on the same side of the neck as the cancer, to lymph nodes on one or both sides of the neck, or to any lymph node that measures more than six centimeters (over two inches). If cancer has spread to any other part of the body, it will also be Stage IV.

What factors are considered in treating cancer of the larynx?

The doctor will try to prescribe treatment that will preserve the voice. Many small cancers of the larynx are successfully treated by radiation or surgery, including laser excision surgery. Some doctors reserve surgery for secondary treatment in the event that radiation is not successful. More advanced stages of cancer of the larynx are treated by combining radiation and surgery.

Is it important for a patient to stop smoking during treatment for cancer of the larynx?

Studies have shown that patients who smoke while receiving radiation for cancers of the larynx do not respond as well to the treat-

TREATMENT CHOICES FOR CANCER OF THE LARYNX

STAGE	SUPRAGLOTTIS	GLOTTIS	SUBGLOTTIS
Stage 1	External radiation preferred; or surgery to remove supraglottis; or total laryngectomy.	Radiation; or surgery to remove vocal cord; or surgery to remove part or all of larynx; or laser surgery.	Radiation; or hemilaryngectomy.
Stage II	External radiation preferred; or surgery to remove supraglottis; or total laryngectomy and radiation. *Clinical trials*: Hyperfractionated radiation; or isotretinoin daily for year.	Radiation; or surgery to remove part of larynx or total laryngectomy; or laser microsurgery. *Clinical trials*: Hyperfractionated radiation; or isotretinoin for prevention.	Same as Stage I. *Clinical trials*: Hyperfractionated radiation; or isotretinoin.

Stage			
Stage III	Surgery with or without radiation; or radiation followed by surgery or *Clinical trials:* Hyperfractionated radiation; or chemotherapy followed by radiation (laryngectomy reserved for those who do not respond); or chemotherapy, radiation sensitizers or particle beam radiation; or isotretinoin for prevention.	Same as Stage II.	Surgery to remove larynx, surrounding tissue and lymph nodes in neck, usually followed by radiation; or radiation if surgery not possible; or *Clinical trials:* Hyperfractionated; radiation and radiosensitizers; or chemotherapy or isotretinoin for prevention.
Stage IV	Total laryngectomy followed by radiation; or *Clinical trials:* Hyperfractionated radiation; or induction chemotherapy followed by radiation; or chemotherapy, radiation sensitizers or particle beam radiation; or isotretinoin daily for a year to prevent further cancers.	Total laryngectomy followed by radiation; or *Clinical trials:* See Stage II.	Laryngectomy plus total thyroidectomy and radical lymph node dissection, usually followed by radiation or radiation alone; or *Clinical trials:* Hyperfractionated radiation; or simultaneous chemotherapy and hyperfractionated radiation; or chemotherapy, radiation sensitizers; particle beam radiation; or isotretinoin as prevention.

Recurrent: Treatment will depend on previous treatment. If surgery was used alone, you may have surgery again or radiation treatment. If you had radiation alone, surgery may be used. If you had surgery and radiation therapy, chemotherapy may be given to relieve symptoms. *Clinical trials:* New chemotherapy drugs.

ment and therefore do not live as long as those who stop smoking. However, there are people with larynx cancer who are so addicted to smoking that they wish to continue to smoke even while receiving treatment for a problem in this sensitive area of the throat. Persons who wish to get help in stopping smoking can call the Cancer Information Service at 1-800-4-CANCER. A trained person will talk with you about ways you might use to quit.

Do cancers of the larynx recur?

Sometimes they do. The most likely time of recurrence is in the first two to three years. Recurrences after five years are quite rare.

Is there a change in the voice when radiation is used for treating cancer of the larynx?

In all probability you will be able to continue talking in much the same way as before radiation treatment. The treatment may change the way your voice sounds. Your voice may be weaker at the end of the day and may be affected by changes in the weather.

Will my voice change as a result of a partial laryngectomy?

Sometimes a change in voice occurs. Usually it sounds like you are slightly hoarse. However, most people are able to continue talking as they did before the operation.

What changes occur as the result of a total laryngectomy?

In a total laryngectomy the entire larynx is removed. Before the operation, breathing and food passages had a common opening in the throat. Farther down, they divided into the windpipe for breathing and the esophagus for carrying food to the stomach. The voice box controlled the entry of air and guarded against the entry of food particles. When the voice box or larynx is removed, the end of the air passage is relocated as an opening at the front of the neck. This is called a stoma. It is a permanent opening in the front of the neck. You will breathe, cough and "sneeze" through the stoma.

How are people who have had a larygectomy able to communicate?

A speech pathologist usually meets with the patient before surgery to explain the various methods that can be used. There are a number of methods that are available. Esophageal speech instruction will usually begin before you leave the hospital. You will be taught to use air forced into the esophagus to produce your new voice. The sound may be low-pitched and gruff. It takes practice and patience to learn to speak understandably. A mechanical larynx may be used until you are able to learn esophageal speech or if esophageal speech is too difficult. The device may be powered by batteries (electrolarynx) or by air (pneumatic larynx). The speech pathologist can help you determine what method is best for you.

What is a tracheoesophageal puncture (TEP)?

A tracheoesophageal puncture is one-day surgery which can be done as long as ten years after larynx surgery. Its purpose is to give people who find it difficult to learn esophageal speech an opportunity to regain the use of their voices. The operation is performed to provide an opening. A small silicone prosthesis is inserted to provide a source of air. The patient diverts air into the esophagus and uses it to resonate in the pharynx. Careful training is given by a speech pathologist to help the patient regain good speech.

Where can I get more information about living without my larynx?

You can call the nearest office of the American Cancer Society or the Cancer Information Service in your area. They can direct you to literature and groups that can be of help to you. The American Cancer Society sponsors Lost Cord Clubs, sometimes called New Voice Clubs, which are groups of laryngectomees and their families dedicated to helping new members get used to the same physical and emotional changes they have experienced. The International Association of Laryngectomees is another organization with excellent resources. Many of the groups offer speech therapy as part of scheduled meetings. It is reassuring to participate with others who have had the same experience. (See Chapter 26, "Where to Get Help," for more information.)

PHARYNX

What is the pharynx?

The pharynx is the passage between the larynx and the esophagus. It is subdivided into the nasopharynx, oropharynx and hypopharynx. Air and food pass through the pharynx on the way to the windpipe (trachea) or the esophagus.

What is the hypopharynx?

The hypopharynx is the bottom part of the throat. It is a hollow tube about five inches long that starts behind the nose and goes down to the neck to become part of the esophagus. The pyriform sinuses are part of this structure.

What are the symptoms of cancer of the hypopharynx?

Symptoms of cancer of the hypopharynx usually include difficulty swallowing and pain on swallowing, a sore throat that does not go away, a lump in the neck, a change in your voice or pain in your ear.

How is cancer of the hypopharynx treated?

Since this is a very difficult cancer to treat, it is most important that you be treated by a surgeon and/or radiation oncologist who is highly skilled in the multiple procedures and techniques available and who is actively and frequently treating patients who have this type of cancer. If the cancer has not spread to the lymph nodes, the larynx and the pharynx will usually be surgically removed in an operation called a laryngopharyngectomy, often followed by radiation. Unless a partial laryngopharyngectomy can be performed with some vocal function being preserved, this means that speech as well as eating and breathing may all be affected by the operation. Some clinical trials are testing the use of chemotherapy to shrink tumors as the initial treatment so that the tumor can be more treatable with either surgery or radiation. Cancers of the oropharyngeal wall are similar to those of the hypopharynx.

What is the oropharynx?

The oropharynx is the middle part of the throat, also called the pharynx. It is a hollow tube about five inches long that starts behind the nose and goes down to the neck to become part of the esophagus, which connects to the stomach. Cancer in the oropharynx is usually a squamous cell type cancer that starts in the cells that line this tube. If your cancer starts in the lymph cells of the oropharynx, it is considered to be non-Hodgkin's lymphoma (see Chapter 17).

How is cancer of the oropharynx treated?

Managing oropharyngeal cancer is very complex and, especially if the tumor is more than four centimeters (about two inches), requires a highly skilled multidisciplinary team. Where radiation is to be the treatment, it is essential that it be done by a radiotherapist who is experienced in treating head and neck cancers. Treatment depends on where the cancer is in the oropharynx—whether it is in the back of the tongue, tonsil, posterior pharynx or soft palate—as well as your age and state of health. Both surgery and external and internal implant radiation are used. In treating the tongue base, radiation may be preferred because it allows more function to be preserved. New surgical techniques developed in the last ten years, including micrographic surgery, make it possible for the cancer to be removed with the least possible tissue being lost. Often, surgery is combined with radiation therapy. Clinical trials are under way to test these various methods.

MOUTH

Cancers of the mouth include those on the lips, in the membrane lining the inside of the cheeks and lips (buccal mucosa), the gums (gingivae), the small area behind the wisdom teeth, the hard palate, the floor of the mouth and what is known as the oral tongue, which is the front two-thirds of the tongue.

Who is likely to get cancer of the mouth?

Cancer of the lip and oral cavity are more common in men than in women. It usually is found in people over the age of 45. People with light-colored skin who have been exposed to the sun are more susceptible to cancers of the mouth. It is also more common in people who chew tobacco or smoke pipes. Early cancers of the lip and oral cavity are highly curable by surgery or by radiation.

What are the symptoms of cancer of the mouth?

A lump on the lip, mouth or gums or a sore in the mouth that does not heal should be checked by the doctor. Bleeding or pain in the mouth or dentures that no longer fit may signal the need to have the mouth checked. Many times, cancers of the lip and oral cavity are found by dentists when they examine the teeth.

NASAL AREA

For the layman, the nose is what protrudes from the middle of the face. To the medical expert, it is a very complex structure that lies within the facial cavity and extends to the ears and the neck. It is divided, from a cancer expert's point of view, into the **nasal cavity,** which is the passageway behind the nose where air passes on the way to the throat, and the **nasopharynx,** which is located behind the nose and becomes the upper part of the throat. Cancers in the two areas are treated differently, so it is important to know exactly what the location of the cancer is before you can understand what will be done.

TREATMENT CHOICES FOR LIP AND ORAL CANCERS

LOCATION	STAGE I	STAGE II	STAGE III	STAGE IV
	No larger than 2 cm, about 1 inch; no spread to lymph nodes	Larger than 2 cm but less than 4 cm, about 2 inches; no spread to lymph nodes	No larger than 4 cm; or any size which has spread to one lymph node no more than 3 cm, on same side as cancer. NOTE: micrographic surgery followed by radiation being tested in clinical trials for all Stage III oral cancer locations. Also testing isotretinoin for prevention.	Spread to tissues around lip and oral cavity. Lymph nodes may or may not be affected; or any size cancer spread to lymph nodes on one or both sides of neck; or any lymph node that measures more than 6 cm or over 2 inches; or if spread to other parts.
Lip	Surgery; or radiation.	Surgery; or external and/or interstitial radiation.	Surgery and/or radiation; orthovoltage, electron beam, radioactive needles, wires or seeds; or external beam; or *Clinical trials:* Chemotherapy followed by surgery or radiation; or surgery followed by chemotherapy; or surgery, radiation and chemotherapy; or superfractionated radiation.	

Tongue	Surgery; **or** surgery followed by radiation to neck; **or** interstitial radiation and/or external radiation.	Radiation; **or** surgery; **or** both.	External radiation with or without interstitial radiation; **or** surgery followed by radiation.	Surgery to remove tongue and possibly voice box (larynx) maybe followed by radiation; **or** radiation to relieve symptoms; **or** *Clinical trials:* Chemotherapy followed by surgery or radiation; **or** adjuvant chemotherapy; **or** combination of treatments.
Buccal mucosa (lining inside cheek and lips)	Surgery; **or** radiation; **or** for larger lesions surgery with skin graft or radiation.	Radiation; **or** surgery; **or** both.	Radical surgery; **or** radiation; **or** surgery plus radiation; **or** *Clinical trials:* Chemotherapy followed by surgery or radiation; **or** surgery followed by chemotherapy; **or** surgery, radiation and chemotherapy.	Surgery to remove cancer and tissue around it and/or radiation; **or** radiation before surgery; **or** *Clinical trials:* Chemotherapy followed by surgery or radiation; **or** surgery followed by adjuvant chemotherapy; **or** surgery, radiation and chemotherapy.

(continued)

TREATMENT CHOICES FOR LIP AND ORAL CANCERS (cont.)

LOCATION	STAGE I	STAGE II	STAGE III	STAGE IV
Floor of the mouth	Surgery; or radiation.	Surgery; or radiation; or surgery followed by interstitial or external radiation.	Surgery to remove cancer and lymph nodes in neck as well as part of jawbone if needed; or external radiation with or without interstitial radiation; or *Clinical trials*: Chemotherapy followed by surgery; chemotherapy followed by radiation; or adjuvant chemotherapy after surgery; or combination of treatments.	Surgery followed by radiation; or radiation followed by surgery; or *Clinical trials*: Chemotherapy followed by surgery or radiation; or surgery followed by chemotherapy; or surgery, radiation and chemotherapy.
Lower gum (gingiva)	Surgery with skin graft; and/or radiation.	Surgery; or radiation.	Radiation given before or after surgery to remove cancer; or radiation alone.	Surgery and/or radiation; or *Clinical trials*: Chemotherapy followed by surgery or radiation; or surgery followed by adjuvant chemotherapy; or surgery, radiation and chemotherapy.

Retromolar trigone (behind wisdom teeth)	Limited surgery to part of jawbone; **or** radiation followed, if needed, by surgery.	Same as Stage I.	Surgery followed by radiation; **or** *Clinical trials*: Chemotherapy followed by surgery or radiation; **or** surgery followed by adjuvant chemotherapy; **or** combination of treatments.	Surgery followed by radiation; **or** *Clinical trials*: Chemotherapy followed by surgery or radiation; **or** surgery followed by adjuvant chemotherapy; **or** surgery, radiation and chemotherapy.
Upper gums and hard palate	Surgery; **or** surgery followed by radiation. *Clinical trials*: Microscopic surgery (MOHS) and postoperative radiation.	Surgery followed by radiation. *Clinical trials*: Microscopic surgery (MOHS) and postoperative radiation or isotretinoin for prevention.	Radiation; **or** surgery and radiation. *Clinical trials*: Microscopic surgery (MOHS) and postoperative radiation or isotretinoin.	Surgery plus radiation; **or** *Clinical trials*: Chemotherapy followed by surgery or radiation; **or** surgery followed by chemotherapy; **or** surgery, radiation and chemotherapy.

Recurrent lip and oral cancers: Treatment will depend on previous treatment. If radiation, may have surgery; if surgery, possibly more surgery, radiation therapy or both. *Clinical trials*: Chemotherapy or hyperthermia.

What are symptoms of cancers in the nasal cavity?

Cancers in this area can affect many parts of the head and neck. Symptoms may include hearing impairment, headache, facial pain, double vision, blocked sinuses, bleeding through the nose, a sore or lump that doesn't heal inside the nose, pain in the upper teeth or problems with dentures.

What kinds of cancer occur in the nasal cavity?

Cancers can occur in the paranasal sinuses (which include maxillary sinuses in the upper part of either side of your upper jawbone, the thymoid sinuses just behind either side of your upper nose and the sphenoid sinus in the center of the skull). The cancers can be of different types. If they start in the melanocytes, the tanning cells of the body, they are called melanomas. If they start in the muscle or connecting tissue, they are called sarcomas. An inverting papilloma, a very slow growing type of cancer, is another variety of cancer that starts in these cells. Cancers called midline granulomas may also occur in the paranasal sinuses or nasal cavity. They cause the tissue around them to break down.

What kind of treatment is usually recommended for cancers in the nasal area?

Treatments vary depending upon where the cancer is located and what type of cancer is involved. For nasopharyngeal cancer, high-dose external radiation to the cancer and the lymph nodes in the neck, sometimes boosted with internal implants, is the usual treatment. Surgery is usually reserved for later treatment in the event that lymph nodes fail to respond or for nodes that reappear after treatment. For cancers in the paranasal sinus and nasal cavity, treatment varies considerably, depending on the type of cancer and where it is found. The chart shows the various therapies.

Where does nasopharyngeal cancer occur?

Cancer of the nasopharynx occurs in the area behind the nose and in the upper part of the throat, called the pharynx. The holes in the nose through which you breathe lead into the nasopharynx and two openings on the side of the nasopharynx lead into the ear.

Who is most likely to get nasopharyngeal cancer?

This type of cancer is relatively rare in the United States. It is most common in the southeastern provinces of China, where there is a high consumption of salted fish. Exposure to the Epstein-Barr virus, heavy cigarette smoking and alcohol use appear to raise the risk.

What are symptoms of cancer of the nasopharynx?

The most common symptom is painless, enlarged lymph nodes in the neck. Other symptoms include trouble in breathing or speaking, frequent headaches, a lump in the nose or neck, pain or ringing in the ear (tinnitus) or hearing problems.

What is the usual treatment for nasopharyngeal cancer?

Radiation is the primary treatment for this type of cancer. Surgery may be used if the enlarged nodes fail to respond to radiation or for nodes that occur after treatment. Presently chemotherapy given to shrink tumors prior to radiation is being studied in clinical trials for Stage III and IV nasopharyngeal cancer.

SALIVARY GLANDS

Where are the salivary glands located?

Salivary glands make saliva, the fluid released into your mouth to keep it moist and to help in food digestion. Major clusters of salivary glands are found just below your tongue, on the side of the face just in front of the ear, and under the jawbone. Smaller clusters are found in other parts of the upper digestive tract and the smaller glands, called the minor salivary glands.

What are the symptoms of cancer in the salivary glands?

Any swelling around or under the chin or around the jawbone, facial numbness, muscles in the face that seem "frozen," or pain that does not go away in the face, chin, or neck should be checked by a physician.

Are most tumors in the salivary glands cancerous?

Many growths in the salivary glands are not cancerous. Only about one-quarter of parotid gland tumors are found to be cancerous. Thirty-five to 40 percent of submandibular tumors are cancerous, while 50 percent of palate tumors and 95 percent of tumors of the sublingual gland are found to be malignant.

What are the different types of low- and high-grade salivary gland cancers?

Tumors considered to be low-grade include acinic cell tumors and Grade I or II mucoepidermoid cancers. Grade III mucoepidermoid, adenocarcinomas, poorly differentiated, anaplastic and squa-

TREATMENT CHOICES FOR CANCERS OF THE PARANASAL SINUS AND NASAL CAVITY

LOCATION	STAGE I	STAGE II	STAGE III	STAGE IV	RECURRENT
Maxillary sinus	Surgery, may be followed by radiation.	Surgery and radiation either before or after.	Same as Stage II.	Radiation; **or** *Clinical trials:* Chemotherapy before surgery or radiation **or** following radiation.	More extensive surgery, followed by radiation; **or** radiation; **or** if radiation already used, surgery and/or chemotherapy. *Clinical trials:* Chemotherapy.
Ethmoid sinus	Radiation if cannot be removed surgically; **or** surgery and radiation.	Radiation; **or** surgery followed by radiation.	Surgery followed by radiation; **or** *Clinical trials:* Chemotherapy either before or after surgery with or without radiation.		Same as for recurrent maxillary sinus.
Sphenoid sinus	Radiation.	Radiation.	Radiation.	Radiation.	Radiation; **or** chemotherapy.

Nasal cavity (squamous cell)	Surgery; or radiation; or both.	Surgery; or radiation; or both.	Surgery; or radiation; or both; or Clinical trials: chemotherapy either before or after surgery, without or with radiation.	Same as Stage IV maxillary sinus.
Inverting papilloma	Surgery; radiation if surgery fails.	Surgery. If recurs after surgery, more surgery and/or radiation.		
Melanoma or sarcoma	Surgery (for certain sarcomas, surgery, radiation and chemotherapy).	Surgery. If cancer cannot be removed, radiation; or combination surgery, radiation and chemotherapy.	Surgery; or chemotherapy.	
Midline granuloma.	Radiation.			
Nasal vestibule (inside nose)	Surgery; or radiation.	External and/or interstitial radiation; or Surgery if cancer returns; or Clinical trials: Chemotherapy before or after surgery.	Surgery if prior radiation; or radiation if prior surgery; or more surgery followed by radiation; or Clinical trials: Chemotherapy.	

mous cell carcinomas are all treated as high-grade. Early, low stage tumors are usually curable with surgery.

How is cancer of the salivary glands treated?

Treatment for cancer of the salivary glands depends upon the size of the cancer and upon whether it is a fast- or slow-growing type. Surgery is usually the treatment, with or without radiation following the surgery. Neutron radiation and radiosensitization are being tested in clinical trials. New chemotherapy drugs are also being tested. Because salivary glands help digest your food and are close to your jaw, treatment may require that plastic surgery be done if a large amount of tissue or bone is removed around the salivary glands.

Where is the incision made for salivary gland tumors?

The incision placement depends upon which glands are affected. For the parotid gland, the incision is usually in front of the ear and along the angle of the jaw. For sublingual gland tumors, the incision will usually be in the mouth or in the skin just below the chin.

THYROID

What is thyroid cancer?

This cancer occurs in this ductless gland located in the front of the throat, below the Adam's apple and just above the breastbone. It is U-shaped and has two lobes—one on each side of the windpipe. Cancer of the thyroid accounts for less than 1 percent of all cancers. It is also one of the least frequent causes of death from cancer.

What are the symptoms of thyroid cancer?

You may become aware of a growth in the neck—or a growth may be discovered during a regular examination. There may also be enlargement of one or a number of nearby lymph nodes either above or below the thyroid nodule. The lump usually is not painful or tender. A hard, irregular lump that does not seem to move is the most suspicious. Softness, mobility, the indication of more than one lump, and slow growth usually indicate a benign tumor. Only about 10 to 20 percent of thyroid lumps prove to be cancerous.

Who usually gets thyroid cancer?

Cancer of the thyroid is found twice as often in women as in men and more often in whites than in blacks. It is frequently found in young adults and occasionally in teenagers. Interestingly, thyroid cancers have been found on autopsy in large numbers of people who never were aware of having cancer. Adults who were *treated* with x-ray (*not* those who had x-rays for diagnostic purposes) for conditions such as ringworm of the scalp, enlargement of the thymus glands in infants, various types of ear inflammations, deafness due to overgrowth of lymphoid tissue, enlargement or inflammation of tonsils and adenoids and acne, should have this fact noted on their permanent medical records, since these cancers may not occur until twenty years or longer after the treatment. People who have had such treatments are at slightly higher risk for thyroid cancers, but only a small percentage of the people irradiated at an early age develop thyroid tumors.

Is it unusual for children to have cancer of the thyroid?

Cancer of the thyroid does occur in children and young adults. In contrast to cancers of some other organs, however, the statistics show that most continue to live normal lives. Even when the disease is locally advanced with extensive involvement of the lymph nodes, this still holds true.

How is the thyroid scan performed?

After you swallow a radioactive iodine liquid, a probe is used to determine how actively your thyroid tissue is absorbing the substance. If it is quite active, the lump is called "hot." If it does not absorb the substance, the lump is called "cold." Cold lumps may be cancerous, slow-growing and slow to spread. Hot spots usually indicate a benign growth. Even if your scan shows that you have a cold spot, 80 percent of the time, cold spots, upon biopsy, prove **not** to be cancerous. Sometimes two thyroid scan readings are taken—usually at 2 and 24 hours after administration of the radioactive material. There is more detailed information on diagostic tests in Chapter 4, "How Cancers Are Diagnosed."

What are the different kinds of thyroid cancers?

There are a number of different varieties of thyroid cancers. Well-differentiated papillary cancers are very curable, but they can recur and grow rapidly, so follow-up is important. Follicular and medullary cancers are slow growing. Poorly differentiated or anaplastic thyroid cancers grow rapidly and may spread. The thyroid may occasionally be the site of other primary tumors, including sarcomas, lymphomas, epidermoid cancers and teratoma. Lung, breast and kidney tumors sometimes metatasize to the thyroid.

TREATMENT CHOICES FOR THYROID CANCER

STAGE	PAPILLARY	FOLLICULAR	MEDULLARY*	ANAPLASTIC*
Stage I—Localized to one or both thyroid glands.	Near-total thyroidectomy; **or** lobectomy and hormone treatment (radioactive iodine sometimes used after surgery).	Near-total thyroidectomy; **or** lobectomy followed by hormone therapy (radioactive iodine may be given after surgery).	Total thyroidectomy and biopsy of tissues around thyroid to see if they contain cancer. If cancerous, lymph node dissection. If spread to other parts of body, chemotherapy.	Surgery to remove thyroid and tissues around it; trachea may be removed. Airway in throat may be needed (tracheostomy); **or** external radiation; **or** chemotherapy; **or** *Clinical trials:* New drugs.
Stage II—Spread to nodes around thyroid.	Same as above but cancerous lymph nodes also removed.			
Stage III—Spread outside thyroid but not outside neck.	Total thyroidectomy plus removal of tissues around thyroid where cancer has spread; **or** total thyroidectomy plus radioactive iodine and/or external radiation.			
Stage IV—Spread to other parts of body.	Radioactive iodine; **or** external radiation; **or** hormone therapy; **or** *Clinical trials:* Chemotherapy.			
Recurrent	External radiation or chemotherapy.			

* There is no staging system for medullary and anaplastic thyroid cancers.

How is cancer of the thyroid treated?
Surgery is the most common treatment for cancers of the thyroid, although radiation, hormone therapy and chemotherapy are also used.

What are the operations performed for thyroid cancer?
Lobectomy (or hemithyroidectomy) means that one lobe of the thyroid (and sometimes the isthmus, or tissue connecting the two lobes) has been removed. Lymph nodes in the area may be removed and biopsied. A near-total thyroidectomy removes all of the thyroid except for a small part. The total thyroidectomy includes removal of both lobes. Because anaplastic thyroid cancer (unlike follicular and medullary thyroid cancer) often spreads very quickly to other tissues, it may be necessary to also remove the trachea (the tube through which you breathe). A tracheostomy will be done so that there is a permanent airway in the throat for breathing.

What kind of follow-up checkups do I need after being treated for cancer of the thyroid?
You should see your doctor every six months for the first and second year and every twelve months thereafter.

What are the parathyroid glands?
The parathyroids are four small glands which are attached to the thyroid gland. They secrete a hormone, parathormone, which is involved with the balance of the body and the excretion of calcium and phosphorus necessary for bone growth and maintenance. They are part of the endocrine system.

What are other parts of the endocrine system?
Other parts include the adrenal glands and the pituitary glands.

Can cancer grow in any of the parts of the endocrine system?
It is possible to have cancer of the parathyroid glands, the adrenal glands or the pituitary glands. Cancer of the endocrine system is relatively rare and is complex to diagnose. (For information on adrenal gland cancer, see Chapter 14, "Gastrointestinal and Urinary Cancers." Pituitary cancers are discussed in Chapter 20, "Brain and Spinal Cord Cancers.")

OCCULT NECK CANCER

What is metastatic squamous neck cancer with occult primary?
Sometimes cancer starts in other parts of the body and spreads to the lymph nodes in the neck. When the cells are studied, the

pathologist can determine whether these cells are from another part of the body. Sometimes, even with this information, it is impossible for the doctor to find the source of the original cancer. When this happens, the cancer is called metastatic squamous neck cancer with occult primary. *Occult* means unseen and *primary* refers to the original cancer. In other words, the source of the original cancer cannot be found, but the lymph node cells are cancerous. The doctor will continue to try to determine where the original cancer is, but meanwhile, treatment may be started. It is imperative that long-term repeat examinations be made so that the primary tumor can be found and treated. The neck should not be biopsied until the possibility of a primary cancer in the head and neck area has been excluded. Fine needle aspiration may be done for early diagnosis. Treatments include surgery and/or a variety of radiation techniques. Chemotherapy is being studied in clinical trials.

chapter 22

Childhood Cancers

Learning that your child has cancer is devastating. It is one of the greatest challenges any parent can face, laden with intense emotions and intensified by fear. Just a decade or two ago, the chances of surviving childhood cancer were extremely slim. However, you can take comfort in the fact that in the last thirty years, the statistics on children's cancers have been reversed—from 70 percent of children who *did not* survive to 70 percent who *do*.

In the United States, about 8,000 youngsters, out of a total population of 50 million between the ages of birth to 14, will be diagnosed with pediatric cancers each year. Almost one-third of these pediatric cancers are leukemias. The remaining are divided among brain tumors, childhood lymphomas, Hodgkin's disease, Wilms' tumors, neuroblastomas, osteogenic sarcomas, Ewing's sarcomas, retinoblastomas, and rhabdomyosarcomas. It has been estimated that by the turn of the century, 1 in 900 young adults in the United States will be a survivor of childhood cancer.

One of the hardest things to comprehend, when your child is diagnosed with cancer, is that something like this can actually happen to your family. The depth of pain is indescribable. But reality must be faced. It is important for you and your family to take charge of the situation. You will find that children can cope and accept illness as well as adults, sometimes better. Try to channel your anxiety to fuel your quest to understand the nature of the child's specific illness so that your family can deal with it in the most effective way.

WHAT YOU NEED TO KNOW ABOUT CHILDHOOD CANCERS

- Treatment at a major medical center where a team approach, using the skills of radiation therapists, pediatric medical oncologists or hematologists, pediatric surgeons, radiation therapists, rehabilitation specialists and social workers, is employed is essential to ensure that your child receives the best treatment.

- Acute lymphocytic leukemia accounts for 80 to 85 percent of childhood leukemia. Thirty years ago, the survival of newly diagnosed children was about 5 percent. Today, nearly 75 percent of these children can be expected to be cured.

- In almost all cases of childhood cancer, its appearance in one child does not mean that a brother or sister is more likely to develop it.

- Diagnosis of pediatric cancers can be difficult due to the rarity of the diseases and the complexity of making a diagnosis.

- Even children who are diagnosed with unusually high white blood cell counts are often found to have something other than cancer.

- Young children, especially girls in their eighth year, may develop a mildly tender swelling in one or both breasts with an underlying mass. This need not alarm you. The mass usually regresses and disappears within six to twelve months. Breast malignancies are rare in children. The enlargement should be observed by a physician. Biopsies or surgical intervention should be postponed and the mass should be removed only if significant enlargement or symptoms occur.

- The possibility of entering your child into a clinical trial through a major medical center or of getting a second opinion from the National Cancer Institute in Bethesda, Maryland, should be explored. Children who are treated on clinical trials have the advantage of getting the latest available therapy.

What type of doctor should be treating my child?

Ideally, an oncological pediatrician should be responsible for coordinating your child's treatment. Pediatricians who do not specialize in childhood cancer and family practitioners may see fewer than half a dozen cases of a specific type of childhood cancer in their careers. Therefore, your own physician will usually refer you to an oncologist, who may suggest that you take your child to one of the major medical centers for treatment. If you decide you will take this treatment route, you will find that total patient care—all of the disciplines, including medical and other subspecialties, nursing and social service—are orchestrated and individualized for the child's care. It may also be possible to arrange to have some of the treatment closer to home. Specialists from many of the comprehensive cancer centers designated by the National Cancer Institute work with local physicians in planning and coordinating follow-up treatment. You need to assess your own situation and decide what will work best for you and your family. However, implementing the latest treatment methods requires teamwork among medical oncologists, pediatric oncologists, surgeons, radiologists, hematologists, physiotherapists, nurses, and social workers.

Can I get a confirming second opinion on my child's treatment from the National Cancer Institute?

You can call the National Cancer Institute's Clinical Center yourself and request a second opinion appointment. **Cases of childhood cancer are the only ones which are accepted by the Center directly from someone who is not a physician.** (The National Cancer Institute's Clinical Center has a childhood cancer disease department as well as a hotel facility, the Children's Inn, which provides housing for children and their parents who are being treated at the Center. Treatment, however, is not available at the Center for all forms of cancer.) The Clinical Center provides nursing and medical care without charge for children who have been diagnosed as having a particular kind or stage of cancer being studied in its clinical research programs. The Clinical Center also gives second opinions after seeing the child. Treatment may then be delivered, in many cases, in the area where the family lives.

Should I consider entering my child in a clinical trial?

This is something you should discuss with your doctor. There are two major cooperative groups in the United States that organize clinical trials for childhood cancers—the Children's Cancer Study Group and the Pediatric Oncology Group. Doctors who belong to these groups or who take part in clinical trials can be found by calling the National Cancer Institute's Cancer Information Service (1-800-4-CANCER). About two-thirds of children with cancer in the United States are treated on a clinical trial at some point in their illness.

Should children be told they have cancer?

Openness and honesty are usually the best approach, depending, naturally, upon the age and understanding of the child. Toddlers can be told that they are sick and need to take medicine to get better. Terms such as *bad cells* for a tumor should be avoided since a child may consider the tumor a punishment for bad behavior. Older children need to know that cancer is a serious but treatable illness. Many of them may have the mistaken impression from watching television that everyone who has cancer dies. They need reassurance that there are successful treatments and that new treatments are being used with very hopeful results. Do not avoid the subject for fear of saying something wrong. As awkward as your response may be, it is better to deal with questions in a matter-of-fact and honest manner so that you keep communication open.

Should the other children in the family be told when a brother or sister has cancer?

Other children in the family can't help but be worried and concerned about the disruption in their sibling's and their lives. Naturally, the age of the child dictates how much needs to be told. A three- or four-year-old can be told that a sibling is sick, needs to go to the hospital and will be taking medicine for a long time. Older children can be given more detailed information. Young children may feel guilty and need to be reassured that they are not responsible for the illness. Children also worry that they may also become ill. Being aware of the many fears and jealousies that are awakened and talking about them will help keep the sibling from becoming resentful about the time you must spend with your sick child. Most children's hospitals have liberal visitation policies for siblings of children with cancer so it is often possible for brothers and sisters to participate in their sibling's hospital life.

Is it normal for my child to be angry over the inconveniences that the treatments impose?

Anger is a very normal reaction—and the child should be allowed to vent some of it. You can let your child know that you understand his feelings but that the treatment is essential to get well.

How do you keep from overprotecting a child with cancer?

Finding a balance for your child's life at this time is a daily challenge. You will need to assess the question regularly, because cancer cannot be ignored, but neither can other important aspects of the young person's life. Special treatment at home or in the classroom can create resentment among peers. Although the diagnosis of cancer will change your child's life for a time, overprotection encourages dependency that prevents the child from learning how to use his own resources. Learning the boundaries for behavior and activity is a valuable part of growing up and is doubly important for the child who may be faced with more uncertainty in the future.

Where can I get more information about childhood cancer?

The Cancer Information Service 1-800-4-CANCER phone service can provide you with information about the specific type of cancer which has been diagnosed, can tell you what hospitals in your local area are participating in the latest treatments and can send you booklets and specific printed information on the subject. There is a wealth of information available for parents of children with cancer.

What kind of doctor is best for dealing with a child with cancer?

To maximize the chance of cure, the first treatment your child receives must be the best available to totally eradicate his cancer. Cancer centers designated by the National Cancer Institute and major medical institutions have teams that specialize in treating cancer in children. A team approach, incorporating the skills of the family physician, radiation therapists, pediatric medical oncologists and hematologists, rehabilitation specialists and social workers, ensures the best treatment. (For information on cancer centers, see Chapter 26, "Where to Get Help.")

QUESTIONS TO ASK YOUR DOCTOR ABOUT YOUR CHILD'S CANCER AND TREATMENT

- Exactly what kind of cancer does my child have and what stage is it in?
- Has this diagnosis been confirmed by other experts?
- Have you treated other children with this type of cancer? How many?
- What kind of treatment are you advising?
- Is it possible to receive treatments locally?
- Is it advisable to go to a cancer center or specialized hospital for treatment? If no, why not?
- Where, in your opinion, is the best place for my child to be treated?

- Can you help me check out clinical trials that might be appropriate?
- Do you have the latest PDQ data base information on my child's cancer?
- Will you help me get a second opinion from the National Cancer Institute?
- How long do you think my child will be hospitalized?
- What treatment choices are there and what have past results been?

LEUKEMIA

What is leukemia?

Leukemia is a form of cancer of the blood. Malignant cells are found in the blood and bone marrow. Normally, the bone marrow makes cells called blasts that mature into several different types of blood cells. In leukemia, the blood cells do not mature, are released into the circulatory system, crowding out normal white cells, platelets and red blood cells and are found in the blood and bone marrow. Leukemia is found in both children and adults. It can be acute, progressing quickly with many immature cancer cells, or chronic, progressing slowly with more mature-looking leukemia cells.

What is the difference between acute and chronic leukemia?

If leukemia affects a young person suddenly, it is called acute because it comes on quickly and progresses rapidly unless it is treated. Almost all childhood leukemias are acute, but the disease may sometimes be of the chronic type. In chronic leukemia, the bone marrow is able to produce a good number of normal cells as well as leukemic cells so that, compared to acute leukemia, the actual course of the disease is milder for a period of time.

Are there different types of leukemia that affect children?

Leukemia is not just one disease. There is actually a type of leukemia for each of the three major kinds of white blood cells—neutrophils, lymphocytes and monocytes. There are two major types of leukemia which are found in children—acute lymphocytic leukemia and acute myeloid leukemia. **Acute lymphocytic leukemia, also called ALL and sometimes referred to as lymphoblastic or lymphoid, accounts for about 80 percent of all childhood leukemias.** Acute myeloid leukemia (also called AML and ANLL as well as myelogenous, granulocytic, myelocytic and myeloblastic) accounts for the remainder of childhood leukemias but is primarily seen in adults. Other kinds of leukemia such as chronic lymphocytic leukemia (CLL), chronic myelogenous leukemia (CML), monocytic, myelomonocytic, progranulocytic, erythroleukemia and hairy cell leukemia are very rare, but still behave similarly to the more common kinds. (For more information on leukemias other than ALL, see Chapter 16.)

Who usually gets ALL?

Most children who have ALL are between 2 and 8 years of age when diagnosed, but ALL can also occur in people in their twenties and thirties. For reasons yet to be understood, slightly more boys get ALL than girls, and it occurs more frequently among white children than black children.

Are electromagnetic fields the cause of leukemia?

The cause of leukemia is unknown. The controversy over the role of electromagnetic fields is still being studied. (Electromagnetic fields are the electric and magnetic fields created by electric charges in the alternating current supplied to U.S. households.) A number of studies are presently being done to determine if there is a possible link between cancer and low-level electromagnetic fields from power lines and household sources.

SYMPTOMS OF ACUTE LYMPHOBLASTIC LEUKEMIA (ALL)

- Fever.
- Tendency to bleed or bruise easily.
- Listlessness.
- Lack of appetite.
- Intermittent or low-grade fever.
- Bone or joint pain.
- Abdominal pain.
- Frequent infections.
- Tiny red dots or purple spots on skin.

What tests are used to diagnose ALL?

The diagnosis of leukemia requires blood tests and examination of the cells in the bone marrow. Early symptoms can mimic diseases such as mononucleosis, anemia from other causes, tonsillitis, rheumatic conditions, meningitis, mumps, or other kinds of cancer. In order to examine the cells, a bone marrow aspiration is usually done. This test requires that a needle be inserted into a bone in the hip so that a small amount of bone marrow can be withdrawn for inspection under the microscope. Spinal taps are done to remove fluid surrounding the child's brain and spine to see if leukemia cells are present. X-rays may also be needed.

Why are so many tests needed?

It is necessary to determine which type of white blood cell has become leukemic, since treatment and response are different for each kind. Usually the type of leukemic cell can be determined from microscopic inspection, but sometimes special tests of the chromosomes and cell chemistry may be needed before treatment can begin. In rare instances, the cells are too young to be classified. Such cases are called acute stem cell leukemia or acute undifferentiated leukemia.

How is ALL staged by doctors?

Unlike most other cancers, there is no numbered staging system for acute lymphocytic leukemia. Staging depends upon clinical and laboratory findings, such as age, biochemistry, numerous blood counts, whether or not there is evidence of spread to the brain, and DNA content. ALL is categorized as low risk, average risk or high risk. In addition, in remission means treatment has been given and white blood cell counts are normal. There are no signs or symptoms of leukemia. Relapsed indicates that the leukemia has come back after having gone into remission. Refractory means the leukemia did not go into remission after being treated.

How is ALL usually treated?

The primary treatment for ALL is chemotherapy. Radiation therapy to the brain may also be used in certain cases where there is evidence that the leukemia cells have spread to the brain.

Does it make a difference where my child is treated?

Where the child is treated is as important as the kind of treatment given. Much research and many trials have been done to determine the best treatments for the various types of leukemia. There are numerous different protocols which must be carefully selected and coordinated to achieve control of the disease. The treatments are intense. The major cancer centers have well-trained, fully integrated staffs on hand to help with all aspects of dealing with the medical and emotional crisis of leukemia.

TREATMENT CHOICES FOR ALL	
STAGE	POSSIBLE TREATMENTS
Low- and average-risk ALL	Chemotherapy, given in phases: induction, consolidation plus radiation to brain if central nervous system involvement; **or** intrathecal chemotherapy without radiation to brain.
High-risk ALL	Chemotherapy with radiation to brain, with or without intrathecal chemotherapy during maintenence. *Clinical trials:* High-dose and intrathecal chemotherapy; **or** intrathecal chemotherapy in induction and consolidation and periodically during maintenance.
In remission Treatment will continue for 2 to 3 years.	Intrathecal and/or high doses of systemic chemotherapy.
Relapsed or refractory	Intensive systemic combination chemotherapy; **or** *Clinical trials:* New chemotherapy drugs or allogeneic or autologous bone marrow transplantation.

What can I expect to happen during the initial treatment period?

The first phase of treatment is called induction therapy. The purpose of induction therapy is to kill as many of the leukemia cells as possible. The initial treatment is designed to make all signs of leukemia disappear. At that time, your child will be in remission. Treatment, of course, will vary with the severity of symptoms, the treatment plan, the doctor and the hospital. Since the child may be anemic, susceptible to infection and at risk of bleeding, the period of initial treatment can be very difficult.

What is remission?

Remission means the decrease or disappearance of the disease. A remission is a temporary—and potentially permanent—arrest of the leukemic process. Remissions can occur as early as seven to fourteen days after induction therapy is begun. When a complete remission occurs, there is a complete return to a state of good health—the symptoms are gone, the physicial findings are normal, and abnormal cells are no longer found in the bone marrow and peripheral blood. Sometimes the remission is only partial, which means that the tumor is reduced by at least 50 percent, but the cancer is still present. With the new combinations of drugs, more than 90 percent of patients with ALL can be expected to achieve remission. Examination of the blood at frequent intervals and of the bone marrow from time to time enables the doctor to follow the course of the disease and to select the proper dosage of the appropriate chemotherapeutic drugs.

Does remission mean that the leukemia is cured?

A remission means that the leukemia is being controlled. At this point, the second phase of treatment, called consolidation therapy, begins. This treatment is used to try to kill any remaining leukemia cells in the body. If the leukemia cells have spread to the brain, or if the doctor feels further preventive therapy is called for, central nervous system (CNS) therapy, usually chemotherapy with radiation therapy to the brain, will be prescribed.

Is bone marrow transplantation used for leukemia?

Bone marrow transplantation is being used for relapsed childhood ALL and childhood acute myeloid leukemia (AML) in first remission. High doses of chemotherapy with or without radiation therapy are given to destroy all of the bone marrow in the body. Healthy marrow is then taken from a donor whose tissue is the same as, or almost the same as, the patient's. The donor may be a twin (the best match), a brother or sister, or another person not related (called an allogeneic bone marrow transplant). The healthy marrow from the donor is given to the patient through a needle in a vein, and the marrow replaces the destroyed marrow. (More information about bone marrow transplants can be found in Chapter 9, "New Advances and Investigational Trials.")

What is an autologous bone marrow transplant?

During this transplant, bone marrow is taken from the patient and may be treated with drugs to kill any cancer cells. The marrow is then frozen and high-dose chemotherapy with or without radiation therapy is given to the child to destroy all the remaining marrow. The marrow that was taken out is then thawed and given intravenously, by needle in a vein, to replace the marrow that was destroyed. (See Chapter 9 for more information on bone marrow transplants.)

What is a relapse?

Relapse occurs when leukemic cells reappear in the bone marrow, blood, central nervous system, or any other site. The symptoms of relapse are usually similar to those at the time the disease was first diagnosed. Children who relapse can usually be reinduced into remission. However, third and subsequent relapses are more difficult to control, because the cells become resistant to chemotherapy.

Do all cases of leukemia progress in the same way?
No two cases are alike—and exact predictions are impossible to make. A great deal depends on the type of leukemia, the treatment given and the way in which the individual body reacts to treatment.

Is it dangerous for my leukemic child to be vaccinated?
IMPORTANT: Your child should not receive live-virus medicine—such as that used in Sabin polio vaccine and measles vaccinations. The child and anyone else in the household should receive Salk (killed) vaccine. Always check with your child's doctor before allowing any such procedures on a child with leukemia. Chickenpox vaccine is live vaccine and may be given under the supervision of an oncologist to children with ALL who are in remission.

How can I help my child deal with hair loss and other changes in appearance?
Encourage your child and others in the family to ask questions and be prepared to answer them as honestly as possible. Siblings, as well as classmates, should be prepared for physical changes in the patient, such as hair loss. Many children and adolescents solve the hair loss problem with caps or more exotic headgear, instead of wigs. Sometimes, siblings or classmates will tease your child. It is best to prepare your child for such occasions. You may also wish to discuss these issues with the health care team. In some institutions there are programs in which classroom visits are made by hospital personnel. A social worker may also be available who can discuss the problems with the child.

Where can I get information and help about the medical aspects of leukemia, as well as the social and psychological issues?
Fortunately there is a great deal of help available on many different levels. An unusual amount of well-written literature is available from the National Cancer Institute, the American Cancer Society, Leukemia Society of America, and Candlelighters Foundation. (See Chapter 26, "Where to Get Help," for addresses and telephone numbers.)

CHILDHOOD BRAIN TUMORS

There are many different types of brain tumors in children and the outlook for recovery varies according to the type of tumor and where it is located in the brain. For best results, you should seek out treatment at a large center with an experienced team of pediatric specialists in neurosurgery, radiation therapy, oncology, neuroradiology, neurology, and psychology. As a first step, review of the diagnostic tissue by a neuropathologist who has particular expertise in this area is strongly recommended. (For more information on brain tumors, also see Chapter 20, ''Brain and Spinal Cord Cancers.'')

SYMPTOMS OF CHILDHOOD BRAIN TUMORS

- Seizures.
- Morning headaches.
- Vomiting.
- Irritability.
- Behavior problems.
- Changes in eating or sleeping habits.
- Lethargy.
- Changes in muscular coordination.

How are childhood brain tumors classified?

Brain tumors are classified by their location within the brain, rather than by stage. Infratentorial tumors are found in the lower part of the brain, usually the cerebellum or brain stem. The cerebellum is the most common site of brain tumors in children. Supratentorial tumors are found in the upper part of the brain. Even physicians agree that the terminology used in classifying brain tumors is confusing.

What is the most common type of childhood brain tumor?

Almost half of all brain tumors in children are found in the lower part of the brain (infratentorial) and about three-quarters of them are located in the cerebellum or fourth ventricle.

CHILDHOOD HODGKIN'S DISEASE

Hodgkin's disease in children under the age of 13, those who are still growing and have not attained sexual maturity, is quite rare

TYPES OF CHILDHOOD BRAIN TUMORS

Type	Characteristics	Possible Treatment
Medulloblastoma	Fast-growing, found almost exclusively in children and young adults, tendency to spread to other parts of nervous system.	Surgery to remove bulk of tumor. *Standard risk patients:* Radiation. *High risk:* Radiation and chemotherapy. *Recurrent disease:* Chemotherapy.
Cerebellar astrocytoma	Slow-growing; does not usually spread.	Surgery to remove all or part of tumor. Possible radiation if all not removed. Chemotherapy may be used to delay radiation in very young children if tumor progresses and further surgery not possible.
Infratentorial ependymoma	Arises from lining of lower part of brain. May spread to other parts of brain or spinal cord.	Radiotherapy; **or** surgery to remove as much of tumor as possible. *Under 3:* Chemotherapy to delay radiation. *Recurrent disease:* Surgery and chemotherapy.
Brain stem glioma	Begins in bottom part of brain that connects to spinal cord. May grow rapidly or slowly but rarely spreads.	Radiotherapy; **or** surgery. *Under 3:* Chemotherapy to delay radiation. *Recurrent disease* (low grade): Surgery, radiation (especially if not already given) and chemotherapy).
Low-grade cerebral astrocytoma	Slow-growing tumor that does not usually spread.	Surgery; **or** surgery and radiation; **or** radiation may be delayed until tumor progresses; **or** chemotherapy. *Clinical trials: For children under 5:* Chemotherapy. *Recurrent disease:* Chemotherapy. *(continued)*

TYPES OF CHILDHOOD
BRAIN TUMORS *(cont.)*

TYPE	CHARACTERISTICS	POSSIBLE TREATMENT
High-grade cerebral astrocytoma (anaplastic astrocytoma glioblastoma multiforme)	Fast-growing tumor that may spread to other parts of brain.	Surgery, radiation and/or chemotherapy. *Clinical trials:* Postoperative chemotherapy with or without radiation. *Under 3:* Chemotherapy after surgery to delay or modify radiation. *Recurrent disease:* If radiation used before, chemotherapy or *being studied:* Chemotherapy, radiosurgery, interstitial implants.
Supratentorial ependymoma (ependymoblastomas usually found in children: rare)	Tumor in upper part of brain. May grow rapidly or slowly. May spread to other areas of brain or spinal cord.	Surgery followed by radiation. *Under 3:* Chemotherapy to delay or modify radiation. *Clinical trials:* Radiation with or without chemotherapy. *Recurrent disease:* Cisplatin or clinical trials.
Cranio-pharyngioma	Located in pituitary region, often curable. Nonmalignant but may cause pressure on nearby structures.	Surgery and/or radiation.
Central nervous system germ cell tumor (germinoma, embryonal carcinoma, choriocarcinoma, teratoma)	Tumors in center of brain, tend to be malignant, usually cannot be totally removed; can spread.	Surgery performed for biopsy. Radiation usually given. *Clinical trials:* Chemotherapy. *Recurrent disease:* Chemotherapy or clinical trials.
Optic tract glioma (neurofibromatosis)	Slow-growing tumor, starts in brain cells, grows along optic nerve or optic tract.	If no symptoms, may be observed. If growing, radiation; **or** surgery **or** *Clinical trials:* Chemotherapy to delay radiation.
Pineal parenchymal tumor	Found in center of brain near pineal gland, can spread to other parts of central nervous system.	Surgery to biopsy tumor followed by radiation therapy. *Under 3:* Chemotherapy to delay radiation.
Supratentorial primitive neuroectodermal tumor	Found in upper part of brain, can spread to other parts of central nervous system.	Radiation; **or** *Clinical trials:* Chemotherapy to delay radiation.

and is treated differently than Hodgkin's disease which appears more commonly in young adults and adults over 65. Hodgkin's disease involves the lymph nodes near the surface of the body. These nodes can be felt as painless swelling in the neck, armpit or groin. Children who have reached full growth will probably be treated according to the treatments set up for adults. (Please see Chapter 17, "Lymphomas and Multiple Myeloma," for more detailed background information on Hodgkin's disease and for treatments used for adults with Hodgkin's disease.) More than 75 percent of all newly diagnosed children with childhood Hodgkin's disease are curable with modern radiation therapy and/or combination chemotherapy. The selection of treatment is influenced by the stage of the disease, the age of the child, and the potential long-term effects of treatments. Because the child is in the growing stage, every attempt is made in planning treatment to preserve the integrity of bony and connective tissues.

SYMPTOMS OF CHILDHOOD HODGKIN'S DISEASE

- Fever.
- Weight loss. For young children, failure to gain weight may carry the same significance as weight loss. Teenagers may attribute weight loss to dieting without realizing that it was easier than usual for them to lose unwanted pounds.
- Night sweats that soak the body.
- Swollen glands that don't go away after a few weeks.
- Finding of Reed-Sternberg cells in blood.

What kind of doctor should be treating a child with Hodgkin's disease?

Since it is so important to have treatment planned so that the child's growth is affected as little as possible, it is of primary importance that your child's treatment be overseen by a pediatric oncologist and a treatment team that understands childhood Hodgkin's disease. Radiation should be given by specialists in radiation oncology with experience in treating children with cancer. Check to see that modern megavoltage equipment will be used. Linear accelerators of 4 to 10 MV energy and treatment-planning simulators will insure optimum treatment. Individually shaped blocks should be fabricated to shield normal tissues.

What kind of testing is needed to determine and stage childhood Hodgkin's disease?

Complete, careful clinical, laboratory and diagnostic imaging evaluations are needed to determine the extent of the disease. Lab studies should include a complete blood count, sedimentation rate, routine liver and renal function tests and bone marrow biopsy. CT scans and MRI may be used. In some cases, in order to properly stage the extent of the disease, a laparotomy (surgery to examine lymph nodes, liver and bone marrow) and the removal of the spleen may be needed, especially when the disease is localized and if there is a probability that subsequent treatment decisions may be altered by the findings.

What are the stages of childhood Hodgkin's disease?

There are four stages, I, II, III and IV, which are further divided into A or B categories. A means there are no symptoms. B means that symptoms include one or more of the following: loss of more than 10 percent of body weight in the previous six months (or for young children, failure to gain weight); fever without any other known cause; or night sweats that leave the child's body soaked.

Are there possible aftereffects to the treatments for childhood Hodgkin's disease?

With young children in the growing stages of their lives, the necessarily rigorous treatments can present problems for the future. The risks of sterility and second cancers are taken into consideration by the treatment team and this is why it is so important that the child be properly staged by a knowledgeable team before any treatment is undertaken.

If my child has radiation and the Hodgkin's disease recurs, can chemotherapy then be used?

Chemotherapy is being used effectively for patients who have had radiation and then had a relapse.

How are bone marrow transplants used in treatment of Hodgkin's disease?

Bone marrow transplants are sometimes used when Hodgkin's disease becomes resistant to treatment with radiation therapy or chemotherapy. Because very high doses of chemotherapy can destroy the bone marrow, marrow is sometimes taken from the bones before treatment. The marrow taken is frozen and high-dose chemotherapy with or without radiation therapy is given. The marrow that was removed is then thawed and returned to the body.

TREATMENT FOR CHILDHOOD HODGKIN'S DISEASE

DESCRIPTION	STAGE	TREATMENT
Stage I: Cancer found in only one lymph node area or in only one area or organ outside lymph nodes. IA means there are no symptoms. IB means there are symptoms.	**Stage IA**—when cancer is above diaphragm and does not involve large part of chest.	Radiation to mantle field and lymph nodes in upper abdomen; **or** radiation therapy to mantle field only (in selected patients with minimal disease); **or** chemotherapy plus lower dose radiation to areas that contain cancer.
	Stage IA—when cancer is above diaphragm but involves large part of chest.	Chemotherapy plus radiation therapy to chest or mantle field; **or** radiation therapy to mantle field, lymph nodes in upper abdomen and spleen; **or** *Clinical trials:* Chemotherapy followed by radiation.
	Stage IB—when cancer is above diaphragm but **does not involve large part of chest.**	Radiation therapy to mantle field, lymph nodes in upper abdomen and spleen; **or** chemotherapy plus radiation to areas with cancer.
	Stage IB—when cancer is above diaphragm but **involves large part of chest.**	Chemotherapy plus radiation to chest or mantle field; **or** radiation to mantle field, lymph nodes in upper abdomen and spleen; **or** *Clinical trials:* Chemotherapy followed by low-dose radiation.
Stage II: Cancer found in two or more lymph node areas on same side of diaphragm, or cancer found in only one area or organ outside lymph nodes and in lymph nodes around it. Other lymph node areas on same side of diaphragm may also have cancer.	**Stage IIA or IIB:** when cancer is above diaphragm but **does not involve large part of chest.**	Radiation to mantle field, lymph nodes in upper abdomen and spleen; **or** chemotherapy plus low dose radiation to areas that contain cancer.

(continued)

TREATMENT FOR CHILDHOOD HODGKIN'S DISEASE (cont.)

DESCRIPTION	STAGE	TREATMENT
IIA means there are no symptoms. IIB means there are symptoms.	**Stage IIA or IIB:** when cancer is located above diaphragm **but involves large part of chest.**	Chemotherapy plus radiation therapy to chest or mantle field; **or** radiation therapy to mantle field, lymph nodes in upper abdomen and spleen; **or** *Clinical trials:* Chemotherapy plus low-dose radiation therapy.
Stage III: Cancer found in lymph node areas on both sides of diaphragm. May have spread to areas near affected lymph nodes and/ or to spleen.	**Stage IIIA** (no symptoms).	Chemotherapy; **or** chemotherapy plus radiation to areas with large amounts of cancer; **or** *Clinical trials:* Chemotherapy with or without total nodal radiation.
	Stage IIIB (with symptoms)	Chemotherapy; **or** chemotherapy plus radiation to areas with large amounts of cancer.
Stage IV: Spread in more than one spot to organ or organs outside lymph system. Nearby lymph nodes may or may not be affected, or spread to one organ outside lymph system but distant lymph nodes involved.	**Stage IV**	Chemotherapy; **or** chemotherapy plus low-dose radiation to areas with large amounts of cancer; **or** *Clinical trials:* Chemotherapy with or without total lymph node radiation.
Relapsed	Cancer has recurred after treatment either in same area or another part of body.	If radiation given before, chemotherapy may be used; **or** if chemotherapy given before, different drugs. If returns only in lymph nodes, radiation therapy; **or** if chemotherapy successful in achieving second remission, *Clinical trials:* Chemotherapy and bone marrow transplant.

This type of transplant is called autologous ("awe-ta-low-gus") transplant. If the marrow given is taken from another person it is called an allogeneic ("al-low-jen-a-ik") transplant. (For more information on bone marrow transplants, see Chapter 9, "New Advances and Investigational Trials.")

CHILDHOOD NON-HODGKIN'S LYMPHOMA

How does non-Hodgkin's lymphoma differ from Hodgkin's disease?

The cells that are found in children with non-Hodgkin's lymphoma are different from those found in Hodgkin's disease. Non-Hodgkin's lymphoma develops in the lymph system but can spread to organs other than lymph nodes, such as the liver or the bones. There are two major types of childhood non-Hodgkin's lymphomas: nonlymphoblastic lymphoma and lymphoblastic lymphoma. The type is determined by the way the cancer cells look under a microscope. This is known as the "histology" of the cancer. The nonlymphoblastic type of lymphoma is more common in children than lymphoblastic lymphoma. Although childhood non-Hodgkin's lymphomas are treated differently (see charts) from adult non-Hodgkin's lymphomas, see Chapter 17 for additional general background information.

What are the symptoms of childhood non-Hodgkin's lymphoma?

Abdominal pain or swelling, breathing and/or swallowing difficulties as well as swelling of the face and neck are common symptoms. Swollen lymph nodes may appear in the head and neck as well as in the groin. They are usually painless and firm. If the tumor is in the chest area, respiratory distress may signal a medical emergency. Gastrointestinal tumors may produce symptoms of obstruction or appendicitis.

Where do most nonlymphoblastic lymphomas occur?

Nonlymphoblastic lymphomas, the most common type of non-Hodgkin's lymphoma, most frequently occur in the bowel, particularly in the area near the appendix, and in the upper midsection of the chest. They are also found in the lymph nodes, liver, testicles, spleen, bone marrow, central nervous system, nasal sinuses, skin and bones.

How is non-Hodgkin's lymphoma diagnosed?

The doctor will examine the child carefully and check for swelling or lumps in the neck, underarms, groin and abdomen. If chest swelling is found, a chest x-ray will be required. If lymph nodes are abnormal or a lump is found in the chest or abdomen, a biopsy will be done to determine if there are any cancer cells. Before starting therapy, a complete staging workup should be done, including a careful physical examination, a complete blood count, urine and liver testing, chest x-ray, CT scan, examinations of bone marrow and spinal fluid, and a bone scan to determine the disease extent. The diagnosis should be verified before treatment begins.

Are childhood non-Hodgkin's lymphomas difficult to diagnose?

Especially if there is bone marrow involvement, there may be a question about whether the child has lymphoblastic lymphoma with bone marrow involvement or leukemia. Usually, if less than 25 percent of the cells are lymphoblasts, the child will be treated for lymphoma rather than leukemia.

It is important in the early stage of diagnosis that the child be referred to a treatment center with experience in this type of can-

TREATMENT CHOICES FOR NONLYMPHOBLASTIC CHILDHOOD NON-HODGKIN'S LYMPHOMA	
STAGE	TREATMENT
Stage I: Cancer found in one area outside abdomen or chest. Stage II: Cancer found in two or more lymph nodes or other areas on same side of diaphragm or found in digestive tract with or without lymph node involvement.	Systemic chemotherapy with or without intrathecal chemotherapy.
Stage III: Cancer found in lymph nodes on both sides of diaphragm or in many places in chest or abdomen or in area around spine but not in brain or its coverings.	Systemic chemotherapy plus intrathecal chemotherapy. *Clinical trials:* New drug combinations.
Stage IV: Spread to bone marrow, brain, brain coverings or spinal cord.	Same as above, but if cancer is in brain, radiation to brain. *Clinical trials:* New chemotherapy combinations.
Recurrent: Recurred either where it first started or in another part of body.	Systemic chemotherapy not used before; **or** allogeneic or autologous bone marrow transplant; **or** *Clinical trials:* New treatments.

cer. There, a multidisciplinary team can be certain that the diagnosis is verified before treatment begins.

What kinds of treatments are recommended for non-Hodgkin's lymphoma?

Treatments differ for the two types—nonlymphoblastic and lymphoblastic. Treatments include chemotherapy, radiation and bone marrow transplants, which are being tested in clinical trials. There are treatments for all patients with this disease and a large percentage of children are cured. The tables detail staging and treatment choices.

TREATMENT CHOICES FOR LYMPHOBLASTIC CHILDHOOD NON-HODGKIN'S LYMPHOMA	
STAGE	TREATMENT
Stage I: Cancer found in only one area outside abdomen or chest.	Systemic plus intrathecal chemotherapy.
Stage II: Cancer found in only one area and in lymph nodes around it or in two or more lymph nodes or other areas on same side of diaphragm or in digestive tract where lymph nodes may or may not be involved.	Same as above.
Stage III: Cancer found in lymph nodes on both sides of diaphragm or in many places in chest and/or abdomen or in area around spine but not in brain or brain coverings.	Same as above. Radiation also given if large mass in chest. *Clinical trials:* New drug combinations.
Stage IV: Cancer spread to bone marrow, brain or brain coverings or to spinal cord.	Same as above. If in brain, radiation also given to brain.
Recurrent: Cancer has recurred either where it first started or in another part of the body.	Allogeneic bone marrow transplant; **or** systemic chemotherapy with different drugs; **or** clinical trial of new treatments.

WILMS' TUMOR OR NEPHROBLASTOMA

Wilms' tumor, a cancerous kidney tumor sometimes referred to as nephroblastoma, is usually found in children between the ages of 1 and 4, rarely after age 7. It is curable in the majority of children who are affected, if found in its early stages. Two cell types—ana-plastic cells and sarcomatous cells—found in a small proportion of childhood kidney tumors, are more difficult to cure.

WHAT YOU NEED TO KNOW ABOUT WILMS' TUMOR

- Wilms' tumor has both hereditary and nonhereditary forms. The hereditary type usually appears at an earlier age, and it is likely to affect both kidneys or several sites in one kidney.
- It has been found that gene mutations on the short arm of chromosome 11 are associated with Wilms' tumor as well as with other mutations that sometimes occur in Wilms' tumor patients. A gene that causes a child to be born without an iris in the eye (aniridia) is located nearby.
- The risk of Wilms' tumor among offspring of persons who have had unilateral Wilms' tumors is quite low.
- Siblings of children with Wilms' tumor have little likelihood of developing Wilms' tumor.
- Wilms' tumor is one of modern medicine's success stories. Experience has shown that children treated for Wilms' tumor can be considered cured if they survive for two years without any signs that the disease has returned. In the early part of the century, Wilms' tumor was almost invariably fatal.
- It is wise to take advantage of clinical trials at a major medical center to assure the best possible treatment.

SYMPTOMS OF WILMS' TUMOR

- A swelling on one side of the upper abdomen.
- Blood in the urine.
- Low-grade fever, loss of appetite, paleness, weight loss, and lethargy.
- The absence of the iris of the eye (the colored portion of the eye), called aniridia.
- A condition called hemihypertrophy, which means the abnormal enlargement of a part of the body—often in the development of the genitals or the urinary system.

How is Wilms' tumor diagnosed?

The diagnosis is usually made through the use of ultrasound or CT scan. These studies are able not only to outline the tumor but to clarify whether there is regional spread or whether the opposite kidney is involved.

STAGES OF WILMS' TUMOR

STAGE	DESCRIPTION
Stage I (UH and FH)	Limited to kidney and completely removed by surgery.
Stage II (UH and FH)	Extends beyond kidney but can be removed by surgery.
Stage III (UH and FH)	Cancer spread to areas near kidneys; cannot be completely removed during surgery.
Stage IV (UH and FH)	Spread from kidney to bones, lungs, liver, brain or other parts.
Stage V (UH and FH)	Cancer involves both kidneys.
Recurrent	Cancer returned after treatment either where started or in another part of body.

TREATMENT CHOICES FOR WILMS' TUMOR

STAGE	TREATMENT
Stage I (FH)	Surgery plus chemotherapy.
Stage I (UH)	Surgery plus chemotherapy and/or radiation depending on cell type.
Stage II (FH)	Surgery plus chemotherapy.
Stage II (UH)	Surgery, radiation, and chemotherapy.
Stage III (FH)	Surgery, radiation, and chemotherapy.
Stage III (UH) If very large tumor or tumors located near large blood vessels	Surgery, radiation, and chemotherapy. Chemotherapy or radiation to shrink tumor followed by surgery plus radiation.
Stage IV (FH and UH)	Surgery and chemotherapy with or without radiation.
Stage V (FH and UH)	Surgery to remove some cancer in both kidneys and surrounding nodes followed by chemotherapy to remove remaining cancer. May be followed by chemotherapy and/or radiation.
Recurrent	Surgery, radiation, if indicated, plus chemotherapy.

NOTE: Clinical trials available for all patients.

What are the stages of Wilms' tumor?

The staging indicates whether the tumor is confined to the kidney or has spread to other parts of the body and the other kidney. In addition, the pathologist will designate whether the tumor has favorable histology (FH) or unfavorable histology (UH). While all cancer cells lack the orderly arrangement of normal cells, those designated UH are especially primitive and lacking in organized microscopic structure. The vast majority of children with kidney cancer (about 90 percent) have cell types described as favorable. Kidney tumors that contain elements of sarcoma—cancer that arises from supportive or connective tissue rather than from lining tissue—are also designated UH, although most specialists believe that these cancers are another disease rather than Wilms' tumor. One type of kidney sarcoma, clear cell sarcoma of the kidney, has a tendency to spread to the bone.

What kind of treatments are usually undertaken for Wilms' tumor?

The first order of business is usually surgery to remove the kidney, if possible. Then, depending upon the type of cells found in the tumor, the treatment will depend upon whether the histology (cell type) is considered favorable or unfavorable, designated as FH for favorable histology and UH for unfavorable histology.

NEUROBLASTOMA

Neuroblastoma is a cancer of the nervous system, usually found in certain nerve fibers of the body. These very young nerve cells, for unknown reasons, develop abnormally. A swelling can appear anywhere but is most commonly found in the abdomen, adrenal gland, chest or eye. It usually affects infants and children under the age of 3. The older the child, the more difficult the disease is to treat. Neuroblastomas sometimes disappear spontaneously or may revert to a benign state.

SYMPTOMS OF NEUROBLASTOMA

- Lump or mass in abdomen, adrenal gland, chest or eye.
- Listlessness.
- Persistent diarrhea.
- Pain in the abdomen or elsewhere.

TREATMENT CHOICES FOR NEUROBLASTOMA

STAGE	TREATMENT
Localized resectable–negative nodes (CCG I, II or III resectable or Stage POG A)	Surgery to remove cancer; **or** surgery plus adjuvant chemotherapy; **or** surgery plus radiation.
Localized unresectable (CCG I, II or III unresectable–negative nodes or POG Stage B)	Surgery may be done to remove as much cancer as possible, may be followed by chemotherapy. Surgery may be done again following chemotherapy. May be followed by radiation.
Regional (CCG Stage II and III—nodes positive or POG Stage C)	*Under 1 year:* surgery, **or** chemotherapy with or without surgery. *Over 1 year of age:* Surgery; **or** chemotherapy with or without surgery to remove remaining cancer; **or** chemotherapy with or without radiation followed by surgery or chemotherapy. *Clinical trials:* For children over 1 year, high-dose chemotherapy and radiation followed by bone marrow transplant; **or** chemotherapy and radiation given at same time.
Disseminated (CCG Stage IV or POG Stage D)	Chemotherapy; **or** chemotherapy plus surgery and radiation therapy. *Clinical trials:* High doses of chemotherapy and radiation followed by bone marrow transplant; **or** new methods of treatment.
Stage IVS (very young infants—may regress)	Treatment is controversial. May require little or no therapy unless early complications develop.
Recurrent	Depends upon site, previous treatment and extent of recurrence or progression.

What is the meaning of the staging used for neuroblastoma?

It may be difficult or confusing for you to sort out exactly what stage your child's cancer is in, since a number of different staging methods are used by different groups. The Children's Cancer Group (CCG) uses Stages I, II, III, IV and IVS. The Pediatric Oncology Group (POG) uses Stages A, B, C, and D, and St. Jude Children's Research Hospital uses I, IIA, IIB, IIIAN and IIIA, B, or C. The International Union Against Cancer has a TNM staging method. An International Neuroblastoma Staging System has been developed, combining the elements of these staging systems along with important biological factors. This system is presently being validated. The following stages are used for neuroblastoma:

- **Localized resectable**—the cancer is found only in the place where it started and can be removed by surgery.
- **Localized unresectable**—the cancer is found only in the place where it started but cannot be totally removed during surgery.
- **Regional**—the cancer has spread from where it started to the tissues around it or to lymph nodes in the abdomen not close to the original cancer.
- **Disseminated**—the cancer has spread to lymph nodes outside the abdomen or to the bone, liver, skin, bone marrow or other organs.
- **Stage IVS**—the cancer is in the place where it began and has spread only to the liver, skin and/or bone marrow.
- **Recurrent**—the cancer has come back after it has been treated. It may come back in the area where it first started or in another part of the body.

SOFT TISSUE SARCOMA ·

Although rhabdomyosarcoma is the most common soft tissue sarcoma in children, a number of other soft tissue sarcomas, known as **non-rhabdomyosarcomas**, occur in children. They include fibrosarcoma, synovial sarcoma, hemangiopericytoma, mesenchymal tumors, neurofibrosarcoma, leiomyosarcoma, liposarcoma, alveolar soft part sarcoma and malignant fibrous histiocytoma. In young children, these soft tissue sarcomas are more curable than in adults. Treatments are similar to those for rhabdomyosarcomas. Fibrosarcoma and hemangiopericytoma in infants and young children are less aggressive cancers than the others and can usually be cured with surgical removal. Because of the grave consequences of misdiagnosis, all soft tissue tumors should be reviewed by a pathologist with special expertise in the area. (See Chapter 19, "Bone and Soft Tissue Sarcomas," for other information.)

RHABDOMYOSARCOMA

Rhabdomyosarcoma, where cancer cells begin growing in striated muscle tissue, is the most common type of soft tissue sarcoma found in children. It can occur anywhere in the body but is most frequently found in the head, neck, genitourinary area, arms, legs, chest and abdominal cavity. It occurs most frequently between the ages of 2 and 6 and in the teens. It is considered to be curable in the majority of children who are treated according to the latest methods. As with most cancers, the spread to lymph nodes and other parts of the body makes it more difficut to cure.

SYMPTOMS OF RHABDOMYOSARCOMA

- Swelling in the eye.
- Ear pain or discharge from ear.
- Bloody nasal discharge.
- Mass in an extremity.
- Vaginal bleeding.
- Obstruction of urinary outlet or recurrent urinary tract infection or incontinence.
- Unexplained lump.

Are there different types of rhabdomyosarcoma?

This cancer can be divided into several types, according to the type of cancer cell that is found. These types include: embryonal, embryonal-botryoid, alveolar, pleomorphic and mixed. The embryonal and embryonal-botryoid are the most common. These usually grow in the head and neck or genitourinary tract but can also be found at other sites in the body.

What is the treatment for rhabdomyosarcoma?

All children with rhabdomyosarcoma require multimodality treatment. Following surgery to remove as much of the tumor mass as possible, chemotherapy will usually be prescribed. Radiation may also be given if there is cancer left following the surgery. In performing surgery, the physician will, where possible, try to completely remove the tumor as well as a surrounding "envelope" of normal tissue. The quantity, type and duration of therapy depends upon many factors.

How is rhabdomyosarcoma that has spread treated?

Clinical trials are available for those with metastatic disease, using intensive chemotherapy followed by autologous bone marrow reinfusion. (See Chapter 9, "New Advances and Investigational Trials,"

STAGES OF RHABDOMYOSARCOMA	
STAGE	**DESCRIPTION**
Group I	Localized disease surgically removed. No regional node involvement.
Group IIA	Large tumor, surgically removed, some residual disease, no regional node involvement.
Group IIB	Regional disease with involved nodes, surgically removed, no residual disease.
Group IIC	Regional disease with involved nodes, surgical removal, but evidence of residual involvement of most distal regional node.
Group III	Incomplete surgery or biopsy only of primary site, gross residual disease.
Group IV	Distant metastatic disease at time of diagnosis.

for more information on bone marrow transplants.) Clinical investigations are also being done with the use of intracavitary or interstitial radiation implants and appears to be successful, especially for girls with vaginal or vulval rhabdomyosarcomas.

Is rhabdomyosarcoma genetic?

Research indicates there may be a chromosomal basis for some types of alveolar and embryonal rhabdomyosarcoma. Rhabdomyosarcoma has been associated with neurofibromatosis, fetal alcohol syndrome and Gorlin's basal cell nevus syndrome.

RETINOBLASTOMA

Retinoblastoma is an eye cancer which affects children under the age of 4. The identification of the retinoblastoma gene now makes it possible for physicians to study the differences between hereditary and nonhereditary retinoblastoma. In children with nonhereditary retinoblastoma the cancer is usually found only in one eye. Retinoblastoma is curable in most patients. In hereditary cancer, one or both eyes may be affected. Brothers and sisters of children with retinoblastoma should be checked to see if they have a tendency to develop the disease. Vision can be preserved in many cases. However, secondary cancers may develop (primarily bone and soft tissue sarcomas), sometimes many years after diagnosis and treatment.

Can retinoblastoma be detected in the fetus?

It is possible to predict the possibility of retinoblastoma in pregnant women where there is a family history of this cancer. The infant's eyesight can be saved by prompt use of radiation on tumors that would not ordinarily be detected at an early age.

SYMPTOMS OF RETINOBLASTOMA

- **White light detected in the pupil behind the lens of the eye.**
- **Eye may appear to have a "cast" or squint.**
- **Loss of vision. (Since young children usually are not aware of vision changes, this symptom may not be identified.)**

Who is best qualified to treat retinoblastoma?

Since this is an unusual cancer, treatment planning should be done by a multidisciplinary team of cancer specialists with experience in treating childhood ocular tumors. Especially important is the need to seek out expertise in pediatric radiation therapy and ophthalmology. The treatment should be planned after the extent of the tumor within and outside the eye is known.

What staging systems are used for retinoblastoma?

There are a number of staging systems used. Reese-Ellsworth classification uses five groups, based upon possibilities of maintaining sight. St. Jude's Children's Research Hospital uses a system with four stages which attempts to relate the extent of the disease within and outside the eye to the possibilities of keeping vision and for freedom from spread of the cancer. These systems can be confusing if you are attempting to relate one to the other. In the Reese-Ellsworth classification, about 90 percent of patients fall into the Group V category. In the St. Jude system, 80 percent of patients are classified as Stage I or II. However, for the purposes of treatment, the most reliable system is the categorization of intraocular or extraocular disease, which is listed in the treatment choices chart on page 702.

How is retinoblastoma treated?

Surgery is the most common treatment. If retinoblastoma is found in only one eye and the other eye has normal sight, the diseased eye may be removed. Cryosurgery is sometimes used for very small cancers. Photocoagulation uses a beam of very strong light to kill blood vessels that feed the tumor. Radiation and chemotherapy are also used.

TREATMENT CHOICES FOR RETINOBLASTOMA

TYPE	TREATMENT
Intraocular: one eye (unilateral), has not spread	Surgery to remove the eye; **or** external beam radiation; **or** photocoagulation, with or without radiation; **or** cryosurgery with or without radiation; **or** brachytherapy with radioactive placcques.
Intraocular: both eyes (bilateral), has not spread	Surgery to remove eye with most cancer, plus radiation to remaining eye; **or** radiation therapy to both eyes if there is potential for vision in both eyes.
Extraocular: spread to other eye or other parts of body	Radiation to eye with or without intrathecal chemotherapy; **or** intrathecal chemotherapy alone; **or** systemic chemotherapy. (Radiation to brain if meningeal involvement.) *Clinical trials:* Systemic chemotherapy: **or** intrathecal chemotherapy.
Recurrent	If returns in eye, surgery or radiation. If appears in other part of body, clinical trials.

OSTEOSARCOMA

Osteogenic sarcoma, sometimes called osteosarcoma, is the most common type of bone cancer in children. The bones most frequently involved are the large bones of the upper arm (humerus) and the leg (femur and tibia). This type of cancer is more common among boys than girls and usually occurs between the ages of 10 and 25. Pain and swelling are the most common symptoms—and because they are such everyday complaints, they may be ignored. Diagnosis can be difficult because the symptoms can suggest injury, local infection, glandular deficiencies, arthritis, vitamin deficiencies or benign tumors. The final diagnosis needs a biopsy to confirm the presence of cancer, and since osteogenic sarcoma spreads to other parts of the body, chest x-rays and CAT scans as well as bone scans are usually necessary before treatment is staged.

WHAT YOU NEED TO KNOW ABOUT OSTEOSARCOMA

- **Children with osteosarcoma should be evaluated before biopsy by an orthopedic surgical oncologist.**
- **If saving a limb is a possibility, the biopsy should be performed by the surgeon who will do the future bone tumor removal, since placement of incision is crucial.**

What treatment is usually used for localized osteogenic sarcoma?

Localized osteosarcoma is a highly treatable, often curable disease, although a great deal depends on where the tumor is located. Surgery and chemotherapy are the most common treatments.

What treatment is prescribed for metastatic osteogenic sarcoma?

Metastatic osteosarcoma, which means the disease has spread beyond the bone, is treatable and can sometimes be cured when a combination of therapies is used.

STAGE	TREATMENT
Localized	Surgery to remove tumor, either limb-sparing or amputation, followed by adjuvant chemotherapy; **or** preoperative chemotherapy followed by surgery to remove tumor, either limb-sparing or amputation, and postoperative chemotherapy. *Clinical trials:* Intensive combination chemotherapy and high-dose local radiation.
Metastatic osteosarcoma	Surgery to remove primary tumor and, if possible, metastases, followed by combination chemotherapy; **or** preoperative chemotherapy followed by surgery to remove primary tumor and lung metastases, followed by postoperative chemotherapy.

TREATMENT CHOICES FOR OSTEOSARCOMA

Are some tumors of the bone not really bone tumors at all?

Malignant tumors in other parts of the body sometimes metastasize to the bone. In some cases, the metastases are discovered before the primary tumor is found. A biopsy can often give a clue to the source of the metastasis.

Is it sometimes possible to save the child's limb and spare amputation?

The question of avoiding amputation is always a major one when making decisions about treatment for osteogenic sarcoma. The use of limb-sparing techniques, through the removal of the bone tumor without amputation and replacement of bones or joints with bone grafts or artificial devices, is being evaluated for both immediate and future results. The amount of surgery required to remove the entire tumor is a major consideration. **If saving of the limb is a possibility, the biopsy should be performed by the surgeon who will do the future bone tumor removal, since the placement of the incision is crucial.** There is additional information on osteosarcoma in Chapter 19, "Bone and Soft Tissue Sarcomas."

EWING'S SARCOMA

Ewing's sarcoma is a cancerous tumor of the bone which affects children and young adults. It differs from osteosarcoma in that it tends to be found in bones such as the ribs rather than the long bones of the arm and leg. It is uncommon before age 5 and after age 30. It may involve almost any part of the bony skeleton and may extend into the soft tissue around the bones. It may metastasize to the lungs or other bones. Fever, chills and weakness, intermittent pain, and later swelling are initial symptoms. When it is found outside the bones it is known as "soft-tissue or extra-osseous Ewing's sarcoma." This type of Ewing's sarcoma is usually treated like rhabdomyosarcoma. For many years Ewing's sarcoma was considered fatal, but with present treatment methods it is highly treatable and in many cases curable.

Is Ewing's sarcoma difficult to diagnose?

Ewing's sarcoma can be difficult to diagnose because the small, round cells resemble those in other cancers such as neuroblastoma, non-Hodgkin's lymphoma or rhabdomyosarcoma. Any diagnosis for Ewing's sarcoma should be carefully checked by a pathologist with experience in the diagnosis of small round cell tumors of childhood. Evaluation of fresh tissue by electron microscopy and immunocytochemistry make it possible for the pathologist to recognize features that sometimes lead to reclassification of the tumor as peripheral neuroepithelioma or primitive sarcoma of bone. Every effort should be made at the start to be certain that it is correctly identified.

How is Ewing's sarcoma staged?

The two most important factors to be identified are the location of the primary site of the tumor and whether the disease has spread. A localized Ewing's sarcoma is a tumor that has not spread beyond the original site. The tumor may invade directly into adjacent tissues and still be considered to be localized. The most curable Ewing's sarcomas are those found in the lower jaw, skull, face, scapula (shoulder blade), vertebra or clavicle, and those below the elbow or knee. Other sites such as ribs, upper arm or upper leg and the pelvis or sacrum are more difficult to cure.

What kind of treatment is usually recommended for Ewing's sarcoma?

Surgery, chemotherapy and radiation are all used in treating Ewing's sarcoma. The way in which they are used depends upon the location of the tumor and whether the disease has metastasized to other parts of the body. Surgery is usually limited to the initial diagnostic biopsy of the tumor. However, surgery may be used to remove the entire tumor following chemotherapy. Surgery may also be used to remove the entire tumor if disability can be avoided. When Ewing's sarcoma is found in a very young child, surgery may be used rather than radiation therapy because of the retardation of bone growth side effects caused by radiation. Whenever radiation is used, it should be done in a hospital that uses stringent planning techniques and by a physician who is experienced in the treatment of Ewing's sarcoma. A number of new approaches are being evaluated in clinical trials.

CHILDHOOD LIVER CANCER (HEPATOMA)

Cancers that start in the liver (which are different from those that have spread to the liver from some other location) can occur in both infants and older children. There are two general types—hepatocellular, which is similar to the adult version of liver cancer, and hepatoblastoma, which is most frequently found in children. Liver cancers classified as hepatoblastomas usually occur before 3 years of age. Hepatocellular cancers most often occur between the ages of infant to 4 or at the later age of 12 to 15. When the tumor is totally confined to the liver and can be removed with surgery, it is highly curable. Babies with a high cholesterol level in the first year of life may be at high risk for hepatoblastoma. Many children with liver cancer have a tumor marker (serum alpha-fetoprotein) in their serum that indicates the presence of the disease. Because of the rarity of this disease, children with hepatoma should be considered for entry in a clinical trial.

TREATMENT CHOICES FOR CHILDHOOD CANCER OF THE LIVER	
TYPE	TREATMENT
Group I: Tumor removable by surgery	Surgery followed by chemotherapy.
Group II: Tumor removable after radiation and chemotherapy	Surgery followed by radiation and chemotherapy; **or** preoperative chemotherapy and radiation to reduce tumor followed by surgery and chemotherapy.
Group IIA: Tumor remaining after surgery confined to one lobe	Same as above; **or** *Clinical trials:* Additional chemotherapy agents; **or** nonoperative arterial embolization.
Group III: Tumor involves both lobes	Surgery followed by radiation and chemotherapy; **or** surgery followed by radiation and chemotherapy to reduce tumor followed by further surgery; **or** preoperative chemotherapy and radiation to reduce tumor followed by surgery and chemotherapy. *Clinical trials:* Preoperative chemotherapy and radiation followed by second-look surgery to remove residual disease; **or** intensification of chemotherapy along with radiation and/or surgery; **or** nonoperative arterial embolization; **or** intrahepatic arterial infusions of chemotherapy; **or** chemotherapy with cisplatin and doxorubicin to make tumor operable.
Group IV: Distant metastases	Same as above.

TREATMENT SIDE EFFECTS IN CHILDHOOD CANCERS

Do children sometimes encounter other health problems after being successfully treated for cancer?

Numerous studies have been done—and more are ongoing—to determine what the long-term effects are of some of the aggressive treatments that have cured many childhood cancers. Studies have shown that there seem to be a higher risk for second cancers developing in children who were previously treated for cancer. Radiation treatment to the head, used to destroy leukemic cells that had infiltrated the central nervous system, which extended lives, also was found to affect intellectual development, early puberty, and growth. With the ever-increasing number of persons entering adult life who are now being cured of cancer, the adverse effects of treatments that have saved lives are now being studied. These studies are also being reflected in the management of present treatment so that as the next generation of cured cancer patients age, the statistics will, it is hoped, reflect fewer aftereffects than earlier treatments.

Do cancer treatments have an effect on the children of adults who had cancer as children?

Studies to determine complete answers to this question are ongoing. However, one recent study showed that there was no evidence of increased risk of abnormalities in the children of adults who had childhood cancer and had received therapy which was potentially mutagenic. There was a very small increase in miscarriages in women treated with radiation.

> **Many long-term survivors of childhood cancer remain dangerously ignorant of their need to take preventive measures such as having regular checkups. It is important to keep a complete record of treatments so that any child who has had cancer is fully informed of the original diagnosis, surgery, radiation site, specific types of chemotherapy drugs and any other treatment information that may be helpful in the future.**

What is Candlelighters?

The Candlelighters Childhood Cancer Foundation, which is the oldest and largest of the networking organizations for families with children who have cancer, has established links with 250 family support groups nationally and internationally. The self-help groups share practical information and ways of dealing with common problems, provide an outlet for the frustrations of those under stress, offer a social outlet for parents and siblings, and offer information through meetings featuring medical speakers, psychologists or in-

POSSIBLE TREATMENT SIDE EFFECTS IN CHILDHOOD CANCER

SIDE EFFECT	TREATMENT BELIEVED RESPONSIBLE
Early puberty	Cranial radiation.
Scoliosis	Spinal radiation (current radiation practices which include whole vertebral body in radiation have decreased, but still not eliminated, incidence).
Gonadal damage, infertility and hormonal dysfunction	Chemotherapy and radiation.
Thyroid disfunction (laboratory values may normalize over time)	Radiation to the neck.
Neuropsychological—intellectual, verbal, fine-motor, attention; severity varies	Cranial radiation therapy and chemotherapy.
Heart damage—left ventricular dysfunction, congestive heart failure, coronary heart disease, arrhythmias	Chemotherapy—anthracyclines, high-dose cyclophosphamide, mitoxantrone—and radiation.
Pulmonary function abnormalities, reduced exercise tolerance	Whole lung or thoracic radiation, bone marrow transplants.
Renal dysfunction	Abdominal radiation, chemotherapy, antibiotic therapy.
Gastric or duodenal ulcers, small bowel obstruction, severe gastritis	Radiation, laparotomy.
Liver damage	Low-dose methotrexate and 6-mercaptopurine therapy.
Eye problems, including cataracts	Cranial radiation.
Dental problems	Head and neck radiation, chemotherapy.
Second cancers	Radiation and chemotherapy—mainly alkylating agents.
Weight gain after treatment	Reason is poorly understood. May be psychological but appears to have other explanations.

surers. Candlelighters also publishes newsletters, operates a telephone hotline, provides training materials for long-term survivor and youth leadership groups and is involved in advocacy issues such as education, medical leave policies, employment and insurance. (Not all groups are called Candlelighters.) For information see Chapter 26, "Where to Get Help."

What is the Ronald McDonald House?

The Ronald McDonald House facilities provide comfortable, accessible quarters for families of children undergoing treatment with long hospital stays away from the family's home. (See Chapter 26, "Where to Get Help," for information on where these are located and how they operate.)

What is Children's Hospice International?

Although treatment is successful for many children with cancer, sometimes cancer cannot be cured. When the disease becomes terminal, some parents wish to have their child die at home rather than in the hospital. Information on home care is available from Children's Hospice International (see Chapter 26, "Where to Get Help"), which provides referrals for home and hospice care in your area. In addition, most pediatric oncology programs provide hospice-type support for their patients.

Where can I get information on the organizations that make wishes come true for children with cancer?

There are a number of organizations across the country which make it possible for children's wishes to be fulfilled. Information is available through the Cancer Information Service, the American Cancer Society, or Candlelighters.

Where can I get information about summer camps for children with cancer?

There are a growing number of summer camps for children with cancer. The camps are medically staffed, and many of the programs are free. See Chapter 26, "Where to Get Help," for information. Further information about camps in your locality is available from the Cancer Information Service, Candlelighters or the American Cancer Society.

chapter 23

Dictionary of Unusual Cancers

So often, in talking with physicians and other health professionals, we, as laymen, stumble upon words that we do not understand. This is particularly true when unusual types of cancer, or unusual subtypes of cancer, are being discussed. It's frustrating to have your cancer described, and then not be able to find any information about it in the normal texts. To help gain a little perspective and shed a little light, this chapter seeks to further define, in the most basic manner, some of the less common types and designations of cancers and to give you clues that will help you to seek out further information.

Acinar cell cancer: A form of exocrine pancreatic cancer.

Acral-lentiginous melanoma: A type of melanoma which appears as a dark spot on palms, soles or nails.

Acute erythroleukemia: A form of acute myelogenous leukemia (AML) characterized by overproduction of immature red cells mixed with a variety of immature white cells.

Acute promyelocytic leukemia: A subtype of acute nonlympho-cytic leukemia (ANLL) characterized by the overproduction of primitive granulocytes.

Adamantinoma: Cancer of the long bones in the body, usually the shinbones.

Adenoid cystic carcinoma: Cancer of one of the minor salivary glands.

Adrenal cancer: Cancer of the adrenal glands located above the kidneys.

Adrenocortical cancer: Cancer of the outer shell of the adrenal glands, located above the kidneys.

Alveolar cell lung cancer: See Brochioloalveolar lung cancer.

Alveolar soft part sarcoma: A soft tissue sarcoma that occurs primarily in thighs of adults and neck area of children.

Anaplastic thyroid cancer: An aggressive, difficult-to-treat thyroid cancer.

Androma: See Sterloi-Lydig tumor

Angiosarcoma: A soft tissue sarcoma originating in a blood vessel.

Arrhenoma: See Sterloi-Lydig tumor

B-cell acute lymphocytic leukemia: A type of acute lympyhocytic leukemia that affects immature stem cells that have started to mature along the B-cell line of development.

Basaloid cancer: Type of anal cancer.

Bile duct cancer: Cancer in the tube system that drains bile from the liver to the intestine. May be distal or proximal.

Bowen's disease: Skin cancer that occurs on areas unexposed to sun. Sometimes considered a precancerous condition.

Bronchioloalveolar lung cancer: A type of adenocarcinoma of the lung, not associated with smoking; affects bronchioles and alveolar walls of the lung. Treated as a nonsmall cell lung cancer.

Bronchogenic cancer: Type of lung cancer that starts in the bronchial tubes.

Burkitt cell acute lymphocytic leukemia: See B-cell acute lymphocytic leukemia.

Burkitt's lymphoma: Fast-growing form of non-Hodgkin's lymphoma. Seen in children as well as AIDS patients.

Cancer en cuirasse: A cancer of the skin of the thorax also called corset cancer and jacket cancer.

Carcinoma mucocellulare: See Krukenberg tumor.

CGL: Another name for chronic myelogenous leukemia. Stands for chronic granulocytic leukemia.

Cholesteatoma: See Congenital brain tumor.

Chondroblastic or **Chondrosarcomatous:** Refers to a subtype of osteosarcoma.

Chordoma: A bone cancer that usually grows in the spinal column, most often at the ends of the spine or the base of the skull.

Choroid plexus tumor: Brain tumor originating in choroid plexus epithelial cells. More benign form is called choroid plexus papilloma. More malignant form is called anaplastic choroid plexus papilloma.

Cloacogenic cancer: Type of anal cancer.

Congenital brain tumor: A tumor that has existed in the brain since birth. Includes dermoids or cystic teratomas, cholesteatomas and craniopharyngiomas.

Connective tissue cancer: Soft tissue sarcoma.

Craniopharyngioma: See congenital brain tumor.

Cushing disease: Fat buildup in face, back and chest while legs and arms become thin, resulting from buildup of ACTH-producing hormones associated with pituitary tumors, many of which are noncancerous.

Dedifferentiated chondrosarcoma: A type of malignant chondrogenic bone tumor.

Desmoplastic fibroma: A primary fibrosarcoma of bone.

DHL: Diffuse histiocytic lymphoma.

Diffuse large cell lymphoma of bone: Usually a sign of disease that has spread but sometimes may be a solitary lesion.

DiGugliemo's syndrome: See Erythroleukemia.

Eaton Lambert syndrome: See Myasthenic syndrome.

En cuirasse: See Cancer en cuirasse.

Eosinophilic granuloma: See Histiocytosis X.

Eosinophilic leukemia: A form of leukemia affecting the eosinophils or granular leukocytes.

Ependemoblastoma or **Ependymoma:** Tumor composed of ependymal cells that line passageway in brain where special fluid that protects brain and spinal cord is made and stored.

Epidermoid cancer: Any tumor appearing in a part of the body other than the skin that is made up of skinlike elements.

Erythroleukemia: Type of acute nonlymphocytic leukemia (ANLL) affecting both red and white cells.

Fibrosarcoma of bone: Bone tumor, most often found in long bones, sometimes found in head and neck. Usually appears in middle age, characterized by interlacing, herringbone-patterned bundles of collagen fibers.

Fibrosarcoma of soft tissue: Sarcoma derived from fibroblasts that produce collagen.

Fibrous histiocytoma: See Malignant fibrous histiocytoma.

Giant cell tumor of bone (GCT): An aggressive bone tumor that may recur locally but has a low potential for metastasizing.

Glomus tumor: A noncancerous small tumor of the neural tissue usually occurring in the head and neck.

Glucagonoma: A cancer of the endocrine pancreas.

Grawitz's tumor: A type of kidney cancer known as cancer of the renal parenchyma.

Hand-Schüller-Christian syndrome: See Histiocytosis X.

Hemangiopericytoma: A type of soft tissue sarcoma originating in the blood vessels of arms, legs and trunk.

Hepatoblastoma: A type of liver cancer which consists chiefly of embryonic hepatic tissue. Occurs in infants and young children.

Histiocytosis X: A generic term which includes three related disorders, eosinophilic granuloma, Letterer-Siwe disease and Hand-Schüller-Christian syndrome, characterized by large histiocytes (macrophages).

Indolent non-Hodgkin's lymphoma: A group of slow-growing non-Hodgkin's lymphomas.

Infantile hemangiopericytoma: A type of soft tissue sarcoma originating in the blood vessels in the arms, legs, trunk, head, and neck of infants up to age 1.

Islet cell cancer: A form of pancreatic cancer that originates in the endocrine glands that produce hormones.

Juxtacortical osteosarcoma: See Parosteal osteogenic sarcoma.

Krukenberg tumor: Also called carcinoma mucocellulare. A type of cancer of the ovary which has usually metastasized from the gastrointestinal tract.

Lacrimal gland tumor: A growth in the tear gland which may be malignant.

Lentigo maligna melanoma: Also known as melanotic freckle of Hutchinson. A brownish pigmented spot on the skin that is considered to be noninvasive.

Leptomeningeal cancer: Cancer that has metastasized from another part of the body to the tissue lining the spinal canal.

Letterer-Siwe disease: See Histiocytosis X.

Leukemic reticuloendotheliosis: Hairy cell leukemia.

Macroglobulinemia: A condition characterized by increase in macroglobulins in the blood.

Malignant fibrous histiocytoma (MPH): A high-grade bone tumor usually found in adult long bones, especially around knee.

Medulloblastoma: A brain tumor composed of undifferentiated neuroepithelial cells.

Melanoma sarcoma: Rare clear cell sarcoma sometimes referred to as malignant melanoma of soft parts.

Meningeal carcinomatosis: Cancer that has spread over the surface of the brain and its lining.

Merkel cell tumor of the skin: A type of primary skin cancer characterized by peculiar distinctive granules. Appears in elderly persons.

Mesenchymoma: Soft tissue, mixed cell sarcoma.

Mucinous breast carcinoma: Slow-growing breast cancer that appears in ducts and produces mucus.

Mullerian tumor: A cancer of the uterus, ovary or fallopian tubes that arises from remnants of embryonic tissue. Occurs usually in women 55 to 60.

Multiple endocrine neoplasia (MEN): An endocrine system cancer that may be inherited.

Myasthenic syndrome: A condition, with symptoms similar to myasthenia gravis, associated with small cell lung cancer.

Null cell acute lymphocytic leukemia: An undifferentiated form of leukemia in which grossly immature stem cells that exhibit no differentiation are affected.

Osteochondroma: Cartilage tumor, usually benign.

Pancoast tumor: A form of small cell lung cancer in which a slow-growing tumor is found in the groove along the top edge of the lung.

Parosteal osteogenic sarcoma: Also called juxtacortical osteosarcoma. A slow-growing sarcoma that involves the midshaft of the long bones.

Periosteal osteosarcoma: A type of osteosarcoma that grows on the cortex of the bone, usually the tibia.

Peripheral neuroepithelioma: A non–central nervous system sarcoma found in children and young adults. Treated like Ewing's sarcoma.

Pheochromocytoma: Cancer of the inner core of the adrenal glands.

Pineal gland tumor: A benign tumor located near the center of the brain. Occurs most often in children and young adults.

Plasmacytoma: A tumor of the plasma cells, multiple myeloma.

Reticulum cell sarcoma of bone: See Diffuse large cell lymphoma of bone.

Round cell sarcomas: Two most common types of round cell sarcomas are Ewing's sarcoma and non-Hodgkin's lymphoma.

Signet-rina cell: A highly malignant, muscus-secreting tumor.

Small cell osteosarcoma: A variant of round cell osteosarcoma that resembles Ewing's sarcoma, but may be treated differently.

Spindle cell lung cancer: Terminology used for squamous cell lung cancer, also called epidermoid.

Sterloi-Lydig tumor: A cancer of the ovary. Also called androma, andreioma, arrhenoma and arrhenoblastoma.

Superior sulcus tumor: See Pancoast tumor.

Telangiectatic: A subtype of osteosarcoma.

Thymoma: A cancer of the tissues of the thymus.

von Hippel Lindau syndrome (VHL): Rare familial disorder which can result in cancer in patients who have visceral lesions. (See Chapter 26, ''Where to Get Help,'' for organization which offers information on disease.)

Waldenstrom's macroglobulinemia: A cancer of the white blood cells which behaves like myeloma. Most often seen in males over 50.

chapter 24

Living with Cancer

> Going back to the well world after you have been through the cancer olympics isn't easy. But there are lots of practical tips that can help, and a great deal of advice from others who have been through it to help you along the way.

This chapter deals with the many practical aspects of living with cancer on a day-to-day basis. It also covers information on feelings and the emotions which are encountered. Consequently, some of the questions apply to all patients, while some may be relevant to only a few. You'll find helpful information about eating well, exercise, about sexual problems that may arise, dealing with pain, and about money matters and insurance. Since dying is part of living, this chapter deals frankly with that subject and includes some information on wills, care at home, hospice care, euthanasia, dying, death and autopsies. Much of the information should be of interest to the healthy as well as to those who are ill.

EATING WELL

Can I go to my doctor for information about what diet is best for me?

Many doctors, realizing the heightened public interest in nutrition as it relates to health, are advising patients to seek nutritional help.

Many traditional doctors still are not educated in nutrition and some can be quite antagonistic about the whole subject. Although you will want to let your oncologist know your concerns about improving your diet, don't be surprised if your request is met in a noncommittal, halfhearted or even hostile way. However, you can ask the doctor or nurse to arrange for you to consult with a dietitian at the hospital where you have been treated or you can find a professional nutritionist to give you advice.

Are there special nutrition requirements for people undergoing treatment?

Good nourishment is essential for healing and building new tissues. People who eat well during treatment, especially foods high in protein and calories, are better able to stand the side effects of treatment. Some researchers feel it may even be possible for these patients to withstand higher doses of certain treatments. There are nutrition experts who believe that during chemotherapy, for example, you may need as much as 50 percent more protein than usual and 20 percent more calories.

What happens when you don't feel like eating?

When a person eats less, for whatever reason, the body uses its own stored-up fat, protein and other nutrients, such as iron. When this happens, your natural defenses are weakened and your body cannot fight infection as well. It is not unusual to lose interest in food during treatment, but you must try to eat a diet that is high enough in calories to keep up your normal weight, if at all possible. Eat any time you are hungry. Try to keep a supply of nutritious, caloric, high-protein foods on hand. Protein can help repair the body if the body is getting enough calories. If it is not, the body will use the protein for energy instead of repair.

What can be done about sore mouth or a sore throat that is a side effect of treatment?

First of all, check with your doctor to be sure the soreness is a treatment side effect and not an unrelated problem. The doctor or dentist can give you medication that will help ease throat and mouth pain. Foods that are difficult to chew can irritate a tender mouth or throat. Try eating soft foods that are easy to chew and swallow such as soups, cottage cheese, pastas, pureed meats and vegetables, mashed potatoes, eggs, milkshakes, bananas, applesauce, fruit nectars, watermelon, oatmeal, custards, puddings and gelatins. Mix food with butter, thin gravies and sauces to make them easier to swallow. Avoid foods that can irritate such as citrus fruit or fruit juices, spicy or salty foods, rough, coarse, or dry foods such as raw vegetables, granola and toast. Rinse your mouth with water often to remove food and bacteria and to promote healing. If swallowing is difficult, you may find it helpful to tilt your head back or move it forward to change the position of the swallowing mechanism to make it more comfortable.

Do treatments sometimes change your sense of taste?

Many people find that chemotherapy, radiation or the cancer itself can alter taste sensations. Sometimes called mouth blindness or taste blindness, this side effect can leave you with a sense that food is tasteless or with a feeling of a bitter, metallic taste in your mouth, especially when eating meat or other protein foods. Usually, this is a short-term problem that eventually resolves itself. To help make foods taste better, you may find that adding flavorings such as bacon, onions, lemon, basil, oregano or rosemary helps. If red meat is a particular problem, you may want to switch to chicken, turkey, eggs, dairy products or bland fish. If you don't have a sore mouth or throat, you may find that tart foods such as oranges, lemons, limes and grapefruit help to bolster your taste buds.

What can be done to relieve a dry mouth or a lack of saliva?

Chemotherapy and radiation therapy in the head or neck area can reduce the flow of saliva and cause you to feel that your mouth is very dry. To help combat this feeling you may find it helpful to suck on hard candy or lollipops (there are many sugar-free types on the market) or chew sugar-free chewing gum. Popsicles are handy to have on hand to help produce more saliva. Keeping a glass of water close by that you can sip on every few minutes helps you to swallow and talk more easily. Lip salves help to moisten your lips. If they can be tolerated, very sweet as well as hot, spicy or tart and sour foods and beverages may help encourage the production of saliva. Lemonade works well but is not advised if you are also suffering from a tender mouth and sore throat. If the problem is very severe, you can ask your doctor or dentist to prescribe products now on the market that coat and protect your mouth and throat.

What can I eat when my mouth and throat are sore from treatment?

Many people who are having chemotherapy or radiation treatments complain of soreness which makes eating difficult.

- Be sure to have the doctor examine the area to see whether or not special medication will help.

- Make sure to see your dentist for special care during this period.
- Put your cooked food into a blender so that it is easier to eat.
- Cold foods can sometimes help to soothe the soreness. Add ice to milk and milkshakes.
- Stews and casseroles can be softened with extra liquids and longer cooking times.
- Mashed potatoes, scrambled and poached eggs, egg custards, ricotta cheese, puddings, gelatins, creamy cereals, all kinds of pastas and milkshakes are easy to eat and good for you.
- Stay away from foods that sting and burn such as citrus fruits and tomatoes; hot spicy foods with pepper, chili powder, nutmeg, and cloves; rough and coarse foods such as raw vegetables and bran; and dry foods like toast and hard bread.
- Do not use hot water or commercial mouthwash to rinse your mouth. A mixture of one teaspoon salt or baking soda to a quart of water or equal parts of glycerin and warm water can be soothing. Rinsing with club soda can relieve dry mouth or thick saliva. Oragel, available at the pharmacy, can help deaden the pain.
- If you wear dentures and have sores under them, remove them and do not wear them when you do not need them for eating.
- If your problem is severe, your doctor can prescribe medication to numb your gums and tongue. Artificial saliva is also available.

Are there ways to help control nausea caused by treatments?

Nausea, with or without vomiting, is a common side effect of chemotherapy, and can also occur as a result of surgery, radiation therapy and immunotherapy. Whatever the cause, nausea can be a serious problem because it keeps you from getting the nutrients you need. Ask your doctor about medications that can be prescribed to help control nausea. Most nausea and vomiting can be prevented or controlled with antiemetic medicines taken before treatment. Foods that are fatty, greasy or fried or hot and spicy, as well as sweet foods such as candy, cookies or cake, should be avoided. Foods like toast and crackers, yogurt, sherbet, pretzels, angel food cake, oatmeal, skinned baked or broiled chicken, ice chips, soft bland fruits and vegetables usually can be most easily tolerated. Drink or sip liquids through a straw throughout the day but avoid drinking liquids with meals. Eat small amounts of food often and slowly. Some people find that hot foods can add to nausea, so eat foods at room temperature or cooler. Try to rest after meals. Rest sitting up, if possible, for about an hour after meals. If nausea is a problem in the morning, try eating dry toast or crackers before getting out of bed.

What are some ideas for how to deal with vomiting?

Vomiting may be brought on by treatment, food odors, motion or gas in the stomach or bowel. You should let your doctor know if vomiting is severe or lasts for more then a few days. Some people find that certain situations or surroundings (such as the hospital setting) may trigger vomiting. Very often, if you can control nausea, you may prevent vomiting. But there may be times when you may not be able to control either nausea or vomiting. To help you deal with vomiting, you should not drink or eat until you have the vomiting under control. Once your stomach seems to have settled down, try taking small amounts of clear liquids. Begin with a teaspoonful every ten minutes, gradually increasing the amount to a tablespoonful every twenty minutes. Then, try two tablespoonfuls every thirty minutes. Once you are able to keep down clear liquids, you can slowly begin to try a full-liquid diet. Continue taking small amounts as often as feels comfortable. Once you are functioning on a full-liquid diet, you can start returning to a regular diet, starting with soft, bland foods. Be sure to discuss any vomiting problems with your doctor and nurse, and if they cannot be brought under control, ask about medications designed to deal with the problem.

Are there guidelines on amounts of protein and calories required during recuperation?

During illness, treatment and recovery, it is estimated that women need about 80 grams of protein (compared to a normal daily need of 44 grams) and men require 90 grams (compared to a normal daily need of 46 grams). An additional 200 to 300 calories should also be added to the diet. Of course, if your weight is stable, you may not need to increase your intake. If you are losing weight, you should definitely try to add extra nourishment.

How can I add protein to my diet?

You can add protein to the diet in several ways without increasing the amount of food you eat. (Some of these are a dieter's dream come true.) For example:

- Add grated cheese, chunks of cheese or melted cheese to sauces, vegetables, soups, sandwiches and casseroles.

- Add cottage cheese or ricotta cheese with vegetables, fruits, eggs, and desserts.
- Add diced or ground meat or fish to soups, salads, omelets, sauces, and casseroles. Calf or chicken livers are good sources of protein, vitamins and minerals and are a good addition to your diet.
- Cook and use dried peas and beans and bean curd (tofu) in soups, casseroles, pastas and grain dishes that also contain cheese or meat.
- Add cream cheese or peanut butter as well as butter to your bread.
- Choose dessert recipes that contain eggs—custards, bread puddings, or rice puddings.
- Use milk in beverages and in cooking. Add skim milk powder to your regular milk.
- Use peanut butter—on crackers, waffles or celery sticks—or eat it out of the jar.
- Add ice cream, yogurt and frozen yogurt to other beverages such as ginger ale and milkshakes, as well as to cereals, fruits and pies.
- Increase your nut, seed, and wheat germ intake by adding them to casseroles, breads, pancakes, waffles or anywhere a crunchy topping would taste good.

How can I add calories?

- Add butter and margarine to soups, potatoes, hot cereals, rice, noodles, cooked vegetables, sauces and gravies.
- Use mayonnaise in salads or on sandwiches. Mayonnaise adds 100 calories per tablespoon.
- Use peanut butter on fruits, vegetables and sandwiches. One tablespoon of peanut butter has 90 calories and is also rich in protein.
- Use sour cream for vegetable dip and on vegetables. Add to gravy, soups, casseroles, sauces, and salad dressings. One tablespoon of sour cream adds 70 calories.
- Add whipping cream to pies, fruit, puddings, hot chocolate, Jell-O or other desserts. One tablespoon adds 60 calories.
- Add raisins, dates, or chopped nuts and brown sugar to hot cereals or to cold cereals for a snack.
- Have nuts, dried fruits, popcorn, crackers and cheese, and ice cream on hand so you can have a quick snack whenever you feel hungry.

- Add jam, honey, and sugar to bread, cereal, and milk drinks.
- Milkshakes add calories and are easy to make with a blender.
- In food preparation, sauté and fry foods when possible because these methods add more calories than baking or broiling.

Should I worry about how much fat I am eating?

Fats are the most concentrated source of energy. They give about twice the number of calories as do an equal weight of protein or carbohydrates. Therefore, nutritionists believe that if you need additional calories, the most efficient way to get them is by adding fat to the diet.

Doesn't fat cause cancer?

There is research which shows that eating too much fat may increase your chance of getting cancers of the colon, breast, prostate, and endometrium. However, you need to look at the requirements your body has while you are undergoing treatment versus the diet you might want to follow for the rest of your life. You need to consider the importance of making sure your body is receiving enough nourishment during treatment.

Is it a good idea for me to go on the higher-fiber, lower-fat diet recommended by the National Cancer Institute while I am having treatment?

No. For individuals under treatment for cancer, the highest priority is a diet adequate in calories, protein, and vitamins. After you complete treatment, you may wish to consider modifying your diet in order to lower fat intake and raise fiber levels.

Should I also be taking extra vitamins and minerals?

Some researchers suggest adding vitamins and minerals to the nutritional regimen to help protect the body, during and following surgery, while taking chemotherapy and radiation treatments and to help improve the functioning of the immune system. It's important to distinguish between reasonably large doses of vitamins and vitamin megadosing. Injectable vitamins are another way of boosting vitamin efficiency. Your doctor or a nutritionist should be consulted about dosages.

What vitamins and minerals and in what amounts are best for you?

Though the government has come up with a set of standards, the role of many vitamins and minerals is still not fully understood. However, it is known that people recovering from injuries or surgery have greatly increased requirements for certain vitamins. People who smoke, drink moderate amounts of alcohol, or take oral contraceptives also need more vitamins than they otherwise would and may undergo vitamin depletion even when their vitamin intake is normal. The B-complex vitamins are essential in the process by which food is used for energy, repair and all the other essentials of life. Vitamin C is necessary, among other things, for the body to make collagen, a major component of skin, tendons, and bones. The body depends on vitamin A for healthy epithelial tissue—that is, the tissue that forms the covering or lining of all body surfaces, including the lining of the digestive tract, lungs and blood vessels. Vitamin E is an antioxidant. It protects lipids (water-soluble fats) from the attack of oxidizing agents. Potassium deficiencies can result from diarrhea or vomiting. Attention should be paid to increasing potassium either through supplements or by adding potassium-rich foods like potatoes, molasses, apricots, raisins or bananas to the daily diet. Checking through your dietary and vitamin needs with a qualified nutritionist (see information in this chapter) is important since self-prescribing of vitamins can be dangerous because of possible toxic side effects.

Is there a difference in nutritional needs once treatment is completed?

During treatment, your body needs extra protein and calories to help in the healing process. Once that is all behind you, you'll want to learn about diet and nutrition as it relates to cancer prevention. Although there is little research on whether or not nutrition can prevent recurrence, more and more evidence is being gathered through animal studies and studies of large population groups that correlates lifestyles with cancer, showing that there is a strong connection between good nutrition and good health. Both the American Cancer Society and the National Cancer Institute recommend a diet low in fat and high in fiber. The National Cancer Institute is also involved in a research program to test the effects of vitamin A, beta-carotene, vitamins C and E, and selenium, among others, to see whether they have an impact on cancer.

What can I do about diarrhea problems?

Some kinds of cancers and some kind of treatments can cause diarrhea, excessive gas, or a bloated feeling. To dealt with this problem:

- Drink liquids between meals instead of with them. Liquids are important since diarrhea causes loss of fluids and salts that must be replaced.

- Eat small amounts of food more often. Applesauce, bananas, white rice, tapioca and plain tea are helpful. Fatty foods and foods that are highly spiced should be avoided.
- If your intestines are irritated, lower the amount of fiber, using only cooked fruits and vegetables and avoiding those with tough skins and seeds such as beans, broccoli, corn, onions and garlic.
- Be aware of your potassium and salt intake. These important elements are lost in great quantities when you have diarrhea, and the result is that you may feel weak. Add foods that are high in potassium but won't worsen diarrhea. Bouillon or fat-free broth are good liquid choices. Bananas, apricot or peach nectar, and potatoes are all good sources of potassium that don't cause diarrhea.
- Limit foods and beverages that contain caffeine, such as coffee, strong tea, some sodas, and chocolate.
- Diarrhea may be caused by lactose intolerance, which means you are having problems digesting the lactose in milk or milk products. Buttermilk, sour cream, and yogurt may be easier for your body to handle.
- If you have cramps, stay away from foods that may encourage gas or cramping, such as carbonated drinks, beer, beans, cabbage, broccoli, cauliflower, and highly spiced foods.
- If your diarrhea is persistent or has blood in it, or if you start to lose weight, see your doctor.

What can be done about constipation?

Constipation may result from treatment with some drugs.

- Make sure your regular diet includes a variety of fruits and vegetables, breads, cereals, bran, dried fruits and nuts. If you cannot chew or swallow these, grate them or put them in a blender to make them easier to eat.
- Drink plenty of liquids—eight or ten glasses each day.
- Drink prune juice, heated, to stimulate bowel activity.
- Add extra bran to other foods such as cooked cereals or casseroles.
- Eat high-fiber snack foods such as sesame sticks, date-nut or prune bread, oatmeal cookies, Fig Newtons, date or raisin bars, granola.
- Try doing some light exercise daily.
- Schedule time to concentrate on bowel movements each day.
- Check with the doctor or nurse before taking a laxative or stool softener.

What kind of nutritional supplements can I use to boost my diet?

Many people find, when they cannot get enough calories and protein from their diets, that it is helpful to add commercial nutrition supplements, such as formulas and instant breakfast powders that are available in supermarkets and drugstores, to their diets. These supplements are high in protein and calories and have extra vitamins and minerals. They come in liquid, pudding, and powder forms. Since these products need no refrigeration until after they are opened, they're handy to have on hand. They can be carried with you so they can be used when you feel hungry or thirsty. They make a good between-meal or bedtime snack and they require no preparation.

Is it unusual to have weight gain as a result of treatment?

Sometimes patients gain extra weight during treatment even though they are not adding extra calories. Some anticancer drugs, such as prednisone, can cause the body to hold on to fluid and, thus, to add extra weight. The extra weight is actually water and does not mean you are overeating. It is important not to go on a diet if you notice a gain in weight without discussing it with your doctor or nurse. If the reason for the extra weight is due to the anticancer drugs, you may be advised to limit the salt you eat because salt causes your body to retain water. Diuretic drugs may be prescribed to help reduce the water.

OUTSIDE HELP

Many kinds of services are available to help you deal with some of the problems that you are likely to face. From homemaker services through nurses and nutritionists, you can call upon a whole battery of people who have specialized training to help you through difficult times and specific problems.

What do homemaker services provide?

Homemaker services provide well-trained, adaptable, mature women to help keep a household running. Homemaker services may be available in your area through a community health or welfare agency, a church, a club or some other nonprofit organization. Look in the yellow pages under "Homemaker Services" or check with the American Cancer Society in your area.

How can visiting nurses help?

Visiting nurse associations or city health departments provide part-time nursing help to patients at home and offer advice and guidance to help the family and others with care. A visiting nurse will give health instructions and referrals to other agencies that may be of help. You can contact the visiting nurses either directly or through your doctor. If you have health insurance which covers nursing care, the charges (which are adjusted to the patient's ability to pay) may be payable under the policy. Medicare covers some part-time public health nursing in the home if it is ordered by your doctor. Many public health nursing organizations use practical nurses, who attend to all general health needs of the patient and work under the direction of a professional nurse.

How can I find a physical therapist?

Physical therapists can be recommended by your doctor or are available through the rehabilitation department of your hospital or visiting nurse associations. They are usually listed in the phone book yellow pages under "Physical Therapists." Whether disabilities are temporary or permanent, and whether they are caused by the cancer or its treatment, there is therapy available. The role of the physical therapist is to help maintain and increase normal body function, to prevent loss of function where possible, to help teach you how to substitute when loss occurs and to help you become as independent as possible. One of the most common problems which physical therapists deal with is loss of strength or paralysis. With simple exercises designed to strengthen muscles or improve balance and coordination, normal movement can often be regained.

Should I schedule extra visits with my dentist?

Cancer and cancer treatment may cause tooth decay and other problems with your teeth and gums, so be sure to schedule followup visits with your dentist. Patients who are receiving treatment that affects the mouth, such as those who are having radiation to the head and neck, may need to see the dentist more often than usual. If your gums are very sensitive, clean your teeth with a very soft toothbrush, cotton swabs or mouth swabs made especially for this purpose. Rinse your mouth with warm water to sooth sore gums and mouth.

How can I find a good nutritionist?

Since only thirteen states license or certify nutritionists, finding a good one on your own can be a problem. Most of the legitimate ones are registered dietitians (RDs), which means they have been certified by the American Dietetic Association. There are about 47,000 registered dietitians in the United States, some of whom are employed by hospitals, clinics and beauty spas. There are also

M.D.s with postgraduate training and clinicians with Ph.D.s in nutrition. They are usually members of the American Society of Clinical Nutrition and certified by the American Board of Nutrition. A lack of registered credentials does not necessarily mean a lack of competence. It does mean, however, that you should check out reputation by other means.

- Ask a doctor, nurse or local hospital for a recommendation. Many food counselors work in conjunction with the medical profession. If you have been a patient at the hospital, you can get a referral to a dietitian there.
- Look in the yellow pages of your telephone directory under "Nutrition." Listed there, you will probably find a number of names, only a few of whom will be Ph.D.s or registered dietitians. Some counselors will have M.S. after their names, indicating an advanced degree in science. Nutrition counselors and clinical nutritionists are common listings, but do not give you information as to qualifications—except by omission.
- Questionable credentials include a degree in nutrition counseling from unaccredited correspondence schools or degree initials such as N.D., Doctor of Naturopathy; C.H., Certified Herbologist; or R.H., Registered Healthologist. Listings offering nutritional and metabolic evaluation service such as hair analyses and cytotoxic blood tests for determining food sensitivities are questionable.
- You can learn a great deal quickly by making telephone calls to those listed. Ask questions about qualifications and background, how long they have been counseling, what types of patients they usually work with, what kind of treatment and testing, if any, is used. Be sure to ask what the charges will be and how many visits most patients average. Usually two visits are sufficient for nutrition counseling. Few people need more than six sessions unless there are complex problems. Services may vary from $30 to $100 an hour.
- Be wary of counselors who suggest megadoses of vitamins and minerals or who sell the remedies they prescribe. Most reputable nutritionists prescribe vitamins and minerals sparingly, concentrating on sharpening your nutritional skills instead.

How can I find a professional sex therapist or counselor?

Many people have sexuality problems following cancer surgery or treatment. Some doctors find it uncomfortable to discuss this subject. However, it is reasonable for you to explain to your doctor that you have concerns about the sexual part of your life. Ask if it is a problem the doctor can help you with or a recommendation can be made. You could also ask a nurse or another health professional or minister to make a referral. (See the section in this chapter on sexuality for more information.)

How do I find appropriate support groups?

There are two general kinds of support groups available—support groups led by health professionals, and self-help groups which are run by people who have cancer. Some groups offer support, some education, some are for patients alone, some for family members and some for both. Some are less traditional and focus on alternative techniques such as visualization, relaxation and meditation. All offer encouragement, information, strategies for coping and a wonderful place to form friendships with others who understand your problems. The national American Cancer Society provides local units with resource materials for setting up a variety of support groups. Cansurmount brings together the patient, family member, Cansurmount volunteer and health professional. Upon referral from your physician, a trained Cansurmount volunteer, who is also a cancer patient, meets with the patient and family in the hospital or home. The I Can Cope program addresses the educational and psychological needs of people with cancer and their families. A series of classes is set up to discuss cancer, how to cope with daily health problems, how to express feelings, living with limitations and available local resources. You can check with your doctor, the social services department of your hospital, or call the American Cancer Society in your area for more information about available groups. (Chapter 26, "Where to Get Help," lists other support group information.)

Is rehabilitation help available for cancer patients?

Until about ten years ago, most rehabilitation services were prescribed for persons with physical handicaps. Today emotional assistance as part of rehabilitation efforts has been extended to patients with cancer and heart disease. Nearly all cancer patients can benefit from rehabilitation services. The focus is on physical, social, psychological, and vocational needs. It has been found that about 30 percent of people recovering from cancer need assistance with activities involved in daily living and in coping with pain. About 15 percent are deeply concerned about their physical appearance. Arm and leg swelling or breathing problems are of concern to about 10 percent, and about 7 percent have needs in communication and transportation.

What kinds of help are available from a rehabilitation team or physiatrist?

Depending on the needs, team members will vary, but the goal is to help you to readapt and to live as normal and full a life as possible. In some cases, a *physiatrist–a doctor who specializes in rehabilitation techniques,* including the strengthening of muscles, the use of artificial limbs, and retraining in day-to-day activities—may be required. Physical therapists or occupational therapists often work together to teach patients the skills needed to allow them to perform their daily tasks. For mastectomy patients, the physical and occupational therapists sometimes work together to teach arm exercises that will help overcome swelling and weakness. Oncology nurses are often helpful in assisting the family to help the patient become more independent. Social workers, members of the clergy, and lay volunteers can be called upon to provide assistance and advice in both personal and religious matters. Psychologists and other mental health professionals, speech pathologists, dietitians, pharmacists, all play a role in helping with readjustment.

Is individual therapy a good idea?

A growing number of psychologists, psychiatrists or licensed clinical social workers specialize in counseling people affected by cancer. Many people find it helpful to explore feelings with a professional who, without judging them, will help them to find ways to deal with the upset in their lives.

What is family counseling?

Family counseling can be valuable if the family group is having problems in dealing with feelings. It can be difficult to discuss the many emotions that changes have brought about. Major shifts in family responsibilities can cause resentment within a family. The loss of accustomed responsibility or authority can cause misunderstandings mingled with anxiety over a loss of power. Children are especially vulnerable as they find their usual roles no longer are defined clearly. If a family has trouble discussing its problems, talking them through in the nonjudgmental atmosphere offered by a professional counselor can be helpful. Besides private counseling services, there are many county health departments and neighborhood or community mental health clinics.

How can I go about getting help?

Though help is available, it can come to you only at your request and with your consent. Many people suffer needlessly because they are afraid to ask for the help they need. Many are reluctant to discuss problems such as changes in sexual or body functioning or in appearance. It is wise to discuss any of your needs frankly with your physicians, nurses, social workers or psychologist at the hospital where you were treated. Home health-care agencies and services such as the American Cancer Society, Visiting Nurses, and public health departments are helpful in pinpointing the specific services that can be utilized. Many county health departments include psychological services, and neighborhood or community mental health clinics are becoming common in cities. Community service organizations such as the United Way usually support mental health facilities. Most of them can be reached with a simple phone call and most of them are more than willing to help you determine what help you need and who is best to call to obtain help.

EXERCISE

What kind of exercise or relaxation should I consider doing?

There are many kinds of exercise or relaxation that you can practice depending upon your energy level. Choose a way of exercising that is something you enjoy. Do it until you are relaxed and pleasantly tired. Don't turn it into another stress in your life. Many people find that walking is one of the best ways to exercise. Consider, if it's convenient, doing your walking in an indoor shopping mall. Many people find it a perfect place to walk because you don't have to worry about the traffic, ruts or holes. Any kind of repetitive exercise, such as walking, running, swimming, rowing or dancing, gives you a chance to relax, because you don't have to think about what you are doing.

What if exercise seems like it's too strenuous for me?

Of course you must pace yourself and listen to your body. What's important is finding things to do that you enjoy. Relaxation means different things to different people. People who are physical become filled with tension unless they are active. Aerobics, swimming, bicycle riding, rowing, sailing, tennis, racquetball, golf or volleyball are all ways of relieving physical tension. Or yoga, massage, sauna or soaking in the hot tub or Jacuzzi may be your idea of pleasure. Someone else may find relaxation in meditation, mental relaxation techniques, reading, doing crossword or jigsaw puzzles, playing chess or card games, watching TV or playing computer games. Or perhaps knitting, needlepointing, carpentry or some other craft activity is your idea of a good escape. Try to give yourself the time to do whatever it is that makes you happy. Pleasure is a powerful prescription for health.

Is it is a good idea to combine meditation and exercise?

Studies show that the effects of meditation are multiplied when combined with exercise. Meditation also has physical effects on the body. Like exercise, it tends to lower blood pressure and pulse rates. Brain wave patterns change, showing less excitement. The blood has fewer stress hormones in it. There is even some indication that there may be a connection between meditation and the immune response.

RELAXATION TECHNIQUES

Relaxation techniques are being used in many different ways by many different people. The various techniques embrace the entire field of biofeedback, relaxation, visualization and meditation. Each method uses its own formula to expand the mind and to allow the body to enter a new dimension. We will cover only the basic information needed for you to begin to try the various methods to see if they appeal to you.

Some of the most common techniques used include:

- Relaxation.
- Hypnosis.
- Visualization.
- Meditation.
- Prayer.
- Biofeedback.
- Verbal therapy.
- Therapeutic touch.

Most of these techniques involve a creative growth process, not a rigid or formal therapy, and you must involve yourself to make them work. At first, you may find the experience confusing and frustrating. But once you learn to concentrate, you may find the whole experience relaxing and rewarding. The information in this section is a very simplified overview of the subject. There are many books, videotapes and cassettes that deal specifically with each technique.

What are the basic steps in learning relaxation?
Learning relaxation can be very helpful in daily life—but many people with cancer have found that it is helpful in dealing with the stresses of treatment and daily living with cancer. There are several simple methods that you can learn quickly.

- **Inhale/tense, exhale/relax.** Breathe in deeply. At the same time, tense all your muscles or a group of muscles of your choice. For example, you can squeeze your eyes shut or you can frown, or clench your teeth, or make a fist, or stiffen your arms or legs, or draw up your arms and legs as tightly as you can. After doing any of these, hold your breath and keep the muscles tensed for a second or two. Then let go and breathe out. Let your body go totally limp. Then relax.
- **Slow rhythmic breathing.** Stare at an object, or close your eyes and concentrate on your breathing or on a peaceful scene. Take a slow, deep breath and, as you breathe in, tense a set of muscles (your arms, for example). As you breathe out, relax and feel the tension draining. Now, remain relaxed and begin breathing slowly and comfortably, concentrating on your breathing. Take about six to nine breaths a minute. Do not breathe too deeply. To maintain a slow, even rhythm as you breathe out, you can say silently to yourself, "IN, one, two, OUT, one, two." If you feel out of breath, take a deep breath and then continue the slow-breathing exercise. Each time you breathe out, feel yourself relaxing and going limp. Try tensing a different set of muscles each time. Continue slow rhythmic breathing for a few seconds or up to ten minutes, depending on your need. To end, count silently and slowly to three. As you open your eyes, say silently to yourself: "I feel alert and relaxed."

What can I do if I find it hard to get into a relaxed state?
Learning to relax yourself completely may be hard at first. Practice the simple forms of relaxation several times during the day. You may try doing relaxation exercises sitting up in a comfortable chair or lying down. Try to choose a quiet spot where you will not be disturbed. Do not cross your arms and legs because that may cut your circulation and cause numbness or tingling. If you are lying down, be sure you are comfortable. Place small pillows under your neck and under your knees if you find that comfortable.

Is there a quick relaxation theme that I can try?
One that has been found to be almost universally helpful is the beach scene. Think of your favorite beach spot. Recall the pleasant

warmth of the sun and the tranquilizing sound of the waves. Imagine yourself basking in the warmth and let the sound of the waves lull you into relaxation. Always try putting yourself inside the scene, rather than being on the outside looking in.

What is imagery and how does it work?

Imagery means using your imagination to create mental pictures of situations. It is like deliberate daydreaming that uses all your senses—sight, touch, hearing, smell and taste. Some believe that imagery is a form of self-hypnosis. To practice the technique, close your eyes. Breathe slowly until you feel relaxed. Then imagine a ball of healing energy forming in your lungs or on your chest. You might imagine it as a white light. Watch it form and take shape. When you are ready, imagine that the air you breathe in blows this healing ball of energy to the area where you have cancer. Once there, it heals and relaxes you. When you breathe out, imagine that the air is blowing the ball away from your body, taking the cancer cells with it. Continue to breathe in, bringing the ball of energy to the spot. Breathe out and watch the ball of energy take the cancer cells away. To end this exercise, count slowly to three, breathe in deeply, open your eyes, and say silently to yourself: "I feel alert and relaxed."

What is visualization?

Visualization is a technique in which the mind is given a strong mental experience that it almost cannot distinguish from an actual physical experience. It has been used in a variety of ways over the last few decades. Carl and Stephanie Simonton adopted some of the techniques used by Silva Mind Control after learning that users of biofeedback often were able to communicate with their bodies more effectively by means of an image than by directly trying to influence a certain organ or function. Dr. Bernie S. Siegel has used a similar technique with his patients and has written several books on the subject.

How does visualization work?

No one understands precisely how it works, but psychologist Charles Garfield studied cancer patients who recovered at the University of California Medical Center in San Francisco and concluded that most of them had the ability to enter states of mind that enabled their bodies to perform at extraordinary levels—much as trained athletes do. Garfield found similarities between their behavior and the behavior of athletes who had used visualization techniques. It is possible that visualization takes advantage of the way the mind works, using a strong mental image that cannot be distinguished by the mind from something that actually happens.

How is visualization taught to athletes?

It is instructive to know how this technique is used in the sports field, because it gives you insights into how you might adapt it for your own use. Most athletes are taught to visualize in a step-by-step process. First they are instructed to write down the entire scenario in three different ways. They write about preparing to compete, about the actual competition, and about their action and feelings when they win. Goals are set for each part, focusing on what the person wants to achieve and the end result. The athletes are told to describe as vividly as possible the details of each phase of their participation—the excitement of being part of the event, the crowds, the weather, the sounds and smells. The written description includes feelings of being in control of their physical and mental state, imagining relaxation, and detailing smooth performance at each point in the match or event. Next, they are taught how to review their written material, looking for flaws and making changes until it satisfies them. They are then instructed in relaxation techniques and in the use of visualization of what they have written. This step-by-step process allows the athletes to make the program a part of themselves, feeling it, seeing it in written form and internalizing it. Some athletes report they actually see the movements and all that goes along with them in their minds. Others say they "see" only through strong feelings in their bodies, while still others may hear only the sounds or the rhythms. However, in rigorous athletic training, visualization tries to use all the senses, concentrating them in the brain to foster confidence and achievement. Many do a final visualization before they go to sleep and the next day "play the film back" as they get ready to compete.

How can I make visualization work for me?

The first step is to learn the art of relaxation. Then you can start perfecting the mental picture that addresses your problem in your own way. You can imagine your brain turning off the valve that directs the flow of blood to your tumor. Some people picture the cancer cells as crabs. One person said he could imagine a fisherman scooping them up in the net. Another pictured the crabs shriveling up and disappearing. You might choose to think in more medical terms—of your white cells attacking cancer cells and destroying them. The important point, in visualization, is to learn to focus your attention on directing your body to do something positive about changing your cancer situation. Many patients make a point of spending some quiet time each day facilitating the healing process by concentrating on the healing energy in their bodies.

Are there any techniques for making me relaxed enough to do visualization?

Some people find it hard to learn the techniques for reaching relaxation. You may find it helpful to use a tape recorder with a relaxation tape you've bought or made yourself. Making your own tape can be helpful. You may want to ask a friend to help you investigate the technique. It's important, in making your own tape, to go at your own speed. Give yourself images that you enjoy, talking slowly and in a relaxed manner. Repeated use of the technique will make the images more and more vivid. You can do this several times, each time telling yourself that you'll be even more relaxed when you close your eyes again. Use the tape recorder as long as you feel comfortable with it. Once you've learned the techniques, you may find that the tape is confining and that you can be more creative and relaxed without it. Relaxation becomes easier each time you practice.

How are pictures or drawings used in visualization?

The technique of using drawings was first used successfully with children with leukemia. Many therapists are using the technique to identify conflicts and then using visualization techniques to reprogram the unconscious. Dr. Siegel explains that the most common conflict is in the patient's attitude toward treatment. The patient often says, "I know this treatment is good for me," but unconsciously feels, "This stuff is poison." He works with patients to change the attitude through visualization—making the patient conscious on an intellectual level that this is what may be blocking his progress. He feels that the drawings are a way to get people to open up and think and talk about things they would otherwise conceal, even from themselves.

Where can I find more information on relaxation and visualization?

There are many books that deal with the mind and medicine. Among them are: *Healing and the Mind* by Bill Moyers (Doubleday, 1993); *Cancer as a Turning Point* by Lawrence LeShan (Dutton, 1989); *Love, Medicine and Miracles,* and *Peace, Love and Healing* by Bernie Siegel (HarperCollins, 1986, 1989); *The Relaxation Response* by Herbert Benson (W.R. Morrow, 1975); *The Relaxation and Stress Reduction Workbook* by Martha Davis, Elizabeth Eshelman, and Matthew McKay (New Harbinger Publications, 1988); and *Anatomy of an Illness* by Norman Cousins (W.W. Norton and Company, 1979).

How does biofeedback work?

Biofeedback uses electronic signals to teach you how to master the control of your body's automatic functions, such as heartbeat, blood pressure, and muscle tension. The electronic machinery is wired to you and your involuntary functions are monitored and reported through light or sound signals. Through observation of the results, you learn to regulate your body. In learning how to relax muscles, for example, patients are wired to a machine that picks up the electrical current produced by a muscle when it contracts. The machine converts this signal to a light or sound. The person learns how to turn off the signal by relaxing the muscle. With practice, muscle relaxation can then become a conscious action. Biofeedback means getting immediate, ongoing information about one's own biological processes or conditions. Biofeedback training means using the information to change or control voluntarily the specific response being monitored.

Can you do biofeedback on your own?

Biofeedback is best taught with professional supervision. If you want to continue biofeedback on your own, once you have learned the technique, several home devices are available for under $100. The most common is the digital thermometer, which may be purchased with sensors that attach to the body. It should have a continuous readout and be sensitive to differences of 0.1 degree. Another device involves galvanic skin response (GSR), which measures the amount of perspiration on the skin. Because you perspire more when you are tense, GSR is a widely used measure of tension. Wristwatches that continuously read out pulse rate can also be used. Biofeedback is a tool. You train your body to achieve the relaxation results that the device is measuring. The device serves as a graphic demonstration that you can regulate your hand temperature or your pulse rate. To locate people in your area who are working with biofeedback look under "Biofeedback" in the yellow pages of your telephone directory.

Is hypnosis used in healing?

Many of us think of stage hypnosis when we hear the word—where an otherwise inhibited, reserved person changes character and behaves in an out-of-character manner. The American Medical Association approved hypnosis as a tool in 1957 and it is being taught to students as a technique in medical schools. Your local medical center may be able to provide you with referrals. Many medical centers are using hypnosis for treatment of pain and many people have used it successfully to help stop smoking. You might consult a doctor, a psychologist, or a hospital-affiliated social worker who has experience with hypnosis rather than going to someone who is simply billed as a hypnotist. The county medical society or American Society of Clinical Hypnosis may be of help in locating a qualified hypnotist (see Chapter 26, "Where to Get Help").

Can I practice self-hypnosis?

There are many different ways of achieving a self-hypnotic state and there are numerous books that cover these methods. Most people start out by going to a qualified hypnotist before they try it on their own. We will outline one basic way in which you can achieve a state of relaxation to induce self-hypnosis.

STAGE 1

Sit comfortably with your feet on the floor or lie down on a couch or mat. You can direct yourself to relax, or you can repeat a prayer or phrase; you can fix your eyes on one spot or object or listen to a monotonous sound, such as the ticking of a clock or dripping water. Any of these can be used to prepare you so you are ready to progress to the next state. Once you feel ready to relax fully through one of these methods, close your eyes, breathe deeply, and feel your muscles becoming loose, limp, and relaxed.

STAGE 2

Some people can become profoundly relaxed with one of the Stage 1 self-hypnosis methods. For most people, however, a second stage of relaxation is necessary to go deeper. You can use any or several of these methods to help you sink into deep relaxation:

- Deep-breathing method: Start breathing deeply, counting slowly from one to ten, feeling yourself becoming more and more relaxed. Suggest to yourself that by the time you reach twenty, you'll be in a state of deep relaxation.
- Staircase method: Imagine yourself standing barefooted at the top of a beautiful staircase that leads down, down, down. The stairs are covered with a thick, luxurious carpet that gets thicker and more luxurious as you go down the stairs. You begin thinking of yourself walking down the carpeted steps, one step at a time, moving slowly. Each step down makes you feel more and more relaxed. Suspended above the stairs as you descend are numbers from 1 to 5. As you pass each number, you feel more and more relaxed and you know that when you reach number 5, you will feel completely relaxed.

STAGE 3

Now you are ready to take yourself into the third stage, from the staircase in Stage 2 into your own special environment. Imagine a comfortable space that is your very own. It is furnished to your own taste. It could be a beautiful room, an exquisite garden, a spot by a babbling brook. Make it a safe neutral spot where you can pause and luxuriate. After experiencing the quiet for a few moments, find a place where you can mentally sit or lie down. Now you can begin to focus on your visualization, seeing your treatment and your immune system removing cancer cells from your body. Try to form active pictures of how this happens. Tell yourself how wonderful you will feel, how well you will be as the cancer disappears from your body.

STAGE 4

When you feel ready, you can gradually begin to return from your hideaway, walking to the stairs, climbing the stairway upward, passing level five, then four, then three, then two, and finally one. Take some deep breaths, each breath making you feel better and more alert. Realize that when you open your eyes, you'll feel wonderful and refreshed.

After doing these exercises several times a day, you'll be able to do them more quickly and easily each time. No two people do them in exactly the same way, but it can be satisfying and productive.

How is meditation used by cancer patients?

Meditation, like relaxation and self-hypnosis techniques, is another way of disengaging your mind from everyday thoughts and focusing it in a different direction. Many people use it to help relieve stress.

Do many people find religion helpful in coping with cancer?

Many people find that their religious beliefs, faith and prayer are a great comfort, especially during times of crisis. A study of 50 patients at the University of Alabama Comprehensive Cancer Center found that 80 percent felt their religious beliefs helped them in coping with their cancer. This same study also noted that half felt the overall quality of their lives was better after cancer than before their diagnosis. They worried less about material things, they appreciated friends and family more, and their religious beliefs became clearer. These people were realistic yet hopeful, and were combining this hope with renewed interest in their daily lives and involvement with people.

What is verbal therapy?

Verbal therapy is the use of words and voice to effect changes. We've all talked to ourselves at one time or another and we all know that talking to ourselves is a way of preparing ourselves mentally, physically, and emotionally for some event. We tell ourselves to slow down or hurry up. We admonish ourselves to calm down when we're about to lose our temper. We all do it, and we do it because it works. You can try this technique concentrating it on a specific part of your body, or on the whole body. Think of your mind and body as a computer that needs positive commands given to it. One helpful exercise calls for programming a statement which represents what you wish to happen, such as "I feel better and better every day." Take a few minutes to repeat it over and over, imagining how good you will feel and the positive results of the improvement. Do this whenever you have a few spare minutes—while waiting in line, driving to work, folding the laundry, mowing the lawn. Get into the habit of verbally giving yourself positive suggestions when talking with others. Listen to how you answer when people ask how you are doing. Do you describe yourself as sick, weak, tired? These words can act as self-suggestions, which can react internally. There are positive affirmation or motivational tapes that can be used to help you in perfecting the technique.

How is therapeutic touch used in healing?

Everyone has the latent ability to use their own natural energy in healing. The technique is being taught at many nursing schools across the country. Scientifically, it is believed that electron-transfer resonance explains what happens when hands are used to transfer energy to another part of the body. Some people unconsciously are able to focus their natural bioenergy field and become known as "healers." But most people can learn the technique and use it on themselves.

- Start by taking three deep breaths to relax your muscles.
- Rub your hands together in a circular, clockwise motion for fifteen to thirty seconds.
- Hold your palms six inches to a foot apart for a few seconds and imagine there is an energy field between them, growing stronger and stronger.
- Cup your fingers inward, place your hands just above the area to be treated, and imagine the energy entering the area and healing. It may help to imagine the energy as a bright color.
- Rub your hands again and repeat.

What's the best way to decide which relaxation technique is best for me?

- Try all the different methods, then use the one that suits you best on a regular basis, once or twice a day for five or ten minutes at a time until it becomes easy and routine.
- You should not use these techniques for more than one hour a day.
- Remember that your ability to use relaxation techniques may vary from day to day.
- Take a deep breath if you have a sensation of shortness of breath or of suffocation. Sometimes, however, this feeling may be caused by breathing too deeply. If this is the problem, take shallower breaths and breathe more slowly.
- If the technique puts you to sleep and you don't want to go to sleep, try sitting in a hard chair, and set a timer or alarm clock.

FEELINGS

People deal with their feelings in many different ways. Some people find that talking about their feelings with others is a good way for them to cope. Others find that discussing their disease only with those closest to them works best for them. Normal is what feels right for you. But there are many feelings that are expressed over and over again by people who have been through cancer and it is reassuring to know that you are not alone in your emotional responses.

What should I do if I feel that the treatment is worse than the disease?

In the midst of treatments, many people feel like giving up. You would be wise to voice this feeling to your doctor or nurse. Don't discontinue taking your treatments without a frank discussion with your health care team. They can explain the pros and cons and alternatives to you, you can think through the reasoning and you can then make the decision about how you wish to proceed.

Why should I stick with a treatment that is difficult and depressing?

Treatments like chemotherapy or radiation can be extremely difficult, drawn out and depressing. However, in most cases, they are set up so that you know when they begin and when they end. If you skip out on treatments, you are cutting yourself off from the full benefits of the treatment. You'll increase your chances of being cured if you can keep your sights on the future. Counting down the treatments, and being especially good to yourself while they are going on, can help to make it easier for you to deal with the day-to-day difficulties.

What if I decide to refuse further treatment?

It is your right to refuse further treatment. If you make this decision, treatment will be given only to relieve pain and other symptoms and to keep you as comfortable as possible. If your condition stabilizes, treatment can always be started again. Your doctors will be able to advise you, but they cannot act against your wishes. You are entitled to have complete information about your illness and prognosis, as well as to withhold this information from others if you wish. A federal law requires all medical facilities receiving Medicare and Medicaid payments to inform patients of rights and options about type and extent of medical care. This law, The Patient Self-Determination Act, also requires medical care facilities to provide information about wills and power of attorney. (See information on Living Wills in this chapter.)

How can I deal with the idea that I might be dying?

A serious illness like cancer makes you examine your own mortality. There are no simple ways to deal with the question of dying except to try to put it into perspective. Simplistic as it sounds, everyone is one day closer to dying every day of life. You may find it helpful to talk with a good friend, a clergyman, or someone in your family about your fears.

What should I tell relatives, friends, neighbors and others about my cancer illness?

Knowing what to tell others, and how much, is something that each patient or family must deal with. Experience indicates that it is better to discuss the subject than to try to hide it. However, the way in which this is done depends upon your own lifestyle. You may prefer to share problems with those around you fully or it may suit you better to keep discussions about your cancer to a minimum.

Shouldn't children be protected from knowing that a parent has cancer?

It really is best not to try to hide the illness from children. You'll find that intuitively they know what is happening. It is frightening and confusing for them not to be told the reason for the concerns within the household. Children need support and reassurance that whatever happens, they will continue to be loved and nurtured. It is better to tell them as much as they are able to understand, depending on their ages, and give them a chance to share and to help. It may be a good idea to notify the child's teacher or school of the illness in the family.

Is it common for cancer patients to have a hard time concentrating on what they are doing?

Anxieties can create mental disorganization, confusion, and memory disturbances, and give you a feeling of being constantly distracted. You may experience a general feeling of loss of motivation. Even simple tasks like writing a check, dealing with routine business tasks, cooking a meal, or making necessary phone calls can seem overwhelming. Once you concentrate on the fact that the reason for the feeling is because of your underlying health concerns, you can begin to focus your energy on calming yourself and getting past your distractions. You'll find that the passage of time will help to put your anxieties into perspective.

How should I deal with postconvalescence letdown?

The time immediately following the end of treatments can be difficult because it is a cutoff point that leaves you without the routine that had occupied you following diagnosis. This may increase worrying and anxiety levels. Getting back to your normal routine as quickly as possible is wise. Taking up a new hobby, starting a new class, getting involved in something that allows you to be completely absorbed will help you to feel alive again. The numbness gradually disappears as you invest yourself in living.

How long does it take for energy level to return to normal?

Many people report that they feel their energy level takes a long time to return to normal—often a year or two after treatment. Studies have shown that some people are still struggling with being tired two or three years after treatment has ended. There is strong evidence that a type of enjoyable exercise, such as walking or swimming, can be helpful in combating these side effects.

Is it unusual to feel that the loss of a part of my body is more difficult to accept than having cancer?

Many people, especially women who have lost their breasts, express this feeling. Any loss of a part of the body, even the extraction of a tooth, is likely to bring about such feelings. Therefore, it's not surprising that the loss of a major body part or function may be more devastating than the fear of cancer. It takes time for these feelings to diminish. Awareness of them can be the first step in developing acceptance.

Are most co-workers supportive of a person with cancer?

Attitudes naturally vary. Some studies have found that co-workers can be among the strongest support networks. However, blue-collar workers were less supportive than white-collar workers. Those people who had cancers that were most visible, such as on the face or neck, had more problems with co-workers than did those whose cancer was not as easily seen. People who had long absences, took off many extra days, or were tired and weak and unable to complete their work had more work-related problems. On the other hand, in the study of white-collar workers, it was found that co-workers willingly took on extra duties and gave moral support and encouragement.

SEXUALITY

Why does the anger I feel at having cancer affect my most personal relationships?

It is not unusual for deep feelings of anger to surface after cancer diagnosis and treatment. Most people feel some form of anger at having a disease over which they feel they have no control. The feeling of helplessness about the situation, the indignities and difficulties of treatment all combine to bring about feelings of anger. Those who are close to you also may have these feelings. Because there is a close connection between anger and sexual feelings, problems in sexual expression may result. Though anger reactions may be different for each partner and each couple, they often exist and are sometimes repressed. An important part of the healing process is to allow these feelings to be expressed. Once the anger has been confronted and understood, steps can be taken toward accepting it and other emotions triggered by a cancer diagnosis.

Is it common for couples who never had sexual problems to develop problems when one of them has cancer?

Since 50 percent of the general population has sexual problems caused by stress, it's certainly understandable why cancer and cancer treatments may put stress on sexual relationships. In addition, as people age, changes take place in response and performance as well as in attitudes toward sexuality. These changes may not be noticed until a crisis occurs. Open, honest communication between partners is essential. Try to express your feelings and concerns honestly.

Why is it that since I've had cancer I have little or no sex drive?

The way you feel is quite normal, but can be expected to change as stress decreases. There can be physical reasons, such as decreased desire caused by treatments. Lessening of sex drive can occur during many different stages of the disease: during diagnosis, at various times during treatment, when new treatments need to be undertaken, or when you feel ill or in pain. At these times, there is a great need for physical contact, though not necessarily for sexual intercourse. Partners should be aware that the special warmth of a loving touch conveys feelings in a very direct way. Sitting or lying together, holding each other, cuddling, and giving a warm, spontaneous hug, a kiss on the cheek, gentle stroking of hair, or a relaxing back rub are all ways of being sexual and fulfilling the need to be physically close. You need to tell your partner how important it is for you to be touched and held even if you do not want to have intercourse. Try not to make your partner guess at your feelings.

Is it possible that my partner thinks my cancer could be contagious?

There is a great deal of anxiety about sexual transmission of disease, due largely to herpes and AIDS. However, there is no evidence to show that cancer is contagious. Sexual contact will not cause your partner to "catch" your cancer or to develop cancer of the sexual organs, mouth, or any other body part. Nor will you develop a recurrence or spread your cancer as a result of having sexual intercourse. If this is a problem, you need to talk openly with your partner about this fear.

Will my body responses ever be the way they once were?

Some people complain that they feel sad and frightened because their body does not respond as it once did. By accepting the lonely and fearful feelings, acknowledging them to someone else and having your feelings accepted, you begin an important process. Try giving yourself the freedom to explore and perhaps to define what gives you sexual pleasure. You can help bring new closeness by talking about the changes with people you love. Examining alternatives is, in itself, an important step.

Why is it so hard for me to talk to my doctor about intimacy and sexual feelings?

Many people tend to be afraid that others will be shocked or embarrassed if we bring up sex when they feel we should be concentrating on our health and well-being, as though sex weren't a natural part of well-being. Fortunately, an increasing number of people (doctors included) will respond to direct questions about sexuality without embarrassment or shock. And if you make it a habit to try to have a continuing dialogue with your partner, you will be keeping communication lines open so that you can continue to express yourself and your needs.

If my doctor won't discuss my sexual problems with me, who should I see?

It's reasonable for you to say to your doctor, "I have concerns about sex. Is this something you can help me with, or can you refer me to someone else?" Some doctors are uncomfortable with questions that pertain to personal relationships. It may be tempting to give up when you've been rebuffed, but remember that your concerns are legitimate and that support and information *are* available. There are many people trained to deal with the problems you are experiencing.

What does a sex therapist do?

Usually, a sex therapist wants to hear from both partners about problems and how each partner views them. Just bringing problems into the open and discussing them with a professional can be a big help.

How do I find a professional sex therapist or counselor?

Your own doctor may find it uncomfortable to discuss your sexual problems with you. Ask if it is a problem the doctor can help you with or can recommend someone for you to see. The professionals most qualified to deal with your sexuality problems include psychiatrists (medical doctors who specialize in mental health), psychologists (people with a Ph.D. or master's degree in psychology), licensed marriage and family therapists, and social workers. Those who specialize in marriage or family counseling usually are best qualified to deal with the kinds of problems you may be experiencing. Those who are most highly trained usually belong to one or more of the following organizations:

- American Association of Sex Educators, Counselors and Therapists.
- National Association of Oncology Social Workers.

If your physician or other health professional or minister cannot make a referral, you can locate members of these organizations by looking in the yellow pages under "Marriage and Family Counseling" or by consulting the American Cancer Society, Cancer Information Service, local Family Service, or United Way agencies.

(Chapter 26, "Where to Get Help," lists national addresses and numbers.)

What questions should I ask the therapist before starting therapy?

Some questions you might want answered include:

- What is your professional training?
- Have you had training and experience in dealing with sexual problems relating to cancer?
- Do you usually see partners together or as individuals? (It is advisable if both partners are together when advice is given.)
- How frequently will we meet?
- How long are the sessions?
- What does each session cost?
- Does insurance cover the cost?

Why is it so difficult to start an intimate relationship after cancer surgery?

Before you can expect someone else to become accustomed to the changes in your body due to cancer surgery, you must come to grips with your own feelings of self-rejection. These very normal feelings hamper your self-image and make it hard for you to move into new intimacies. You may find it necessary to risk rejection as part of your emotional healing process. You will learn, through this risk, that you are still desirable and attractive. Take time to become accustomed to the way your changed body looks. It is helpful to study yourself nude in front of a mirror. Once you become more comfortable with the way you look, you'll be able to move toward a new intimate relationship with more confidence.

How can I get my partner to start talking about sexual feelings?

Sometimes it's hard to discuss intimate feelings. Yet it can be dangerous to second-guess what your partner is thinking. The questionnaire on the next pages was designed so that each partner could fill it out separately. Make a second copy for your partner. You can then compare notes and use what you learn about each other to gain greater understanding. This is not a test. There are no passing or failing scores. The statements merely highlight what is happening in your sexual life and may help you to understand each other better.

PUTTING YOUR RELATIONSHIP INTO PERSPECTIVE

	True or False	Don't Want to Discuss	Does Not Apply
I want to share intimacy but am not up to sexual intercourse.			
She/he doesn't seem interested in sex.			
I don't seem to get sexually aroused.			
I'm afraid it will hurt or I will hurt my partner.			
I'm not interested anymore.			
I purposely avoid sex.			
Sex is unsatisfying for me.			
I'm satisfied just being held and cuddled.			
I feel failure and inadequacy about sex.			
I wish we could be more open and frank.			
I get excited but don't reach a climax.			
I'm getting too old to enjoy sex.			
I can't seem to get an erection/climax so I avoid sex.			
My partner won't try anything different.			
My illness has changed the way I see myself as a person.			

Statement						
I'm not sure whether he/she is avoiding me, doesn't feel up to it, or just isn't interested.						
I think it's time we faced the fact that we cannot have intercourse and should discuss other means of physical interaction.						
I would be happy if he/she would talk with me honestly about how he/she feels about making love.						
He/she is afraid of catching cancer.						
I'm embarrassed about the changes in my body.						
I think my partner is unfair to want sex when I'm so ill.						
I think it's inappropriate to be thinking about sex in the midst of a life-threatening illness.						
I'm ready to give up the sexual factor in our relationship, but I'd like to talk about it.						
I've never tried masturbation.						
I find self-stimulation is a good sexual outlet for me.						
I'm turned off by changes in his/her body.						
I think masturbation is abnormal.						
Sex is still good, even though we have problems.						
I'd be willing to try some different ways of making love.						
Our love has developed into deeper love.						

After you have discussed your checklists together, you may want to talk about the following questions:

- How satisfied are you with the quality of closeness you share?
- How important is sexual intercourse to you as an expression of intimacy?
- What makes you feel most loved and appreciated?
- What was one recent circumstance that made you feel close?
- What keeps you from becoming closer?
- What would make you happier?
- What does your partner think makes you happiest in your physical relationship?

How can a single person deal with telling a potential partner about a cancer history?
This is a difficult question with different answers for different people. Much, of course, depends upon your own medical situation. To help you with your perspective, try to think about how you would tell someone about yourself if you had heart disease or diabetes rather than cancer. Usually, discussion in an honest and open manner is best. This does not mean that you need to discuss your problems with everyone you meet in a casual way. If the subject should arise in the course of conversation, then you can contribute insights from your own personal experience. This question is one that is often discussed in support groups. It might be possible for you to find a group in your area where there are other people with the same concerns with whom you could share your thoughts.

How can a single person without a partner fulfill needs to be touched and held?
It is difficult to be alone during times of stress, and the need to have real contact with others is one that needs to be recognized and fulfilled. It is important, especially in time of crisis, to have the support of friends, neighbors, family, and religious or social groups.

- Reach out to friends, co-workers and neighbors, letting them know your needs. Greet them with a warm embrace. Take the time to include them in your life.
- Find a cancer support group where you can discuss your problems with others who understand.
- Massage can give real relief from depression, stress, anxiety and pain. Perhaps a friend can give you a simple back rub. Check with local YMCAs, health clubs, or beauty salons for names of qualified massage therapists.
- Giving pleasure to yourself, through masturbation, is a possible avenue for some to explore.

What does the doctor mean when he tells me to find "other means of sexual expression"?

Genital intercourse is only one way of expressing physical love. If your cancer problems no longer make this possible, there are other alternatives. People find that using hands, fingers, tongues, lips and mouths can provide exciting and pleasurable alternatives to "normal" intercourse. A sexual therapist can help you and your partner to explore possibilities.

Is masturbation a solution?

If your religious, social and cultural background permits it, masturbation is a form of sexual activity that can be a satisfactory form of gratification when sexual intercourse is not possible or not desired. Some people have found that mechanical vibrators can be used, either alone or along with other sexual activities with their partners.

PAIN

People who have cancer may have pain for a number of reasons. It may be due to the cancer itself or may be the result of treatment. It can depend on the type of cancer, the stage of cancer and personal tolerance for pain. Many people put up with pain, thinking that nothing can be done. Some people have concerns about side effects of pain medications because they think they can become addicted. As a matter of fact, addiction is extremely rare in people taking medication for cancer pain. When pain is not well controlled, it can lead to depression, fatigue, anger or isolation. Almost all pain caused by cancer can be relieved. However, a team effort is important when managing cancer pain. Patients and families need to talk with doctors, nurses and pharmacists about pain and its treatment.

Is it true that most cancer patients do not experience any pain?

Most people think of cancer as a painful disease. The truth is that most cancers cause no pain in their early stages. Therefore, the people whose cancers are found and treated in an early stage usually have only the pain and discomfort that is part of any operation or treatment. This pain is temporary and can be easily tolerated and controlled with medication. However, pain can be more of a problem with some advanced cancers.

What can be done for pain that is caused by cancer?

The best way to manage pain is to treat the cause. If you have a cancer that has spread, then your doctor will probably recommend surgery, radiation therapy, or chemotherapy to remove the tumor or decrease its size. When none of these procedures can be done, or when the cause of the pain is not known, then other pain-relief measures are needed—and there are many available. Together, you, your doctor, and your nurse can decide which methods are best for you.

Is pain more of a problem with advanced cancers?

Pain occurs more often in people with advanced cancers. But even among people with advanced disease, more than half have little or no pain or discomfort. Some advanced patients require light medication. For those who experience severe pain, there are modern methods of pain relief which can be prescribed.

Is cancer pain different from pain of other illnesses?

Some recent studies seem to indicate that when cancer pain occurs, it has different characteristics, since it may be both severe and of long duration. And since it is a reminder of the disease, the pain of cancer patients is also believed to have some psychological aspects.

Do some people feel more pain than others?

Some people are more sensitive to pain than others. Response to pain depends upon a number of factors: a person's general makeup, whether there are especially sensitive nerves at the point of pain, how long the pain has persisted and how much pain can be endured (called pain tolerance or threshold of pain).

Can worry, unhappiness, or fear intensify pain?

Studies have shown that worry, unhappiness or fear can make pain feel more intense. This does not mean that the pain does not exist—it means that if you can learn how to keep yourself from worrying about it, it can be lessened and tolerated more easily.

What are the main causes of pain for patients with advanced cancer?

Pain can result from any of the following causes:

- Pressure on a nerve caused by a tumor.
- Infection or inflammation.
- Poor blood circulation because of blocked blood vessels.
- Blockage of an organ or tube in the body.

- Bone fractures caused by cancer cells that have spread to the bone.
- Aftereffects of surgery, stiffness from inactivity, or side effects from medications.
- Nonphysical responses to illness—such as tension, depression, or anxiety.

What methods are available for controlling pain?

There are a variety of methods available for helping to control pain:

- Simple medications like aspirin and much stronger prescription pain medications are available. Always check with your doctor to be sure they are safe for you to use if you are taking other medications or treatment.
- A number of methods can be combined with medication, such as skin stimulation, distraction, relaxation, biofeedback and imagery.
- Nerve blocks or neurological pain relief can be used to block pain messages that are sent by nerves to the brain. Surgery or injection of a local anesthetic into the nerve sometimes works.
- Radiation therapy is often used to relieve pain when cancer has spread to other sites.

Is it wise to do something about pain as soon as it begins?

It is important to try to prevent pain from becoming chronic. Don't wait for pain to get worse before doing something about it. Learn which methods of pain relief work best for you. Plan on varying and combining pain-relief methods. Try each method more than once. If it doesn't work the first time, try again before giving up on it.

What if my doctor says that nothing more can be done to help relieve my pain?

Cancer pain almost always can be lessened or relieved. And it is important to remember that it takes less pain medication to keep pain away than to break an acute, established pain cycle. If your doctor feels you cannot be helped, ask to see a pain specialist. The following sources can help you locate a pain program or specialist:

- Call the Cancer Information Service at 1-800-4-CANCER. They will be able to help you find pain-related services in your area and can help you with tracking and describing your pain to your health care team.
- The local American Cancer Society unit in your area is listed in your telephone directory and is another source of information for pain specialists. For more information you may call the American Cancer Society at 1-800-ACS-2345.
- There are several national associations of pain specialists. See Chapter 26, ''Where to Get Help.''

Is it a good idea for me to keep a record of my pain?

Keeping a record of when you have pain and how bad the pain is is the first step in dealing with it.

How can I describe how intense the pain is?

A pain scale has been devised to assign a number to the intensity of the pain:

0 = no pain
1 = discomfort
2 = mild pain
3 = distress
4 = severe pain
5 = the worst pain

What should a record of my pain include?

Included should be: The number on the rating scale that describes your pain before and after using a pain-relief medication or technique; the time you take medication; any activity that seems to increase or decrease pain; any activity that you cannot do because of pain; the name of the pain medicine taken and dose; how long the medication works; any other techniques used beside pain medication. The chart shows you one way of organizing your pain diary.

Is there some way to describe pain besides saying "It hurts"?

There is specific information you can tell your doctor or others who are helping you with pain, such as:

- Where do you feel the most pain?
- What does it feel like? Is it sharp, dull, throbbing or steady?
- When did it begin?

DAILY PAIN DIARY FOR _____ (NAME)				
DATE:				
TIME	**PAIN RATING**	**MEDICATION USED**	**OTHER PAIN RELIEF METHODS TRIED**	**ACTIVITY**
Set up hour by hour or for specific times of day	Use scale numbers 1–5 as suggested or set up your own scale	List type of medication taken and dosage	List anything tried— relaxation, etc., and success rating	List whether resting, sitting, standing, walking, etc.

- Does it keep you from doing your daily activities? Which ones?
- What relieves the pain?
- What makes it worse?
- What have you tried for relief?
- What helped? What did not help?
- Have you been successful in the past in relieving pain? How?
- Is the pain constant? If not, how many times a day (or week) does it occur? Does it occur when you are lying down, standing, walking, etc.?
- How long does it usually last?
- Does it interfere with sleeping?
- Does it interfere with eating?
- Does it affect you emotionally?

Only when health professionals know exactly how pain is affecting you can they help you to find the right type of pain control.

What are the usual nonprescription pain relievers used?

These include **aspirin** sold under brand names like Bufferin, Ascriptin, Ecotrin, etc.; **acetaminophen,** sold over the counter as Anacin-3, Tylenol, Datril, etc.; and **ibuprofen,** such as Advil, Motrin, Nuprin, etc. Other brand names also contain one of these three medicines which are effective for relief of moderate and mild pain.

You can check the labels or your druggist can help you to find a generic product that may be less expensive than the brand name ones. (Be sure to check with your doctor or nurse to be certain they are safe to take if you are having treatment.)

Do aspirin, acetaminophen and ibuprofen help solve different problems?

- Aspirin and ibuprofen reduce inflammation. Acetaminophen does not.
- Aspirin and ibuprofen are often used to reduce the pain of swollen joints and other inflamed areas. Acetaminophen is not.
- Acetaminophen does not irritate the stomach. Aspirin and ibuprofen can irritate and cause stomach bleeding.
- Acetaminophen has no effect on blood clotting. Aspirin and ibuprofen can affect blood clotting and cause bleeding.
- Ibuprofen can make existing kidney problems worse. In normal doses, aspirin and acetaminophen usually do not cause kidney problems.
- Aspirin, when used to treat children with viral diseases such as the flu or chicken pox, may cause Reye's syndrome, a rare brain and liver disease. Acetaminophen and ibuprofen can be used to treat viral diseases without causing Reye's syndrome.
- Aspirin should be avoided by people who are on anticancer drugs that may cause bleeding, and steroid medicines, such as prednisone, are taking blood-thinning medicine, have stomach ulcers, are taking prescription drugs for arthritis or are taking oral medicines for diabetes or gout.
- Some nonprescription drugs also contain aspirin—such as Excedrin, Coricidin and Alka-Seltzer.
- Be sure to check with your pharmacist to be certain there is no aspirin in prescription pain relievers.
- There are usually few side effects from the usual dose of acetaminophen. But kidney or liver damage may result from use of large daily doses or drinking large amounts of alcohol with the usual dose.
- Ibuprofen has few side effects. Some people say it upsets the stomach. When used for long periods of time or when used in combination with steroid medications there may be an increased risk of stomach bleeding. It may be dangerous for patients with low platelet counts because it can interfere with the ability of blood to clot.

What are safe daily dosages of aspirin, acetaminophen and ibuprofen?

You should always check with your doctor, nurse or pharmacist about taking any medication because doses of these pain relievers react differently in different people. However, in general, here are some guidelines.

Aspirin: The usual safe dose is two to three tablets (325 milligrams or 5 grains each) taken three or four times a day. Eight aspirins a day is average, but many adults can take twelve a day. Any higher dose should be taken only if prescribed.

Acetaminophen: The same as aspirin. Extra-strength forms, such as extra-strength Tylenol, which are 500 milligrams or 7½ grains, should be limited to eight tablets every 24 hours.

Ibuprofen: One 200-milligram tablet every four to six hours is the usual dose. No more than six tablets should be taken in 24 hours. Larger doses should be taken only if they are prescribed by the doctor.

Aren't prescription medications stronger and more effective than nonprescription pain relievers?

Nonprescription pain relievers are stronger analgesics than people realize. Research has shown that for most people the usual dose of nonprescription pain relievers provides as much pain relief as prescription medications, such as codeine or Darvon—and with fewer side effects.

Are both nonprescription and prescription drugs sometimes ordered?

Many doctors find that patients who need prescription pain medicine also can benefit from continuing to take regular doses of nonprescription drugs. The two types relieve pain in different ways, attacking pain on two levels. It is a good idea to discuss with your doctor whether you should continue taking aspirin, acetaminophen or ibuprofen in addition to prescribed drugs.

What are the different kinds of high-powered pain relievers?

There are a number of different kinds. Narcotics, also called opiods or opiates, may be natural or synthetic products. They may be taken by mouth, intramuscularly by injection, through a vein or by rectal suppository (not all are available in each of these forms).

They include:

- Codeine.
- Hydromorphone (Dilaudid).
- Levorphanol (Levo-Dromoran).
- Methadone (Dolophine).
- Morphine.
- Fentanyl.
- Oxycodone (in Percodan).
- Oxymorphone (Numorphan).

Another group are the nonsteroidal anti-inflammatory drugs, useful for moderate to severe pain, and especially helpful in treating the pain of bone metastasis. They are similar to ibuprofen, which also requires a prescription when given in large doses. This group is nonnarcotic:

- Motrin.
- Naprosyn.
- Nalfon.
- Trilisate.

Won't I become addicted if I use narcotics for pain relief?

Narcotic addiction is dependence on the regular use of narcotics to satisfy physical, emotional and psychological needs rather than for medical reasons. Addiction is a common fear of people who take narcotics for pain relief. Drug addiction in cancer patients is rare. It is important to realize that if narcotics are the only effective way to relieve pain, the patient's comfort is more important than a remote possibility of addiction. If you have concerns about addiction, share them with your doctor or those who are caring for you. Other people's concerns about addiction are often due to lack of information.

If pain becomes severe, will I need shots for pain relief?

Probably not. Intramuscular injections or "shots" are rarely used for relieving cancer pain. Narcotic rectal suppositories can be effective, and new methods of giving narcotic pain relievers have been developed. Long-acting morphine tablets are now available and some narcotics provide quick pain relief when they are given under the tongue (sublingually). One narcotic drug, fentanyl, is now available as a skin patch which continuously releases the medicine through the skin for 48 to 72 hours.

What is patient-controlled intravenous medication?

With this method, a portable computerized pump containing the medication is attached to a needle that is placed in a vein. The patient controls the pain medication and presses a button on the pump that delivers a preset dose of pain medicine into the vein.

Isn't there a method that dispenses the medication under the skin?

A new simple, safe and effective method, called continuous subcutaneous infusion, uses a small electronic pump to dispense the drug automatically through a small needle placed under the skin.

How does an ambulatory infusion pump work for relieving pain?

An ambulatory infusion pump makes it possible to have medication, such as continuous morphine infusions, away from a hospital setting and while continuing usual activity. The pump operates on a seven-day rechargeable power pack. It fits into a pocket so that continuous medication and ongoing pain relief are possible.

What about medication injected into the spine?

Another way of treating cancer pain is to inject pain medicine into the spine, called intrathecal, or into the space around the spinal cord, called epidural.

What is the special injectable radioactive medication for bone metastases?

Strontium-89 (Metastron) is sometimes used in treating the pain of bone metastases. More information on this medication is found in Chapter 25, ''When Cancers Recur or Metastasize.''

Is heroin available for pain relief?

Heroin is not legally available in the United States. Strong narcotics like morphine and Dilaudid usually relieve very severe pain. In fact, the body converts heroin to morphine. Even in England, where heroin is available, morphine is being used routinely because it has been shown to be just as effective as heroin.

Are there other drugs that can be used along with narcotics to relieve cancer pain?

There are several classes of drugs that are used along with—or instead of—narcotics to relieve cancer pain.

- Antidepressants, such as Elavil, Tofranil, or Sinequan, are used to treat pain that results from surgery, radiation or chemotherapy.
- Antihistamines, such as Vistaril or Atarax, relieve pain, help control nausea, and help with sleeping problems.

- Antianxiety drugs, such as Xanax or Ativan, may be used to treat muscle spasms that may go along with severe pain. They are also helpful in treating anxiety.
- Dextroamphetamine (Dexedrine) increases the pain-relieving action of narcotic pain relievers and also reduces the drowsiness they cause.
- Anticonvulsants, such as Tegretol or Klonopin, are helpful for pain from nerve injury caused by the cancer or cancer therapy.
- Steroids, such as prednisone or Decadron, are useful for some kinds of both chronic and acute cancer pain.
- Nonsteroidal antiinflammatory drugs, such as Motrin, decrease inflammation and lessen pain from bone metastases.

Can nerves be severed to relieve pain?

A neurosurgeon can cut nerves close to or in the spinal cord to block the pain impulses to the brain. When the nerves that transmit pain are destroyed, the sensations of pressure and temperature can no longer be felt. For this reason, after such an operation, patients can easily be injured as they no longer have the protective reflexes of pain, pressure, or temperature. A rhizotomy means that a nerve close to the spinal cord has been cut. A cordotomy means that bundles of nerves in the spinal cord itself have been severed.

What are nerve blocks?

Local anesthetics, sometimes combined with cortisone, are sometimes injected into or around a nerve to stop pain. For longer-lasting pain relief, phenol or alcohol may be used. There can be side effects to nerve blocks. Muscle paralysis may result or the affected area may lose all feeling.

What is electric nerve stimulation?

Sometimes called TENS, for Trancutaneous Electric Nerve Stimulation, this is a technique that uses mild electric currents which seem to interfere with pain sensations. A small power pack connected to two electrodes is applied. The current can be adjusted so that the sensation is pleasant—a buzzing, tingling feeling is how it's usually described. Pain relief lasts beyond the treatment. Your doctor or physical therapist should be able to tell you where to get a TENS unit.

What is acupuncture?

This ancient Chinese method of treatment has been used in the Orient for thousands of years. To perform the treatment, special needles are inserted into the body at certain points and at various depths and angles. Particular groups of acupuncture points are believed to control specific areas of pain sensation. The patient usually feels no pain from the insertion of needles. Treatments are generally given in a series—sometimes every day for a week or more. Although its usefulness for cancer patients has not been proven, most doctors believe it is not harmful as long as the needles are sterile. People who are getting chemotherapy should be cautioned against acupuncture because of the danger of increased bleeding where the needles are placed. Acupuncturists are usually listed in the yellow pages of the telephone directory.

What is acupressure?

Acupressure is based on principles similar to those of acupuncture, but it can be performed by anyone or on yourself without using anything except fingertip pressure. The method concentrates on stimulating trigger points in the body. The most popular pressure point is above the thumb, in the fleshy area between the thumb and the first finger. The technique is simple and involves probing deeply with the tip of the forefinger or thumb until a sharp twinge is felt, and then stimulating as deeply as possible for from a few seconds to a few minutes. The same spot on the opposite side of the body is then given the same treatment for the same amount of time. Applying steady circular-motion pressure appears to relax the tenseness and relieve the pain. It is worth trying, since it is free of any harm and you can do it yourself. There are a number of books that detail this method. It is a technique that has been used in China for centuries, and which is taught to Chinese children by their mothers.

Is hypnosis helpful?

Some patients have learned methods of self-hypnosis that they use to control pain. There are many different ways of achieving a self-hypnotic state and there are numerous books available that cover these methods. (See information on relaxation techniques earlier in this chapter.) Many people start out by going to a qualified hypnotist before they try it on their own.

Are there any benefits to hypnosis over other kinds of pain management?

Hypnosis seems to offer many benefits and few drawbacks, mainly because hypnosis does not usually have any unpleasant side effects. Some doctors have found that hypnosis is so effective that some patients are able to give up painkilling drugs.

How does hypnosis work on cancer pain?

It depends upon the techniques being used. Hypnosis has been used to block awareness of pain, to substitute another feeling for the pain, to move the pain to a smaller or less significant area of the body, to change the sensation to one that is not painful, and in extreme cases to dissociate the body from the awareness of the pain. Although no one knows exactly how hypnosis works to control real physical pain, there are cancer patients who feel they have been helped by this treatment.

Is hypnosis dangerous?

Hypnosis can be dangerous if it is not being done by a trained professional. A trained hypnotist will not usually attempt to remove pain unless the cause has been fully probed and definitely known, because hypnosis can conceal real pain and conceal an underlying condition.

Is marijuana helpful?

Marijuana is not legally available. Therefore, the quality of marijuana is not consistent. Though marijuana has been reported to reduce anxiety or control nausea, some patients have reported that, rather than decreasing pain, smoking marijuana increased pain. (There is a prescription drug, called Marinol, which is a synthetic form of the active marijuana constituent THC which is available and is sometimes prescribed to reduce nausea and vomiting.)

Is a drink before dinner or with meals a good idea?

Drinking small amounts of alcoholic beverages with meals or in the evening may help you to relax. However, check with your doctor to make certain that the combination of alcohol with other pain-relieving drugs, chemotherapy, or other medications you are taking is not dangerous to you, since many drugs have serious effects when combined with alcohol.

What options do I have if pain is not relieved?

You can ask for a consultation with a pain specialist. Many of the larger hospitals now have pain clinics, devoted to helping patients cope with pain. There are many different techniques being used to relieve pain and many professionals feel that much suffering can be eliminated through the use of proper pain control techniques. You can also call the Cancer Information Service at 1-800-4-CANCER for local resources you can contact for help with pain.

MONEY MATTERS

Bills, insurance forms and money matters are part of all our lives. But they are especially important when they involve hospitalization and medications. If you are like most cancer survivors, the costs of initial treatment and continuing care are a major concern. What happens to insurance coverage and costs during and after treatment for cancer is something you can't help worrying about. We hope that new national initiatives will help to ease some of the burden. But meanwhile, the problems of the present must be addressed. People who had life and health insurance before treatment are usually able to keep it, although costs and benefits may change. However, those who change jobs or apply for new policies may find it more difficult. Understanding your rights and how the system works can help you to get the most out of your coverage.

What is the best way to set up my records concerning doctor visits, hospitalizations, medications, etc.?

The most efficient way seems to be with a loose-leaf notebook divided into sections. A sheet at the beginning of the book can be used to keep an ongoing record of every visit to a doctor or hospital. An individual section in the notebook can be set up for each doctor, for hospital information and for insurance information. In the section under each doctor, you may want to have a sheet that is divided to list the date, the reason for the visit, treatment recommended, complications, prescriptions, cost of visit, how paid, and reimbursement information. You should add copies of any bills received from the doctor in the same section. You may even wish to add a sheet with the date of visit, the questions asked and the answers given. You can set up the rest of the notebook in the same manner. Keep a chart of your insurance claims. This information will also be helpful in determining if you can deduct medical expenses on your tax returns. You will find that if you keep all of the information about your case in one spot, you'll have everything you need right at hand when a new bill or reimbursement statement arrives.

What kinds of items and services should my insurance cover?

Health insurance policies differ in what they cover, so it's a good idea to check your policy before a procedure, test or treatment, to see what items and services will be reimbursed. Without that information, you may be cheating yourself because you are unaware of what can be claimed.

INSURANCE POLICY CHECKLIST

ITEM OR FEATURE	COMMENTS	YOUR POLICY
Number of days of hospitalization	Least should be 30 days; many offer 90 days.	
Coinsurance/copayment	Check to see how much insurer pays and how much you pay—usually insurer pays 75% to 85% of covered cost, you pay rest.	
Outpatient services	Important since vital cancer treatments such as chemotherapy and radiation given on outpatient basis.	
In-hospital services	Make sure anesthesia, x-rays, laboratory tests, drugs, CT scans, blood and blood components, nursing care are covered.	
Home health benefits	Check whether services of visiting nurses, homemakers, aides are covered.	
Deductibles	First $100, $500 or $1,000 may not be covered. Many policies with higher deductibles give better long-range coverage. For long illnesses, like cancer, this type may be preferable.	
Who is covered	Wise to check, especially if you have stepchildren or foster children.	

Retirement benefits	Check limitations regarding age or place of employment. Can benefits be converted to individual policy or Medicare supplement at retirement?
Cancellation	Check to be sure you will be covered even if health deteriorates or you have severe or repeated need for treatment.
Maximum lifetime or benefit limits	Check to see what maximum figure refers to. Is it paid in full for each illness or all illnesses in course of a year? Is it paid only once in life of policy?
Stop loss provision	Many major medical plans provide that you share (with copayments) the cost of care up to a specified amount. After that, insurance pays full costs.
Inside limits	This refers to payment of a fixed amount for hospital room or surgical conditions, etc., with the policyholder paying the difference.
Preadmission certification	Some health plans require certification before procedures are performed and indicate maximum length of hospital stay. Stay can be extended only at direction of physician and will be paid for by insurance company only if company agrees that a longer stay is indicated.

(continued)

INSURANCE POLICY CHECKLIST (cont.)

ITEM OR FEATURE	COMMENTS	YOUR POLICY
Elimination period	For disability policies. Specifies length of time at beginning of disability during which no benefits are available.	
Preexisting conditions	If there is an exclusion, should never go back longer than 1 year.	
Waiting period	If buying a new policy, check waiting period. The shorter the waiting period (30 to 60 days) the better.	
Guaranteed renewable	Policy stays in effect up to specified age as long as premium is paid. Premium rate cannot be raised for any one individual, but only for all policyholders with same type of benefits.	
Noncancellable—guaranteed renewable	Safest type. Cannot be canceled and premium rate cannot be changed.	
Physician/surgeon services	Check to see if these are covered.	
Second opinions	Many policies cover these to insure against unnecessary surgery. May need referral from primary physician.	

Diagnostic tests	Check to see exactly what is covered.
Physical therapy	Check to see if covered on an outpatient basis.
Oxygen/oxygen supplies	Check to see if and how covered.
Prescription drugs	Check type of coverage.
Prosthetic devices	Check coverage.
Rehabilitation services	Check coverage.
Respiratory therapy	Check coverage.
Ambulance services	Check coverage.
Transfusions	Check coverage.
Outpatient mental health services	Check coverage.
Rental of hospital bed/wheelchair, etc.	Check coverage.
Experimental treatment	Check to see if there is a specific exclusion.
Nursing home care	Special insurance is now available to cover this, not usually part of regular policy.

What does Medicare cover?

Medicare is the health insurance program of the federal government provided through Social Security or Railroad Retirement. It comes in two parts: Medicare Hospital Insurance, Part A, covers room and board in a semiprivate room, nursing care, supplies and equipment, x-ray, radiology, operating room, medical supplies and lab tests. Part B, which must be applied for separately and is an optional plan, covers 80 percent of the allowable charges. It is intended to fill some of the gaps left in medical insurance coverage under Part A. The major benefit under Part B is payment for physician's services. Covered by Plan B are: medical and surgical services of physician in the hospital, nursing home, office, clinic, or patient's home. (Plan B, for example, covers the administration of chemotherapy at a physician's office.) It covers radiology and pathology costs as well as services prescribed by the physician in connection with diagnosis and treatment. Emergency room and clinic services, physical therapy, lab tests, radiology services, casts, surgical dressings and rental or purchase of medical equipment such as oxygen, wheelchairs, and colostomy equipment are covered. Medicare will also help pay for transportation by an approved ambulance service to a hospital or skilled nursing facility if used to avoid endangering the patient's health. Some items not covered are: prescription drugs that do not require administration by a physician, routine physical checkups, custodial care, eyeglasses, hearing aids, cosmetic or dental services.

Is insurance to supplement the Medicare A and B plans available?

Some companies offer plans (sometimes referred to as Medigap plans) with an annual premium based on age, sex and number in the family. Most of these are guaranteed renewable and offer hospital benefits. These are in addition to Medicare benefits.

If I have Medicare do I need any other insurance?

As good as Medicare is, it was never meant to cover all the health care expenses of older people. Medicare, Plan B, helps to cover major medical expenses. However, as with all health care insurance, there are deductible amounts and percentages of charges for various services which you must pay before becoming eligible for payment. Whatever type of basic health insurance you have—Medicare or other—adding some supplemental protection is a good idea. Some companies offer special Medicare supplemental insurance that fills the gaps in Medicare A and B.

What is Medicaid?

Medicaid is a federally sponsored plan which is administered by the state, with each state setting its own rules of eligibility and coverage. It is a public assistance program for people of all ages and usually pays hospital and doctor bills and covers additional services as well.

Is cancer insurance a good buy?

Most insurance experts feel that good general medical and surgical policies are a better investment than specialized cancer insurance. Cancer insurance, as a supplement to existing health insurance, is available in most states. Many of the benefits offered are similar to those available through most major medical plans. The regular plans, however, cover the family in other medical emergencies and usually give more economical coverage. Cancer insurers require the buyers to sign a pledge that they do not have cancer and have never had it. Payments are made in addition to claims paid by basic health insurance. Some of the policies specifically state that they do not cover diagnostic x-ray and laboratory examinations.

Should I consider buying a mail order insurance policy?

As with every other type of product, there are good and poor buys in mail order policies. Check the company and policy carefully before buying. Buyers should bear in mind that any omission of pertinent health information will be held against them when they try to collect. At claim time, some companies have been known to find some preexisting condition to justify nonpayment of claims. Furthermore, the benefits in some policies are based on the number of days of hospitalization. Usually they are advertised as having a maximum payment of $400, $800 or $1,000 a month. The payment is usually a direct cash payment. One thousand dollars a month breaks down to $33.33 a day, far less than daily hospital costs and far less coverage than most people require. This type of policy is a very inadequate one as a basic protection plan, but might be a useful supplement.

What should I know about filing for insurance benefits?

In order to make the most of the insurance benefits you have paid for, it is important that you understand what benefits are covered. You need to read your policy and have a general record of what is covered. Many times because of lack of knowledge, items that are covered are not claimed. It's a good idea to have a family member or friend familiarize themselves with your policies and records so that claims can be handled if you are unable to do so yourself.

- Understand the language insurance companies use. For example, ask your doctor to write a prescription for a hairpiece.

Be sure the prescription specifically uses the term "hair prosthesis," since this is what is reimbursable under many insurance policies. Be sure the receipt for the hairpiece also calls it a hair prosthesis rather than a wig. This is important, since this documentation will be the basis for your claim for reimbursement.

- Keep a chart of your claims. Accurate records are essential not only for insurance but for tax returns.
- Make copies of all bills and correspondence and use copies when filing claims or questioning charges. Never send original bills to the insurance company unless they insist on it. If you are required to send originals, make good copies to keep for your own records.
- Get all information in writing, if possible. Make notes concerning telephone conversations. Always get the names of people with whom you are talking. Follow up, if possible, with a written note confirming the conversation.
- Use the insurance company's claim forms and fill them out completely. Using the doctor's form, or failing to complete the insurer's form, can delay payment.
- Submit your claims in the correct order. The patient's insurance should be filed first. Wait to receive payment and an Explanation of Benefits. Then, if you have a secondary policy, submit the claim to that insurer and include a copy of the Explanation of Benefits from the patient's insurer. The second insurer will pay only on the amount not covered by the first insurance company, not on the total original claim. This is called coordination of benefits and is designed to assure that the patient collects no more than 100 percent of the original claim.
- Read your Explanation of Benefits (called the EOB) carefully. Every medical treatment has a corresponding numerical code, which is filled in by your doctor. The wrong codes translate into incorrect reimbursements. Check this statement carefully to be certain that your care is recorded correctly.
- If your claim is denied for insufficient information reasons, submit additional information.
- If your claim is denied or you think the insurer should have paid more, ask to have the case reviewed and ask your doctor to supply additional information. If you are turned down again, check to see what the company's appeal process is.
- Don't hesitate to call the insurance company and talk to a supervisor in the claims department. Follow up any phone

call with a letter recapping the conversation and restating your claim. Include background information, even if you have sent the same information before.

- Many policies have time limits on appeals—often six to twelve months—and the disputed amount must usually be over $100.
- If you still feel you have been treated unfairly by your insurance company, you can report the case to the state insurance commission. (See Chapter 26, "Where to Get Help," for a list of state insurance commissions.) Send a copy of your letter to your state representative and senator.

What is involved in making an insurance appeal?

The first step is to notify the insurance company that you are dissatisfied with your reimbursement. If possible, make your appeal in person. Usually, however, it is more convenient to appeal by mail. Send the insurer:

- A short letter explaining why your claim should be covered.
- A copy of the doctor's bill you submitted with your original claim (always keep an extra copy in your files).
- A copy of the Explanation of Benefits (EOB).
- If a mistake by your doctor's office was responsible for the underpayment, you should also enclose a note from your doctor stating that your insurance claim was filled out incorrectly.

If you do not receive a response within a month, call to ask what the status of your claim is. You may be told that your claim was sent to medical peer review.

How long does peer review take?

Peer review can take six to eight weeks. During this time, your insurance company submits your appeal to one or more physicians specializing in the area of your appeal.

Is there anywhere else to turn if the insurance company turns down my case?

If your appeal is denied you may want to bring your case to the attention of your state insurance commissioner. If your complaint involves Medicare, contact your Social Security office or check your telephone book or your state information center to see if there is a state Medicare Advocate who can help you. Send copies to your state and U.S. senator and representatives. For more information about insurance complaints, you may wish to call the National Insurance Consumer Hotline at 800-942-4242.

Should hospital bills for outpatient or inpatient services be checked and questioned?

One study shows that more than 90 percent of hospital bills have errors in them—and 75 percent of the errors are in favor of the hospital. One reason for this is that hospitals usually charge patients for goods and services when the physician orders them, rather than when they are received. To help you in checking your bill, request an itemized bill, which most hospitals provide only upon request. Ask for a bill you can understand, not one with indecipherable computer codes. If it is not ready when you leave the hospital, ask to have it sent to you. Check the bill carefully to make sure you were billed correctly for:

- The kind of room you used (private or semiprivate).
- The correct number of days.
- The correct time spent in specialized units.
- Specific treatments (radiation, chemotherapy, inhalation, etc.).
- The x-rays and tests that were actually given.
- The medications, dressings, injections, etc., that you received.
- Make sure that any bedpans, humidifiers, thermometers, or other personal items listed were items you were allowed to take home.
- The correct number of daily hospital visits by your doctor.

If there is anything on the bill that you do not understand, ask for an explanation. Don't pay for any charge that is under dispute until the hospital has shown proof that the item or service was provided. If the bill is being paid by the insurance company and you feel that there are unexplained charges that cannot be justified, contact the fraud division of the insurance company.

Where can I get help in keeping track of my insurance claims and hospital bills?

This can become almost a full-time job, and can be very draining if you are also trying to deal with treatments and recovery. Perhaps a family member or friend may be willing to take over this task. Sometimes help can come from an American Cancer Society volunteer (in some areas, volunteers are trained to help with insurance claims) or from your local American Association for Retired Persons chapter (which also trains volunteers in insurance claims). There are also medical claims companies that provide this service for a fee. You can find them in the yellow pages under "Insurance Claim Processing Services."

Will insurance cover costs for legitimate clinical trials or investigational treatments?

Some insurers will not cover certain costs when a new treatment is under study. Although some clinical trials offer some part of care free of charge, there usually are other expenses involved. Before becoming involved in the treatment, be sure to check your insurance policy or health care provider to see if there is a specific exclusion for experimental or investigational treatment. Also ask your doctor:

- What has been the experience of other patients in the trial?
- Have insurers paid for their care?
- Have there been recurring problems with insurance payment?
- Is it possible to describe the procedure in a way that would help chances of getting insurance coverage?

Where can someone who is hard to insure because of serious medical conditions go for health insurance coverage?

A number of states currently sell comprehensive health insurance to state residents with serious medical conditions who can't find a company to insure them. These are often referred to as "risk pools." A list of the states which offer these programs can be found in Chapter 26, "Where to Get Help," under "Health Coverage for the Hard-to-Insure." If your state is not listed, you should contact your state department of insurance to find out if such programs are being made available in your state.

Are prescription drugs available free of charge to patients who are unable to pay for them?

Many prescription drug manufacturers make their medications available free of charge to patients who do not have the means to pay for them. Call the Cancer Information Service, 1-800-4-CAN-CER, for further information. Usually the physician must certify that you are unable to afford the cost of the drug and are unable to obtain assistance elsewhere.

How does the Family and Medical Leave Act work?

If you are an eligible employee, this national law allows you to take up to twelve weeks of unpaid leave from your job each year to care for children, spouses or parents who have serious health conditions or to recover from your own serious health condition. (It allows the same coverage for care of newborn or newly adopted babies.) After the leave, the law entitles you to return to your previous job or an equivalent job with the same pay, benefits and other conditions. You are covered if you work for an employer that has 50 or more employees within 75 miles of the workplace, the federal government, or state or local government. You must have worked for your employer for one year and at least 1,250 hours the previous year. Your employer must continue to pay health benefits at the same rate while you are on leave. But if you do not return to work your employer may try to recover the cost of the premiums, unless the reason you didn't return was continuation of serious health conditions or other circumstances beyond your control.

Should I give up my company's group plan when I leave for a new job?

Cancer patients are advised not to leave a job with insurance benefits until they have a new job with good coverage or have made other plans for insurance. Your partner, if you have one, should keep this in mind if you are covered under his or her policy. Consider continuing to take part in your current company's group plan after you leave. If a new job does not work out, you could be left with no coverage. Federal law (Public Law 99-272, COBRA or the Consolidated Omnibus Budget Reconciliation Act) requires many employers to allow employees who quit, are let go, or whose hours are reduced to pay their own premiums for the company's group plan. This protection lasts 18 months for employees (and up to 29 months if they lose their jobs due to disability and are eligible for Social Security disability benefits at the time they leave the job) and 36 months for their dependents. If an employee leaves a company and takes a new job, continuation coverage by the former company can be kept for up to 18 months if the new company's coverage is limited or excludes a pre-existing condition, such as cancer. It pays to look for work in a large company whose group insurance plans rarely exclude employees with a history of illness.

What are other ways of qualifying for insurance when you have cancer?

Some people are able to obtain dependent coverage under a partner's insurance plan. Sometimes it is possible to join a plan during open enrollment periods when you may be accepted regardless of your health history. Professional, fraternal, membership and political organizations sometimes have group plans that you can join. An independent insurance broker can sometimes locate a reasonable insurance package for you. Seek out an agent who specializes in finding policies for high-risk individuals, but be sure to do your homework before you accept a policy, checking to make certain it is financially sound and has a reputable service record. When filling out an application, think about how much you need to divulge. Many cancer survivors divulge superfluous information that may wave a red flag unneccesarily. Unless you call attention to special circumstances regarding your health, your application is likely to go through in routine fashion.

Are cancer patients discriminated against when seeking employment?

Having cancer can sometimes be a hurdle to returning to work. Although no comprehensive federal cancer survivor bill of rights has been written, national lawmakers have expressed their concern about discrimination based on cancer history. Federal and many state laws provide protection for those who are termed physically handicapped—a stereotype most cancer patients feel does not apply to them. Be that as it may, the laws which protect those who have had cancer from employment discrimination are most often contained in provisions protecting the physically handicapped. (These laws include The Rehabilitation Act of 1973—Sections 501, 503 and 504; The Americans with Disabilities Act of 1990; as well as state laws prohibiting employment discrimination.) For more information, you can contact the American Cancer Society and the National Coalition for Cancer Survivorship, two organizations that are taking leadership roles in organizing on behalf of those who are faced with discrimination because of cancer.

Why do employers discriminate against people who have had cancer?

Many discriminate because of their own fears and lack of information about cancer. They maintain that they are hesitant to invest in an employee who, in their minds, may die. They consider their judgments to be business ones, citing fears that insurance companies will increase their rates or refuse to insure them. They fear that the employee will become less and less productive because of medical problems. Of course, the facts all prove just the opposite. Half of all individuals in the United States diagnosed with cancer this year will overcome the disease. For people under the age of 55, survival rates are even higher. There are eight million cancer survivors in the United States, five millon of whom have lived more than five years since their diagnosis. Decades of studies confirm that cancer survivors have the same productivity rates as other workers. Millions of individuals remain as productive or more productive after a cancer diagnosis than they were before. Furthermore, cancer accounts for only 20 percent of deaths in the United States. Cardiovascular disease kills twice as many people as cancer.

How honest should I be in filling out an application for a new job?

You can be honest without disclosing your entire health history. You should be aware that your employer needs to know your health history only as it affects your ability to do the job for which you are applying. Moreover, that knowledge is needed only after you have been given serious consideration as an applicant.

What can I say during a job interview if I am asked about my health?

Answer in a straightforward manner. Remember that it is not necessary to completely explain or dwell on your cancer history. Be positive and assertive. Stress your strengths and capabilities. Bring a letter from your doctor to the interview, attesting to your health status. Don't forget that you are selling the employer on your ability to do the job. You have no obligation to talk about your cancer unless it has some bearing on job performance. Leave the interviewer with the impression that you want the job and that you intend to be a faithful, hardworking employee. If you have had an attendance record at your last job that reflects the fact that you were absent because of your cancer experience, you can stress your attendance average in terms of how many days per month you were absent over the entire period of your last employment. Phrases like "I like to work and I give my best to every job I've ever done" can help present you in a positive way and change the focus of the question.

HOME CARE

Where can I look for information on the different kinds of health care services in my community?

Many communities, even small ones, have a directory of health agencies available in the community. Ask at the public library. You'll be amazed to find agencies you never knew existed. Other sources of information include the yellow pages, your doctor, the social services department at your hospital, the Cancer Information Service, the American Cancer Society and the local visiting nurse association.

What kind of help will be needed to care for a patient at home?

Often a patient can be cared for at home with little more professional assistance than a periodic visit by a nurse. If the patient is more seriously ill, part- or full-time nursing care may be necessary. If round-the-clock nursing care is performed by registered nurses, the cost can be almost as much as hospital care. Often, a nurse can be retained for a few hours a day or several days a week. Many tasks can be performed by licensed practical nurses (LPNs) or nurse's aides. If family members are willing and able to perform bedside duties, an agency-supplied part-time homemaker may be able to relieve the family of domestic duties so they can spend time with the patient.

Where can I get information about how I can learn to care for a patient at home?

The American Red Cross offers a course which teaches home-nursing skills as well as first aid. Learning the basics and following the guidance of available health personnel can make it possible for you to bring comfort and peace to convalescence.

What are some guidelines for setting up a comfortable space for convalescence?

A restful, comfortable atmosphere is the goal.

- Make sure the room is near a bathroom.
- Give the patient a handbell or get a small intercom so that the patient can call when needed.
- A hospital bed is convenient if much time will be spent in bed. (Hospital beds may be rented and the monthly fee may be covered by your medical insurance or Medicare.)
- A low bed is best for someone who is not confined to bed. Be sure the bed is firmly anchored and will not slip.
- Mattresses can be protected with a waterproof pad. Rubberized pads available in baby sections of stores work well, are inexpensive and can be reused and cleaned. Placing a drawsheet on the bed under the patient's hips provides added protection. Disposable waterproof bed pads are a great innovation.
- A visitor's chair encourages relaxed visiting.
- A bedside table with space for tissues, drinking water, a radio, extension telephone and reading and writing material should be provided.
- A good light, firmly attached and within easy reach, is a must.
- A pull-up device can be made to help if the patient has trou-

ble rising from bed or changing position. A strong rope, tied to the end of the bed, knotted at intervals, is very useful.

- Other special items such as bathtub handrails, a commode or a raised seat in the bathroom, bed tables and such items available at surgical supply houses should be considered.
- Whenever possible, help the patient to enjoy a change of scenery by making it possible, through the use of a wheelchair or walker if necessary, to spend part of the day sitting up or resting in the family living room or kitchen, with the rest of the family.

How can I keep track of medicines that need to be taken?

Keep a daily written record of the type and amount of medicine and the time it was given, along with a record of the patient's temperature and pulse, etc., as recommended by the doctor. This is especially important if more than one person is helping care for the patient. Remember that you must give only the medications prescribed by the physician at the time and in the amounts specified. One helpful idea for pills is to set out the amount needed for the day. This makes it easy to check to see that all medications are taken each day. There are compartmentalized plastic containers available at pharmacies and by mail order for this purpose.

What do abbreviations mean on prescriptions?

The typical prescription gives the dosage strength in milligrams (mg), usually notes the type of medicine such as capsule or tablet, how many times a day it should be taken, and how much of the medicine is prescribed. How many times the prescription can be refilled is also noted. Some of the common terms used are:

- a.c. (*ante cibos*): before meals.
- ad lib. (*ad libitum*): take drug freely as needed.
- d. (*die*): day.
- dur. dolor (*durante dolor*): while the pain lasts.
- g: gram.
- h. (*hora*): hour.
- h.d. or h.s. (*hora somni*): at bedtime.
- mg: milligrams.
- omn. hor. or omn. noct: every hour or every night.
- p.c. (*post cibos*): after meals.
- p.o. (*per os*): by mouth.
- p.r.n. (*pro re note*): whenever necessary.
- q. (*quaque*): every.

- q. 2 h (*quaque 2 hora*): every 2 hours, etc.
- q.d. (*quaque die*): every day.

What should I tell the doctor when I call to report a change in the patient's condition?

Always give your name and the patient's name, address and telephone number. Explain that you are calling because of changes in the patient's condition. Before calling, write down all the pertinent information, such as:

- What has happened to prompt you to call the doctor—rise in temperature, heavy breathing, weak pulse, bleeding, etc.
- The time when the changes took place and how the patient's condition has changed.
- If you want the doctor to visit the patient, be sure to say so.
- Listen carefully and write down any instructions you are given.
- If the doctor is not available and you are told to expect a call back, ask what time the doctor usually makes these calls so that you are certain that you or someone else will be available to give the information.

Is it possible to arrange for intravenous therapy at home?

Many visiting nurses associations and other nursing services now have programs which provide intravenous therapy to patients at home. The nurses' association will train patients and their families to administer the medication, but nurses are usually available for visits on a 24-hour-a-day basis.

Can tube feeding be done at home?

Tube feeding, called parenteral feeding, is used for patients who, as a consequence of surgical or radiation treatment, are unable to eat normally or for patients who need to build up their bodies nutritionally before surgery, chemotherapy, or radiation treatments. A hollow plastic tube is inserted surgically into a central vein. The fluids, a mixture of amino acids, fat, sugar, vitamins and other essential nutrients, are slowly infused into the tube by means of a small pump which the patient operates. It takes ten to fourteen hours to infuse a full day's nourishment, but the patient can usually rest or sleep while the food is being injected. Any patient who requires parenteral feeding and who does not otherwise require being in a hospital can be cared for at home.

How can incontinence be handled in the home setting?

This problem often looms as a barrier to providing home care for a patient. The doctor and visiting nurse will be helpful in the decision as to how the patient can be handled. Incontinence is an embarrassment to the patient, and often comes as such a shock that the patient becomes depressed, and even may insist that he or she would rather die than be a bother. Organizing the changing process so that it is done quickly and simply helps to alleviate guilt feelings. The use of adult toss-away diapers, sanitary napkins, and bed pads makes it easier. In the case of the male patient, a plastic bag filled with absorbent toweling or tissues, secured to the patient with masking tape, can be an easy solution. The visiting nurse can be most helpful in teaching techniques for handling this difficult job.

Is there any treatment for incontinence?

If you leak urine when you laugh, cough, sneeze, run or lift heavy objects—which the doctors call *stress urinary incontinence*—there is a treatment that has been approved by the Food and Drug Administration. Collagen can be injected into the tissue at the neck of the bladder. This can increase the bulk in the walls of the urethra, allowing tigher closure and less leakage. The treatment can be done under local anesthesia and you can go home the same day.

What is the best way to help the patient with bathing and keeping clean?

- The first rule is to allow the patient to do as much for himself or herself as possible.
- Shaving someone, if you've never done it before, takes skill. If the patient wears dentures, they should be worn for shaving. Use an electric razor if possible. If not, soften the whiskers by leaving a towel wrung out in hot water on the face for a few minutes. Stretch the patient's skin tight at all times to prevent cutting skin. Shave by stroking upward and returning downward over the same area.
- A shower is less strain on a patient than a tub bath and often recommended by the doctor. A shower chair, a small straight chair with locking wheels, is best. Soap on a string around the patient's neck is another convenience. It is helpful to arrange a ramp so that the shower chair can be wheeled into the shower.
- Be sure to check the strength, direction and temperature of

the water before the patient enters. Aim the spray to reach below shoulder level.

- Never leave the patient alone in the shower.

How can bedsores be prevented?

Bedsores often occur when a patient is bedridden or sitting in one position on a couch or recliner for a period of time. They can be prevented by changing the patient's position frequently. Pillows of various sizes, both hard and soft, can be used to change the patient's position. Rolled-up pillows can also be used to keep the weight of bedclothes off the toes, knees or other parts of the body. Bed pads of real or synthetic sheepskin and egg crate foam mattresses also help to deter bedsores. If you see a red spot or a bedsore developing, discuss it with the visiting nurse. There are special medications and medicated patches that can be used to treat bedsores. The sooner they are medicated, the better the chance for healing.

How do you give a back rub?

Heat body lotion or alcohol by placing the container in a pan of warm water. Then, starting at the patient's neck, move gently with long, firm strokes down to the lower spine and buttocks and up again to the neck. Repeat several times. Circular motions can also be used. Back rubs are a wonderful way to promote relaxation and to help stimulate circulation.

Is it unusual for friends to stop visiting when someone is very ill with cancer?

Prolonged illness seems to have a profound effect on relationships. The fault lies with society's being uncomfortable with the whole subject of dying—which has been a taboo subject for so long. Coupled with what has always been thought of as a dreaded disease, the idea of cancer sometimes makes people withdraw because they cannot handle the situation emotionally. Even doctors and nurses sometimes have a difficult time. The patient and family can help by encouraging people to visit, by letting friends know the best times to visit, by discussing the illness and by letting others share the concern and needs.

THINKING ABOUT DYING

We debated whether or not to include this whole subject in the book since so many people are living with cancer as a chronic disease for longer and longer periods of time. But we decided that this subject needed to be openly discussed, since it is a topic that is on the mind of every cancer patient. Besides, the time to face wills and Living Wills and the decisions about prolonging life is when you are well enough to make those decisions in a rational way. So, we will share with you questions and insights we have gathered from the many people we know who have had to find answers to their questions on this very sensitive subject.

Should I be thinking about writing a will?

Everyone should have a will. A lawyer can help you with all the intricacies of your own special situation. For a small set fee, you may have an initial office consultation to review your needs, discuss fees, and determine whether you wish to have the attorney draw up a will. If your will is a simple one, it can be drawn up for $100 or less. If you wish, you can call a lawyer on the phone, outline your needs, explaining your property worth, and ask about the charge. Of course, the more complicated your situation, the higher the cost.

Can I write my own will?

If there are any complicated trust or tax situations, this can be risky. However, in every state, you can buy a standard will form from a stationery store. Many people have a will drawn up by a lawyer and a handwritten will for their personal possessions. Some states will accept an unwitnessed will in the form of a letter or note written entirely in your own handwriting. However, most states require at least two witnesses, while some require three.

What is a Living Will?

A Living Will is a legal document that lets you specify exactly how much you want done to prolong your life. The Living Will is now valid in most states. The document is designed to permit you to specify in writing your wishes regarding the use of life support systems to keep you alive if you become terminally ill or enter a permanent coma or persistent vegetative state. The document takes effect only if you become incapacitated and can no longer actively decide and direct your physician as to the medical care you desire. In most states, a physician who is presented with a copy of your Living Will must either comply with your wishes or take all reasonable steps to transfer your medical care to another physician or health care provider who is willing to comply with your wishes. As a practical matter, you may want to inform your regular physician, while you are in good health, that you have completed a Living

Will and provide your physician with a copy of it. You can get a copy, in the form preferred in your state, from Choice in Dying. (See Chapter 26, "Where to Get Help.")

What other legal documents are recommended?

In addition to a will and a Living Will, you may want to discuss with your attorney the advisability of appointing someone as your Health Care Agent (who is empowered to convey your decisions about withholding or withdrawal of life support systems), Power of Attorney for Health Care Decisions (which allows the appointed to make a wide variety of health care decisions but does not extend to making decisions regarding the withholding or withdrawal of life support systems), as well as Power of Attorney for money matters. Some people also like to leave a document outlining their wishes for funeral arrangements and services.

How can I arrange to donate my body or body organs?

A uniform anatomical gift act or similar law has been passed in all states. Persons can become donors by signing a card in the presence of two witnesses. The card allows the person to specify what donation is desired. You may contribute any organs or parts, restrict donation to certain organs or parts, or give the entire body for anatomical study. More information can be obtained from Living Bank. (See Chapter 26, "Where to Get Help.")

Will I be allowed to make a decision about whether I plan to die at home or in the hospital?

It is important to let your feelings be known to your doctor so that everything possible can be done to see that your wishes are followed. For those who prefer to spend their last days at home, the Hospice program, which in most communities is run by the hospital, a skilled care facility or the visiting nurses association, has instituted home-care programs with medical supervision in the home under trained medical staff. Hospice emphasizes the management of pain and other comfort measures, providing help for the family as well as the patient. Hospice makes the family the unit of care, centering much of the caring process in the home with the support of a team of medical professionals and trained volunteers. It seeks to enable the patient to carry on an alert and pain-free existence. The decision of how your illness will be managed depends on many different factors, but if you feel strongly about your desire to die at home, you should discuss it with your family and doctor so that when the time comes, your wishes can be carried out.

What services does Hospice offer?

The primary concern of hospice care is quality of life, not cure. Hospice seeks to prolong life, not prolong dying. The goal is to control pain and other symptoms so the patient can remain as alert and comfortable as possible. Hospice offers many kinds of care. Most will help with home care, some provide services in a special hospice center, others are located within a hospital or skilled nursing facility. Many Hospice programs offer a combination of these services, tailored to patient and family needs.

How can I find out about Hospice in my area?

For information on hospices, contact the National Hospice Organization (see Chapter 26, "Where to Get Help"). The Cancer Information Service (1-800-4-CANCER) or the American Cancer Society may also be able to guide you to Hospice service in your area.

FOR THE CAREGIVER

Isn't it best if everyone just pretends that the patient isn't dying?

When death is imminent, pretending that a patient isn't dying is very difficult both for the patient and for family and friends. It puts a tremendous burden on the patient, who can be plunged into depression. It takes a great deal of energy, which is exhausting. Accepting the fact that the patient is going to die opens the way for the patient to dissipate loneliness and depression by allowing a verbalization of feelings from both the patient and the family members. Naturally, if stoicism is a family's way of life, members can deal with this in the accustomed way. But stoicism is not denial, and pretense really does not make it easier for the patient.

What if I am not able to care for the patient at home at the end even though the person wishes to be there?

Circumstances sometimes make it impossible to continue to give care at home. But there is no reason to feel guilty. Many people who have been able to take part in care during the course of the illness find that circumstances make it impossible to cope with the final stages of illness. This is a very painful time, and each family must find its own answers. If the patient is hospitalized, arrangements can usually be made for some member of the family to stay at the hospital, helping as much or as little as he or she chooses.

How can a person be helped to die in comfort?

When it is determined that the patient is dying and there is no reasonable hope for recovery, the patient, family and doctor can make plans to help the patient die comfortably. Either at home or in the hospital, all testing, transfusions, etc., can cease. This means that temperature no longer needs to be taken at the usual intervals, and the obtaining of blood samples, etc., can be curtailed so that the patient will not be disturbed. Morphine, or whatever drugs are most effective, should be prescribed to be given continuously to relieve pain. Glucose and water can be given intravenously if the patient cannot eat or drink and complains of thirst. Oxygen may be used if there is shortness of breath. A catheter can be inserted in the bladder for comfort. Lips can be kept moist with Vaseline, ice chips or glycerin sponges. The important thing for everyone to keep in mind is that any measures that are taken are for the purpose of maintaining the patient's comfort.

What kind of care must be given to the dying patient?

Being with the patient as much as possible is the most important consideration. Remember that even if the patient does not seem to be able to hear what is happening, awareness may be very acute. Professionals say that it is helpful to give the dying person your permission to "let go." The patient may want to talk about dying, and those close to the patient can help to do so. Do not be afraid if the patient seems to be in physical distress and frightened, restless, gasping for breath, and disoriented. Keep the patient warm. Most important, keep the mouth moist. Special oiled swabs which can be used to remove mucus from inside the mouth and which help keep the mouth and lips moist are most helpful. Placing the patient on his side helps drain mucus from mouth and nose. Every effort should be made to reduce irritating conditions and provide an atmosphere that is peaceful and comfortable.

What are the specific signs of impending death?

People in the health care field who see death almost every day tell us that although many people think of death as being a traumatic time for the patient, in reality, most people die very peacefully, in their sleep or while at rest. The signs of death will vary from patient to patient. It is very important to note changes in the patient's normal status. Some of the significant changes to be aware of include:

- Marked changes in breathing: labored, spasmodic, heavy breathing, followed by quiet or shallow breathing or a decreased number of breaths per minute (sometimes referred to as Cheyne-Stokes respiration).
- Heartbeat rate either faster or slower than usual.

- Change in skin texture and temperature; though the patient feels cold to the touch, may perspire profusely.
- Lapsing in and out of consciousness, being confused, or going into a coma.
- Loss of sensation, power of motion, and/or loss of reflexes first in legs, then in arms.
- Tendency to turn the head toward the light as a result of failing sight and hearing.
- When breathing ceases, be sure the body is laid flat on its back with one pillow under the head. Close the eyes and mouth. If necessary clean the patient. Put any dentures or artificial parts in place.

Why are autopsies necessary?

Autopsies are not always necessary, but this final examination may be requested by the patient, family or the physician to determine the cause of death and to allow data to be gathered on the effects of the disease. By comparing findings, treatment for others with the same disease may be improved in the future. The medical profession treats an autopsy as a surgical procedure with full respect of the individual. However, if you do not wish to allow an autopsy, it is your right to withhold permission.

Why is there a feeling of relief after a prolonged illness?

When an illness is prolonged, often the grieving process is completed before the actual death. It is not uncommon for the family to feel relief that the pain, suffering, and uncertainty have ended. Some people may misinterpret this acceptance and think you are unfeeling. You must not feel guilty, for this has been found to be a perfectly normal reaction. People experience grief in different ways, and often the deepest grief may be felt by those who do not show grief outwardly.

chapter 25

When Cancers Recur or Metastasize

The first question many people ask their doctors after cancer surgery is "Did you get it all?" assuming that surgical removal of a cancer is a guarantee of cure. "Getting it all" may be impossible if cancer cells have already started their journey in the body. That's why many treatments and strategies have been developed that include chemotherapy and other measures that try to destroy all cancer cells at the original site, as well as trying to stem the silent movement of cancer cells to other parts of the body. Cancer can recur, that is, it can come back again. It might come back in the same place as before (local recurrence), somewhere close to the first area (regional recurrence) or it may spread far from where it was first found. When cancer cells spread, it is referred to as metastasis or metastatic cancer.

If it should happen in your case that some cells were able to escape and do their damage elsewhere in your body and you are faced with the fact that the cancer which you hoped had been cured has recurred or spread, you must be prepared to deal with it as a chronic disease.

THINGS TO REMEMBER:

- **A recurrence is not a death sentence. It is a crisis to be faced.**
- Many of your concerns may be unfounded, so rather than worry unnecessarily, ask your doctor exactly what the recurrence means and whether this is a chronic problem that can be treated. Medical skills and advances now make it possible to deal with many problems and crises in very positive ways.
- There are many appropriate treatments available. You may want to investigate a clinical trial—many are designed especially for persons with cancer that has recurred or spread.
- Some recurrences are inherently less a cause for alarm than others.
- Cancer that recurs is very much like the first cancer in the way that it starts. If not stopped, cancer cells will continue to replace normal cells. Cancer that has metastasized may be found in places far from the original site.
- Not every cancer cell that breaks away is able to start a growth elsewhere. Most are stopped by the body's natural defenses or can be destroyed by treatment.
- Be sure to use the resources discussed in Chapter 5, "Treatment," to make certain you are getting the very newest treatment. Renew your use of the toll-free 1-800-4-CANCER number so that you will have the latest information and help in dealing with your present problems. Your past knowledge, your familiarity with the medical system, and your ability in dealing with the original cancer give you an advantage in this area.

**DON'T HESITATE TO CALL
1-800-4-CANCER
FOR THE LATEST INFORMATION ON
TREATMENT**

Is it normal to think that every ache and pain is a sign that my cancer has recurred?

This is a perfectly normal reaction. Many people who have had cancer have gone through the routine of fearing every cough, every bone ache, every headache, every change, thinking it might be a sign that they might have a recurrence. Since about 50 percent of all cancers are cured with the first treatment, you may be worrying without reason. To help you to deal with this, you should talk over your fears with your physician. Though no one, not even your doctor, can predict your future, you may find it helpful to know if there is very little chance of recurrence with your kind of cancer, where metastases might occur, and what symptoms you should watch for.

Does having a recurrence mean there's no hope for me?

Some people make that assumption—and they couldn't be farther from the truth. Don't try to make any assumptions about the meaning of the recurrence until you have had plenty of time to have all the tests that need to be run completed and analyzed. So many people, during this crisis time, assume that nothing can be done. Many people try to make critical family and personal decisions during an emotionally charged period. Families often are even more discouraged than the patient and mistakenly begin to prepare themselves mentally for a future without their loved one. This can be disastrous for everyone concerned. If you are faced with a recurrence, though it is difficult to do, take time to wait for a full diagnosis. Discuss the situation fully with your doctor. Check out all the newest treatments. Ask enough questions to make sure you are getting clear information.

What if I just can't face the thought of going back through treatment again?

This is a normal reaction. It is certainly easy to understand your reluctance to undergo further discomfort and disability. You need to ask your doctor for a frank assessment of the possible outcome of the treatment. If you feel it would be helpful, arrange for a second opinion from another doctor. In many cases, the treatment will be successful. Your attitude toward the treatment is an important factor in a return to health, and if it is possible for you to think of cancer as a chronic disease, much as you would if you had diabetes or heart disease, it is easier to deal with facing what is happening to you.

Isn't it true that sometimes the risks and side effects of further treatment aren't worth the benefits?

The point at which this begins to be true is always debatable. Some people feel that once they've been through the initial treatment, that is all they care to deal with. Of course, with the fast-moving progress of medicine, it's important not to come to this conclusion too hastily. It is up to each patient to weigh the pros and cons, the side effects and aftereffects, to determine what is right in each case. In this highly personal area of decision making, it is possible only to suggest some avenues that should be considered. Here are some things to think about:

- Have you gotten another opinion so that you are certain what your alternatives are?
- Have you been to a major cancer center for information and consultation?
- Have you checked the PDQ (you can do this by calling the toll-free 1-800-4-CANCER information service phone number) to see what investigational treatments are available for you?
- Are you most interested in **quality** or **quantity** of life or a compromise of the two?
- Have you asked your doctor what benefits are expected from the treatment? What side effects? What risks? What will happen if you don't have treatment?
- Are you ready to stop treatments altogether?
- What is it you are most afraid of? Try to isolate what your biggest fears are—pain, isolation, leaving things undone, being unable to take care of yourself, dying—and discuss them with your doctor or other competent counselors for advice and guidance.

Is it unusual for me to be angry at my doctor?

Most of us have expectations for our doctors that can be quite unreasonable and impossible. Quite frankly, we expect our doctors to cure us. When cancer recurs, we often feel that the doctor has failed. We know it's irrational, but sometimes we just need to blame someone or something for our illness. This anger is rooted in our mistaken feelings about a doctor's infallibility. Doctors do not have all the answers. Cancer is a very elusive disease and even with all the advances, it can still be very unpredictable. If you find yourself with angry feelings about your doctor, you should examine the reasons for your feelings and discuss them with your doctor. Schedule an extra fifteen minutes at your next appointment to talk over the problems as you see them. Discussion will help to dissipate some of the frustration and anger, and should make communication easier. The doctor's business is to help you. This cannot be done unless the doctor knows what is bothering you. Clear the air.

Be honest and share your feelings. If that doesn't help, then perhaps it's time for you to make the break and start using another physician. After all, you need someone who is supportive and willing to communicate with you so you can approach your problems in a positive fashion.

Why does cancer recur?

When cancer recurs it means that disease that was thought to be cured, or was at least inactive for a period of time, has become active again. Sometimes cancer recurs after several months, sometimes it may remain dormant for many years. It is always hoped that the original treatment will destroy the original cancer and any of the cells that may have become detached from it. Sometimes, however, microscopic cells, too small to be detected, may survive and eventually start to grow in the same or in another location.

What is a local recurrence?

Local recurrence means that the cancer has come back in the same place as the original cancer. The term "local" also means that there is no sign of cancer in nearby lymph nodes or other tissues. For example, someone who has had breast cancer could later have a local recurrence in or around the area of the original surgery. The same is true of colon or bowel cancer, where sometimes recurrences occur in the scar area or nearby tissues.

What is a regional recurrence?

A regional recurrence involves growth of a new tumor in lymph nodes or tissues near the original site, but with no evidence of growth at distant sites. For instance, a woman treated for cervical or ovarian cancer may have a regional recurrence in the abdomen.

What is a metastatic recurrence?

In the case of a metastatic recurrence, cancer has spread to organs or tissue at some distance from the original site, such as in the lung, bone, liver or brain.

How does metastasis occur?

Metastasis is a complex course of events that is still not completely understood. However, the term "metastasis" or "metastatic" means that the cancer has spread from one part of the body to another, from the primary or original site to another part of the body. Under the microscope the metastatic cancer cells usually resemble the cancer cells from your original disease. Metastases start from cells that break away from the original tumor and travel through the lymph system or bloodstream to start new cancer growths. The cancer that reappears is the same type as the original cancer—no matter where it appears. This means, for example, that if breast cancer recurs in the lung, it is not lung cancer, it is breast cancer that has spread to the lung. The physician might refer to it as "breast metastasis in the lung." In other words, what you have is not a second cancer, not lung cancer, but a recurrence of the breast cancer you had before.

How do cells become metastatic?

The avenues leading to uncontrolled growth of a cell are varied and distinctive and not fully understood even by scientists. Cancer involves changes in genetic information—the DNA—but damage in some cases is a mere blip and in others involves a total reshuffling of the information. Some cells become malignant by losing the function of tumor suppressor genes, while others do it by turning on cancer-causing genes. The cancer cells are influenced by the organs in which the original tumors occur. There is more detailed information on how cancer starts in Chapter 3, "What Is Cancer?"

Why is it that the first treatment sometimes fails to kill all the cancer cells?

If only the answer to that were known, we wouldn't have to deal with metastasis. The goal of treatment is always to remove all of the cancer cells. However, a single cancerous tumor might itself be composed of a mixture of cells having different properties. Cell subpopulations can vary in their ability to spread to other sites in the body, as well as in their susceptibility to treatment. They also vary in the ease with which they provoke or avoid an immune attack and in their ability to produce chemical markers that are used to detect the presence of particular cancers. It is no wonder that sometimes a few cells escape from the original tumor and form new tumors at other sites in the body without medical science presently being able to forecast or circumvent their spread.

Which cancers are the least likely to metastasize?

Cancers that rarely spread from where they begin include basal cell and squamous cell skin cancers, cancers of the salivary gland and cancers of the thyroid.

Which cancers most often spread to nearby lymph nodes and may go to distant areas much later?

These include cancers of the cervix and many of the cancers of the face, mouth and neck.

Which types of cancer spread most often to other parts of the body?

Cancers that often spread early to other parts of the body include some of the sarcomas, choriocarcinoma (a rare cancer of the uterus) and small cell lung cancer.

Which cancers are most unpredictable in their ability to spread?

There is a large group of common cancers which show a great deal of variation from one person to another. These include cancers of the breast, lung, bowel, stomach and melanoma of the skin.

Are there places where specific cancers commonly recur?

Some primary cancers have a tendency to recur more often in specific places. The most common locations for metastases to occur are in the lungs, bones, liver and brain.

COMMON AREAS OF SPREAD	
ORIGINAL SITE	**WHERE IT USUALLY SPREADS**
Bladder	Bone, liver, brain
Breast	Bone, lung, brain
Colon/rectum	Lung, liver, ovary, brain
Kidney	Bone, liver, lung, brain
Leukemia/lymphoma	Liver, lung, membranes of brain and spine
Lung	Brain, liver, bone
Melanoma	Brain, liver, bowel, lung, bone
Prostate	Bone, brain
Sarcomas	Lung, brain
Thyroid	Bone

What kinds of cancer are likely to spread to the lung?

Spread of cancer to the lung is quite common in breast cancer, gastrointestinal cancer, kidney cancer, melanoma, sarcomas, lymphomas and leukemias, and germ cell tumors. A few cancers, like sarcomas, metastasize almost exclusively to the lung and can, in some cases, be cured with surgery. Some tumors, like kidney cancers, metastasize to the lungs with a few slow-growing spots that can be surgically removed. Most of the metastasized tumors that grow in the lung are quite small, round and sharply demarcated.

Usually if there is an irregular border, this indicates a primary lung cancer or infection. Calcified lung metastases are seen in osteogenic sarcoma, chondrosarcoma and synovial sarcoma and less frequently in thyroid, ovarian, gastrointestinal and breast tumors. Urinary tract cancers often metastasize to the lungs, but when surgically removed, allow for good long-term survival. Head and neck cancers including the nose, nasopharynx, larynx, mouth, tongue, salivary glands and oropharynx sometimes spread to the lung.

What are the symptoms when cancer has spread to the lung?

Many people who have cancer which has spread to the lung have no symptoms. Shortness of breath may be a sign that there is some involvement in the lung. CT scans and MRI may be used to detect these cancers.

What is the treatment for cancers that have spread to the lung?

Treatment will depend on a number of factors, including the tumor type, the length of time from treatment of the primary tumor to lung metastases, how quickly the tumor is growing, whether there are other metastatic growths in other parts of the body, and, of course, your own health status.

What kinds of cancers are most likely to metastasize to the bone?

Metastases to the bone are seen most often in patients with breast, lung, or prostate cancer. Metastatic bone cancer rarely is life-threatening, and many patients live for years after the discovery of bone metastases. However, pain from these cancers sometimes can be debilitating and fractures can impair mobility. Some metastases occur singly, some are multiple. They are usually small and well defined, though tumors in the hip and pelvis may be larger. It has been found that the denser the pattern, the slower the growth. Seventy percent involve the cranium, ribs, spine or sacrum.

How are bone metastases diagnosed?

CT scans and MRIs are used to detect metastatic bone cancer when pain suggests there might be metastatic disease.

What kind of treatment is used for bone metastases?

Patients with breast cancer and those with multiple myeloma may be treated with hormonal agents or combination chemotherapy. Prostate cancer patients are usually treated with hormonal manipulation. If the metastatic cancer is found in a long bone, radiation is usually used. Radiation is also used to relieve pain from metastases in the bones.

What is Strontium-89 (Metastron)?

Strontium-89 (often referred to as Metastron) is a new type of medication used for cancers that metastasize to the bone. It is not recommended for patients with cancer that does not involve bone. It is injected and goes directly to the sites of metastatic bone disease where, like calcium, it is absorbed in the bones. The injection contains small amounts of a specially selected form of radioactive strontium, chosen because almost all of its radiation is given to the area where it is absorbed, allowing it to deliver therapy precisely where it is needed. A single outpatient injection generally provides pain relief for an average of six months and has minimal effect on normal bone and surrounding tissues. The effects of Strontium-89 are confined within your body. Other people cannot receive the effects of radiation through bodily contact with you. However, for the first week after injection, Strontium-89 will be present in your blood and urine and your doctor will discuss simple precautions that should be taken.

What are the side effects of Strontium-89 (Metastron)?

Some people experience a mild facial flushing immediately after injection. This may happen when the medication is administered too quickly (in thirty seconds rather than in a one- or two-minute time frame). Some people have a mild but temporary increase in pain several days after the injection that may last for two or three days. Doctors usually prescribe an increase in painkillers until the pain is under control. After one or two weeks, sometimes a little longer, the pain begins to diminish and continues to diminish, with effects lasting for up to six months. You may be advised to reduce the dose of other pain medications gradually. Eventually, you may not need painkillers at all. You can eat and drink normally. There may be a slight fall in your blood cell count. Your doctor will probably ask you to have routine periodic blood tests. Repeated dosages can be given if the doctor feels this is the most appropriate treatment.

Are bone fractures from metastasized bone cancer hard to heal?

Fractures and forced immobility are two of the most difficult side effects of metastatic bone cancer. Bone metastases from breast cancers and multiple myelomas are known to have the highest rate of healing. Metastases from lung and colorectal cancers and melanomas have been found to be more difficult to heal following bone fractures. It has also been shown that patients who have had high-dose postoperative radiation (greater than 3,000 to 3,500 rads) may have greater difficulty in healing. Cryosurgery is useful for metastasized bone tumors that have recurred and those in difficult anatomic locations.

What kind of cancers metastasize to the liver?

Liver metastases occur in many kinds of cancer. Tumors of the colon, rectum, stomach, pancreas, biliary tree and small intestines often metastasize to the liver. Breast and lung cancers sometimes will be found with liver metastasis, as will lymphoma.

What are the symptoms when cancer spreads to the liver?

An enlarged or tender liver is an indication that there may be metastases in the liver. Symptoms may include weight loss, abdominal swelling, a yellowish tinge to the skin (jaundice), a fever or a buildup of fluid in the abdominal cavity (ascites).

What treatment is used when cancer spreads to the liver?

Treatment depends on a number of factors, including the number of metastases, their location in the liver, and the primary site of the cancer. When the entire tumor can be removed, chances of recovery are excellent. The recuperative powers of the liver are amazing, and many people live perfectly normal lives after surgery has removed as much as 80 percent of their livers. Lymphomas and testicular cancer involving the liver can be cured with combination chemotherapy. Breast cancer and small cell lung cancers that spread to the liver often go into partial remission with chemotherapy. Metastasis may sometimes return again in the liver and may be operated on a second time. In cases where surgery of the liver is not possible, regional treatment of the liver with the use of an implantable pump may be used. New techniques using pumps and chemotherapy regimens designed to take advantage of daily variations in chemotherapy metabolism are being evaluated, as are biological response modifiers, palliative radiation and cryotherapy.

What is the outlook for cancer that has spread to the brain?

Today's expectations for patients with cerebral metastatic cancer have gradually improved, with modest benefits for the majority of patients and guarded optimism for selected patients. Sometimes cancer spreads to the brain after it has already spread to another organ, such as the lung or the liver. Melanomas are the most likely cancers to spread to the brain, followed by lung and breast. Lung, melanoma and renal tumors tend to spread more quickly following initial diagnosis. Breast and colon cancers and sarcomas seem to take longer to metastasize.

What are symptoms of metastatic brain cancer?

Headache, usually occurring in the morning or early hours and gradually increasing in duration and frequency, is a common symptom. Focal weakness, seizures, loss of sensation or difficulties with gait or balance may be other symptoms. Many times, family members or friends will notice lethargy, emotional instability, or personality changes.

How are brain metastases diagnosed?

CT and MRI scanning are the most specific and sensitive for evaluating brain metastases. Other conditions can mimic brain metastases, so it is important that careful evaluation be conducted to avoid inappropriate or dangerous and unnecessary treatment.

What treatment is most common for brain metastases?

Radiation therapy is usually the primary treatment. Sometimes surgery is combined with radiation therapy. Steroids may be used along with radiotherapy. Innovative radiation methods including stereotactic radiosurgery and brachytherapy are being used. Interstitial radiation to increase the dose without damaging any more tissue than is necessary is also being studied. In some chemotherapy-sensitive tumors, like lymphoma, small cell lung cancer, breast and testicular cancer, chemotherapy can produce remission of metastases. Laser-assisted surgical excision is also under clinical evaluation.

Are there other areas beside the more common ones of lungs, bone, liver and brain, where cancer may metastasize?

Sometimes cancer can spread to the membranes of the brain and spinal cord (leptomeningeal), or to the membrane lining the chest cavity (pleural cavity), or to the sac surrounding the heart (pericardium).

What type of cancers spread to the membranes of the brain and spinal cord (leptomeningeal metastases)?

These cancers, referred to medically as leptomeningeal metastases, affect the tissue lining the spinal canal. Acute lymphocytic leukemia and high-grade non-Hodgkin's lymphomas as well as breast, small cell lung cancer, melanoma, genital, urinary tract, head and neck and adenocarcinoma of unknown primary are found to metastasize to the membranes of the brain and spinal cord.

What are the symptoms of metastatic spread to the brain and spinal cord membranes?

There may be headaches, uncoordinated movements, mental changes, nausea, vomiting and sometimes seizures. Diagnosis will be made with CT or MRI scans.

What is the treatment for brain and spinal cord membrane metastases?

Treatment varies depending on the original cancer. For solid tumors, intrathecal chemotherapy (where anticancer drugs are injected into the cerebrospinal fluid) and radiation are usually used. In children with acute leukemia, radiation and intrathecal chemotherapy have cut down the incidence of these metastases occurring by a great percentage. This treatment has been less successful for adults with acute lymphocytic leukemia. For those with acute non-lymphocytic leukemia, standard treatments include chemotherapy and radiation or chemotherapy alone. Treatment for those with lymphomas is radiation with a short course of chemotherapy. This type of metastasis is rare in those with Hodgkin's disease and low-grade non-Hodgkin's lymphoma.

What types of cancers spread to the lung cavity?

The types of cancers most likely to spread to the membranes that cover the lungs and interior walls of the chest cavity are lung, breast, gastrointestinal tract, pancreas, uterus or ovary.

What are the symptoms of metastatic spread to these membranes surrounding the lungs (pleural effusion)?

Cough, labored breathing, and chest pain are typical symptoms. Usually fluid begins to accumulate in the space between the lung and the interior walls of the chest, making breathing difficult. Doctors refer to this as "pleural effusion." In 50 percent of cases, these symptoms are not caused by metastatic spread, but rather by infection or heart problems. Sometimes these symptoms may be due to poor lymph drainage rather than to further spread. Pleural effusions are classified as transudative (meaning they have a low protein content) or exudative (high protein content). Exudative (often bloody) effusions often suggest that they are caused by metastasis. But careful evaluation is necessary to make a positive diagnosis. Diagnosis is usually done with thoracentesis, or pleural tap, with a small amount of fluid removed for analysis as well as to relieve symptoms.

What is the treatment for metastatic spread to the membrane surrounding the lungs?

If the final diagnosis is malignant pleural effusion, treatment depends on the tumor type and prior treatment. Small and stable effusions may require no further treatment after the fluid has been removed. Malignant effusions caused by lymphomas, breast cancer, small cell lung cancer or ovarian cancer may respond to systemic chemotherapy or hormonal therapy.

What types of cancers spread to the membranes surrounding the heart (pericardial effusion)?

The heart and the area surrounding it can become involved with metastases in patients with cancers of the lung, breast, leukemia, Hodgkin's and non-Hodgkin's lymphoma, melanoma, gastrointestinal cancers and sarcomas.

What are the symptoms of heart involvement due to metastasis?

Symptoms can be quite vague and include labored breathing, difficult breathing except when upright, cough, palpitations, weakness, fatigue, dizziness and chest pain.

What is the treatment for pericardial effusion?

Some patients whose echocardiograms or CT scans show effusions do not require any specific therapy. However, if the heart becomes compressed ("tamponade" is the medical term) an emergency situation exists and pericardiocentesis (needle used to remove fluid for examination) may be done for diagnosis. Treatment can include drainage followed by chemotherapy, radiation or surgical procedures, depending on many factors. Being clinically evaluated is sequential intrapericardial chemotherapy.

What causes severe swelling of the abdomen (ascites)?

It is not unusual for fluid containing cancer cells to be found in the lining of the wall of the abdomen in advanced cancers. Ascites (pronounced "ah-si-tease") is a medical term for severe swelling of the abdomen.

What types of cancers metastasize and cause ascites?

Malignant ascites is seen most commonly in patients with ovarian, endometrial, colon, gastric and pancreatic cancer.

What treatments are used for malignant ascites?

A variety of treatments may be used. Intraperitoneal chemotherapy, delivered through a surgically implanted catheter, makes it possible for higher doses of some drugs to be delivered to the tumor than other methods.

Do some cancers regress spontaneously?

There are a few kinds of cancer that sometimes disappear spontaneously. These include low-grade lymphomas, melanomas and kidney cancer. How that happens is a mystery.

Can you have a metastasis without ever having cancer?

Sometimes a metastasis is discovered first, such as when pain is experienced in the bone before any symptoms of a primary cancer are seen. If the original site of the cancer cannot be found, it is known as "cancer of unknown primary."

What if the primary tumor can't be found?

A small number of cancer patients have tumors which clinically and pathologically can be proven to be cancer metastases, yet tests and examinations do not reveal where the first cancer is located. Even after extensive diagnostic studies, some of these primary cancers are impossible to detect. There are a number of ways in which such cases are managed, depending on the history, the site of the metastatic cancer and where the doctor suspects the primary cancer might be located. In such cases, it is especially important that your pathology be completely reviewed by a skilled pathologist who understands cancers of unknown primary. Be sure to report any previous problems with what were thought to be harmless symptoms— such information as any skin tumors that were removed, benign polyps of the colon, D&C or conization procedures, biopsies of the prostate, etc. The tissue that was removed may have been considered benign, but could explain the location of the original tumor. Think carefully about your past medical history—changes in bowel habits or voiding pattern, vaginal or other unusual bleeding, pelvic discomfort, or pain—that might give the doctor clues that will help determine where the original cancer is located. It is sometimes necessary to start treatment before the original cancer is found—and many times the original site is never pinpointed.

What are some of the medical emergencies that can occur as the result of cancers that have spread or from treatments used to try to control the cancer?

There are a number of medical emergencies that can occur as the result of the cancer or from treatments. As more effective and aggressive treatments are used, patients have a greater likelihood of encountering complications. Awareness of symptoms, prompt reporting and diagnosis of the problems allows for appropriate treatment. Some of the medical emergencies include:

- **Blood clotting problems,** referred to as DIC by the profession, may include mild to moderate urinary or gastrointestinal bleeding, phlebitis or pulmonary embolism. Any unexplained or unexpected bleeding should be carefully evaluated. Blood clotting problems are most often seen in those with gastrointestinal, pancreas, prostate, lung, breast and ovarian cancers, melanoma, acute leukemia and myeloma. Any early signs of bleeding should be reported so that underlying causes can be treated.

- **Bowel obstruction** resulting in loss of function requires immediate attention. Bowel obstruction may be due to a number of causes—impacted fecal matter, lesions, bands of adhesions or scar tissue from past surgery or spread of cancer to the bowel wall. Abdominal and pelvic radiation can also cause tissue changes, sometimes as long as 20 years after treatment. Many times, fluid and electrolyte inbalances are identified and corrected. Symptoms of bowel problems such as vomiting, abdominal distention and constipation should be reported to the doctor promptly so that preventive measures can be taken to help prevent complications. Following careful investigation and observation, surgery may be required.

- **Superior vena cava syndrome** is the result of an obstruction of the vena cava (the vein that drains blood from the head, neck, upper extremities, and chest). Airway obstruction, cough, neck vein distention, shortness of breath, and facial swelling are most common symptoms. The person often complains of a "tight collar" feeling, swelling of the trunk and upper extremities or that the rings on fingers become tight. If the cause is found to be due to a growth, radiation or chemotherapy are the common treatments used to reduce the tumor and relieve symptoms.

- **Pericarditis** or pericardial effusion is caused by the accumulation of fluid in the pericardial space, the sac which surrounds the heart. It can be the result of radiation to the chest area or be caused by the spread of cancer to the area. The most common symptom is chest pain which can be somewhat relieved by leaning forward but is more severe when the patient is lying down. Other symptoms are shortness of breath, cough, abdominal tenderness, and nausea. It may occur in patients with lung cancer, breast cancer, leukemia, Hodgkin's disease, lymphoma, melanoma, gastrointestinal tumors and sarcomas. Pericardial fluid is withdrawn and treatment is given to prevent reaccumulation of fluid.

- **Septic shock** is a serious infectious complication that can result from treatment that lowers blood count. Symptoms of early septic shock include: fever, shaking, chills, followed by stiffening of muscles, rapid cardiac rate, confusion and hypotension. Any such symptoms should be reported to the doctor immediately so that immediate treatment can be given.

- **Hypercalcemia,** an excess of calcium in the blood, can cause weakness, depression, anorexia, nausea, constipation, confusion, renal failure or coma. It occurs most frequently in patients with multiple myeloma or bone metastases from a wide variety of cancers. Drugs can be prescribed to help control hypercalcemia. If the hypercalcemia is severe, hospitalization may be required so that intravenous methods can be used.

- **Tumor lysis syndrome** is a side effect that can occur as a result of the administration of chemotherapy to certain very bulky tumors. It may occur in patients with high-grade lymphoma or acute lymphoblastic leukemia when abnormally high levels of potassium and phosphorus are released. A large amount of tumor may shrink in days as chemotherapeutic agents destroy tumor cells while the cells are dividing, causing the patient's system to deal with massive tumor burdens. Symptoms include weakness, muscle cramps, nausea, vomiting, diarrhea and lethargy.

- **Spinal cord compression** may occur as the result of a metastasis in the spinal cord. Since the spinal cord contains motor and sensory elements, the severity of the problem depends upon the tumor location within the spinal cord. Symptoms can include back pain from pressure on the spinal cord, foot drop, weakness, balance disturbances, and locomotion impairment. Again, depending upon the location of the tumor, other symptoms such as sensory impairment, incontinence, bowel problems, loss of feeling, etc., can occur. The goal of treatment is to relieve the compression as rapidly as possible to prevent further damage to the spinal cord.

Will I have pain as a result of my recurrent or advanced cancer?

Many people, when their cancer recurs or metastasizes, are afraid that they will have pain. However, some cancer patients, even those with advanced disease, have little or no pain. For those who do have pain problems, new pain therapies are being explored with good results. The many ways of dealing with pain are described in Chapter 24, "Living with Cancer."

chapter 26

Where to Get Help

> ## QUICK REFERENCE FOR ESSENTIAL NUMBERS
>
> **CANCER INFORMATION SERVICE**
> 1-800-4-CANCER
> 1-800-422-6237
>
> **AMERICAN CANCER SOCIETY**
> 1-800-ACS-2345
> 1-800-227-2345
>
> **CANCERFAX**
> 301-402-5874
>
> **CANCERNET**
> Use Internet electronic mail
>
> **NATIONAL HOSPICE ORGANIZATION**
> 1-800-658-8898
>
> **NATIONAL LIBRARY OF MEDICINE**
> 1-800-272-4787
>
> **AMERICAN BOARD OF MEDICAL SPECIALTIES**
> 1-800-776-CERT

Contents

NOTE: Listings in this chapter are focused on organizations that operate on a national level. Since there are many local or regional organizations that are too numerous to mention, this listing is just a starting point for your information seeking. The listings in this chapter are up-to-date at the time of publication. You may find that some of your inquiries will be routed to different organizations and individuals.

1. MAJOR INFORMATION SOURCES

CANCER INFORMATION SERVICE

Call 1-800-4-CANCER
(1-800-422-6237)

The Cancer Information Service covers the entire United States. Based on the area code from which you are dialing, you will be connected to the regional center which covers your area.

All offices are open from 9:00 A.M. until 7:00 P.M.

The Cancer Information Service (CIS), a program of the National Cancer Institute (NCI), has a nationwide toll-free telephone service for cancer patients and their families, the public, and health care professionals. The CIS information specialists can provide rapid access to the latest information on cancer and local resources. The staff, located in nineteen regional offices across the country, have extensive training in providing up-to-date and understandable information. They can:

- Explain diagnostic procedures.
- Tell you about state-of-the-art treatments, using PDQ, a computerized data base of the National Cancer Institute.
- Conduct a computer search to give you information on where investigational treatment is being done.
- Help you explore referrals and medical facilities.
- Send free printed material.
- Discuss rehabilitation assistance and home-care assistance programs.
- Help you find financial aid or emotional counseling services.
- Discuss prevention.
- Give you information on causes of cancer.
- Answer questions in English and Spanish.
- Generally help you to get answers to any questions you might have about cancer or treatment.

CIS can tell you what hospitals and doctors in your area are involved in what kinds of investigational treatment. If, for instance, a relative lives in a different part of the country, the staff can explore investigational treatments in that area. In many places, the Cancer Information Service offices are affiliated with comprehensive cancer centers (specialized research and treatment centers designated by the National Cancer Institute) and with the American Cancer Society.

What kind of questions should I ask when I call the Cancer Information Service?

The more specific you can be with your questions, the better the information you will receive. It is wise to think through what you want to know and to write down the questions you want to have answered before you call. You can call as many times as you wish. You do not have to give your name if you do not want to. All calls are kept confidential.

Can the Cancer Information Service send me written information about cancer?

The Cancer Information Offices are supplied with a wealth of printed information about cancer. All of them have brochures which are supplied by the National Cancer Institute. Some also have available brochures from the American Cancer Society. The material will be sent to you free of charge.

Can the Cancer Information Service tell me where different kinds of investigational treatments (clinical trials) are available in the United States? Overseas?

Yes, the Cancer Information Service, through the PDQ data base, has information on the investigational treatments being conducted in the cancer centers and community hospitals around the country and overseas.

What is PDQ?

PDQ is a data-based treatment information system supported by the National Cancer Institute. PDQ offers state-of-the art treatment statements, compiled and updated monthly by panels of the country's leading cancer specialists, giving the range of effective treatment options that represent the best available therapy for a specific type or stage of cancer. PDQ also gives the latest information on clinical treatment trials being offered around the country for each type and stage of cancer. The Cancer Information Service can provide you with printed copies of up-to-date treatment information on your type of cancer. In addition, it can give you information on clinical trials that may be available to you.

What do I need to know in order to have a PDQ search of clinical trials for my kind of cancer?

If you call the Cancer Information Service and request a PDQ search of clinical trials, you will be asked a series of questions to determine the information needed to complete the search for you:

- Whether or not you are currently in treatment. If you are being treated, a clinical trial is probably not appropriate.
- Whether you (or the patient) are interested in participating in a clinical trial.
- Whether you are able or willing to travel to a participating center and how far you are willing to travel for treatment.
- The primary site of your cancer, the stage, and, depending on your cancer site, cell type and grade; for breast cancer patients, hormonal and menopausal status.
- The site of metastases, if any.
- What previous treatments you have had, type of treatment, when and where, including names of drugs previously received and when.
- Major medical conditions that might preclude participation.

What is CancerFax?

This service of the National Cancer Institute enables you to get PDQ treatment information via a fax machine, 24 hours a day, seven days a week for the cost of your fax call. You first need to get instructions and a list of necessary codes (call 301-402-5874). Clinical trial searches are not available through CancerFax.

AMERICAN CANCER SOCIETY

> ### Call 1-800-ACS-2345
> ### (1-800-227-2345)
>
> **In most areas of the country, this number is answered at the state offices of the American Cancer Society. To reach your local unit, look in the white pages of the telephone book under "American Cancer Society." Ask for patient services.**

The American Cancer Society (ACS) is the nationwide, community-based, voluntary health organization (2.5 million Americans volunteer for this organization) dedicated to eliminating cancer as a major health problem by preventing cancer, saving lives from cancer, and diminishing suffering from cancer through research, education and service. It is composed of 57 chartered divisions and nearly 3,000 local units. The national society administers programs of research, medical grants, and clinical fellowships and is charged with carrying out public and professional education at the national level. The divisions are in all states, in addition to six metropolitan areas, the District of Columbia, and Puerto Rico. The units are organized to cover the counties in the United States. Some units have branches which cover smaller geographic areas.

The units of the American Cancer Society conduct basic service programs, including:

- Answering many questions by telephone and offering printed material on cancer.
- Information and counseling for the cancer patient and the patient's family.
- Information and guidance concerning ACS services, community health services, and other resources, such as providing transportation to and from a doctor's office, clinic, or hospital for treatment.
- Arranging for lodging (sometimes donated by hotels and hotel chains) if you need to be treated at a hospital away from home.
- Home health care, blood programs, assistance with employment problems and social work assistance.

Rehabilitation programs, primarily directed toward laryngectomy, mastectomy, and ostomy patients, are an important part of the American Cancer Society service. These include Lost Cord clubs, Reach to Recovery volunteers, ostomy clubs, and Candlelighters, as well as support groups for patients and their families. Sponsors I Can Cope and many camps for children with cancer.

National Office
American Cancer Society

1599 Clifton Road NE
Atlanta, GA 30329-4251
1-800-ACS-2345

Division Offices

Alabama Division, Inc.
504 Brookwood Boulevard
Homewood, AL 35209
205-879-2242

Alaska Division, Inc.
406 West Fireweed Lane
Anchorage, AK 99503
907-277-8696

Arizona Division, Inc.
2929 East Thomas Road
Phoenix, AZ 85016
602-224-0524

Arkansas Division, Inc.
901 North University
Little Rock, AR 72203
501-664-3480

California Division, Inc.
1710 Webster Street
Oakland, CA 94612
510-893-7900

Colorado Division, Inc.
2255 South Oneida
Denver, CO 80224
303-758-2030

Connecticut Division, Inc.
Barnes Park South
14 Village Lane
Wallingford, CT 06492
203-265-7161

Delaware Division, Inc.
92 Read's Way
New Castle, DE 19720
302-324-4227

District of Columbia Division, Inc.
1875 Connecticut Avenue, N.W.
Washington, D.C. 20009
202-483-2600

Florida Division, Inc.
3709 West Jetton Avenue
Tampa, FL 33629-5146
813-253-0541

Georgia Division, Inc.
2200 Lake Boulevard
Atlanta, GA 30319
404-816-7800

Hawaii Pacific Division, Inc.
Community Services Center
  Building
200 North Vineyard Boulevard
Honolulu, HI 96817
808-531-1662

Idaho Division, Inc.
2676 Vista Avenue
Boise, ID 83705-0836
208-343-4609

Illinois Division, Inc.
77 East Monroe
Chicago, IL 60603-5795
312-641-6150

Indiana Division, Inc.
8730 Commerce Park Place
Indianapolis, IN 46268
317-872-4432

Iowa Division, Inc.
8364 Hickman Road
Des Moines, IA 50325
515-253-0147

Kansas Division, Inc.
1315 SW Arrowhead Road
Topeka, KS 66604
913-273-4114

Kentucky Division, Inc.
701 West Muhammad Ali
  Boulevard
Louisville, KY 40203-1909
502-584-6782

Louisiana Division, Inc.
2200 Veteran's Memorial
  Boulevard
Suite 214
Kenner, LA 70062
504-469-0021

Maine Division, Inc.
52 Federal Street
Brunswick, ME 04011
207-729-3339

Maryland Division, Inc.
8219 Town Center Drive
Baltimore, MD 21236-0026
410-931-6868

Massachusetts Division, Inc.
247 Commonwealth Avenue
Boston, MA 02116
617-267-2650

Michigan Division, Inc.
1205 East Saginaw Street
Lansing, MI 48906
517-371-2920

Minnesota Division, Inc.
3316 West 66th Street
Minneapolis, MN 55435
612-925-2772

Mississippi Division, Inc.
1380 Livingston Lane
Lakeover Office Park

Jackson, MS 39213
601-362-8874

Missouri Division, Inc.
3322 American Avenue
Jefferson City, MO 65102
314-893-4800

Montana Division, Inc.
17 North 26th
Billings, MT 59101
406-252-7111

Nebraska Division, Inc.
8502 West Center Road
Omaha, NE 68124-5255
402-393-5800

Nevada Division, Inc.
1325 East Harmon
Las Vegas, NV 89119
702-798-6857

New Hampshire Division, Inc.
360 Route 101, Unit 501
Bedford, NH 03110-5032
603-472-8899

New Jersey Division, Inc.
2600 US Highway 1
North Brunswick, NJ 08902-
  0803
908-297-8000

New Mexico Division, Inc.
5800 Lomas Boulevard, NE
Albuquerque, NM 87110
505-260-2105

New York State Division, Inc.
6725 Lyons Street
East Syracuse, NY 13057
315-437-7025
  Long Island Division
  75 Davids Drive
  Hauppauge, NY 11788
  516-436-7070

New York City Division, Inc.
19 West 56th Street
New York, NY 10019
212-586-8700

Queens Division, Inc.
112-25 Queens Boulevard
Forest Hills, NY 11375
718-263-2224

Westchester Division, Inc.
30 Glenn Street
White Plains, NY 10603
914-949-4800

North Carolina Division, Inc.
11 South Boylan Avenue
Raleigh, NC 27603
919-834-8463

North Dakota Division, Inc.
123 Roberts Street
Fargo, ND 58102
701-232-1385

Ohio Division, Inc.
5555 Frantz Road
Dublin, OH 43017
614-889-9565

Oklahoma Division, Inc.
4323 63rd, Suite 110
Oklahoma City, OK 73116
405-843-9888

Oregon Division, Inc.
0330 SW Curry
Portland, OR 97201
503-295-6422

Pennsylvania Division, Inc.
Route 422 and Sipe Avenue
Hershey, PA 17033-0897
717-533-6144

Philadelphia Division, Inc.
1422 Chestnut Street
Philadelphia, PA 19102
215-665-2900

Puerto Rico Division, Inc.
Calle Alverio #577
Esquina Sargento Medina
Hato Rey, PR 00918
809-764-2295

Rhode Island Division, Inc.
400 Main Street
Pawtucket, RI 02860
401-722-8480

South Carolina Division, Inc.
128 Stonemark Lane
Columbia, SC 29210-3855
803-750-1693

South Dakota Division, Inc.
4101 Carnegie Place
Sioux Falls, SD 57106-2322
605-361-8277

Tennessee Division, Inc.
1315 Eighth Avenue, South
Nashville, TN 37203
615-255-1227

Texas Division, Inc.
2433 Ridgepoint Drive
Austin, TX 78754
512-928-2262

Utah Division, Inc.
941 East 3300 S.
Salt Lake City, UT 84106
801-483-1500

Vermont Division, Inc.
13 Loomis Street
Montpelier, VT 05602
802-223-2348

Virginia Division, Inc.
P.O. Box 6359
Glen Allen, VA 23060-6359
804-527-3700

Washington Division, Inc.
2120 First Avenue, North
Seattle, WA 98109-1140
206-283-1152

West Virginia Division, Inc.
2428 Kanawha Boulevard East
Charleston, WV 25311
304-344-3611

Wisconsin Division, Inc.
P.O. Box 902
Pewaukee, WI 53072
414-523-5500

Wyoming Division, Inc.
2222 House Avenue
Cheyenne, WY 82001
307-638-3331

2. MAJOR NATIONWIDE DIRECT HELP, SERVICES, AND ORGANIZATIONS

(The) American Bone Marrow Donor Registry
Search Coordinating Center
University of Massachusetts Medical Center
55 Lake Avenue, North
Worchester, MA 01655
508-756-6444
Assists those with leukemia, aplastic anemia and other blood-related disorders in finding compatible bone marrow donors.

American Brain Tumor Association
(formerly Association for Brain Tumor Research)
2720 River Road, Suite 146
Des Plaines, IL 60018
708-827-9910
1-800-886-ABTA (patient line)
Offers free services including publications about brain tumors, support group lists, referral information. Supports research.

American Lung Association
1740 Broadway
New York, NY 10019-4374
212-315-8700
212-265-5642 (fax)
Promotes lung health, runs smoking cessation groups, provides literature on lung diseases. Telephone numbers for local offices can be found in white pages of telephone directory.

American Self-Help Clearinghouse
St. Clare's-Riverside Medical Center
25 Pocono Road
Denville, NJ 07834
201-625-7101

Provides current information and contacts for national self-help groups. Gives information concerning any state or local self-help group that may exist. Supports caller in forming group if none exists. Publishes Self-Help Source Book.

Association for Brain Tumor Research
See American Brain Tumor Association.

Association for the Care of Children's Health
Suite 300
7910 Woodmont Avenue
Bethesda, MD 20814
301-654-6549
The association carries out a variety of programs to promote the health of children. It publishes educational materials on child health of interest to parents, educators, and health professionals.

Bone Marrow Transplant Family Support Network
P.O. Box 845
Avon, CT 06001
1-800-826-9376
Offers support to famiies when coping with decisions, daily routines prior to and following transplants, follow-up care.

Bone Marrow Transplant Newsletter
1985 Spruce Avenue
Highland Park, IL 60035
708-831-1931
Newsletter and book on issues, attorney referrals for those having difficulty obtaining reimbursement for treatment.

Breast Implant Information Service (FDA)
1-800-532-4440
Provides latest information on breast implants.

CAN ACT (Cancer Patients Action Alliance)
26 College Place
Brooklyn, NY 11201
718-522-4607
Addresses problems of access to advanced cancer treatments, barriers created by the FDA drug approval process and restrictive insurance reimbursement policies.

Cancer Care, Inc. and National Cancer Care Foundation
1180 Avenue of the Americas
New York, NY 10036
212-302-2400

A nonprofit social service agency helping patients and families cope with emotional, financial, and psychological consequences of cancer. Provides free individual, family and group counseling. Financial counseling is also available as is financial assistance for home care and transportation.

Cancer Information Service
(a program of the National Cancer Institute)
1-800-4-CANCER (1-800-422-6237)
Nationwide telephone service for cancer patients and their families, the public, and health care professionals. CIS information specialists have extensive training in providing up-to-date and understandable information about cancer. They can answer questions in English and Spanish and can send free printed material. CIS offices serve specific geographic areas and have information about cancer-related services and resources in their region.

CANCERVIVE
6500 Wilshire Boulevard, Suite 500
Los Angeles, CA 90048
213-203-9232
A nationwide network that runs support groups to help with everyday concerns of survivors. They will put you in touch with the group nearest you or advise you how to start a group of your own.

Candlelighters Childhood Cancer Foundation
7910 Woodmont Avenue, Suite 460
Bethesda, MD 20814
301-657-8401
1-800-366-2223
301-718-2686 (fax)
Organization formed by parents of young cancer patients. An important goal of the organization is to help families cope with the emotional stresses of their experiences. Can give information on camps for children with cancer. Has an ombudsman program to assist families and survivors with problems in education, employment, insurance, welfare or military enlistment.

CANSURMOUNT
American Cancer Society
1-800-ACS-2345
Group that offers patient and family education and support. It tries to match a volunteer who has had cancer with a patient for hospital visits. Local information available through the American Cancer Society.

Center for Medical Consumers
237 Thompson Street
New York, NY 10012
Provides information and referrals to national health organizations
and maintains a medical consumers' public library.

ChemoCare
220 St. Paul Street
Westfield, NJ, 07090
1-800-55-CHEMO
Support for people undergoing chemotherapy and radiation.
Trained volunteers who have survived treatment.

Children's Hospice International
901 North Washington Street
Alexandria, VA 22314
703-684-0330
1-800-242-4453
Nonprofit agency that encourages use of hospices and home care
programs for children. Serves as clearinghouse for support groups
and offers publications.

Children's Oncology Camps of America
2309 West White Oaks Drive
Springfield, IL 62704
217-793-3949
Organization publishes national directory of children's oncology
camps.

Clinical Center of the National Institutes of Health
Patient Referral Service
Building 10, Room 12N214
9000 Rockville Pike
Bethesda, MD 20892
301-496-5583

Choice in Dying
(formerly Concern for Dying & Society for the Right to Die)
200 Varick Street, Suite 1001
New York, NY 10014
1-800-989-WILL
212-366-5540
Provides latest information on right-to-die, Living Wills, etc.

Corporate Angel Network, Inc.
Westchester County Airport, Building 1
White Plains, NY 10604
914-328-1313
1-800-328-4226 (fax)
A service which matches available space on corporate airplanes with cancer patients in need of transportation to treatment centers.

DES
Registry for Research on Hormonal Transplacental Carcinogenesis
University of Chicago
5841 South Maryland Avenue
Chicago, IL 60637
A worldwide registry for individuals who developed clear cell adenocarcinoma as a result of exposure to DES.

DES Action USA
(West Coast Office)
1615 Broadway, Suite 510
Oakland, CA 94612
510-465-4011
(East Coast Office)
Long Island Jewish Medical Center
New Hyde Park, NY 11040
516-775-3450 (staffed by volunteers Tuesday and Thursday)
Provides counseling, educational materials, and a newsletter about diethylstilbesterol (DES), a synthetic hormone once given to pregnant women to prevent miscarriages.

DES Cancer Network
P.O. Box 20285
Rochester, NY 14610
Provides information about DES-related cancer.

Encore
YWCA of USA
726 Broadway
New York, NY 10003
212-614-2827
For postoperative breast cancer patients. Supportive discussion and rehabilitative exercise. Call national office or your local YWCA branch.

Families Against Cancer (FACT)
P.O. Box 588
Dewitt, NY 13214
315-446-5326 or 315-446-6385

Grass roots coalition of cancer patients, families and friends seeking new and more vigorous national policy on cancer.

Food and Drug Administration
Office of Consumer Affairs HFE-88
Rooms 16–63, 5600 Fishers Lane
Rockville, MD 20857
301-443-3170
MedWatch Program
1-800-332-1088
Provides information on federal regulation of drugs.

Gilda Radner Familial Ovarian Cancer Registry
Roswell Park Cancer Institute
New York Department of Health
Elm and Carlton Streets
Buffalo, NY 14263
1-800-682-7426
716-845-3545 (fax)
Individuals can register; newsletter.

Hereditary Cancer Institute
Creighton University
Omaha, NE 68178
402-422-6237
Nonprofit organization devoted to the study of the genetics of familial cancer. Attempts to assess and verify the nature of cancer patterns in families and the simple or complex modes of inheritance that may help in predicting cancer risk to family members and their offspring. Maintains a registry of families interested in participating in its work.

Hereditary Colon Cancer Registries

Cleveland Clinic Florida
3000 W. Cypress Creek
Fort Lauderdale, FL 33309

Jernigan Cancer Center
Southeastern FAP Registry
1350 Walton Way
Augusta, GA 30910

The Johns Hopkins Hospital
Familial Polyposis Registry
600 N. Wolfe Street
Baltimore, MD 21205

Ferguson Clinic
72 Sheldon Boulevard SE
Grand Rapids, MI 49503

Jewish Hospital
Washington University
Division Colorectal Surgery
216 S. Kings Highway
    Boulevard
St. Louis, MO 63178

Hereditary Cancer Institute
Department of Preventive
   Medicine
Creighton University
Omaha, NE 68178

Roswell Park Memorial
   Institute
666 Elm Street
Buffalo, NY 14263

New York Hospital
Surgical Registry, Room F19-2
528 E. 68th Street
New York, NY 10021

The Graduate Hospital
Cancer Prevention Center
Pepper Pavilion, Suite 100
1800 Lombard Street
Philadelphia, PA 19146

M. D. Anderson Hospital and
   Tumor Institute
1515 Holcombe Boulevard
Houston, TX 77030

Kelsey-Seybold Foundation
6624 Fannin Street
Houston, TX 77030

Mayo Clinic
Department of Medical
   Genetics
Rochester, MN 55905

Cleveland Clinic Foundation
Familial Polyposis Registry
Department of Colorectal
   Surgery
9500 Euclid Avenue
Cleveland, OH 44195

For complete, updated list of all
   registries:
IMPACC (Intestinal Multiple
   Polyposis and Colorectal
   Cancer)
Delores Boone, Administrator
1008 101 Brinker Drive
Hagerstown, MD 21740
301-791-7526

Newsletter information:
Hereditary Colon Cancer
   Newsletter
Department of GI Oncology,
   Box 78
M. D. Anderson Hospital and
   Tumor Institute
1515 Holcombe Boulevard
Houston, TX 77030

Hospice
See National Hospice Organization.

Hospice Link
Hospice Education Institute
Suite 3-B, P.O. Box 713
190 Westbrook Road
Essex, CT 06426
1-800-331-1620
(203-767-1620 in Alaska and Connecticut)
Maintains HOSPICELINK, computerized database of hospice programs in country.

I Can Cope
American Cancer Society
1-800-ACS-2345
A patient education program of the American Cancer Society designed to help patients, families, and friends cope with the day-to-day issues of living with cancer. Look in the telephone directory white pages for your local ACS unit.

International Association of Laryngectomees
c/o American Cancer Society
1599 Clifton Road N.E.
Atlanta, GA 30329
1-800-ACS-2345
Voluntary organization composed of 190 member clubs. Also called Lost Cord, Anamilo, or New Voice clubs. Assists people who have lost their voices as a result of cancer, provides education in skills needed by laryngectomees, and works toward total rehabilitation of patient. Maintains registry of postlaryngectomy speech instructors, publishes educational materials, sponsors meetings and other activities. Look in telephone directory white pages for your local ACS unit.

International Bone Marrow Transplant Registry
Medical College of Wisconsin
P.O. Box 26509
Milwaukee, WI 53226
414-257-8325
Collects and analyzes data about allogeneic bone marrow transplantations. Most BMT teams throughout the world participate in the registry. Staff is available to answer questions about the procedure. Donor matches are not made by this registry. (See National Marrow Donor Program.)

Intestinal Multiple Polyposis and Colorectal Cancer
1008 101 Brinker Drive
Hagerstown, MD 21740
301-791-7526
Specifically designed to provide support for families with either of the forms of hereditary colon cancer. Publishes Hereditary Colon Cancer Newsletter quarterly for professionals and families. Contact Department of GI Oncology, Box 78, M.D. Anderson Hospital and Tumor Institute, 1515 Holcombe Boulevard, Houston, TX 77030, for newsletter information.

International Myeloma Foundation
2120 Stanley Hills Drive
Los Angeles, CA 90046
1-800-452-CURE

Promotes education and research, informs patients about available treatments and provides support to community and patient support groups.

Joint Commission on Accreditation of Healthcare Organizations (JCAHO)
1 Renaissance Boulevard
Oak Brook Terrace, IL 60181
708-916-5800
Hospital accrediting organization. Will tell you if hospital has been accredited by JCAHO.

Komen (Susan G.) Breast Cancer Foundation
5005 LBJ Freeway, Suite 370
Dallas, TX 75244
800-IM-AWARE
Breast cancer organization dedicated to eradicating breast cancer as a life-threatening disease through research, education, screening and treatment.

Let's Face It
P.O. Box 711
Concord, MA 01742-0711
508-371-3186
International information and support organization for people with facial difference and their families. Provides mutual support, educational services and an annual resource listing with biannual updates for individuals who are facially disfigured.

Leukemia Society of America
600 Third Avenue
New York, NY 10016
1-800-955-4LSA
212-573-8484
Focuses on leukemia, the lymphomas, and Hodgkin's disease. Provides referral services to other sources of help in the community. Offers financial assistance for drugs used in care, treatment, and/or control of disease; transfusing of blood, transportation to and from a doctor's office, hospital, or treatment center and x-ray treatment. Supports research and provides printed materials.

Living Bank
4545 Post Oak Place, Suite 315
Houston, TX 77027
1-800-528-2971
713-528-2971
713-961-0979 (fax)
Information on donating body or organ parts.

Look Good . . . Feel Better
American Cancer Society
1-800-395-LOOK
Program developed by Cosmetic, Toiletry, and Fragrance Association in cooperation with American Cancer Society and National Cosmetology Association. It focuses on techniques that can help people undergoing cancer treatment improve their appearance. The Cancer Information Service or local ACS unit, listed in the white pages of the telephone directory, can provide more information about this program.

Lost Cord Club
See International Association of Laryngectomees.

Lymphedema Network
See National Lymphedema Network.

National Alliance of Breast Cancer Organizations (NABCO)
93 E. 37th Street, 10th Floor
New York, NY 10016
212-719-0154
212-689-1213 (fax)
Advocate for needs and concerns of patients/survivors and all women at risk for breast cancer.

National Brain Tumor Foundation
323 Geary Street, Suite 510
San Francisco, CA 94102
415-296-0404
415-296-9303 (fax)
Publishes a resource guide for brain tumor patients and their families. Raises funds to support brain tumor research. Provides information and support services to patients and families.

National Breast Cancer Coalition
PO Box 66373
Washington, D.C. 20035
202-296-7477
202-265-6854 (fax)
A grass roots breast cancer advocacy organization. Seeks funding for research on breast cancer, better access to services for women, and influence by the breast cancer patient in decision making.

National Coalition for Cancer Survivorship
1010 Wayne Avenue, 5th Floor
Silver Spring, MD 20910
301-650-8868

Network of groups and individuals offering support to cancer survivors and families. Provides information and resources on support and life after a cancer diagnosis. Advocates for legal rights of survivors. Holds annual conference on survivor issues. Publishes *Networker* magazine and maintains national data base.

National Consumers League
815 15th Street, NW, Suite 92N
Washington, D.C. 20005
202-639-8140
National nonprofit membership organization offering publications on a range of health issues such as hospice, home health care and insurance.

National Council Against Health Fraud Resource Center
Consumer Health Information Research Institute
3521 Broadway
Kansas City, MO 64111
1-800-821-6671
Provides information on questionable health practices and organizations.

National Hospice Organization
1901 North Moore Street
Suite 901
Arlington, VA 22209
703-243-5900
1-800-658-8898
An association of groups that provide hospice care. Designed to promote and maintain hospice care and to encourage support for patients and family members. Information about hospice concepts also available.

National Institutes of Health Consensus Program Clearinghouse
P.O. Box 2577
Kensington, MD 20891
Voice Mail: 1-800-NIH-OMAR
Fax: 301-816-2494
Electronic Bulletin Board: 301-816-9840
The clearinghouse provides up-to-date official consensus statements developed by nonadvocate, nonfederal panels of experts brought together to evaluate scientific information on biomedical technologies. There are several statements relating to cancer subjects that are useful to the public and to health professionals.

National Kidney Cancer Association
1234 Sherman Avenue, Suite 200
Evanston, IL 60202
708-332-1051
708-328-4425 (fax)
Provides information to patients and physicians, sponsors research on kidney cancer and acts as an advocate on behalf of patients.

National Lymphedema Network
2211 Post Street, Suite 404
San Francisco, CA 94115
1-800-541-3259
Nonprofit network provides printed information and other assistance to those who develop lymphedema as a result of lymph node surgery or radiation therapy. Serves as a resource center for patients and health care professionals, and publishes a newsletter.

National Marrow Donor Program
3433 Broadway Street N.E., Suite 400
Minneapolis, MN 55413
612-627-5800
1-800-654-1247 or 1-800-526-7809 (patient advocacy)
Maintains file of donors, processes searches and matches donors and recipients for transplants. Also maintains listing of centers that perform transplants from unrelated donors.

National Oral Health Information Clearinghouse
Box NOHIC
9000 Rockville Pike
Bethesda, MD 20892
301-402-7364
This is a resource for patients, health professionals and the public seeking information on the oral health of special care patients, such as people whose medical treatment causes oral problems. A service of the National Institute of Dental Research, this Clearinghouse can provide patient education materials, directories and resource guides that provide current information on specialized resources and key organizations, and can generate custom and standard searches from the Oral Health Subfile of the Combined Health Information Database.

National Self-Help Clearinghouse
25 West 43rd Street, Room 620
New York, NY 10036
212-642-2944
Refers callers to regional self-help services.

National Women's Health Network
1325 G Street NW
Washington, D.C. 20005
1-202-347-1140
Provides information on women's cancers and other issues related to women's health.

Ostomy Rehabilitation Program
American Cancer Society
1-800-ACS-2345
Provides mutual aid, emotional support and educational materials to people with ostomies. Program is available from local ACS unit, listed in the white pages of the telephone directory.

PDQ (Physician's Data Query)
1-800-4-CANCER
National Cancer Institute's computerized listing of up-to-date information for patients and health professionals on latest cancer treatments, research studies, clinical trials, promising cancer treatments. Treatment statements and fact sheets may also be accessed by personal computer. See Section 9, Data Base and Publications Sources.

Polyposis and Hereditary Colon Cancer
See Hereditary Colon Cancer Registries.

Quality Care National Resource Center
2 Copley Place, Suite 200
Boston, MA 02116
1-800-645-3633
National provider of home nursing services. Operates toll-free telephone line that provides information about home care and related services such as home nursing services, hospices, skilled nursing, rehabilitation facilities and homemaker services throughout the United States. Two-hundred-office network can provide referral information for these services and also for some specialty programs for cancer patients.

R. A. Bloch Cancer Foundation, Inc.
The Cancer Hotline
4410 Main Street
Kansas City, MO 64111
816-932-8453
Information for people diagnosed with cancer to help them find best ways of treating it.

Reach to Recovery
American Cancer Society
1-800-ACS-2345
Offers assistance to breast cancer patients. Trained volunteers who have had breast cancer lend emotional support and furnish information. In most cases must have physician referral. Call your local American Cancer Society office listed in telephone directory white pages.

Ronald McDonald House
Kroc Drive
Oak Brook, IL 60521
708-575-7418
Nonprofit organization offers home-away-from-home for parents and families of children being treated for serious illness. Found in the United States, Canada and Sydney, Australia. Each Ronald McDonald House is different, created by a team of local citizens to meet needs of community. Each house is owned and operated by local not-for-profit organization comprised of volunteers and is primarily funded by local contributions. Call national coordinator for locations.

(The) Skin Cancer Foundation
245 Fifth Avenue, Suite 2402
New York, NY 10016
212-725-5176
Conducts public and medical education programs to help reduce skin cancer. Major goals are to increase public awareness of the importance of taking protective measures against damaging sun rays, and to teach people how to recognize the early signs of skin cancer.

State Vocational Rehabilitation Service
c/o American Cancer Society
1-800-ACS-2345
Service offers training for another vocation for those physically unable to return to the same work performed prior to surgery. Check "State Services" in telephone directory.

United Ostomy Association
36 Executive Park, Suite 120
Irvine, CA 92714-6744
1-800-826-0826
714-660-8624

Organization which helps people who have had ostomies. Offers a variety of booklets compiled from the experiences of many hundreds of patients, nurses and doctors. Local chapters are located across the country and are listed in the yellow pages under "Associations" or "Social Service Organizations." Contact the American Cancer Society in your area for the location of the nearest chapter.

US-TOO International
930 North York Road, Suite 50
Hinsdale, IL 60521-2993
1-800-82-US-TOO
708-323-1002
708-323-1003 (fax)
A national support network for prostate cancer survivors. Contact them for the chapter nearest you.

VHL Family Alliance
171 Clinton Road
Brookline, MA 02146
1-800-767-4VHL (serving the U.S. and Canada)
Offers information and support to families with the rare familial disorder called von Hippel Lindau Syndrome (VHL), which can result in cancer in patients who have visceral lesions.

WE CAN Weekend Programs
North Cancer Center
North Memorial Medical Center
3300 Oakdale North
Robbinsdale, MN 55422
612-520-5155
Family support weekends held twice a year to help families understand and cope with the impact of cancer on the family. The weekends include workshops, discussions, and other activities for patients and family members of all ages, using volunteer staff. Information on organizing a weekend in your area is available.

Well Spouse Foundation
P.O. Box 801
New York, NY 10023
212-724-7209
212-724-5209 (fax)
A network of support groups and families that provide emotional support to husbands, wives and children of the chronically ill. Foundation also advocates for the families of the chronically ill and publishes quarterly newsletter.

(The) Wellness Community
2716 Ocean Park Boulevard, Suite 1040
Santa Monica, CA 90405-5207
310-314-2555
310-314-7586 (fax)
Provides free psychosocial support to people fighting to recover from cancer, as an adjunct to conventional medical treatment. Has fourteen facilities throughout nation.

Y-ME
212 W. Van Buren, 4th Floor
Chicago, IL 60607
1-800-221-2141
312-986-0020 (fax)
Hotline counseling, educational programs and self-help meetings for breast cancer patients, family and friends.

3. DOCTORS, OTHER HEALTH PROFESSIONALS AND HOSPITALS

PROFESSIONAL ORGANIZATIONS

American Academy of Dermatology
P.O. Box 4014
Schaumburg, IL 60168-4014
708-330-0230
Organization of doctors who specialize in diagnosing and treating skin problems. Provides information and references to dermatologists in your area.

American Association of Sex Educators, Counselors and Therapists (AASECT)
Suite 1717
435 N. Michigan Avenue
Chicago, IL 60611
312-644-0828
Provides names of sex therapists in your area.

American Board of Medical Specialties
1-800-776-CERT
Toll-free telephone line provides verification of physician's certification status. (See Chapter 2, "Choosing Your Doctor and Hospital").

American College of Radiology
1891 Preston White Drive
Reston, VA 22091
703-648-8900
1-800-ACR-LINE
703-648-9176 (fax)
Will provide updated information concerning mammograms. ACR voluntary program evaluates and approves equipment, personnel, procedures and facilities. ACR-accredited facilities are staffed with doctors and personnel trained to perform and interpret mammograms.

American College of Surgeons
55 East Eire Street
Chicago, IL 60611
312-664-4050
Provides list of board-certified surgeons in all specialties. Maintains certification program for hospitals relating to quality of cancer care. Approved status is based on level of excellence in relation to standards established by the College of Surgeons. In order to be certified, the hospital must have a cancer committee, a cancer registry, a clinical education program, and means for evaluating the quality of care in the hospital. Hospitals that have been given approved status are listed in the *College of Surgeons Directory*, published annually and updated twice a year.

American Endocurietherapy Society
1101 Market Street, 14th Floor
Philadelphia, PA 19107
215-574-3158
Promotes highest standards of practice of brachytherapy and clinical and laboratory research in this specialty. Encourages continuing education for radiation oncologists.

American Foundation for Urologic Disease
300 West Pratt Street, Suite 401
Baltimore, MD 21201-2463
800-828-7866
Provides educational opportunities for the public, patients and health care professionals about urologic diseases. Support groups: US-TOO, Bladder Health Council and Prostate Health Council.

(The) American Society of Clinical Hypnosis
2250 East Devon Avenue, Suite 336
Des Plaines, IL 60018
312-297-3317
National organization for clinical hypnotists.

American Society of Clinical Oncology
435 N. Michigan Avenue, Suite 1717
Philadelphia, PA 19107
312-644-0828
Exchange and diffusion of information and ideas relating to human neoplastic diseases.

American Society of Plastic and Reconstructive Surgeons
444 East Algonquin Road
Arlington Heights, IL 60005
1-800-635-0635
708-228-9900
Provides names of board-certified plastic surgeons in your area and free information regarding surgical procedures.

American Society for Therapeutic Radiology and Oncology
1101 Market Street, 14th Floor
Philadelphia, PA 19107
215-574-3180
Extends benefits of radiation therapy to patients with cancer or other disorders, advances scientific basis, provides education.

Association of Pediatric Oncology Nurses (APON)
11512 Allecingie Parkway
Richmond, VA 23235
804-379-9150
804-379-1386 (fax)
Promotes optimal nursing care for children and adolescents with cancer and for their families.

International Union Against Cancer
Union Internationale Contre le Cancer (UICC)
Rue de Conseil-General 3
1205 Geneva
Switzerland
(41-22) 20 18 11
Nongovernmental, voluntary organization devoted solely to promoting research, therapeutic and preventive aspects of cancer throughout the world. Worldwide association with member organizations in 78 countries. Facilities exchange information among national cancer organizations. With NCI support, publishes *International Directory of Specialized Cancer Research and Treatment Establishments.*

National Association of Oncology Social Workers
1275 York Avenue MRI 1107
New York, NY 10021
212-639-7015
National organization of professional social workers in oncology.

National Society of Genetic Counselors
233 Canterbury Drive
Wallingford, PA 19086-6617
Exchange of information on genetic diseases and training of counselors.

Office of Alternative Medicine
Building 31, Room B1C35
National Institutes of Health
Bethesda, MD 20892
Established in 1992 to find practical treatments that may be of use to physicians. Funds research in areas such as acupuncture, biofeedback, hypnosis, music therapy, massage therapy, yoga and prayer, as they relate to many different diseases including cancer.

Oncology Nursing Society
501 Holiday Drive
Pittsburgh, PA 15220-2749
412-921-7373
412-921-6565 (fax)
Professional organization dedicated to providing optimal care to persons with an actual and/or potential diagnosis of cancer. Publishes directory of major bone marrow transplant centers in country.

(The) Society for Clinical and Experimental Hypnosis
128A Kings Park Drive
Liverpool, NY 13090
National organization for clinical hypnotists.

Society of Gynecologic Oncologists
401 North Michigan Avenue
Chicago, IL 60611
312-644-6610
312-527-6640 (fax)
Professional organization dedicated to improving care of patients with gynecologic cancer, advancing knowledge and standards, encouraging research.

STATE PHYSICIAN LICENSING BOARDS

ALABAMA
Alabama State Board
of Medical
Examiners
P.O. Box 946
Montgomery, AL 36102
205-261-4116

ALASKA
Alaska State Medical Board
Division of Occupational
Licensing
3601 C Street Number 722
Anchorage, AK 99503
907-561-2878

ARIZONA

Arizona Board of Medical
Examiners
1651 E. Morten Avenue,
Suite 210
Phoenix, AZ 85020
602-255-3751

ARKANSAS

Arkansas State Medical Board
2100 Riverfront Drive,
Suite 200
Little Rock, AR 72202-1748
501-324-9410

CALIFORNIA

California Board of Medical
Quality Assurance
1426 Howe Avenue
Sacramento, CA 95825-3236
916-263-2499

COLORADO

Board of Medical Examiners
1560 Broadway, Suite 1300
Denver, CO 80202-5140
303-894-7690

CONNECTICUT

Connecticut Department of
Health Service
Medical Quality Assurance
150 Washington Street
Hartford, CT 06106
203-566-1035

DELAWARE

Board of Medical Practice
O'Neill Building
Box 1401
Dover, DE 19903
302-739-4522

DISTRICT OF COLUMBIA

Board of Medicine
605 G. Street NE
Washington, DC 20001
202-727-5365

FLORIDA

Board of Medicine
1940 N. Monroe Street
Tallahassee, FL 32399-0770
904-488-0595

GEORGIA

Composite State Board of
Medical Examiners
166 Proyor Street SW
Atlanta, GA 30303
404-656-3913

HAWAII

Board of Medical Examiners
P.O. Box 3469
Honolulu, HI 96801
808-586-2708

IDAHO

State Board of Medicine
280 N. 8th Street, Suite 202
Statehouse
Boise, ID 83720
208-334-2822

ILLINOIS

Illinois Board of Medical
Examiners
State of Illinois Center
100 West Randolph Street
#9-300
Chicago, IL 60601
312-917-4500

INDIANA
Indiana Health Professionals
  Bureau
402 West Washington Street
Room 041
Indianapolis, IN 46204
317-232-2960

IOWA
Board of Medical Examiners
Capitol Complex Executive
  Hills West
1209 E. Court Avenue
Des Moines, IA 50319
515-281-5171

KANSAS
State Board of Healing Arts
235 S.W. Topeka Boulevard
Topeka, KS 66603
913-296-7413

KENTUCKY
Kentucky Board of Licensure
310 Whittington Parkway,
  Suite 1B
Louisville, KY 40222
502-429-8046

LOUISIANA
Louisiana State Board of
  Medical Examiners
830 Union Street, Suite 100
New Orleans, LA 70112
504-524-6763

MAINE
Maine Board of Registration in
  Medicine
State House Station, 137
Augusta, ME 04333
207-287-3601

MARYLAND
Maryland Board of Physician
  Quality Assurance
4201 Patterson Avenue
P.O. Box 2571
Baltimore, MD 21215-0095
301-764-4777

MASSACHUSETTS
Massachusetts Board of
  Registration in Medicine
10 West Street, 3rd Floor
Boston, MA 02111
617-727-1788

MICHIGAN
Michigan Board of Medicine
611 W. Ottawa Street
P.O. Box 30192
Lansing, MI 48909
517-373-9102

MINNESOTA
Board of Medical Examiners
2700 University Avenue West,
  No. 106
St. Paul, MN 55114
612-642-0538

MISSISSIPPI
Mississippi State Board of
  Medical Licensure
2688-D Insurance Center Drive
Jackson, MS 39216
601-354-6645

MISSOURI
Missouri State Board of Reg.
  Healing Arts
P.O. Box 4
Jefferson City, MO 65102
314-751-0098

MONTANA

Montana State Board of
Medical Examiners
111 N. Jackson
P.O. Box 200513
Arcade Building, Lower Level
Helena, MT 59620
406-444-4284

NEBRASKA

Nebraska State Board of
Examiners in Medicine and
Surgery
P.O. Box 95007
Lincoln, NE 68509-5007
406-471-2115

NEVADA

Nevada State Board of Medical
Examiners
P.O. Box 7238
Reno, NV 89510
702-329-2559

NEW HAMPSHIRE

Board of Registration in
Medicine
2 Industrial Park
Concord, NH 03301
603-271-1203

NEW JERSEY

New Jersey Board of Medical
Examiners
28 W. State Street, Room 602
Trenton, NJ 08608
609-292-4843

NEW MEXICO

New Mexico State Board of
Medical Examiners
P.O. Box 20001
Santa Fe, NM 87504
505-827-7317

NEW YORK

State Board for Medicine
Cultural Education Center,
Room 3023
Empire State Plaza
Albany, NY 12230
800-342-3729

NORTH CAROLINA

North Carolina Board of
Medical Examiners
P.O. Box 26808
Raleigh, NC 27611
919-828-1212

NORTH DAKOTA

North Dakota State Board of
Medical Examiners
418 E. Broadway Avenue,
Suite 12
Bismarck, ND 58501
701-223-9485

OHIO

Ohio State Medical Board
77 S. High Street, 17th Floor
Columbus, OH 43266-0315
614-466-3934

OKLAHOMA

Oklahoma State Board of
Licensure
P.O. Box 18256
Oklahoma City, OK 73154
405-848-6841

OREGON
Board of Medical Examiners
Crown Plaza
1500 SW 1st Avenue, Suite 620
Portland, OR 97201
503-229-5770

PENNSYLVANIA
Pennsylvania State Board of
Medicine
P.O. Box 2649
Harrisburg, PA 17105-2649
717-787-2381

RHODE ISLAND
Board of Medical Licensure
and Discipline
Cannon Building, Room 205
Three Capitol Hill
Providence, RI 02908
401-277-3855

SOUTH CAROLINA
South Carolina Board of
Medical Examiners
101 Executive Center Drive,
Suite 120
Saluda Building
Columbia, SC 29210
803-734-8901

SOUTH DAKOTA
South Dakota Department of
Medical Examiners
1323 S. Minnesota Avenue
Sioux Falls, SD 57105
605-334-8343

TENNESSEE
Tennessee State Board of
Medical Examiners
283 Plus Park Boulevard
Nashville, TN 37219-1010
615-367-6231

TEXAS
Texas State Board of Medical
Examiners
P.O. Box 149134, Capitol
Station
Austin TX 78714-9134
512-834-7728

UTAH
Utah Physicians Licensing
Board
P.O. Box 45802
Salt Lake City, UT 84145-0805
801-530-6740

VERMONT
Vermont Board of Medical
Practice
Secretary of State's Office
109 State Street
Montpelier, VT 05609-1106
802-828-2673

VIRGINIA
Virginia State Board of
Medicine
1601 Rolling Hills Drive
Richmond, VA 23230
804-662-9908

WASHINGTON
Washington State Department
of Health
Board of Medical Examiners
1300 S.E. Quince
Olympia, WA 98504-7866
206-586-3335

WEST VIRGINIA
West Virginia Board of
Medicine
101 Dee Drive
Charleston, WV 25311
304-558-2921

WISCONSIN
Wisconsin Board of Medical
  Examiners
P.O. Box 8935
Madison, WI 53708
608-266-2811

WYOMING
Wyoming Board of Medical
  Examiners
4848 N. Lincoln Boulevard,
  Suite 100
Cheyenne, WY 82002
307-777-6463

4. NATIONAL CANCER INSTITUTE PROGRAMS

NATIONAL CANCER INSTITUTE

Samuel Broder, M.D., Director
National Cancer Institute
National Institutes of Health
Bethesda, MD 20892
301-496-4000

The National Cancer Institute (NCI) is the federal government's principal agency for research on cancer prevention, diagnosis, treatment, and rehabilitation, and for dissemination of information for the control of cancer. It is one of eleven research institutes and four divisions that form the National Institutes of Health (NIH), located in Bethesda, Maryland. As an agency of the Department of Health and Human Services, the NCI receives annual appropriations from Congress. These funds support cancer research in the institute's Bethesda headquarters and in about 1,000 laboratories and medical centers throughout the United States.

The NCI also conducts research and treats a limited number of patients in specific research studies at the NIH Clinical Center located in Bethesda, Maryland.

NCI is responsible for the National Institute Cancer Centers Program, which is made up of 55 NCI-designated Cancer Centers actively engaged in multidisciplinary research efforts to reduce cancer incidence, morbidity, and mortality. Within this program there are four tiers of cancer centers:

- 27 Comprehensive Cancer Centers which emphasize a multidisciplinary approach to cancer research, patient care and community outreach.
- 13 Clinical Cancer Centers which focus on clinical research.
- 1 Consortium Cancer Center which specializes in cancer prevention and control research.
- 14 Basic Science Cancer Centers which engage primarily in basic cancer research.

Many people choose to go to one of these major centers either for treatment or for a second opinion. See Chapter 2, "Choosing Your Doctor and Hospital."

COMPREHENSIVE CANCER CENTERS

The 27 comprehensive cancer centers are designated as "centers of excellence," having met specific NCI criteria established for "comprehensiveness." It is the top designation given by the National Cancer Institute after vigorous review. The centers conduct research to provide the latest scientific information in the prevention and treatment of cancer. Comprehensive cancer centers have teams of experts working together on research, teaching, and treating cancer patients. They are carrying out the newest investigational treatments for cancer, using clinical trials as described in Chapter 9, "New Advances and Investigational Trials."

ALABAMA
University of Alabama at
  Birmingham
Comprehensive Cancer Center
Basic Health Sciences Building
1918 University Boulevard
Birmingham, AL 35294
205-934-5077

ARIZONA
University of Arizona Cancer
  Center
1501 North Campbell Avenue
Tucson, AZ 85724
602-626-6372

CALIFORNIA
USC/Norris Comprehensive
  Cancer Center
University of Southern
  California
1441 Eastlake Avenue
Los Angeles, CA 90033-0804
213-226-2370

Jonsson Comprehensive
  Cancer Center
University of California at Los
  Angeles
100 UCLA Medical Plaza
Suite 255
Los Angeles, CA 90024-1781
1-800-825-2631

CONNECTICUT
Yale Cancer Center
Yale University School of
  Medicine
P.O. Box 208028
333 Cedar Street
New Haven, CT 06510-8028
203-785-4095

DISTRICT OF COLUMBIA
Lombardi Cancer Research
  Center
Georgetown University
  Medical Center
3800 Reservoir Road NW
Washington, D.C. 20007
202-687-2192

FLORIDA

Sylvester Comprehensive
  Cancer Center
University of Miami Medical
  School
1475 Northwest 12th Avenue
Miami, FL 33136
305-545-1000

MARYLAND

The Johns Hopkins Oncology
  Center
600 North Wolfe Street
Room B156
Baltimore, MD 21287-8915
410-955-8964

MASSACHUSETTS

Dana-Farber Cancer Institute
44 Binney Street
Boston, MA 02115
617-632-3476

MICHIGAN

Meyer L. Prentis
  Comprehensive Cancer
  Center of Metropolitan
  Detroit
110 East Warren Avenue
Detroit, MI 48201
313-745-4329

University of Michigan
Comprehensive Cancer Center
101 Simpson Drive
Ann Arbor, MI 48109-0752
313-936-9583

MINNESOTA

Mayo Comprehensive Cancer
  Center
200 First Street Southwest
Rochester, MN 55902
507-284-3413

NEW HAMPSHIRE

Norris Cotton Cancer Center
Dartmouth-Hitchcock Medical
  Center
2 Mynard Street
Hanover, NH 03756
603-646-5505

NEW YORK

Kaplan Cancer Center
New York University Medical
  Center
462 First Avenue
New York, NY 10016-9103
212-263-6485

Memorial Sloan-Kettering
  Cancer Center
1275 York Avenue
New York, NY 10021
1-800-525-2225

Roswell Park Cancer Institute
Elm and Carlton Streets
Buffalo, NY 14263
1-800-767-9355

NORTH CAROLINA

Duke Comprehensive Cancer
  Center
P.O. Box 3814
Durham, NC 27710
919-684-2748

UNC Lineberger
  Comprehensive Cancer
  Center
University of North Carolina
  School of Medicine
Chapel Hill, NC 27599
919-966-4431

Cancer Center of Wake Forest
University at Bowman Gray
School of Medicine
300 South Hawthorne Road
Winston-Salem, NC 27103
919-748-4354

OHIO

Ohio State University
Comprehensive Cancer
Center
Arthur G. James Cancer
Hospital
410 West 10th Avenue
Columbus, OH 43210
1-800-638-6996

PENNSYLVANIA

Fox Chase Cancer Center
7701 Burholme Avenue
Philadelphia, PA 19111
215-728-2570

University of Pennsylvania
Cancer Center
3400 Spruce Street
Philadelphia, PA 19104
215-662-6364

Pittsburgh Cancer Institute
200 Meyran Avenue
Pittsburgh, PA 15213-2592
1-800-537-4063

TEXAS

The University of Texas
M.D. Anderson Cancer Center
1515 Holcombe Boulevard
Houston, TX 77030
713-792-3245

VERMONT

Vermont Regional Cancer
Center
University of Vermont
1 South Prospect Street
Burlington, VT 05401
802-656-4580

WASHINGTON

Fred Hutchinson Cancer
Research Center
1124 Columbia Street
Seattle, WA 98104
206-667-5000
(Primary treatment offered is
bone marrow
transplantation)

WISCONSIN

University of Wisconsin
Comprehensive Cancer
Center
600 Highland Avenue
Madison, WI 53792
608-263-8090

CLINICAL CANCER CENTERS

There are thirteen National Cancer Institute–designated clinical
cancer centers which conduct both basic and clinical research. Clinical cancer centers have also been given thorough review by the
National Cancer Institute. Although they have not met all the criteria to qualify as comprehensive centers, they qualify to provide
state-of-the-art treatment for cancer patients, including investigational treatments.

CALIFORNIA

City of Hope National Medical
Center
Beckman Research Institute
1500 East Duarte Road
Duarte, CA 91010
818-359-8111

University of California at San
Diego Cancer Center
225 Dickinson Street
San Diego, CA 92103
619-543-6178

COLORADO

University of Colorado Cancer
Center
4200 East 9th Avenue
Box B188
Denver, CO 80262
303-270-3007

ILLINOIS

Robert H. Lurie Cancer
Center
Northwestern University
303 East Chicago Avenue
Olson Pavilion, Room 8250
Chicago, IL 60611
312-908-8400

University of Chicago Cancer
Research Center
5841 South Maryland Avenue
Chicago, IL 60637
312-702-9200

NEW YORK

Albert Einstein College of
Medicine
Cancer Research Center
Chanin Building

1300 Morris Park Avenue
Bronx, NY 10461
718-920-4826

Columbia University Cancer
Center
College of Physicians and
Surgeons
630 West 168th Street
New York, NY 10032
212-305-6905

University of Rochester Cancer
Center
601 Elmwood Avenue
Box 704
Rochester, NY 14642
716-275-4911

OHIO

Ireland Cancer Center
at Case Western Reserve
University
University Hospitals of
Cleveland
2074 Abington Road
Cleveland, OH 44106
216-844-5432

TENNESSEE

St. Jude Children's Research
Hospital
332 North Lauderdale Street
Memphis, TN 38101-0318
901-522-0306

TEXAS

San Antonio Cancer Institute
4450 Medical Drive
San Antonio, TX 78229
210-616-5798

UTAH
Utah Cancer Center
University of Utah Medical
Center
50 North Medical Drive
Room 2C110
Salt Lake City, UT 84132
801-581-4048

VIRGINIA
Massey Cancer Center
Medical College of Virginia
1200 East Broad Street
Richmond, VA 23298
804-371-5116

CONSORTIUM CANCER CENTER

The consortium cancer center works with state and local public health departments to provide effective prevention and control techniques learned from its research findings to those institutions responsible for implementing population-wide public health programs. The center is heavily engaged in collaborations with institutions that conduct clinical trials to investigate new treatments and to coordinate community hospitals into a network of cooperating institutions in these research efforts.

TENNESSEE
Drew-Meharry-Morehouse Consortium Cancer Center
1005 D. B. Todd Boulevard
Nashville, TN 37208
615-327-6927

BASIC SCIENCE CANCER CENTERS

Basic science cancer centers engage almost entirely in basic research. However, some centers collaborate with outside clinical research investigators and with industry to generate medical applications from new discoveries in the laboratory. These centers are located as follows:

CALIFORNIA
Armand Hammer Center for
Cancer Biology
Salk Institute
San Diego, CA

La Jolla Cancer Research
Foundation
La Jolla, CA

INDIANA
Purdue Cancer Center
Purdue University
West Lafayette, IN

MAINE
The Jackson Laboratory
Bar Harbor, ME

MASSACHUSETTS

Center for Cancer Research
Massachusetts Institute of
  Technology
Cambridge, MA

NEBRASKA

Eppley Institute
University of Nebraska Medical
  Center
Omaha, NB

NEW YORK

American Health Foundation
New York, NY

Cold Spring Harbor
  Laboratory
Cold Spring Harbor, NY

PENNSYLVANIA

Fels Research Institute
Temple University School of
  Medicine
Philadelphia, PA

Wistar Institute
Philadelphia, PA

VIRGINIA

Cancer Center
University of Virginia Health
  Sciences Center
Charlottesville, VA

WISCONSIN

McArdle Laboratory for
  Cancer Research
University of Wisconsin
Madison, WI

CLINICAL TRIALS COOPERATIVE GROUPS

The Clinical Trials Cooperative Group Program is sponsored by the
National Cancer Institute. It is designed to promote and support
clinical trials of new cancer treatments, to explore methods of cancer prevention and early detection, and to study quality-of-life issues
and rehabilitation during and after treatment. There are 14 major
cooperative groups. The program involves more than 2,200 institutions that contribute patients to group-conducted trials. More than
16,000 individual investigators also participate in NCI-supported
cooperative group studies.

   The list contains the various clinical cooperative groups and institutional projects funded by NCI, with the names and institutions
of the chairmen of the groups. (Groups are *not* confined to the
area indicated by the address.) Information on the kinds of cancers
being studied by these groups is available through PDQ (Physician
Data Query). If you want to know whether a doctor or an institution
in your area is participating in clinical trials being run by any of
the groups, call the Cancer Information Service.

   There are groups, both in Canada and Europe, which are studying various treatments, some in collaboration with U.S. scientists,
researchers, and doctors. Information about them is available by
calling the 1-800-4-CANCER.

Brain Tumor Cooperative Group
William R. Shapiro, M.D., Chair
Barrow Neurological Institute
St. Joseph Hospital and Medical Center
350 West Thomas Road
Phoenix, AZ 85013

Cancer and Leukemia Group B
O. Ross McIntyre, M.D., Chair
Central Office of the Chair
444 Mount Support Road, Suite 2
Rural Route 3, Box 750
Lebanon, NH 03766

Children's Cancer Group
W. Archie Bleyer, M.D., Chair
Department of Pediatrics, Box 87
University of Texas M.D. Anderson Cancer Center
1515 Holcombe Boulevard
Houston, TX 77030

Eastern Cooperative Oncology Group
Douglass Tormey, M.D., Chair
AMC Research Center
1600 Pierce Street
Denver, CO 80214

European Organization for Research on Treatment for Cancer
Francoise Meunier, M.D., Director
EORTC Central Office—Data Center
Avenue E. Mounier 83, BTE 11
1200 Brussels
Belgium

Gynecologic Oncology Group
Robert C. Park, M.D., Chair
GOG Central Office
Suite 1945
1234 Market Street
Philadelphia, PA 19107

Intergroup Rhabdomyosarcoma Study
Harold M. Maurer, M.D., Chair
Dean's Office
University of Nebraska College of Medicine
600 South 42nd Street
Omaha, NE 68198-6545

National Surgical Adjuvant Breast and Bowel Project
Ronald Heberman, M.D., InterimChair
University of Pittsburgh
914 Scaife Hall
3550 Terrace Street
Pittsburgh, PA 15261

National Wilms' Tumor Study Group
Daniel M. Green, M.D., Chair
Roswell Park Cancer Institute
Elm and Carlton Streets
Buffalo, NY 14263

North Central Cancer Treatment Group
Michael J. O'Connell, M.D., Chair
Mayo Foundation
200 First Street, SW
Rochester, MN 55905

Pediatric Oncology Group
Sharon B. Murphy, M.D., Chair
Suite 910
645 North Michigan Avenue
Chicago, IL 60611

Quality Assurance Review Center

Arvin S. Glicksman, M.D., Chair
Quality Assurance Review Center
Roger Williams General Hospital
825 Chalkstone Avenue
Providence, RI 02908

Radiation Therapy Oncology Group

James Cox, M.D., Chair
University of Texas M.D. Anderson Cancer Center
1515 Holcombe Boulevard
Houston, TX 77030

Southwest Oncology Group

Charles A. Coltman, M.D., Chair
14980 Omicron Drive
San Antonio, TX 78245-3217

COMMUNITY CLINICAL ONCOLOGY PROGRAMS

The Community Clinical Oncology Program (CCOP) was established by the NCI in 1983. Through this program, community physicians work with scientists conducting NCI-supported clinical trials. Clinical trials are research studies conducted with patients or with healthy people. (See Chapter 9, "New Advances and Investigational Trials.") The program helps in the transfer of the latest research findings to the community level. Many CCOPs affiliate with hospitals and physician offices that cross state lines; addresses are for administrative offices. For further information call 1-800-4-CANCER.

ALABAMA

University of South Alabama Minority-Based CCOP
USA Cancer Center Room 414
307 University Boulevard
Mobile, AL 36688
205-460-7194

ALASKA

Virginia Mason Medical Center CCOP
1100 9th Avenue
Seattle, WA 98111
206-223-6193

ARIZONA

Greater Phoenix CCOP
925 East McDowell Road, 2nd Floor
Phoenix, AZ 85006-2726
602-239-2413

Scottsdale CCOP
Mayo Clinic Scottsdale
13400 East Shea Boulevard
Scottsdale, AZ 85259
602-301-8294

CALIFORNIA

Bay Area Tumor Institute
CCOP
2844 Summit Street, Suite 204
Oakland, CA 94609-3637
510-465-8570

Central Los Angeles CCOP
St. Vincent Medical Center
Post Office Box 57992
2131 West Third Street
Los Angeles, CA 90057
213-484-7086

San Diego Kaiser Permanente
CCOP
Department of Oncology
4647 Zion Avenue
San Diego, CA 92120
619-528-5888

DELAWARE

Medical Center of Delaware
CCOP
P.O. Box 1668
Wilmington, DE 19899
302-731-8116

FLORIDA

Florida Pediatric CCOP
Florida Association of Pediatric
Tumor Programs, Inc.
P.O. Box 17757
Tampa, FL 33682-7757
813-632-1310

Mount Sinai Community
Clinical Oncology Program
Mount Sinai Medical Center
4300 Alton Road
Miami Beach, FL 33140
305-674-2625

GEORGIA

Atlanta Regional CCOP
St. Joseph's Hospital
5665 Peachtree Dunwoody
Road NE
Atlanta, GA 30342-1701
404-851-7114

Grady Hospital Minority-Based
CCOP
P.O. Box 26149
Atlanta, GA 30335-3801
404-616-5975

Southeast Cancer Control
Consortium CCOP
Suite 220
2150 Country Club Road
Winston-Salem, NC 27104-4241
919-777-3036

ILLINOIS

Carle Cancer Center CCOP
Carle Clinic Association
602 West University Avenue
Urbana, IL 61801
217-383-3010

Central Illinois CCOP
Memorial Medical Center
800 North Rutledge Street
Springfield, IL 62781-0001
217-788-4178

Illinois Oncology Research
Association CCOP
Suite 780
900 Main Street
Peoria, IL 61602
309-672-5783

Kellogg Cancer Care Center
  CCOP
Evanston Hospital
2650 Ridge Avenue
Evanston, IL 60201
708-570-2109

University of Illinois Minority-
  Based CCOP
Section of Medical Oncology
Room 720N CSB
840 South Wood Street
Chicago, IL 60612
312-996-5958

IOWA

Cedar Rapids Oncology
  Project CCOP
525 10th St. SE
Cedar Rapids, IA 52403
319-363-8303

Iowa Oncology Research
  Association
Suite 19
1223 Center Street
Des Moines, IA 50309-1014
515-244-7586

KANSAS

Wichita CCOP
P.O. Box 1358
929 North Saint Francis Street
Wichita, KS 67201
316-262-5784

LOUISIANA

Ochsner CCOP
Ochsner Cancer Institute
1514 Jefferson Highway
New Orleans, LA 70121
504-838-3708

MICHIGAN

Grand Rapids Clinical
  Oncology Program CCOP
Butterworth Hospital
100 Michigan Street NE
Grand Rapids, MI 49503
616-774-1230

Kalamazoo Community
  Clinical Oncology Programs
1521 Gull Road
Kalamazoo, MI 49001
616-383-7007

Minority-Based Community
  Clinical Oncology Program
  of Metropolitan Detroit
27211 Lahser Road, Suite 200
Southfield, MI 48034-9998
313-356-2828

MINNESOTA

Duluth CCOP
400 East Third Street
Duluth, MN 55805
218-722-8364, ext. 3308

Metro-Minneapolis CCOP
5000 West 39th Street
Minneapolis, MN 55416-2699
612-928-1517

Scottsdale CCOP
Mayo Foundation
200 First Street SW
Rochester, MN 55905
507-284-2511

MISSOURI

Kansas City CCOP
Baptist Medical Center
6601 Rockhill Road
Kansas City, MO 64131
816-276-7834

Ozarks Regional CCOP
1235 East Cherokee Street
Springfield, MO 65804-2263
417-883-2610

St. Louis–Cape Girardeau
  CCOP
Mercy Doctors Building
Suite 3018, Tower B
621 South New Ballas Road
St. Louis, MO 63141
314-569-6959

NEVADA
Southern Nevada Cancer
  Research Foundation CCOP
501 South Rancho Drive, Suite
  C-14
Las Vegas, NV 89106
702-384-0013

NEW JERSEY
Bergen-Passaic CCOP
Northern New Jersey Cancer
  Center
5 Summit Street
Hackensack, NJ 07601
201-996-5900

Saint Michael's Medical Center
  Tri-County CCOP
Saint Michael's Medical Center
268 Dr. Martin Luther King
  Boulevard
Newark, NJ 07102
201-877-5000

South Jersey Oncology Group
  CCOP
3 Cooper Plaza, Suite 220
Camden, NJ 08103
609-963-3572

NEW YORK
Brooklyn CCOP
Cancer Institute of Brooklyn
927 49th Street
Brooklyn, NY 11219
718-972-5816

Kings County Minority-Based
  CCOP
SUNY Health Science Center,
  Brooklyn
450 Clarkson Avenue, Box 55
Brooklyn, NY 11203
718-780-1419

North Shore University
  Hospital CCOP
North Shore University
  Hospital-Cornell Medical
300 Community Drive
Manhasset, NY 11030
516-562-8910

Syracuse Hematology-
  Oncology CCOP
100 East Genessee Street
Syracuse, NY 13210
315-472-7504

NORTH CAROLINA
Southeast Cancer Control
  Consortium CCOP
2150 Country Club Road
Winston-Salem, NC 27104-4241
919-777-3036

NORTH DAKOTA
Merit-Care Hospital CCOP
820 4th Street North
Fargo, ND 58122
701-234-2397

OHIO

Allegheny CCOP
Allegheny General Hospital
320 East North Avenue
Pittsburgh, PA 15212-9986
412-359-6191

Columbus CCOP
1151 South High Street
Columbus, OH 43206
614-443-2267

Dayton Clinical Oncology
  Program
Cox Heart Institute
3525 Southern Boulevard
Kettering, OH 45429
513-296-7278

Toledo Community Clinical
  Oncology Program
3314 Collingwood Boulevard
Toledo, OH 43610
419-255-5433

OKLAHOMA

St. Francis Hospital/Natalie
  Warren Bryant CCOP
6161 South Yale Avenue
Tulsa, OK 74136
918-494-5139

OREGON

Columbia River CCOP
4805 Northeast Glisan Road
Portland, OR 97213
503-230-6008

Northwest CCOP
Tacoma General Hospital
314 Martin Luther King Lane,
  Suite 204
Tacoma, WA 98405-0986
206-552-1461

PENNSYLVANIA

Allegheny CCOP
Allegheny General Hospital
320 East North Avenue
Pittsburgh, PA 15212-9986
412-359-6191

Geisinger Clinical Oncology
  Program
Department of Hematology/
  Oncology
Geisinger Medical Center
North Academy Avenue
Danville, PA 17822-2001
717-271-6544

Mercy Hospital CCOP
General Services Building,
  Suite 205
743 Jefferson Avenue
Scranton, PA 18501
717-342-3675

PUERTO RICO

Florida Pediatric CCOP
Florida Association of Pediatric
  Tumor Programs, Inc.
P.O. Box 17757
Gainesville, FL 33682-7757
818-632-1310

San Juan City Minority-Based
  CCOP
G.P.O. Box 70344
Centro Medico Mail Station 54
San Juan, PR 00936-7344
809-758-7348

SOUTH CAROLINA
Southeast Cancer Control
  Consortium CCOP
2150 Country Club Road,
  Suite 200
Winston-Salem, NC 27104-4241
919-777-3036

Spartanburg CCOP
Spartanburg Regional Medical
  Center
101 East Wood Street
Spartanburg, SC 29303
803-560-6812

SOUTH DAKOTA
Sioux Community Cancer
  Consortium CCOP
Central Plains Clinic, Ltd.,
  Suite 2000
1000 East 21st Street
Sioux Falls, SD 57105
605-331-3160

TENNESSEE
Southeast Cancer Control
  Consortium CCOP
2150 Country Club Road, Suite
  200
Winston-Salem, NC 27104-4241
919-777-3036

TEXAS
San Antonio Minority-Based
  CCOP
Santa Rosa Hospital
519 West Houston Street
San Antonio, TX 78215
210-224-6531

South Texas Pediatric
  Minority-Based CCOP
Department of Pediatrics
Division of Hematology/
  Oncology
University of Texas Health
  Science Center
7703 Floyd Curl Drive
San Antonio, TX 78284-7810
210-567-5265

VERMONT
Green Mountain Oncology
  Group
Rutland Regional Medical
  Center
160 Allen Street
Rutland, VT 05701
802-747-1655

VIRGINIA
Fairfax CCOP
Fairfax Hospital, Suite 206
3301 Woodburn Road
Annandale, VA 22003
703-560-7210

Medical College of Virginia
  Minority-Based CCOP
Box 37, MCV Station
Richmond, VA 23298-0037
804-786-0450

Southeast Cancer Control
Consortium CCOP
2150 Country Club Road, Suite
200
Winston-Salem, NC 27104-4214
919-777-3036

WASHINGTON
Columbia River CCOP
4805 Northeast Glisan Road
Room 5F 40
Portland, OR 97213
503-230-6008

Northwest CCOP
Tacoma General Hospital
314 Martin Luther King Lane
Suite 204
Tacoma, WA 98405-0986
206-552-1461

Virginia Mason Medical Center
CCOP
1100 9th Avenue, P.O. Box
900
Seattle, WA 98111
206-223-6194

WISCONSIN
Marshfield Medical Research
Foundation CCOP
Marshfield Clinic
1000 North Oak Avenue
Marshfield, WI 54449
715-387-5134

NIH CLINICAL CENTER

Warren Grant Magnuson Clinical Center

The National Institutes of Health has a medical research center and hospital—the Warren Grant Magnuson Clinical Center located in Bethesda, Maryland, just outside of Washington, D.C. The hospital portion of the Clinical Center, with room for 540 patients, is especially designed for medical research. The number of beds available for a particular project and the length of the waiting list of qualified patients are important in determining whether and when you can be admitted. Research on a particular disease may allow only one or two patients to be studied at any given time. The Clinical Center provides nursing and medical care without charge for patients who are being studied in a clinical research program.

You can be treated at the Clinical Center only if your case fits into a research project. Each project is designed to answer scientific questions and has specific medical eligibility requirements. For this reason you must be referred by your own doctors, who can supply the Clinical Center with the needed medical information, such as your diagnosis and details of your medical history. If your doctor feels that you might benefit by participating in a cancer research study at NIH, the doctor should call the National Cancer Institute's Public Inquiries Office at 301-496-5583 or write to the Clinical Director, National Cancer Institute, Building 10, Room 12N214, Bethesda, MD 20892.

The Pediatric Branch of the Clinical Center is the only branch that accepts patients without a physician referral. The kinds of cancers treated and the protocols change periodically. Current clinical treatment protocols include brain tumors, leukemia, lymphomas, sarcomas, neuroblastomas, supportive care and HIV disease. You can call at 301-402-0696 or write Pediatric Branch/Clinical Center, Building 10, Room 13N240, Bethesda, MD 20892. (Also see Chapter 22, "Childhood Cancers.") Children and their families may be eligible to stay at the Children's Inn (1-800-644-4660).

5. PAIN CONTROL

Pain is a common problem among cancer patients and they and their families should be aware that cancer pain can be relieved, that they have the right to demand adequate pain relief, and that they need not fear addiction and the side effects of potent analgesics. (See Chapter 24, "Living with Cancer.")

The National Institutes of Health (NIH) has established a multidisciplinary pain clinic at the Clinical Center in Bethesda, Maryland, to improve the understanding of pain mechanisms and to develop better ways of assessing and treating pain. Scientists and research physicians in the pain clinic are available to the medical community for consultation regarding special difficulties in pain management.

PAIN ASSOCIATIONS

Agency for Health Care Policy and Research
Publications and Informations Branch
Parklawn Building, Room 18-12
Rockville, MD 20852
1-800-358-9295
Develops guidelines for caring for patients, including pain.

American Academy of Pain Medicine
5700 Old Orchard Road, 1st Floor
Skokie, IL 60077-1057
708-966-9510

Official organization representing physicians in pain field in U.S. Publishes membership directory listing primary care and specialty physicians with interest in pain medicine.

American Pain Society
5700 Old Orchard Road, 1st Floor
Skokie, IL 60077-1057
708-966-5595
708-966-9418 (fax)
Not-for-profit educational and scientific organization whose mission is to serve people in pain by advancing research, education, treatment and professional practice.

Commission on Accreditation of Rehabilitation Facilities
101 N. Wilmot Road, Suite 500
Tucson, AZ 85711
602-748-1212
List of facilities with accredited pain programs.

Committee on Pain Therapy and Acupuncture
American Society of Anesthesiologists
515 Busse Highway
Park Ridge, IL 60068
Publishes a directory of pain clinics.

International Association for the Study of Pain
909 NE 43rd Street, Suite 306
Seattle, WA 98105
206-547-6409
206-547-1703 (fax)
Fosters and encourages research of pain mechanisms and pain syndromes. Helps to improve the management of patients with acute and chronic pain by bringing together health professionals who have interest in pain research and management. Publications and information are available.

National Chronic Pain Outreach Association
7979 Old Georgetown Road
Suite 100
Bethesda, MD 20814-2429
301-652-4948

Society of Clinical Hypnosis
2250 East Devon Avenue, Suite 336
Des Plaines, IL 60018
312-297-3317
Provides lists of trained personnel who use hypnotism to control pain.

Biofeedback Research Society
University of Colorado
Medical Center
Denver, CO 80262
303-270-7960
Society is researching the use of biofeedback to control cancer pain.

STATE PAIN CONTACTS

Wisconsin Cancer Pain Initiative
Room 3675
University of Wisconsin Medical School
1300 University Avenue
Madison, WI 53706
608-262-0978
Clearinghouse of resource materials. Works to improve management of cancer pain. Educational material available.

Thirty-two states now have pain initiative programs, patterned after the Wisconsin Pain Initiative, which began in 1986. Their goal is to make cancer pain relief a high priority. You can contact them directly for information and help.

ALABAMA
John J. Marsella, M.D.
1504 Tacoma Street
Dothan, AL 36303
205-793-8105

ARIZONA
Eugenie A. Obbens, M.D.
222 West Thomas Road, Suite 415
Phoenix, AZ 85013
602-650-6306
602-650-7161 (fax)

Cheryl Lewis
1225 W. Atlantic Drive
Gilbert, AZ 85234
602-835-0711
602-835-9716 (fax)

ARKANSAS
Jonathan Wolfe, R.Ph.
University of Arkansas for Medical Sciences
4301 W. Markham, Slot 543
Little Rock, AZ 72205-7122
501-686-5140
501-664-4381 (private office)

CALIFORNIA

Pamela J. Haylock, R.N.
220 Ware Road
Woodside, CA 94062
415-851-5620 (phone/fax)

Betty R. Farrell, Ph.D.
Department of Nursing
  Research
City of Hope Medical Center
1500 East Duarte Road
Duarte, CA 91010-0289
818-359-8111
818-301-8941 (fax)

COLORADO

Janelle M. Betley, R.N.
Hospice of Metro Denver
3955 E. Exposition Avenue,
  Suite 500
Denver, CO 80209
303-778-1010

CONNECTICUT

Didi Loseth, R.N., M.S.N.
705 Sport Hill Road
Easton, CT 06612
203-261-6630 (home)
212-639-8708 (Memorial Sloan-
  Kettering)
212-717-3081 (fax)

Rich Gannon, R.P.N.
41 Sunset Avenue
Meriden, CT 06450
203-237-7849 (home)
203-524-2003
203-524-7066(fax)

DELAWARE

Gretchen W. Jones, R.N.
P.O. Box 581
Hockessin, DE 19707
302-658-7468

FLORIDA

Lisa O. Sienon, R.N., O.C.N.
Lee Moffitt Cancer Center
Pain Service
12902 Magnolia Drive
Tampa, FL 33612
813-972-8456
813-972-8495 (fax)

GEORGIA

Anne Marie McKenzie, M.D.
1719 Pine Ridge Drive NE
Atlanta, GA 30324
404-686-2320
404-686-4889 (fax)

HAWAII

Hob Osterlund, R.N., M.S.
The Queen's Medical Center
1301 Punchbowl Street
Honolulu, HI 96813
808-547-4726
808-547-4032 (fax)

Patricia M. Kahua R.N.
St. Francis Hospice
24 Puiwa Road
Honolulu, HI 96817
808-595-7566
808-595-6996 (fax)

ILLINOIS

Carol J. Swenson, R.N., M.S.,
  O.C.N.
Swedish American Hospital
1400 Charles Street
Rockford, IL 61104
815-968-4400 (pager 128)
815-968-3713 (fax)

Mary Cooper, R.N.
St. James Hospice
441 Hay Street, Suite 203
Decatur, IL 62526
217-875-3913
217-428-1243 (fax)

Rita Haines
1058 11th Street
Charleston, IL 61920
217-348-1841/345-3231

Linda Mohaupt
Rockford Memorial Hospital
2400 N. Rockton Avenue
Rockton, IL 61103
815-968-6861
815-961-6716 (fax)

Martha Twaddle, M.D.
Hospice of the North Shore
2821 Central Street
Evanston, IL 60201
708-866-4601
708-866-6023 (fax)

INDIANA
Neil Irick, M.D.
Pain Resource Center
2020 West 86th Street, Suite 310
Indianapolis, IN 46260
317-872-2332
317-872-2889 (fax)

Julie Painter, R.N., O.C.N.
Oncology Clinical Nurse Specialist
Regional Cancer Center
1500 North Ritter Avenue
Indianapolis, IN 46219
317-355-4848
317-351-7739 (fax)

IOWA
Peggy Christ, R.N.
Jennie Edmundson Hospital
933 E. Pierce Street
Council Bluffs, IA 51502
712-328-6000

Eric Goldsmith, D.O.
1440 Grand
Des Moines, IA 50314
515-265-1457

Wendy Gronbeck, R.N.
1017 Bowery Street
Iowa City, IA 52240
319-354-4971 (home)
319-353-8189
319-356-4545 (fax)

Iowa Cancer Pain Relief Initiative
Box 21
Iowa City, IA 52244

KENTUCKY
Lin Edwards, R.N.
Director of Program Development
Hospice of Louisville
3532 Ephraim McDowell Drive
Louisville, KY 40205-3224
502-456-6200
502-456-6655 (fax)

MAINE
Kandyce Powell, R.N.
Executive Director
Maine Hospice Council
295 Water Street, Suite 201
Augusta, ME 04330
207-626-0651

MARYLAND

Rebecca Finley, Pharm.D.
University of Maryland Cancer
  Center
22 South Greene Street
Baltimore, MD 21201
410-328-7683
410-328-6896 (fax)

Beth Gregory, Pharm.D.
Johns Hopkins Oncology
  Center, Carnegie 180
600 N. Wolfe Street
Baltimore, MD 21205
410-955-6591
410-955-0125 (fax)

Julie A. Steele
National Cancer Institute
Office of Cancer
  Communications
9000 Rockville Pike
Building 31, Room 4B43
Bethesda, MD 20892
301-496-6792
301-402-0894 (fax)

MASSACHUSETTS

Margaret Barton Burke, R.N.
c/o American Cancer Society,
  Massachusetts Division
247 Commonwealth Avenue
Boston, MA 02116
617-267-2650
617-469-9549 (home)
617-536-3163 (fax)

MICHIGAN

Josefina Magno, M.D.
International Hospice Institute
Henry Ford Hospital
2799 West Grand Boulevard
Detroit, MI 48202
313-876-9234
313-874-4044 (fax)

Stuart Weiner, D.O.
Academy of Hospice Physicians
G-3371 Beecher Road
Flint, MI 48532
313-733-7270
313-733-0250 (fax)

MINNESOTA

Thomas E. Elliott, M.D.
The Duluth Clinic, Ltd.
400 East Third Street
Duluth, MN 55805
218-722-8364
218-725-3030 (fax)

Paula Sallmen, R.N.
Virginia L. Piper Cancer
  Institute
Abbott Northwestern Hospital
800 E. 28th Street at Chicago
Minneapolis, MN 55407-3799
612-863-4633
612-863-4689 (fax)

MISSISSIPPI

Karen Koch, Pharm.D.
N. Mississippi Medical Center
830 S. Gloster Street
Tupelo, MS 38801
601-841-3778
601-841-3785 (fax)

MISSOURI

Maryann R. Nalley, R.N.
Professional Education
    Director
3322 American Avenue
Jefferson City, MO 63131
314-893-4800
314-893-2017 (fax)

NEBRASKA

Elaine J. Pohren, M.S.N., R.N.
Pain Center
University of Nebraska Medical
    Center
600 S. 42nd Street
Omaha, NE 68198-5640
402-559-4364
402-559-5915 (fax)

NEVADA

Carl R. Noback, M.D.
Noback Pain Center
630 S. Rancho Drive, Suite A
Las Vegas, NV 89106
702-870-1111
702-870-7121 (fax)

NEW HAMPSHIRE

Paul Arnstein, R.N.
% Concord Hospital
250 Pleasant Street
Concord, NH 03301
603-228-4646
603-225-2711

Marion B. Dolan
Heritage Home Health
169 Daniel Webster Highway,
    Suite 7
Meredith, NH 03253
603-279-4700
603-279-1370 (fax)

NEW JERSEY

Donna Bocco
2600 U.S. Highway 1
P.O. Box 2201
New Brunswick, NJ 08902-0803
908-297-8000
908-297-9043 (fax)

Alice Duigon, M.S.N., R.N.
798 Michigan Avenue
Toms River, NJ 08753-4507
908-929-4281
908-288-9480 (fax)

NEW MEXICO

Walter B. Forman, M.D.
    (Chair)
Department of Veteran's
    Affairs Medical Center
2100 Ridgecrest Drive
Albuquerque, NM 87108
505-256-2795
505-256-2882 (fax)

Carol Dolan, R.N., M.S.N.
University of New Mexico
    Cancer Center
900 Camino de Salud NE
Albuquerque, NM 87131
505-277-2858
505-277-2841 (fax)

Antonio Goncalves, Ph.D.
Director, Behavioral Oncology
University of New Mexico
    Cancer Center
900 Camino de Salud NE
Albuquerque, NM 87131
505-277-2858
505-277-2841 (fax)

NEW YORK

Kimberly Calder, M.P.S.
Cancer Care, Inc.
1180 Avenue of the Americas
New York, NY 10036
212-302-2400
212-719-0263 (fax)

Terry Altillo
Memorial Sloan-Kettering
  Cancer Center
Social Work Department
1275 York Avenue
New York, NY 10021

Bruce Kaplan, M.D.
Department of Anesthesia
New York Medical Center of
  Queens
5645 Main Street
Flushing, NY 11355
718-670-1080
718-445-8597 (fax)

NORTH CAROLINA

Jo Ann Dalton, R.N., Ed.D.
Associate Professor
School of Nursing
7460 Carrington Hall
University of North Carolina
Chapel Hill, NC 27599
919-966-1582
919-966-7298 (fax)

NORTH DAKOTA

John G. Harris, M.D.
Dakota Cancer Institute
1702 S. University Drive
Fargo, ND 58103
701-280-3300
701-280-8602 (fax)

LaRae Palmer, R.N.
Hospice of the Red River
  Valley
702 28th Avenue North
Fargo, ND 58102
701-237-4629
701-280-9069 (fax)

OHIO

Warren Wheeler, M.D.
Belinda Reed
Ohio Cancer Pain Initiative
3732 Colentangy River Road
Columbus, OH 43214
614-442-0608

OKLAHOMA

Barbara Bilderback, R.N., M.S.
Department of Education
St. Francis Hospital
6161 S. Yale Avenue
Tulsa, OK 74136
918-494-1193

Ed Wanack
School of Pharmacy
Southwestern Oklahoma State
  University
100 Campus Drive
Wertherford, OK 73096
405-774-3128

Agatha Underhill
Director of Pharmacy
Mercy Hospital
Oklahoma City, OK 73120

OREGON

Kelly Scott, Pharm.D.
Oregon Cancer Pain Initiative
P.O. Box 6313
Portland, OR 97228-6313
503-229-7760
503-790-1208 (fax)

PENNSYLVANIA

Georgia Trostle, R.N.
Hershey Medical Center
P.O. Box 850 C1726
Hershey, PA 17033
717-531-6849
717-531-6916 (fax)

Mary A. Simmonds, M.D.
Cowley Associates
Plaza 21, Suite 22-1
425 N. 21st Street
Camp Hill, PA 17011
717-761-7400
717-761-1796 (fax)

RHODE ISLAND

Phoebe Fernald, R.N., M.S.
Rhode Island Hospital
Dept. Medical Oncology
593 Eddy Street
Providence, RI 02903
401-444-5013
401-444-4184 (fax)

SOUTH CAROLINA

Judith Blanchard, Director
Community Support Services
Medical University of South
 Carolina
Hollins Oncology Center
171 Ashley Avenue
Charleston, SC 29425-2802
803-792-0700

803-792-3200 (fax)

Debbie Seale
Center for Cancer Treatment
 and Research
Richland Memorial Hospital
7 Medical Park
Columbia, SC 29203
803-434-3460
803-434-3095 (fax)

SOUTH DAKOTA

Kris Gaster, R.N.
624 Wiswall Place
Sioux Falls, SD 57105
605-339-8000 ext. 349

TENNESSEE

Dr. Alvin Meaver
U.T. Memphis
3 N. Dunlap, 3rd Floor
Memphis, TN 37203
901-523-5798

K. Mark Hilliard
American Cancer Society
1315 8th Avenue S.
Nashville, TN 37203
1-800-227-2345

TEXAS

Chree Boydstun, Executive
 Director
P.O. Box 980185
Houston, TX 77098-1724
713-745-0957
713-794-1724 (fax)

C. Stratton Hill, Jr., M.D.,
 Director, Pain Service
Deborah Thorpe, R.N., M.S.
UTMD Anderson Cancer
 Center
1515 Holcombe Boulevard,
 Box 82

Houston, TX 77030
713-792-7318
713-794-4999 (fax)

UTAH

Perry G. Fine, M.D.
Department of Anesthesiology
University of Utah Health
  Sciences Center
50 North Medical Drive
Salt Lake City, UT 84132
801-581-6393
801-581-4367 (fax)

Arthur G. Lipman, Pharm.D.
The University of Utah
Department of Pharmacy
  Practice
Salt Lake City, UT 84112
801-581-5986
801-581-6160 (fax)

VERMONT

Jean Harkins, R.N.
Medical Center Hospital of
  Vermont
111 Colchester Avenue
Burlington, VT 05402
802-656-2415

VIRGINIA

Lea Ann Hanson, Pharm.D.
Medical College of Virginia
  Hospitals
Box 533
Richmond, VA 23298-0533
804-786-8331

Patrick Coyne, R.N.
Medical College of Virginia
  Hospitals, Box 7
Richmond, VA 23298-0007
804-755-9189

Susan Robinson, R.N.
Massey Cancer Center, Box 37
Richmond, VA 23298-0037
804-786-0450
804-371-8453 (fax)

WASHINGTON

Nigel Bush, Ph.D.
Fred Hutchinson Cancer
  Research Center
1124 Columbia Street FB600E
Seattle, WA 98104
206-667-PAIN
206-667-3531 (fax)

Judy Kornell, R.N.
Fred Hutchinson Cancer
  Research Center
1124 Columbia Street FB600E
Seattle, WA 98104
206-667-5021
206-667-3531 (fax)

WEST VIRGINIA

Lucille DeFrank, R.N.
Northern WV Pain Center
99 J.D. Anderson Drive, 4
Morgantown, WV 26505
304-598-1969/6313

WISCONSIN

June L. Dahl, Ph.D.
1300 University Avenue, 3675
Madison, WI 53706
608-262-0978
608-262-4014 (fax)

6. HOME CARE ORGANIZATIONS

National Association for Home Care
519 C Street NE
Washington, D.C. 20002
202-547-7424
Provides information about home health services. Free brochure
"How to Select a Home Health Agency" can be requested.

Foundation for Hospice and Home Care
513 C Street NE
Washington, D.C. 20002
202-547-6586
Send a self-addressed stamped business envelope for "Consumers
Guide to Hospice Care." Also publishes other material for home-
makers and home health aides caring for cancer patients.

Amherst H. Wilder Foundation
919 Lafond Avenue
St. Paul, MN 55104
612-642-4000
Publishes "Take Care! A Guide for Caregivers on How to Improve
Their Self-Care," which is available for a small fee to cover shipping
and handling.

Hospice Education Institute
Five Essex Square
P.O. Box 713
Essex, CT 06426-0713
1-800-331-1620
Maintains HOSPICELINK, a computerized directory of hospice
programs in the United States. Call the toll-free number for references to local hospice and palliative care programs. HOSPICELINK
also provides general information about the principles and practices of hospice care.

National Consumers League
815 15th Street NW, Suite 92N
Washington, D.C. 20005
202-639-8140
Home care publications available.

7. MONEY MATTERS

Cancer can impose heavy economic burdens on both patients and their families. For many people, a portion of medical expenses is paid by their health insurance plan. An employer's personnel office or an insurance company can provide information about the types of medical costs covered by a particular policy. Medical costs that are not covered by insurance policies sometimes can be deducted from annual income before taxes.

For individuals who do not have health insurance or who need additional financial assistance, several resources are available, including government-sponsored programs and services supported by voluntary organizations.

Before leaving the hospital, discuss any concerns you may have about medical costs with a hospital social worker or patient accounts representative. There may be appropriate sources of aid and you may be able to negotiate a reasonable payment plan.

- Medicare, a health insurance program that is administered by the Social Security Administration (SSA), is designed for people over 65 or who are permanently disabled. The telephone number of the closest Social Security office is listed in the telephone directory or can be obtained by calling 1-800-772-1213.
- Medicaid is a program for people who need financial assistance for medical expenses. It is coordinated by the Health Care Financing Administration of the Department of Health and Human Services and is administered by individual states. Information about coverage is available from a hospital social worker or a local public health or social services office.
- The federal government also administers the Hill-Burton Program, through which many medical facilities and hospitals provide free or low-cost care. Hill-Burton hospitals receive government construction and modernization funds and are required by law to provide some services to people who cannot afford to pay. For eligibility information call 1-800-638-0742.
- If a cancer patient or his or her spouse is or has been a member of the Armed Forces, the U.S. Department of Veterans Affairs (VA) may be able to help with health care costs. The VA provides hospital care covering the full range of medical services. Treatment is available for all service-related conditions and some non-service-related ones.

- The Civilian Health and Medical Program of the Department of Veterans Affairs is a medical benefits program for dependents of veterans through which the VA provides payment for medical services and supplies obtained from civilian sources. Any VA health care facility can provide information about these programs.

- The federal government's Civilian Health and Medical Programs of the Uniformed Services (CHAMPUS) helps pay for civilian medical care for spouses and children of active-duty Uniformed Services personnel, retired Uniformed Services personnel and their spouses and children, and spouses and children of active-duty or retired active-duty personnel who have died. Information about CHAMPUS is available from the CHAMPUS Advisor/Health Benefits Advisor at your nearest Uniformed Services medical facility, or write to: Information Office of CHAMPUS, Aurora, CO 80045.

- The American Cancer Society (ACS) offers counseling, transportation and rehabilitation programs. Consult your telephone directory for your local office.

- The Leukemia Society of America (LSA) offers service programs and provides some financial aid to eligible patients who have leukemia, lymphoma or multiple myeloma. The local office is listed in your telephone directory.

- Groups such as the Salvation Army, United Way, Lutheran Social Services, Jewish Social Services, the Lions Club, Associated Catholic Charities as well as churches and synagogues sometimes provide financial help.

- There is more information on finances and cancer in Chapter 24, "Living with Cancer."

American Association of Retired Persons (AARP)
601 E Street, NW
Washington, D.C. 20049
1-800-424-3410
202-434-2277
Provides legislative advocacy, programs such as Medicare/Medicaid assistance and the Breast Cancer and Mammography Awareness information campaign for people 50 or older. Wide range of membership benefits including *Modern Maturity* magazine and Medicare supplementary insurance.

Blue Cross and Blue Shield Association
676 North St. Clair Street
Chicago, IL 60601
312-440-6000

Provides information on Blue Cross/Blue Shield coverage offered in every state, including the availability of annual open enrollment periods.

Communicating for Agriculture Inc.
2626 East 82nd Street, Suite 325
Bloomington, MN 55425
1-800-445-1525
612-854-9005
A national rural organization, open to all, offering up-to-date information on high-risk insurance pools. Since 1975 has served as a strong advocate for the establishment of these state-run high-risk pools.

Disabled American Veterans
807 Main Avenue, SW
Washington, D.C. 20024
202-554-3501
202-554-3581 (fax)
A national organization, serving veterans and their dependents. Approximately 3,000 chapters offer counseling, educational materials, support groups, transportation, conferences and a newsletter.

Group Health Association of America
Membership Department
1129 20th Street NW, Suite 600
Washington, D.C. 20036
202-778-3200
202-331-7487 (fax)
A trade association providing information about eligibility for group health plan coverage with commercial insurers. It represents HMOs and sells a national directory of HMOs.

Health Insurance Association of America (HIAA)
1025 Connecticut Avenue, N.W. Suite 1200
Washington, D.C. 20036
1-800-942-4242
202-223-7808
A trade association representing major health insurance companies. Offers consumer publications about health insurance, long-term care insurance and Medicare supplement insurance.

Medical Information Bureau Incorporated (MIB)
P.O. Box 105
Esses Station
Boston, MA 02112
617-426-3660

MIB can send a copy of your medical records so that you can verify the information in them and correct any inaccuracies. Call MIB first to find out the type of information it requires to process your request.

The National Insurance Consumer Helpline
1-800-942-4242
Provides information on all types of insurance.

National Underwriter Company
505 Gest Street
Cincinnati, OH 45203
513-721-2140
Publishes annual guide "Who Writes What in Life and Health Insurance."

Pension and Welfare Benefits Administration
U.S. Department of Labor, Room N-5669
200 Constitution Avenue, NW
Washington, D.C. 20210
202-523-8521
PWBA enforces your rights under COBRA to continued health insurance coverage and provides information about how to enforce your rights to equal job benefits under ERISA.

United States Department of Health and Human Services
Social Security Administration
Baltimore, MD 21235
1-800-772-1213
This office provides information on Medicare.

STATE INSURANCE COMMISSIONS

If you feel you are being treated unfairly by your insurance company, you can contact your state commission.

ALABAMA
Insurance Department
64 North Union Street, Room 504
Montgomery, AL 36130
205-269-3550

ALASKA
Division of Insurance
Commerce and Economic Development Department
P.O. Box D
Juneau, AK 99811
907-465-2515

ARIZONA
Department of Insurance
3030 North Third Street,
   Room 1100
Phoenix, AZ 85012
602-255-5400

ARKANSAS
Insurance Department
400 University Tower Building
Little Rock, AR 72204
501-686-2900

CALIFORNIA
Department of Insurance
770 L Street, Suite 1120
Sacramento, CA 95814
916-445-5544

COLORADO
Division of Insurance
Department of Regulatory
   Agencies
303 West Colfax Avenue, 5th
   Floor
Denver, CO 80204
303-866-3201

CONNECTICUT
Department of Insurance
P.O. Box 816
Hartford, CT 06142
203-297-3802

DELAWARE
Department of Insurance
The Green
Dover, DE 19901
302-736-4251

DISTRICT OF COLUMBIA
Insurance Administration
Consumer and Regulatory
   Affairs

613 C Street, NW, Room 600
Washington, D.C. 20001
202-727-8000

FLORIDA
Insurance Commissioner and
   Treasurer
State Capitol, PL11
Tallahassee, FL 32399
904-922-3100

GEORGIA
Office of Insurance
   Commissioner
Two Martin Luther King Jr.
   Drive
704 West Tower
Atlanta, GA 30334
404-656-2056

HAWAII
Division of Insurance
Commerce and Consumer
   Affairs Department
1010 Richards Street
Honolulu, HI 96813
808-586-2790

IDAHO
Department of Insurance
500 South 10th
Boise, ID 83720
208-334-2250

ILLINOIS
Department of Insurance
320 North Washington, 4th
   Floor
Springfield, IL 62767
217-782-4515

INDIANA
Department of Insurance
311 West Washington Street,
Suite 300
Indianapolis, IN 46204
317-232-2406

IOWA
Insurance Division
Department of Commerce
Lucas State Office Building
Des Moines, IA 50319
515-281-5705

KANSAS
Insurance Department
420 Southwest Ninth Street
Topeka, KS 66612
913-296-3071

KENTUCKY
Department of Insurance
Public Protection and
Regulation Cabinet
229 West Main Street
Frankfort, KY 40601
502-564-6027

LOUISIANA
Department of Insurance
P.O. Box 94214
Baton Rouge, LA 70804-9214
504-342-5900

MAINE
Bureau of Insurance
Professional and Financial
Regulations Department
State House Station #34
Augusta, ME 04333
207-582-8707

MARYLAND
Division of Insurance
Licensing and Regulatory
Department
501 St. Paul Street
Baltimore, MD 21202-2272
410-333-6300

MASSACHUSETTS
Division of Insurance
Executive Office of Consumer
Affairs
280 Friend Street
Boston, MA 02114
617-727-7189

MICHIGAN
Licensing and Regulation
Department
611 West Ottawa
P.O. Box 30220
Lansing, MI 48909
517-373-9273

MINNESOTA
Department of Commerce
113 East Seventh Street
St. Paul, MN 55101
612-296-4026

MISSISSIPPI
Department of Insurance
1804 Sillers Building
Jackson, MS 39201
601-359-3569

MISSOURI
Division of Insurance
Department of Economic
Development
Truman Building, Box 690
Jefferson City, MO 65102
314-751-4126

MONTANA
Insurance Division
Office of State Auditor
Mitchell Building
Helena, MT 59620
406-444-2040

NEBRASKA
Department of Insurance
The Terminal Building
941 O Street, Suite 400
Lincoln, NE 68508
402-471-2201

NEVADA
Insurance Division
Department of Commerce
1665 Hot Springs Road
Carson City, NV 89710
702-687-4270

NEW HAMPSHIRE
Insurance Department
169 Manchester Street
Concord, NH 03301
603-271-2261

NEW JERSEY
Department of Insurance
20 West State Street, CN 325
Trenton, NJ 08625
609-633-7667

NEW MEXICO
State Insurance Board Division
State Corporation Commission
Room 428, PERA Building
Santa Fe, NM 87503
505-827-4297

NEW YORK
Insurance Department
Empire State Plaza
Agency Building #1

Albany, NY 12257
518-474-4550

NORTH CAROLINA
Department of Insurance
430 North Salisbury Street
Raleigh, NC 27603-5908
919-733-7343

NORTH DAKOTA
Insurance Department
5th Floor, State Capitol
600 East Boulevard
Bismarck, ND 58505
701-224-2440

OHIO
Department of Insurance
2100 Stella Court
Columbus, OH 43266-0566
614-644-2651

OKLAHOMA
Insurance Department
408 Will Rogers Building
Oklahoma City, OK 73105
405-521-2828

OREGON
Department of Insurance and
    Finance
21 Labor and Industries
    Building
Salem, OR 97310
503-378-4120

PENNSYLVANIA
Insurance Department
Strawberry Square, 13th Floor
Harrisburg, PA 17120
717-787-6835

RHODE ISLAND
Department of Business
  Regulation
233 Richmond Street, Suite
  233
Providence, RI 02903
401-277-2223

SOUTH CAROLINA
Department of Insurance
1612 Marion Street
Columbia, SC 29201
803-737-6117

SOUTH DAKOTA
Commerce and Regulations
  Department
910 Sioux, State Capitol
Pierre, SD 57501
605-773-3563

TENNESSEE
Department of Commerce and
  Insurance
500 James Robertson Parkway
Nashville, TN 37243
615-741-2241

TEXAS
Board of Insurance
1100 San Jacinto Boulevard
Austin, TX 78701-1998
512-463-6464

UTAH
Department of Insurance
3110 State Office Building
Salt Lake City, UT 84114
801-538-3800

VERMONT
Department of Banking and
  Insurance
120 State Street
Montpelier, VT 05602
802-828-3301

VIRGINIA
State Corporation
  Commissioner
1220 Bank Street, 13th Floor
Richmond, VA 23219
804-786-3603

WASHINGTON
Office of Insurance
  Commissioner
Insurance Building
M/S: AQ-21
Olympia, WA 98504
206-753-7301

WEST VIRGINIA
Division of Insurance
2100 Washington Street, East
Charleston, WV 25305
304-348-3394

WISCONSIN
Office of Commissioner of
  Insurance
123 West Washington Avenue
P.O. Box 7873
Madison, WI 53707
608-266-3585

WYOMING
Insurance Department
Herschler Building
Cheyenne, WY 82002
307-777-7401

Health Coverage for the Hard-to-Insure

A number of states currently sell comprehensive health insurance to state residents with serious medical conditions who are unable to find a company to insure them. If your state is not listed, contact your state Department of Insurance to find out what assistance they can offer.

ALASKA: Short-term insurance program that provides six months of coverage.
Blue Cross of Washington and Alaska
2550 Denali Street, Suite 600
Anchorage, AK 99503
907-258-5065

ARIZONA: Informal program with each case handled separately.
Arizona Department of Insurance
3030 North Third Street, Suite 1100
Phoenix, AZ 85012
1-800-544-9208 or 602-255-2113

CALIFORNIA: Risk pool with waiting list.
California Major Risk Medical Insurance Program
c/o Blue Cross of California
P.O. Box 6666
Oxnard, CA 93031-6666
1-800-289-6574

COLORADO: Risk pool.
Colorado Uninsurable Health Insurance Plan
Blue Cross and Blue Shield of Colorado
700 Broadway
Denver, CO 80273
1-800-423-6174 or 303-831-2391

CONNECTICUT: Risk pool.
Health Reinsurance Association of Connecticut
Travelers' Insurance Company
One Tower Square, 2NB
Hartford, CT 06183-2937
203-527-5369

DISTRICT OF COLUMBIA: Spring and fall yearly. Available to District of Columbia, Montgomery and Prince Georges County, Maryland, and most of northern Virginia. Also see Maryland and Virginia.
Blue Cross and Blue Shield of the National Capitol Area
Department 5853
550 12th Street, SW
Washington, D.C. 20065-5863
202-484-9100

FLORIDA: Risk pool with waiting list.
Blue Cross and Blue Shield of Florida
P.O. Box 45216
Jacksonville, FL 32232-5216
1-800-766-3242

GEORGIA: High-risk program not operational yet.
Georgia Insurance Department
#2 Martin Luther King Drive, SE
Atlanta, GA 30334
404-656-6054

HAWAII: Risk pool provides only basic preventive care.
State Health Insurance Program
1000 Bishop Street, Room 908
Honolulu, HI 96813
808-586-4141

ILLINOIS: Risk pool with waiting list.
Blue Cross and Blue Shield of Illinois
P.O. Box 2401
ICHIP Administrative Unit, 18th Floor
Chicago, IL 60690
1-800-367-6410

INDIANA: Risk pool.
Indiana Comprehensive Health Insurance Association
9525 Delegates Row
P.O. Box 40438
Indianapolis, IN 46240-0438
317-581-1005 or 1-800-552-7921

IOWA: Risk pool.
Iowa Comprehensive Health Insurance Association
Mutual of Omaha
P.O. Box 31746
Omaha, NE 68131
1-800-445-8603

KANSAS: High-risk program not yet operational.
Kansas Insurance Department
Accident and Health Division
420 Southwest 9th Street
Topeka, KS 66612
913-296-3071

LOUISIANA: High-risk program not yet operational.
Louisiana Health Insurance Association
7904 Wrenwood, Suite D
Baton Rouge, LA 70809
504-926-6245

MAINE: Risk pool.
Maine High-Risk Health Organization
Mutual of Omaha
P.O. Box 31726
Omaha, NE 68131
1-800-228-0460

MARYLAND: Spring and fall yearly. Also see District of
  Columbia.
Blue Cross/Blue Shield Open Enrollment Policy
10455 Mill Run Circle
Owings Mills, MD 21117
1-800-544-8703

MASSACHUSETTS: Year-round.
Blue Cross and Blue Shield of Massachusetts
Nongroup Coverage
P.O. Box 9140
North Quincy, MA 02171-9140
617-956-3934 or 1-800-822-2700

MICHIGAN: Year-round.
Blue Cross and Blue Shield of Michigan
600 East Lafayette
Department B613
Detroit, MI 48226
517-322-9470 or 1-800-637-2227

MINNESOTA: Risk pool.
Minnesota Comprehensive Health Association
P.O. Box 64566
St. Paul, MN 55164
612-456-5290 or 1-800-382-2000, ext. 5290

MISSISSIPPI: Risk pool.
Mississippi Comprehensive Health Insurance Risk Pool
  Association
P.O. Box 13748
Jackson, MI 39236
601-362-0799

MONTANA: Risk pool.
Montana Comprehensive Health Association
404 Fuller Avenue
P.O. Box 5683
Helena, MT 59604
406-444-8200 or 1-800-447-7828

NEBRASKA: Risk pool.
Nebraska Comprehensive Health Insurance Pool
Blue Cross/Blue Shield of Nebraska
P.O. Box 3248
Main Post Office Station
Omaha, NE 68180-0001
1-800-356-3485

NEW HAMPSHIRE: Year-round.
Blue Cross and Blue Shield of New Hampshire
2 Pillsbury Street
Concord, NH 03306
603-228-0161

NEW JERSEY: Year-round.
Blue Cross/Blue Shield of New Jersey
33 Washington Street
Newark, NJ 07102
201-491-2729

NEW MEXICO: Risk pool.
New Mexico Comprehensive Health Insurance Pool
Blue Cross/Blue Shield of New Mexico
12800 Indian School Road, NE
Albuquerque, NM 87112
1-800-432-0750

NEW YORK: Year-round.
Empire Blue Cross/Blue Shield
Tradition Plus
622 Third Avenue
New York, NY 10017
212-476-7111

NORTH CAROLINA: Year-round.
Blue Cross and Blue Shield of North Carolina
Access Plan
P.O. Box 2291
Durham, NC 27702
919-490-3829

NORTH DAKOTA: Risk pool.
Comprehensive Health Association of North Dakota
4510 13th Avenue, SW
Fargo, ND 58121
701-282-1100

OREGON: Risk pool.
Blue Cross/Blue Shield of Oregon
P.O. Box 1271
Portland, OR 97207
1-800-848-7280

PENNSYLVANIA: Year-round.
Independence Blue Cross and Pennsylvania Blue Shield
1901 Market Street
Philadelphia, PA 19103-1480
215-568-8204 or 1-800-453-2566

RHODE ISLAND: Fall of each year.
Blue Cross and Blue Shield of Rhode Island
444 Westminister Street
Providence, RI 02903
401-831-7300 or 1-800-527-7290

SOUTH CAROLINA: Risk pool.
South Carolina Health Insurance Pool
P.O. Box 61173
Columbia, SC 29260
803-736-0043 or 1-800-868-2503

TENNESSEE: Risk pool.
Tennessee Comprehensive Health Insurance Pool
P.O. Box 6249
Chattanooga, TN 37401-6249
1-800-533-9892 or 615-755-5918

TEXAS: High-risk program planned.
Blue Cross/Blue Shield of Texas Insurance High-Risk Pool
P.O. Box 655082
Dallas, TX 75265-5082
1-800-338-2227

UTAH: Risk pool.
Utah Comprehensive Health Insurance Pool
P.O. Box 27797
Salt Lake City, UT 84127
801-481-6063 or 1-800-624-6519

VERMONT: Year-round.
Blue Cross and Blue Shield of Vermont
P.O. Box 186
Montpelier, VT 05601
802-223-6131 or 1-800-247-2583

VIRGINIA: Year-round. Also see District of Columbia.
Blue Cross and Blue Shield of Virginia
P.O. Box 13047
Roanoke, VA 24045
1-800-334-7676

WASHINGTON: Risk pool.
Washington State Health Insurance Pool
Mutual of Omaha
P.O. Box 31726
Omaha, NE 68131
1-800-228-4044

WISCONSIN: Risk pool.
Wisconsin Health Insurance Risk-Sharing Plan
Mutual of Omaha
P.O. Box 31746
Omaha, NE 68131
1-800-228-7044

WYOMING: Risk pool.
Wyoming Health Insurance Pool
P.O. Box 2256
Cheyenne, WY 82003
1-800-442-2764

8. DATA BASE AND PUBLICATION SOURCES

There has been an explosion of information on every aspect of cancer. It is suggested that you use the sources listed as a guide and starting point in your search for information.

DATA BASES

Electronic information services have become a convenient, cost-effective method of accessing information. Most hospital and university libraries subscribe to specific on-line data bases, or you can access them from home through your personal computer.

Some of the data bases are in the general health field, such as HealthNet. Others cover special areas, such as those in the cancer field. Some are available only by paying extra charges, such as Health Database Plus, and IQuest Medical Information Center. Still others are people related, such as Cancer Forum, which puts you in touch with other people facing or who have faced cancer.

CancerFax
National Cancer Institute
Bethesda, MD 20892
301-402-5874
301-496-7403 (for technical assistance)
Quick and easy way to obtain cancer information from the National Cancer Institute. Operates 24 hours a day, 7 days a week, with no charge other than telephone call from your fax machine to the Cancer Fax computer in Bethesda, Maryland. Lets you request information statements in English or Spanish from the NCI's Physician Data Query system as well as fact sheets on various cancer topics from the NCI's Office of Cancer Communications.

CancerNet
National Cancer Institute
Bethesda, MD 20892
301-402-5874 or 496-8880
Quick and easy way to get, through electronic mail, cancer information from the National Cancer Institute. Can be accessed through a number of different networks including Internet and BITNET. No charge for the service unless your local computer center charges for the use of e-mail. You can request information statements from the NCI's Physician Data Query system as well as a list of patient publications available from the Office of Cancer Communications, information about PDQ, PDQ distributors and other products and services from the NCI.

International Cancer Information Center
National Cancer Institute
Building 82, Room 107
Bethesda, MD 20892
301-402-5874
Collects, updates and maintains the following data bases which are specifically cancer related:

- The PDQ data base, which contains the latest updated information concerning cancer treatment and clinical trials, is available on-line through the National Library of Medicine's MEDLARS system. NCI is responsible for licensing PDQ to hospitals, universities and other nonprofit institutions
- CANCERLIT, a data base which contains the majority of cancer-related citations from MEDLINE, supplemented with additional citations of books, meeting abstracts, theses, and other publications.

- CANCERFAX, which makes treatment, supportive care and cancer screening statements from PDQ available via fax in either English or Spanish. Statements are available for health professionals as well as for the general public.
- CANCERNET, which makes treatment, supportive care and cancer screening statements from PDQ available via electronic mail.

National Library of Medicine
8600 Rockville Pike
Bethesda, MD 20894
1-800-638-8480 or 1-800-272-4787 (MEDLARS)
The NLM's MEDLARS is a 24-hour-a-day system that allows for cost-effective searching of specialized data bases. Its specific data bases include:

MEDLINE (abstracts of journal articles)
CATLINE (records of books)
AVLINE (records of audiovisuals)
CHEMLINE (information about chemical substances)
HEALTH (information about health care services)
TOXLINE (toxicological information)
DIRLINE (directory of 15,000 information resources)
AIDLINE (AIDS-related references)
PDQ (advances in cancer treatment and clinical trials)

The GRATEFUL MED data base allows for easy access to the NLM's vast collection of medical and health-science information. An average search costs about $3.00.

BRS Search Services
Maxwell Online, Inc.
8000 Westpark Drive
McLean, VA 22102
1-800-289-4277
Comprehensive service with over 200 data bases available with access 24 hours a day, including cancer-related subjects.

Dialog Information Services, Inc.
3460 Hillview Avenue
Palo Alto, CA 94304
1-800-3DIALOG
415-858-3785 (California only)
Has a scope of 380 data bases, including cancer-related subjects.

NONTECHNICAL MAGAZINES

Articles which appear in the most popular nontechnical magazines and journals are listed in the *Reader's Guide to Periodical Literature* or in the Public Affairs Information Service. These two guides are usually available in most public libraries. Look in the index under the subject in which you are interested—or, if you know it, under the author's name.

HEALTH-SCIENCE JOURNALS

The Index Medicus, which is found in medical libraries, most university and college libraries, and some public libraries, lists articles appearing in over 2,400 health-sciences journals. There are also dozens of oncology-related journals and bibliographic resource books. A resource *Medical Health Books and Serials* is available in most medical libraries.

OTHER PUBLICATION RESOURCES

Consumer Product Safety Commission
401 M Street, N.W.
Washington, D.C. 20207
301-492-6800
1-800-638-2772 (hotline)
Commission sets standards on potentially hazardous products, among them carcinogens and other chronic hazards. Single copies of printed materials available free of charge. Order via hotline number.

Department of Labor
Publications Office S-4203
Occupational Safety and Health Administration
Washington, D.C. 20210
Provides information on work-related hazards. Has regional offices.

Environmental Protection Agency
Office of Information Center—PM-215
401 M Street S.W.
Washington, D.C. 20460
Provides information on hazards in the environment, outside of industry.

Food and Drug Administration
Office of Consumer Affairs
5600 Fishers Lane
Rockville, MD 20857
301-443-3170
Serves as clearinghouse for consumer publications including mammography.

Industrial Union of Metal Trades
Department of AFL-CIO
815 16th Street, N.W.
Washington, D.C. 20006
Provides information on asbestos control and insurance matters.

National Health Information Center
Office of Disease Prevention and Health Promotion
P.O. Box 1133
Washington, D.C. 20013-1133
301-565-4167
1-800-336-4797
Central information source. Maintains a computer data base of government agencies, support groups, professional societies and other organizations that can answer questions

National Institute of Neurological and Communicative Diseases and Strokes
Office of Scientific and Health Reports
Building 31, Room 8A06
National Institutes of Health
Bethesda, MD 20205
301-496-5751
Provides information on brain tumors.

National Toxicology Program
National Institute of Environmental Health Services
M.D. B2-04, Box 12233
Research Triangle Park, NC 27709
919-541-3991
Provides information about potentially hazardous chemicals, including those that may cause cancer.

National Cancer Institute
Office of Cancer Communications
National Institutes of Health
Bethesda, MD 20892
301-496-5583
1-800-4-CANCER

Provides information on all aspects of cancer to physicians, scientists, educators, Congress, the Executive Branch, the media and the public. The CIS 800-4-CANCER is located within this office with a network of locations across the country.

Office on Smoking and Health
Mail Stop K-JO
1600 Clifton Road, N.E.
Atlanta, GA 30333
404-488-5705

AUDIOVISUAL MATERIAL

In addition to the sources listed, many universities and medical centers produce audiovisual material that can be purchased or rented. Their film libraries usually contain cancer-related audiovisuals that can be borrowed.

American Cancer Society
1599 Clifton Road N.E.
Atlanta, GA 30029-4251
404-320-3333
1-800-ACS-2345
Has videos, filmstrips, audio tapes and slides with accompanying text available for free loan.

National Audiovisual Center
National Archives
8700 Edgeworth Drive
Capitol Heights, MD 20743-3701
1-800-788-6282
301-763-1896
Center distributes over 8,000 U.S. government–sponsored productions including programs on cancer and the environment, breast cancer, cancer detection and smoking. Free catalog of listings available.

National Cancer Institute
Office of Cancer Communications
Bethesda, MD 20892
301-396-5583
1-800-4-CANCER
Publishes Cancer Patient Education Videotape Directory.

9. CANCER FUND-RAISING ORGANIZATIONS

If you have any questions as to the validity of an individual cancer fund-raising organization, contact one of the following agencies before you make a contribution.

Council of Better Business Bureaus
Philanthropic Advisory Service, Suite 800
4200 Wilson Boulevard
Arlington, VA 22203-1804
703-276-0100

National Charities Information Bureau
19 Union Square West, Dept. 250
New York, NY 10003-3395
212-929-6300
212-463-7083 (fax)

References

ALPHA INSTITUTE. *The Alpha Book on Cancer and Living.* (Brent Ryder, editor); Alameda, California, 1993.

ALTMAN, ROBERTA, AND SARG, MICHAEL J., M.D. *The Cancer Dictionary.* Facts on File Inc., 1992.

AMERICAN CANCER SOCIETY. *Cancer Facts and Figures, 1994.* Atlanta, Georgia, 1994.

——. *Cancer Manual.* (Robert T. Osteen, M.D., editor); Boston, Massachusetts, 1990.

——. *A Cancer Source Book for Nurses, Sixth Edition.* (Susan B. Baird, editor); 1991.

BAIRD, SUSAN B.; McCORKEL, RUTH; AND GRANT, MARCIA. *Cancer Nursing: A Comprehensive Textbook.* W.B. Saunders Company, 1991.

BENSON, RALPH C., M.D., AND PERNOLL, MARTIN L., M.D. *Handbook of Obstetrics and Gynecology.* McGraw Hill, 1994.

BERGER, KAREN, AND BOSTWICH, JOHN III, M.D. *A Woman's Decision.* Quality Medical Publishing, Inc., 1994.

CALABRESI, PAUL, M.D., AND SCHEIN, PHILIP S., M.D., *Medical Oncology: Basic Principles and Clinical Management of Cancer.* McGraw Hill, 1992.

DEVITA, V.T.; HELLMAN, S.; AND ROSENBERG, S.A.. *Cancer: Principles and Practice of Oncology.* J.B. Lippincott Company, 1992.

DOW, KAREN HASSEY, AND HILDERLEY, LAURA J. *Nursing Care in Radiation Oncology.* W.B. Saunders Company, 1992.

FISCHER, DAVID S.; KNOBF, M. TISH; AND DURIVAGE, HENRY J. *The Cancer Chemotherapy Handbook.* Mosby Year Book, 1993.

FISCHBACH, FRANCES. *A Manual of Laboratory and Diagnostic Tests.* J.B. Lippincott Company, 1992.

GROENWALD, SUSAN L., ET AL. *Cancer Nursing: Principles and Practice.* Jones and Bartlett Publishers, 1993.

HARRIS, JAY R., M.D., ET AL. *Breast Diseases.* J.B. Lippincott Company, 1991.

HOLLAND, JAMES F., ET AL. *Cancer Medicine.* Lee and Febiger, 1993.

HOLLEB, A.I.; FINK, D.J.; AND MURPHY, G.P. *American Cancer Society Textbook of Clinical Oncology.* American Cancer Society, 1991.

881

KELLY, P.T. *Understanding Breast Cancer Risk.* Temple University Press, 1991.

LATOUR, K. *The Breast Cancer Companion.* William Morrow and Company, 1993.

LESHAN, LAWRENCE. *Cancer As a Turning Point.* Dutton, 1989.

LIPMAN, LICHTER, DANFORTH. *Diagnosis and Management of Breast Cancer.* W.B. Saunders Company, 1988.

LOVE, SUSAN M., M.D. *Dr. Susan Love's Breast Book.* Addison-Wesley Publishing Company, Inc., 1990.

MOYERS, BILL. *Healing and the Mind.* Doubleday, 1993.

NATIONAL CANCER INSTITUTE. Site Pamphlets and Research Reports.

———. *Chemotherapy and You,* 1993.

———. *Facing Forward: A Guide for Cancer Survivors,* 1992.

THE NATIONAL COALITION FOR CANCER SURVIVORSHIP. *Charting the Journey: An Almanac of Practical Resources for Cancer Survivors.* Consumer Reports Books, 1990.

SIEGEL, BERNIE. *Love, Medicine and Miracles.* Harper & Row, 1986.

———. *Peace, Love and Healing.* Harper & Row, 1989.

SOBEL, DAVID S., M.D. AND FERGUSON, TOM, M.D. *The People's Book of Medical Tests.* Summit Books, 1985.

U.S. DEPARTMENT OF HEALTH AND HUMAN SERVICES. *Healthy People 2000: National Health Promotion and Disease Prevention Objectives.* Washington, D.C., 1991.

———. *Eating Hints,* 1992.

———. *When Cancer Recurs,* 1990.

———. *Management of Cancer Pain,* 1994.

In the process of reading and using this book, questions which are not included in it may come to your mind. The authors would be most pleased if you would share your thoughts with them. Kindly send any comments to:

Eve Potts, Marion Morra
c/o Avon Books
1350 Avenue of the Americas
New York, New York 10019

MARION MORRA is the Associate Director of the Yale Cancer Center in New Haven, Connecticut. She is Associate Research Scientist at the Yale School of Medicine and Associate Clinical Professor at the Yale School of Nursing. Marion is widely published, having written articles and authored books for both the health professional and the public, with emphasis on health, especially in the field of cancer. She serves on major national committees for the National Cancer Institute and the American Cancer Society.

EVE POTTS has been a medical writer for more than 30 years. Her expertise is in making difficult medical information easy to understand. She has served as a medical writer and consultant to the Department of Health and Human Services and to many medical-oriented companies and institutions. Her interest in history is represented by another book, *Wesport, A Special Place, 1987*.

The two authors, who are sisters, have collaborated on five books: *Understanding Your Immune System* (Avon Books, 1986); the first two editions of *Choices* (Avon Books, 1980 and 1987); and *Triumph: Getting Back to Normal When You Have Cancer* (Avon Books, 1990). In 1993, the authors received the Natalie Davis Spingarn Writer's Award from the National Coalition for Cancer Survivors for "their valuable contributions to the literature of survivorship and for their books, *Choices* and *Triumph*."

Index